Anesthesiology and Intensive Care Medicine: Challenges and Concerns

Anesthesiology and Intensive Care Medicine: Challenges and Concerns

Editor: Adam Bowers

AMERICAN
MEDICAL PUBLISHERS
www.americanmedicalpublishers.com

AMERICAN
MEDICAL PUBLISHERS
www.americanmedicalpublishers.com

Cataloging-in-Publication Data

Anesthesiology and intensive care medicine : challenges and concerns / edited by Adam Bowers.
p. cm.
Includes bibliographical references and index.
ISBN 978-1-63927-873-2
1. Anesthesiology. 2. Anesthesia. 3. Critical care medicine. 4. Emergency medicine. I. Bowers, Adam.
RD81 .A54 2023
617.96--dc23

American Medical Publishers,
41 Flatbush Avenue,
1st Floor, New York,
NY 11217, USA

ISBN 978-1-63927-873-2 (Hardback)

Contents

Preface IX

Chapter 1 **Transcutaneous Electrical Acupoint Stimulation Decreases the Incidence of Postoperative Nausea and Vomiting After Laparoscopic Non-Gastrointestinal Surgery** 1
Wei Gao, Linzhong Zhang, Xuechang Han, Lai Wei, Jie Fang, Xiaqing Zhang, Jiaqiang Zhang, Haiyun Wang, Qi Zhou, Chenggang Wang, Wenting Chen, Xinli Ni, Lan Yang, Ruini Du, Ge Wang, Bingyu Liu, Yajuan Li, Shanshan Zhang and Qiang Wang

Chapter 2 **Using RNA-Seq to Investigate Immune-Metabolism Features in Immunocompromised Patients with Sepsis** 11
Po-Liang Cheng, Hsin-Hua Chen, Yu Han Jiang, Tzu-Hung Hsiao, Chen-Yu Wang, Chieh-Liang Wu, Tai-Ming Ko and Wen-Cheng Chao

Chapter 3 **Association Between Epidural Analgesia and Cancer Recurrence or Survival After Surgery for Renal Cell Carcinoma: A Propensity Weighted Analysis** 21
Fang-Yu Yen, Wen-Kuei Chang, Shih Pin Lin, Tzu-Ping Lin and Kuang-Yi Chang

Chapter 4 **Evaluation of the Time Spent by Anesthetist on Clinical Tasks in the Operating Room** 29
Vincent Compère, Emmanuel Besnier, Thomas Clavier, Nicolas Byhet, Florent Lefranc, Frederic Jegou, Nicolas Sturzenegger, Jean Baptiste Hardy, Bertrand Dureuil and Thomas Elie

Chapter 5 **Sequential Organ Failure Assessment Score for Prediction of Mortality of Patients with Rhabdomyolysis Following Exertional Heatstroke: A Longitudinal Cohort Study in Southern China** 35
Ming Wu, Conglin Wang, Zheying Liu and Zhifeng Liu

Chapter 6 **The Effect of Dexmedetomidine as a Sedative Agent for Mechanically Ventilated Patients with Sepsis** 44
Caimu Wang, Qijiang Chen, Ping Wang, Weisheng Jin, Chao Zhong, Zisheng Ge and Kangmin Xu

Chapter 7 **PPV May be a Starting Point to Achieve Circulatory Protective Mechanical Ventilation** 55
Longxiang Su, Pan Pan, Huaiwu He, Dawei Liu and Yun Long

Chapter 8 **Association of Time–Varying Intensity of Ventilation with Mortality in Patients with COVID–19 ARDS: Secondary Analysis of the PRoVENT–COVID Study** 61
Michiel T. U. Schuijt, David M. P. van Meenen, Ignacio Martin–Loeches, Guido Mazzinari, Marcus J. Schultz, Frederique Paulus and Ary Serpa Neto

Chapter 9 **Effects of Dexmedetomidine on Postoperative Nausea and Vomiting in Adult Patients Undergoing Ambulatory Thyroidectomy** **71**
Cuiyu Xie, Caihui Zhang, Hao Sun and Yao Lu

Chapter 10 **Lidocaine and Bupivacaine Downregulate MYB and *DANCR* lncRNA by Upregulating *miR-187-5p* in MCF-7 Cells** **79**
Chiao-Yi Lin, Wen-Ting Tseng, Yao-Yin Chang, Mong-Hsun Tsai, Eric Y. Chuang, Tzu-Pin Lu and Liang-Chuan Lai

Chapter 11 **Case Series: Video-Assisted Minimally Invasive Cardiac Surgery During Pregnancy** **88**
Anyi Lu, Yingxian Ye, Jiaqi Hu, Ning Wei, Jinfeng Wei, Bimei Lin and Sheng Wang

Chapter 12 **A Thrombomodulin Promoter Gene Polymorphism, rs2239562, Influences Both Susceptibility to and Outcome of Sepsis** **94**
Eizo Watanabe, Osamu Takasu, Youichi Teratake, Teruo Sakamoto, Toshiaki Ikeda, Joji Kotani, Nobuya Kitamura, Masaaki Ohmori, Ayako Teratani, Goichi Honda, Masahiko Hatano, Benjamin Mayer, E. Marion Schneider and Shigeto Oda

Chapter 13 **The Amplitude of Diaphragm Compound Muscle Action Potential Correlates with Diaphragmatic Excursion on Ultrasound and Pulmonary Function After Supraclavicular Brachial Plexus Block** **102**
Xiuxia Bao, Tao Liu, Haorong Feng, Yeke Zhu, Yingying Wu, Xianghe Wang and Xianhui Kang

Chapter 14 **Association Between Platelet Levels on Admission and 90-day Mortality in Patients with Exertional Heatstroke, a 10 Years Cohort Study** **112**
Li Zhong, Ming Wu, Jingjing Ji, Conglin Wang and Zhifeng Liu

Chapter 15 **Effectiveness of Combined Strategies for the Prevention of Hypothermia Measured by Noninvasive Zero-Heat Flux Thermometer During Cesarean Section** **119**
Antonella Cotoia, Paola Sara Mariotti, Claudia Ferialdi, Pasquale Del Vecchio, Renata Beck, Simona Zaami and Gilda Cinnella

Chapter 16 **Priorities Towards Fair Allocation of Ventilators During COVID-19 Pandemic: A Delphi Study** **127**
Seyyed-Hadi Ghamari, Mohsen Abbasi-Kangevari, Nasim Zamani, Hossein Hassanian-Moghaddam and Ali-Asghar Kolahi

Chapter 17 **Effect of Serum Phosphate on the Prognosis of Septic Patients: A Retrospective Study Based on MIMIC-IV Database** **135**
Zhaoyang Li, Tingwen Shen and Yi Han

Chapter 18 **The Prognostic Capacity of the Radiographic Assessment for Lung Edema Score in Patients with COVID-19 Acute Respiratory Distress Syndrome—An International Multicenter Observational Study** **144**
Christel M. A. Valk, Claudio Zimatore, Guido Mazzinari, Charalampos Pierrakos, Chaisith Sivakorn, Jutamas Dechsanga, Salvatore Grasso, Ludo Beenen, Lieuwe D. J. Bos, Frederique Paulus, Marcus J. Schultz and Luigi Pisani

Chapter 19 **The Application of a SaCoVLM™ Visual Intubation Laryngeal Mask for the Management of Difficult Airways in Morbidly Obese Patients** 152
Yongtao Sun, Linlin Huang, Lingling Xu, Min Zhang, Yongle Guo and Yuelan Wang

Chapter 20 **A Positive Fluid Balance in the First Week was Associated with Increased Long-Term Mortality in Critically Ill Patients** 158
Tsai-Jung Wang, Kai-Chih Pai, Chun-Te Huang, Li-Ting Wong, Minn-Shyan Wang, Chun-Ming Lai, Cheng-Hsu Chen, Chieh-Liang Wu and Wen-Cheng Chao

Chapter 21 **Tools are Needed to Promote Sedation Practices for Mechanically Ventilated Patients** 168
Tao Wang, Dongxu Zhou, Zhongheng Zhang and Penglin Ma

Chapter 22 **Pathophysiology of Coagulopathy Induced by Traumatic Brain Injury is Identical to that of Disseminated Intravascular Coagulation with Hyperfibrinolysis** 175
Takeshi Wada, Atsushi Shiraishi, Satoshi Gando, Kazuma Yamakawa, Seitaro Fujishima, Daizoh Saitoh, Shigeki Kushimoto, Hiroshi Ogura, Toshikazu Abe, Toshihiko Mayumi, Junichi Sasaki, Joji Kotani, Naoshi Takeyama, Ryosuke Tsuruta, Kiyotsugu Takuma, Shin-ichiro Shiraishi, Yasukazu Shiino, Taka-aki Nakada, Kohji Okamoto, Yuichiro Sakamoto, Akiyoshi Hagiwara, Satoshi Fujimi, Yutaka Umemura and Yasuhiro Otomo

Chapter 23 **Urine Output is Associated with In-Hospital Mortality in Intensive Care Patients with Septic Shock: A Propensity Score Matching Analysis** 187
Tianyang Hu, Zhao Qiao and Ying Mei

Chapter 24 **Extracorporeal Cytokine Removal in Critically Ill COVID-19 Patients** 197
Marcell Virág, Máté Rottler, Klementina Ocskay, Tamás Leiner, Balázs Horváth, Daniel Adam Blanco, Alexa Vasquez, László Bucsi, Ágnes Sárkány and Zsolt Molnár

Chapter 25 **The Effect of General Anesthesia vs. Regional Anesthesia on Postoperative Delirium** 205
Xianlin Zhu, Min Yang, Junying Mu, Zaiping Wang, Liang Zhang, Hongbai Wang and Fuxia Yan

Chapter 26 **Alternative Therapies for the Prevention of Postoperative Nausea and Vomiting** 218
Nicoleta Stoicea, Tong J. Gan, Nicholas Joseph, Alberto Uribe, Jyoti Pandya, Rohan Dalal and Sergio D. Bergese

Chapter 27 **Preventing Ventilator-Associated Lung Injury: A Perioperative Perspective** 223
Satoshi Kimura, Nicoleta Stoicea, Byron Rafael Rosero Britton, Muhammad Shabsigh, Aly Branstiter and David L. Stahl

Permissions

List of Contributors

Index

Preface

Anesthesiology is a branch of medicine involved in the total perioperative care of patients before, during, and after a surgical procedure. It is closely related to intensive care medicine that seeks to provide life support, resuscitation, invasive monitoring, and end-of-life care to critically ill patients. Anesthesiology within the domain of intensive care involves dealing with patients who are suffering from severe trauma or infections, as well as the patients recovering from a major surgery. It also involves assessing the patients in order to determine whether the patient will be able to survive the stress of the surgery and anesthesia. This book unravels the recent studies in the field of anesthesiology and intensive care medicine. It strives to provide a fair idea about the challenges and concerns associated with these fields. With state-of-the-art inputs by acclaimed experts of this field, this book targets medical students and professionals.

This book has been the outcome of endless efforts put in by authors and researchers on various issues and topics within the field. The book is a comprehensive collection of significant researches that are addressed in a variety of chapters. It will surely enhance the knowledge of the field among readers across the globe.

It gives us an immense pleasure to thank our researchers and authors for their efforts to submit their piece of writing before the deadlines. Finally in the end, I would like to thank my family and colleagues who have been a great source of inspiration and support.

Editor

1

Transcutaneous Electrical Acupoint Stimulation Decreases the Incidence of Postoperative Nausea and Vomiting After Laparoscopic Non-Gastrointestinal Surgery

Wei Gao[1], Linzhong Zhang[2], Xuechang Han[3], Lai Wei[4], Jie Fang[5], Xiaqing Zhang[6], Jiaqiang Zhang[7], Haiyun Wang[8], Qi Zhou[9], Chenggang Wang[10], Wenting Chen[11], Xinli Ni[12], Lan Yang[1], Ruini Du[1], Ge Wang[1], Bingyu Liu[1], Yajuan Li[1], Shanshan Zhang[1] and Qiang Wang[1]*

[1] Department of Anesthesiology, Center for Brain Science, The First Affiliated Hospital of Xi'an Jiaotong University, Xi'an, China, [2] Department of Anesthesiology, Second Hospital of Shanxi Medical University, Taiyuan, China, [3] Department of Anesthesiology, The First Affiliated Hospital, College of Clinical Medicine of Henan University of Science and Technology, Luoyang, China, [4] Department of Anesthesiology, Hunan Provincial People's Hospital, Changsha, China, [5] Department of Anesthesiology, The First Affiliated Hospital of Henan University of Chinese Medicine, Zhengzhou, China, [6] Department of Anesthesiology, Affiliated Hospital of Shaanxi University of Chinese Medicine, Xianyang, China, [7] Department of Anesthesiology, Henan Provincial People's Hospital, Zhengzhou, China, [8] Department of Anesthesiology, The Third Central Hospital of Tianjin, Tianjin, China, [9] Department of Anesthesiology, The First Hospital of Hunan University of Chinese Medicine, Changsha, China, [10] Department of Anesthesiology, Shanxi Traditional Chinese Medicine Hospital, Taiyuan, China, [11] Department of Anesthesiology, Shuguang Hospital Affiliated to Shanghai University of Traditional Chinese Medicine, Shanghai, China, [12] Department of Anesthesiology, General Hospital of Ningxia Medical University, Yinchuan, China

***Correspondence:**
Qiang Wang
dr.wangqiang@mail.xjtu.edu.cn

Importance: Postoperative nausea and vomiting (PONV) gives patients a bad experience and negates their good recovery from surgery.

Objective: This trial aims to assess the preventive effectiveness of transcutaneous electrical acupoint stimulation (TEAS) on the incidence of PONV in high-risk surgical patients.

Design: The large sample size, multicenter, evaluator-blinded, and randomized controlled study was conducted between September 3, 2019 to February 6, 2021.

Setting: The 12 hospitals were from different Chinese provinces.

Participants: After obtaining ethics approval and written informed consent, 1,655 patients with Apfel score $\geq$ 3 points were enrolled for selective laparoscopic non-gastrointestinal surgery under general anesthesia.

Interventions: Patients were randomly allocated into the TEAS and Sham group with a 1:1 ratio. The TEAS group was stimulated on bilateral Neiguan and Zusanli acupoints after recovery from anesthesia on the surgical day and the next morning for 30 min, while the Sham group received an identical setting as TEAS but without currents delivered. Electronic patient self-reported scale was used to evaluate and record the occurrence of PONV.

Main Outcomes and Measures: Primary clinical end point is the incidence of PONV which was defined as at least one incidence of nausea, retching, or vomiting after operation within postoperative 24 h.

Results: Compared with the Sham treatment, the TEAS lowered the PONV incidence by 4.8% (29.4 vs. 34.2%, $P = 0.036$) and vomiting incidence by 7.4% (10.4 vs. 17.8%, $P < 0.001$). TEAS also lowered persistent nausea incidence and PONV scores and decreased PONV related complications and Quality of Recovery−40 scores ($P < 0.05$). TEAS lowered the 24 h PONV risk by 20% (OR, 0.80, 95% CI, 0.65 −0.98; $P = 0.032$), and lowered hazard ratio by 17% (HR, 0.83, 95% CI, 0.70–0.99; $P = 0.035$). Both TEAS and palonosetron were the independent PONV risk protective factors for 24 h PONV incidence and cumulative PONV incidence. The combination of TEAS and palonosetron was the most effective strategy to reduce the PONV incidence ($P < 0.001$).

Conclusions and Relevance: TEAS attenuated the PONV incidence and severity in high-risk surgical patients and may be applied clinically as a complement therapy to prevent PONV.

Clinical Trial Registration: https://clinicaltrials.gov/ct2/show/NCT04043247, identifier: NCT04043247.

Keywords: antiemetic drugs, laparoscopic non-gastrointestinal surgery, nausea, transcutaneous electrical stimulation, vomiting

KEY POINTS

- **Question:** Dose transcutaneous electrical stimulation prevent postoperative nausea and vomiting (PONV) in high-risk surgical patients?
- **Findings:** The electrical stimulation significantly reduced the PONV incidence and its severity. Both TEAS and palonosetron were independent PONV risk protective factors for 24 h PONV incidence and cumulative PONV incidence.
- **Meaning:** TEAS may enhance recovery of PONV high-risk surgical patients and should be routinely used clinically as a complementary strategy.

INTRODUCTION

Postoperative nausea and vomiting (PONV), characterized as nausea, retching, or vomiting or any these symptoms in combination after surgery, is one of the most common complaints after surgery with an overall incidence of 30%, but its incidence can be as high as to be 60–80% in high-risk patients who have three or four PONV risk factors (1). Nausea gives patients an extremely afflictive medical experience, induces stomach discomfort including the feeling of keck and poor appetite, and even causes dizziness and headache. Vomiting increases the potential risks of electrolyte imbalances, pain, incision dehiscence or hernia, dehydration, esophageal damage, or airway aspiration (2). PONV prevention has been included in enhanced recovery after surgery (ERAS) management strategy. Even though the incidence of PONV can be decreased by using less opioids and inhalational anesthetics and even using antiemetic drugs, its occurrence is still high, with up to 20% of high-risk patients treated with three antiemetic prophylaxis (1, 3).

Owning to multiple mechanisms triggering PONV, several antiemetic drugs are often used clinically in high-risk PONV patients (4), but their effectiveness is still limited and include unwanted side effects such as headaches, xerostomia, abnormal liver function, and extrapyramidal reactions (5–8). Compared to antiemetic drugs, non-pharmaceutical therapy including acupuncture has considerable advantages, for example, non-toxic effects, which has been widely used in postoperative pain analgesia and gastrointestinal function rehabilitation (9, 10). Indeed, acupuncture, a safe and effective non-pharmacotherapy, can directly or indirectly inhibit the emesis center or regulate gastrointestinal function through multiple regulatory mechanisms, such as modulating gastric motility through somatovisceral reflex and influencing the endogenous opioid system and serotonin transmission (11–14). Acupoint Neiguan (P6) stimulation was reported to be comparable to antiemetic drugs in reducing PONV incidence but its effectiveness in combination with antiemetic drugs is inconclusive (1). Transcutaneous electrical acupoint stimulation

Abbreviations: PONV, Postoperative nausea and vomiting; TEAS, transcutaneous electrical acupoint stimulation; QoR-40, the 40-item Quality of Recovery; P6, Neiguan; ST36, Zusanli; EX-LE5, Xiyan; 5-HT3, 5-hydroxytryptamine 3; PACU, postoperative recovery unit; VAS, visual analog scale score.

(TEAS) with transcutaneous electrical nerve stimulation applied to acupuncture points has been used to prevent PONV occurrence (15, 16). However, its effectiveness in preventing PONV has not been established yet due to small sampling size and being not well controlled in the previous studies (1). Therefore, the large sample size, multicenter, evaluator-blinded, and randomized controlled study was carried out to verify the effectiveness of TEAS on P6 and Zusanli (ST36) in reducing the incidence of PONV.

METHODS

Study Design and Participants

This multicenter randomized controlled trial was approved by the Ethics Committee of the First Affiliated Hospital of Xi'an Jiaotong University (XJTU1AF2019LSK-084) and then registered at ClinicalTrials.gov (NCT04043247). The detailed trial protocol is available online as **Supplementary Material 1**. The study was carried out in accordance with clinical research CONSORT and acupuncture clinical trial STRICTA to provide reliable concrete evidence for clinical application of TEAS in PONV prophylaxis (**Supplementary Material 2**). The following inclusion criteria were included: (1) selective laparoscopic non-gastrointestinal surgery under general anesthesia; (2) age 18–50 years, BMI 15–40 kg/m^2, ASA class I–III; (3) Apfel score $\geq$ 3 points; and (4) ability to understand, sign informed consent, and coordinate intervention and evaluation. The following exclusion criteria were included: (1) pregnant and breast-feeding patients; (2) TEAS contraindications such as skin allergy, breakage, infection or itching of test points, allergic to adhesive tape, pacemaker implanted; (3) history of alcohol, opioids, or other drug abuse; (4) likely admission to ICU after surgery; and (5) participation in other clinical studies within 3 months before admission to this study. All investigators were trained according to the standardized acupoints selection and TEAS manipulation by a senior licensed acupuncturist with 20 years of practicing experience.

Enrolment, Randomization, and Blinding

After written informed consent was obtained, patients scheduled for selective laparoscopic non-gastrointestinal surgery under general anesthesia were screened for potential enrolments from 12 hospitals (listed in the authorship) in China from September 3, 2019 to February 6, 2021. The eligible patients were randomly divided into the Sham and TEAS groups in a 1:1 ratio (with a block size of 4) by Crabyter scientific research system (Xinyu Information Technology Co., Ltd.). All patients, anesthesiologists, surgeons, and evaluators were blinded for group allocation, screening, intervention treatment, and statistical analysis. Designated evaluators who were totally blinded took charge for follow-up data collections.

Clinical End Points

Primary clinical end point is the incidence of PONV, which was defined as nausea, retching, and/or vomiting after operation within postoperative 24 h. Secondary clinical end points were the postoperative 24 h PONV severity and the 40-item Quality of Recovery (QoR-40) and PONV-related complications. The PONV severity was assessed with the time and visual analog scale (VAS) score of first PONV, the cumulative numbers, and VAS score in postoperative 24 h. The specific contents of QoR-40 score include five aspects: physical comfort (12 items, 60 scores), emotional state (9 items, 45 scores), physical independence (5 items, 25 scores), psychological support (7 items, 35 scores), and pain (7 items, 35 scores). PONV-related complications are dizziness and headache, electrolyte imbalances, and pain.

Anesthesia and Surgery

After receiving 0.5 mg pre-medication of anticholinergics drug penehyclidine, atropine, or scopolamine, patients were inducted with propofol (2 mg/kg), sufentanil (0.3 μg/kg), and cisatracurium (0.15 mg/kg), and maintained with remifentanil (0.1 μg/kg/h), cisatracurium (0.1 mg/kg/h), dexmedetomidine (initial dose 1 μg/kg for 10 min, maintenance dose 0.4 μg/kg/h), and sevoflurane (1% in 2 L/min enriched oxygen). Propofol (4–8 mg/kg/h) as necessary was used for anesthesia maintenance to keep BIS 40–60 throughout surgery. Patients were treated with 50 mg non-steroidal anti-inflammatory drug flurbiprofen axeril or 40 mg parecoxib at the end of surgery, and were intravenous injection pumped with sufentanil individualized postoperative analgesia pump to keep the perioperative pain numerical score at <4 points.

Interventions

Both groups received 5 mg dexamethasone (before induction) combined with 0.075 mg palonosetron (before induction) as the first choice. When palonosetron was not available at some hospitals, patients received 5 mg dexamethasone (before induction) combined with 2 mg tropisetron (at the end of surgery) instead. According to the criteria of WHO acupuncture points, P6 and ST36 were selected in this study (**Supplementary Figure 1**). These acupoints are far from the operation site. P6 is located at 2 inches above palm wrist transverse striation, between the palm long tendon and the temporal flexor tendon. ST36 is located at 3 inches below EX-LE5 (the lateral pit of the patella and patellar ligament), and one transverse finger outward lateral tibia. The true or sham TEAS was given to the TEAS or sham group patients, respectively, in the PACU when recovered from anesthesia (to be awake and calm, Richmond Agitation-Sedation Scale = 0) on the same surgical day and on the next morning of surgical ward for 30 min. The bilateral P6 and ST36 were pressed to achieve a tingling sensation called "de qi", and electrode slices were stuck and fixed on those acupoints. Interveners connected electrode slices to electrical stimulator (TEAS stimulator, SDZ-V; Hwato, China) and selected the distant-dense wave with the frequency of 2/10 Hz. After adjusting the intensity to the patient's maximum tolerance, the treatment lasted for 30 min. Patients in the sham group received identical settings and manipulation to the TEAS group, except that the wire between electrode pads and TEAS stimulator was cut so that no current could be delivered. The 5-HT$_3$ receptor antagonists or propofol or haloperidol were used for PONV rescue when necessarily.

Data Collection

Electronic patient self-reported scale (Jiangsu Rehn Medtech Technology Co., Ltd.) was used to evaluate and record the occurrence of PONV, including time and corresponding severity. The severity was evaluated with VAS score which is a psychometric response scale to measure the intensity of subjective characteristics or attitudes and has been widely used for pain quantification. In our study, the severity of nausea and vomiting was rated on the VAS score from 0 to

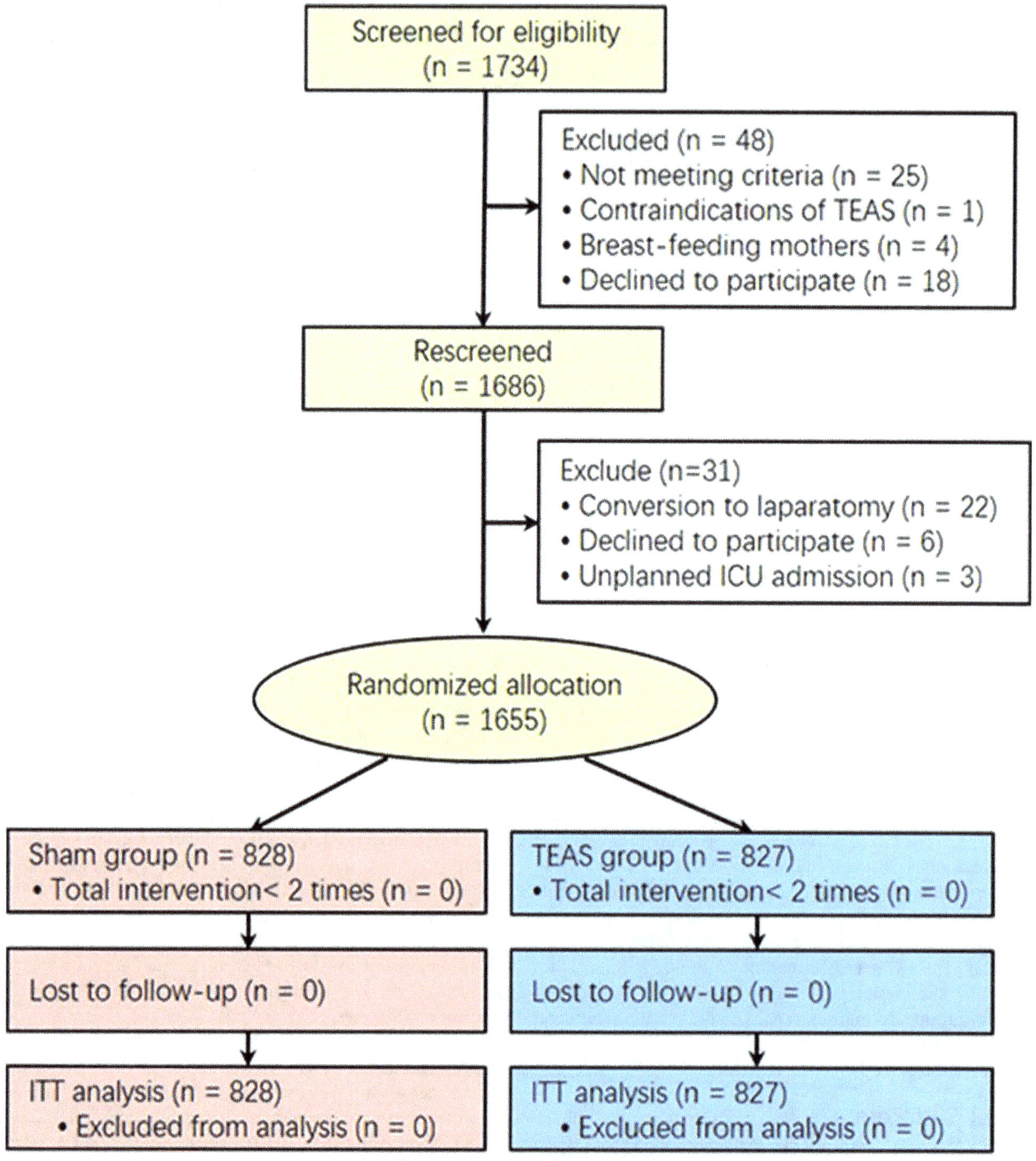

FIGURE 1 | CONSORT diagram for patients enrolled in the study. TEAS, transcutaneous electrical acupoint stimulation; ITT, Intention-To-Treat.

10 (0 = no nausea or vomiting, 10 = maximum severity). Once patients suffered PONV, patients or their caregivers pressed the buttons on an electronic scale and reported the related information (**Supplementary Figure 2**). Postoperative 24 h cumulative PONV incidence refers to the cumulative number of PONV episodes in the postoperative 24 h period. Persistent nausea was defined as continuous nausea lasting over 5 min. To avoid the leakage of allocation, evaluators went to the wards after 12 a.m. at the 1st and 2nd postoperative day to check the electronic patient self-reported system running condition and obtain the information of QoR-40 and complications. The postoperative 30-day complications and adverse events were obtained through telephone follow-ups and were stored in the electronic medical record system.

TABLE 1 | Baseline characteristics.

	TEAS (*n* = 827)	Sham (*n* = 828)	*P*-value
Age, yr	39.0 (31.0, 46.0)	39.0 (31.0, 46.0)	0.693
BMI, kg/m^2	23.1 (21.0, 25.4)	22.7 (20.6, 24.8)	0.001
Education level, *n* (%)			0.154
≤Primary education	223 (27.6)	209 (25.6)	
Secondary education	147 (18.2)	179 (22.0)	
Tertiary education	439 (54.3)	427 (52.4)	
Apfel's score, *n* (%)			
Female	803 (97.1)	803 (97.0)	0.888
Non-smoker	821 (99.3)	818 (98.8)	0.316
Use of postoperative opioids	734 (88.8)	737 (89.0)	0.869
History of PONV or motion sickness	477 (57.7)	485 (58.6)	0.712
4 scores	354 (42.8)	359 (43.4)	0.821
Comorbidities, *n* (%)			
Coronary heart disease	3 (0.4)	5 (0.6)	0.479
Stroke	2 (0.2)	1 (0.1)	0.563
Diabetes	10 (1.2)	5 (0.6)	0.194
Hypertension	40 (4.8)	56 (6.8)	0.094
SAS anxiety score	40.0 (32.0, 45.0)	40.0 (32.0, 45.0)	0.942
The operation types, *n* (%)			0.147
Gynecology	610 (73.8)	587 (70.9)	
Cholecystectomy	142 (17.2)	145 (17.5)	
Urinary	53 (6.4)	57 (6.9)	
Hernia repairment	14 (1.7)	28 (3.4)	
Liver surgery	8 (1.0)	11 (1.3)	
Operation time, hr	1.6 (1.1, 2.3)	1.6 (1.1, 2.3)	0.373
Anesthesia time, hr	2.0 (1.5, 2.8)	2.0 (1.4, 2.8)	0.503
RASS score after extubation	0.0 (0.0, 0.0)	0.0 (0.0, 0.0)	0.144
PACU electrolyte index			
Na^+, mmol/L	139.0 (137.0, 141.0)	140.0 (137.9, 141.0)	0.734
K^+, mmol/L	3.8 (3.5, 4.0)	3.8 (3.6, 4.1)	0.512
Cl^-, mmol/L	109.0 (107.0, 111.0)	109.0 (108.0, 111.0)	0.810
Glu, mmol/L	6.3 (5.4, 7.4)	6.1 (5.3, 7.2)	0.111

ASA, American society of anesthesiologists physical status classification system; RASS, Richmond agitation-sedation scale; PACU, post anesthesia care unit.
Data are presented as median (IQR) or number (%).

Statistical Analysis

Power Calculation

In previous studies, the PONV incidence was reported to be ~40%, and the PONV incidence was reduced by 7% with the TEAS treatment (15). With significance set at 0.05 and power set at 80%, the sample size required to detect differences was 742 patients in each group calculated with the Pass 11 software (NCSS, LLC. Kaysville, Utah, USA). Taking into account a loss-to-follow-up rate of about 10%, 1,634

TABLE 2 | Anticholinergics drugs, antiemetics, and analgesic drug records.

	TEAS (*n* = 827)	Sham (*n* = 828)	*P*-value
Anticholinergics drugs, *n* (%)	461 (55.7)	438 (52.9)	0.245
Penehyclidine	393 (47.5)	383 (46.3)	0.606
Atropine	68 (8.8)	61 (7.6)	0.389
Scopolamine	4 (0.5)	3 (0.4)	0.669
Prophylaxis antiemetic, *n* (%)			
Dexamethasone	770 (93.1)	758 (91.5)	0.233
Palonosetron	431 (52.1)	438 (52.9)	0.750
Tropisetron	396 (47.9)	390 (47.1)	0.750
Dexamethasone+ Palonosetron	407 (49.2)	417 (50.4)	0.640
Dexamethasone+ Tropisetron	363 (43.9)	341 (41.2)	0.265
Rescue medication, *n* (%)	41 (5.0)	36 (4.3)	0.556
Nerve blocking, *n* (%)	81 (9.8)	70 (8.5)	0.344
NSAIDs or cyclooxygenase-2 inhibitors, *n* (%)	274 (33.1)	275 (33.2)	0.972
Flurbiprofen axetil	234 (30.2)	251 (31.2)	0.658
Parecoxib	40 (5.0)	24 (2.9)	0.034
Analgesic pump sufentanil, *n* (%)	597 (72.2)	588 (71.0)	0.596
24 h analgesic pump, μg	33.0 (0.0, 50.0)	30.0 (0.0, 60.0)	0.197
Intraoperative medication			
Sufentanil, μg	30 (30, 40)	30 (30, 40)	0.580
Remifentanil, μg	1,000 (600, 1,200)	1,000 (600, 1,255)	0.908
Propofol, mg	450 (300, 600)	450 (300, 600)	0.936
Sevoflurane, ml	20 (15, 30)	20 (15, 30)	0.798
Intraoperative fluid, ml			
Crystalloid solutions	1,000 (600, 1,500)	1,000 (600, 1,500)	0.149
Solute solutions	500 (500, 500)	500 (500, 500)	0.855

Data are presented as median (IQR) or number (%).

patients in total were enrolled to meet the minimum sample size requirement.

Intention-to-treat analysis was used for all enrolled patients. Continuous variables were presented as mean ± SD if data are normally distributed; otherwise, they were presented as median (interquartile range, IQR). Categorical values were presented as numbers (percentages). The differences between two groups were compared using the Mann-Whitney or Chi-square tests. The Kaplan-Meier log-rank test was used to illustrate the cumulative incidence of nausea and vomiting. Variables with significant differences ($P < 0.10$) in univariate analysis were included in multivariate analysis, which was used to identify the associated risk factors of the PONV occurrence. The comparison of independent risk factors related to PONV was further analyzed by chi-square tests or Kaplan-Meier log-rank test. A 2-sided *P*-value < 0.05 was considered to be of statistical significance. All these statistical analyses were performed using the SPSS software (version 25.0, IBM Corporation, NY, USA). All authors had access to the study data and reviewed and approved the final manuscript.

RESULTS

Characteristics of Study Population

A total of 1,734 patients were scheduled for laparoscopic non-gastrointestinal surgery at 12 hospitals in China between September 3, 2019 and February 6, 2021. At two-step recruitment screenings, 48 patients were excluded at the first screening and of those, 31 patients were excluded at the second screening. A total of 1,655 patients were enrolled and randomly divided into two groups: 828 patients allocated to the Sham group and 827 patients to the TEAS group. All 1,655 patients were included in the intention-to-treat analysis (**Figure 1**). No TEAS-related adverse effects occurred in the study. The demographics, comorbidities, preoperative SAS anxiety score, surgical and anesthesia data, RASS scores after extubation, and PACU electrolyte index between the TEAS and Sham group were presented in **Table 1**. The selective laparoscopic non-gastrointestinal surgery under general anesthesia included gynecology (>70%), cholecystectomy, urinary, hernia repairment, and liver surgery. The anticholinergics, antiemetics, and multimode analgesics used during the perioperative period showed no significant differences between the two groups, except the parecoxib usage was more often higher in the TEAS group than in the Sham group (**Table 2**). The patients with or without parecoxib had no significant difference of PONV incidences.

Primary and Secondary Outcomes

Compared to the Sham group, patients in the TEAS group had significantly lower PONV incidence (29.4 vs. 34.2%, $P = 0.036$) and lower vomiting incidence (10.4 vs. 17.8%, $P < 0.001$). For nausea, the TEAS group showed lower persistent nausea incidence (2.2 vs. 5.1%, $P = 0.003$), lower first-time nausea score, and 24 h nausea highest scores ($P < 0.001$). Specifically, in 827 patients of the TEAS group, 29.4% (243) patients suffered nausea, including 0.7% (6) patients who suffered both persistent nausea and vomiting, 1.5% (12) patients who suffered persistent nausea without vomiting, 9.7% (80) patients who suffered vomiting without persistent nausea, and 17.5% (145) patients who suffered nausea without persistent nausea or vomiting. Correspondingly, in 828 patients of the Sham group, these incidences were, respectively, 2.1% (17), 3.0% (25), 15.7% (130), and 13.4% (111) (**Supplementary Figure 3**).

TABLE 3 | PONV outcomes and related complications.

Outcomes	TEAS (*n* = 827)	Sham (*n* = 828)	*P*-value
24 h PONV, *n* (%)	243 (29.4)	283 (34.2)	0.036
Vomiting, *n* (%)	86 (10.4)	147 (17.8)	<.001
Nausea			
Persistent nausea, *n* (%)			0.003
Persistent nausea	18 (2.2)	42 (5.1)	
Non-persistent nausea	225 (27.2)	241 (29.1)	
Non-PONV	584 (70.6)	545 (65.8)	
First-time nausea score	1.2 (2.3)	1.65 (2.8)	<.001
24 h nausea highest score	1.3 (2.4)	1.7 (2.9)	<.001
Vomiting			
First-time vomiting score	0.6 (1.8)	0.9 (2.0)	0.005
24 h vomiting highest score	0.6 (2.0)	0.9 (2.1)	0.008
24 h vomiting times	0.3 (0.9)	0.4 (1.2)	0.001
Related complications			
Dizzy, *n* (%)	321 (38.8)	363 (43.8)	0.038
Headache, *n* (%)	37 (4.5)	58 (7.0)	0.027
Electrolyte disturbance, *n* (%)	14 (1.7)	20 (2.4)	0.300
24 h pain VAS score	2.0 (1.7)	2.2 (1.8)	0.006

PONV, Postoperative nausea and vomiting; VAS, visual analog scale score.
Data are presented as mean (SD) or patient's number (%).

In the vomiting patients, the TEAS group showed lower first-time vomiting score ($P = 0.005$) and lower highest vomiting scores ($P = 0.008$) together with vomiting times at the postoperative 24 h ($P = 0.001$). TEAS also significantly decreased the PONV-related postoperative 30 days complications including dizziness ($P = 0.038$), headache ($P = 0.027$), and postoperative 24 h Pain ($P = 0.006$) (**Table 3**). Compared to the non-PONV patients, the PONV patients had worse QoR-40 scores in all the five items (all $P < 0.001$). Compared to the 24 h QoR-40 scores in the Sham group, patients in the TEAS group had better physical comfort ($P = 0.003$), emotional state ($P = 0.001$), psychological support ($P = 0.002$), and pain ($P = 0.012$). Compared to the vomiting patients, the non-vomiting patients had significantly better scores in the same items (all $P < 0.001$) (**Supplementary Table 1**).

Multivariate Binary Logistic and COX Regression Analysis for PONV

Both TEAS and palonosetron were independently protective factors of PONV (**Table 4**). Compared with the Sham group, the TEAS group had 20%lower risk of PONV (OR, 0.80, 95% CI, 0.65–0.98; $P = 0.032$) and 48%lower risk of vomiting occurrence (OR, 0.52, 95% CI, 0.39–0.70; $P < 0.001$) by multivariate logistic

TABLE 4 | Multivariates binary logistic and cox regression associated with PONV.

Variable	Multivariate logistic		Cox regression	
	OR (95% CI)	*P*-value	HR (95% CI)	*P*-value
PONV				
TEAS	0.80 (0.65, 0.98)	0.032	0.83 (0.70, 0.99)	0.035
Palonosetron	0.62 (0.50, 0.77)	<0.001	0.68 (0.57, 0.81)	<0.001
Vomiting				
TEAS	0.52 (0.39, 0.70)	<0.001	0.57 (0.43, 0.74)	<0.001
Palonosetron	0.31 (0.23, 0.42)	<0.001	0.34 (0.26, 0.45)	<0.001

regression analysis; the TEAS group delayed PONV occurrence time by 17% (HR, 0.83, 95% CI, 0.70–0.99; $P = 0.035$) and delayed vomiting occurrence time by 43% (HR, 0.57, 95% CI, 0.43–0.74; $P < 0.001$) by COX regression analysis (**Supplementary Figure 4**). Compared with the tropisetron antiemetic, palonosetron reduced risk of PONV by 38% (OR, 0.62, 95% CI, 0.50–0.77; $P < 0.001$) by multivariate logistic regression analysis; the palonosetron delayed postoperative 24 h PONV occurrence time by 32% (OR, 0.68, 95% CI, 0.57–0.81; $P < 0.001$) by COX regression analysis.

The combined TEAS and palonosetron group had the lowest PONV incidence (25.1%), followed with combined Sham and palonosetron (28.8%) and combined TEAS and tropisetron (34.1%), and the combined Sham and tropisetron group had the highest PONV incidence (40.3%) ($P < 0.001$). The similar distribution of cumulative PONV incidences and vomiting among the four groups was noted (**Figure 2**).

DISCUSSION

Our study found that the TEAS significantly decreased the 24 h PONV incidence and also lowered persistent nausea incidence, PONV scores, and postoperative 24 h cumulative PONV incidences. Further, the TEAS also significantly decreased PONV-related complications, and improved postoperative 24 h physical comfort and emotional state, psychological support scores, and pain score in 24 h QoR-40 Scores. We also found that both TEAS and palonosetron were the independent PONV protective factors for 24 h PONV incidence and cumulative PONV incidence.

PONV is triggered by the nerve projected to the vomiting center, which is influenced by the cerebral cortex, vestibular and cerebellar nuclei, and chemoreceptor trigger band (4). The surface of the chemoreceptor trigger band covers various receptors, such as 5-HT_3, 5-HT_4, opioid, cholinergic, cannabis, and dopamine receptor (17). It has been reported that the incidence of PONV can be decreased by 26% for each additional type of antiemetic drug. The incidence of PONV was 52, 37, 28, and 22% in the absence or presence of 1, 2, and 3 types of antiemetic drugs, respectively (3). The Enhanced Recovery after Surgery Society recommended that more than two types of antiemetics should be used for patients undergoing gynecologic procedures (18), while three types of antiemetics did not show improved efficacy over the two agents (19). Thus, two types antiemetics in combination (dexamethasone with tropisetron/palonosetron) were used in our study. Compared to the first-generation 5-HT_3 receptor antagonists of tropisetron, the second-generation 5-HT_3 receptor antagonist palonosetron has a higher binding affinity and longer half-life and duration of action, and a single injection of a 0.075 mg dose of palonosetron for PONV prevention was used for up to 24 h after surgery (20).

However, the combination of two types of antiemetic drugs only inhibited part of the PONV-related receptors, and the prophylaxis effect reached the maximum effect and increasing their doses did not increase antiemetic effects due to receptor occupancy saturation. However, the side effects were increased (7). Correspondingly, the TEAS can modulate comprehensive PONV triggering receptors and reflex pathways to prevent PONV. For example, TEAS stimulates neuronal pathways from the soma splanchnic neurons to the paraventricular nucleus of the hypothalamus (21); TEAS also reduces secretion of 5-HT in the duodenum and suppresses the activation of the nucleus tractus solitarii in the brain-stem (22). TEAS inhibits sympathetic nerve and stimulates parasympathetic nerve and hence increases the activity of acetylcholinesterase (23); TEAS also stimulates receptors such as NO, CCK-A, cannabinoid, opioid receptor, and others and regulates neurotransmitters such as serotonin, GABA, and catecholamines (14). All these result in a decreased incidence of PONV.

Furthermore, the PONV prophylaxis outcome of TEAS might be due to stimulating acupoints of P6 and ST3. P6 is currently recognized as the standard acupoint for the prevention of PONV (24), and its effect was comparable to that of antiemetic drugs (25). Stimulation of P6 and ST36 in laparoscopic radical gastrectomy for gastric cancer significantly reduced the incidence of PONV, decreased early postoperative pain intensity and analgesic dosage, shortened the time of exhaust and excretion, promoted the recovery of gastrointestinal function, and improved patient satisfaction (26). Stimulation of P6 alone or combined with ST36 for 30 min before the lumbar anesthesia of cesarean section decreased PONV, and the mechanism is related to the reduction of plasma 5-HT5 concentration (27). Electroacupuncture at P6 and St36 together was reported to decrease period-dominant frequency in the electrogastrograph, and this effect was abolished by naloxone, indicating a central opioid pathway involvement (12).

It is worth noting that we enrolled the PONV high risk patients who had Apfel $\geq$ 3. The Apfel score includes female gender, non-smoker, history of motion sickness or PONV,

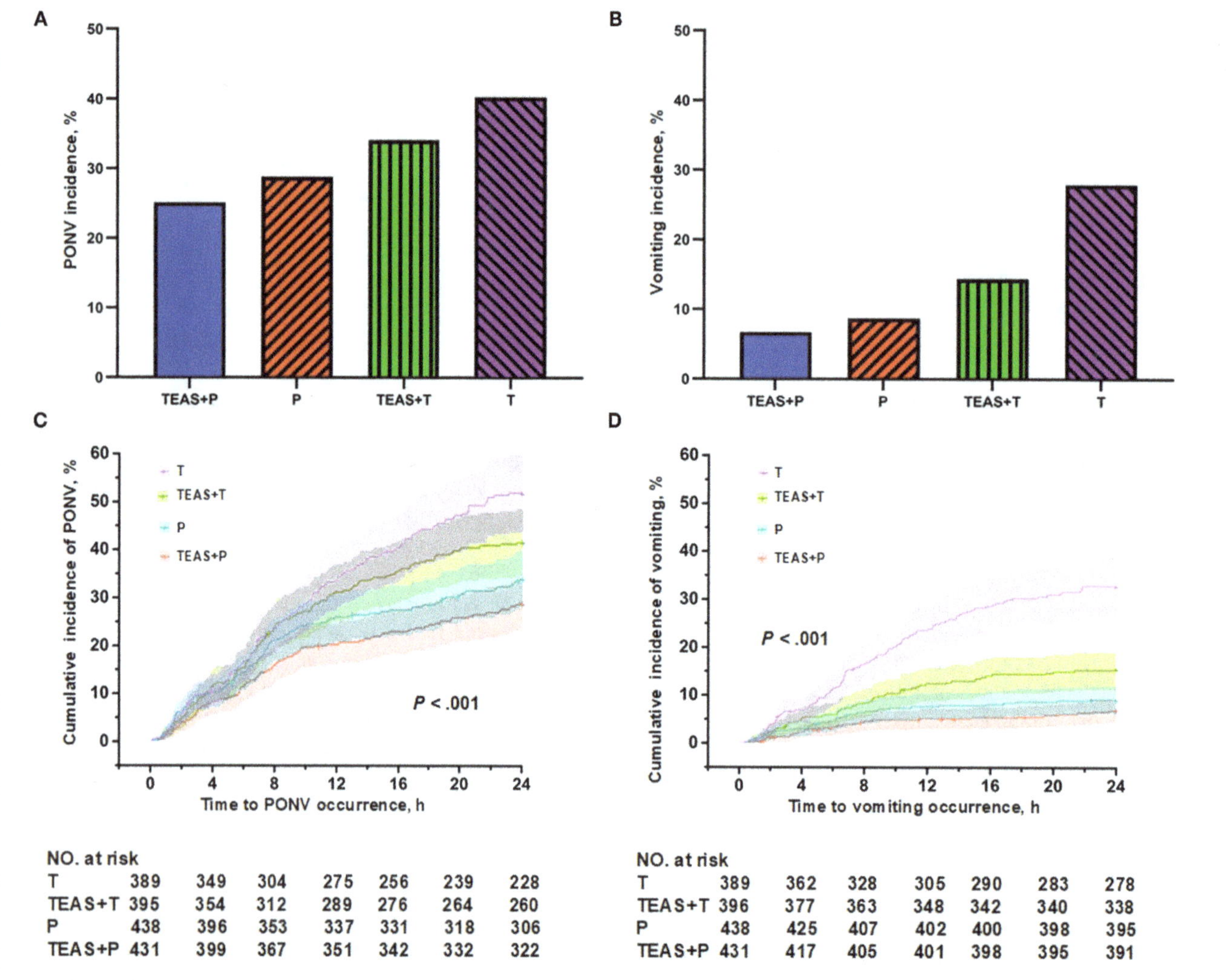

FIGURE 2 | The postoperative 24 h **(A)** PONV incidences, **(B)** vomiting incidences, postoperative 24 h cumulative **(C)** PONV and **(D)** vomiting incidences among combined TEAS and palonosetron (TEAS + P), combined Sham and palonosetron (Sham + P), combined TEAS and tropisetron (TEAS + T), and combined Sham and tropisetron (Sham + T).

and postoperative opioid use. In our study, 97.0% of patients were female. Besides accounting for a quarter of Apfel score, females were more likely to be non-smoking (28) and have motion sickness than males (29). This agreed with the previous epidemiological study, in which females accounted for 93.3% in Apfel score 3 population and 100% in Apfel score 4 population (30). Without any PONV prophylaxis, the estimated probability of PONV in Apfel $\geq$ 2 patients were between 39 and 78%, whereas if Apfel $\geq$ 3 is present, it may rise up to 78% (1). In addition, we enrolled high PONV risk surgical types. The laparoscopic gynecological operation and the laparoscopic cholecystectomy accounts for about 70 and 18% in our study, respectively (**Table 1**). Without any PONV prophylaxis, the PONV incidence of gynecological surgery and cholecystectomy surgery were 69 and 59.6% (31). When PONV prophylaxis with dexamethasone and tropisetron, the PONV incidence of laparoscopic gynecological surgery had been reported even up to 77.4% (32). In contrast, we found that the PONV incidence was much lower. What factors caused these discrepancies between previous studies and the current study remain unknown. However, the study heterogeneity was avoided in our study which may be one of reasons; for example, almost all patients were female and non-smokers and the SAS anxiety score were comparable among patients.

Limitations

The strengths of our trial are its large sample size, multiple centers, high PONV risk patients and surgeries, and the effectiveness of TEAS group in reducing PONV was clearly demonstrated. However, the unavoidable limitation in our study was that patients cannot be blinded to the intervention totally as they can sense the acupoint stimuli in the TEAS group whilst others in the sham group did not. As such, any "placebo" effects of TEAS are unknown. In addition, the balance anesthesia as a potential factor to reduce PONV, the non-standardization of anesthesia management, and the use of different regimens to prevent PONV during surgery may cause potential bias on the results. Antiemetic prophylactic medication used during our study remained similar but not identical due to different medical supplies in various centers. We have narrowed 5-HT_3 receptor antagonists down to two specific drugs (palonosetron or tropisetron). Meanwhile, only 92.3% patients received dexamethasone, although there is no significant difference regarding dexamethasone usage between the TEAS group and Sham group (**Table 2**). Lastly, the sample size calculation was based on the previous publications without any antiemetic prophylaxis medication (15) which might induce sample size bias. However, our study is a large sample size and a multi-centers trial and, therefore, all those limitations were unlikely to have affected our conclusions.

CONCLUSIONS

This multi-center randomized controlled study concluded that the use of postoperative TEAS (at anesthesia recovery arrival and in the following morning) in conjunction with antiemetic prophylaxis may significantly reduce PONV incidence and its severity. Both TEAS and palonosetron were independent PONV risk protective factors for 24 h PONV incidence and cumulative PONV incidence. The combination of TEAS and palonosetron was the most effective strategy to reduce the PONV incidence. Our work may suggest that one should consider implementing TEAS clinically for patients' better and smoother postoperative recovery.

ETHICS STATEMENT

The studies involving human participants were reviewed and approved by the Ethics Committee of the First Affiliated Hospital of Xi'an Jiaotong University (XJTU1AF2019LSK-084). The patients/participants provided their written informed consent to participate in this study.

AUTHOR CONTRIBUTIONS

WG and QW: study conception, critically revised the manuscript for important intellectual content, and obtained funding. WG, LZ, XH, LW, JF, XZ, JZ, HW, QZ, CW, WC, XN, LY, RD, GW, and BL: acquisition or interpretation of data. WG and YL: statistical analyses. WG, LY, and QW: drafted the manuscript. WG, LZ, XH, LW, JF, XZ, JZ, HW, QZ, CW, WC, XN, LY, RD, GW, BL, and QW: provided administrative, technical, or material support.

ACKNOWLEDGMENTS

The authors thank Prof. Daqing Ma, MD, PhD, FRCA, MAE, Imperial College London, Chelsea and Westminster Hospital, London, UK for his critical comments during manuscript preparation. The authors thank the Department of Anesthesiology of the Second Hospital of Hebei Medical University, Department of Anesthesiology of Hebei Hospital of Traditional Chinese Medicine, Department of Anesthesiology of Xiyuan Hospital of China Academy of Chinese Medical Sciences, Department of Anesthesiology of Fujian Provincial Hospital, and Department of Anesthesiology of Ningxia Chinese Medicine Research Center for their guidance in protocol.

REFERENCES

1. Gan TJ, Belani KG, Bergese S, Chung F, Diemunsch P, Habib AS, et al. Fourth consensus guidelines for the management of postoperative nausea and vomiting. *Anesth Analgesia.* (2020) 131:411–48. doi: 10.1213/ANE.0000000000004833
2. Schmitt ARM, Ritto FG, de Azevedo J, Medeiros PJD, de Mesquita MCM. Efficacy of gastric aspiration in reducing postoperative nausea and vomiting after orthognathic surgery: a double-blind prospective study. *J Oral Maxillofac Surg.* (2017) 75:701–8. doi: 10.1016/j.joms.2016.10.002
3. Apfel C, Korttila K, Abdalla M, Kerger H, Turan A, Vedder I, et al. A factorial trial of six interventions for the prevention of postoperative nausea and vomiting. *N Engl J Med.* (2004) 350:2441–51. doi: 10.1056/NEJMoa032196
4. Chandrakantan A, Glass PS. Multimodal therapies for postoperative nausea and vomiting, and pain. *Br J Anaesth.* (2011) 107 (Suppl. 1):i27–40. doi: 10.1093/bja/aer358
5. Cao X, White PF, Ma H. An update on the management of postoperative nausea and vomiting. *J Anesth.* (2017) 31:617–26. doi: 10.1007/s00540-017-2363-x
6. Kovac AL. Comparative pharmacology and guide to the use of the serotonin 5-HT3 receptor antagonists for postoperative nausea and vomiting. *Drugs.* (2016) 76:1719–35. doi: 10.1007/s40265-016-0663-3
7. Gan T, White P, Scuderi P, Watcha M, Kovac A. FDA "black box" warning regarding use of droperidol for postoperative nausea and vomiting: is it justified? *Anesthesiology.* (2002) 97:287. doi: 10.1097/00000542-200207000-00059
8. Kovac A. Prevention and treatment of postoperative nausea and vomiting. *Drugs.* (2000) 59:213–43. doi: 10.2165/00003495-200059020-00005
9. Chen J, Zhang Y, Li X, Wan Y, Ji X, Wang W, et al. Efficacy of transcutaneous electrical acupoint stimulation combined with general anesthesia for sedation and postoperative analgesia in minimally invasive lung cancer surgery: a randomized, double-blind, placebo-controlled trial. *Thorac Cancer.* (2020). doi: 10.1111/1759-7714.13343
10. Zhou D, Hu B, He S, Li X, Gong H, Li F, et al. Transcutaneous electrical acupoint stimulation accelerates the recovery of gastrointestinal function after cesarean section: a randomized controlled trial. *Evid Based Complement Alternat Med.* (2018) 2018:7341920. doi: 10.1155/2018/7341920
11. Wang C, Chen X, Xie PY. Electroacupuncture at PC6 or ST36 influences the effect of tacrine on the motility of esophagus. *Evid Based Complement Alternat Med.* (2014) 2014:263489. doi: 10.1155/2014/263489
12. Streitberger K, Ezzo J, Schneider A. Acupuncture for nausea and vomiting: an update of clinical and experimental studies. *Auton Neurosci.* (2006) 129:107–17. doi: 10.1016/j.autneu.2006.07.015
13. Stoicea N, Gan TJ, Joseph N, Uribe A, Pandya J, Dalal R, et al. Alternative therapies for the prevention of postoperative nausea and vomiting. *Front Med.* (2015) 2:87. doi: 10.3389/fmed.2015.00087
14. Wang C, Zhou D, Shuai X, Liu J, Xie P. Effects and mechanisms of electroacupuncture at PC6 on frequency of transient lower esophageal sphincter relaxation in cats. *World J Gastroenterol.* (2007) 13:4873–80. doi: 10.3748/wjg.v13.i36.4873
15. Chen J, Tu Q, Miao S, Zhou Z, Hu S. Transcutaneous electrical acupoint stimulation for preventing postoperative nausea and vomiting after general anesthesia: a meta-analysis of randomized controlled trials. *Int J Surg.* (2020) 73:57–64. doi: 10.1016/j.ijsu.2019.10.036
16. Fu C, Wu T, Shu Q, Song A, Jiao Y. Acupuncture therapy on postoperative nausea and vomiting in abdominal operation: a Bayesian network meta analysis. *Medicine.* (2020) 99:e20301. doi: 10.1097/MD.0000000000020301

17. Dabbous A, Jabbour-Khoury S, Nasr V, Moussa A, Zbeidy R, Khouzam N, et al. Dexamethasone with either granisetron or ondansetron for postoperative nausea and vomiting in laparoscopic surgery. *Middle East J Anaesthesiol.* (2010) 20:565–70.
18. Nelson G, Altman AD, Nick A, Meyer LA, Ramirez PT, Achtari C, et al. Guidelines for pre- and intra-operative care in gynecologic/oncology surgery: enhanced recovery after surgery (ERAS(R)) society recommendations–part I. *Gynecol Oncol.* (2016) 140:313–22. doi: 10.1016/j.ygyno.2015.11.015
19. Benevides ML, Oliveira SS, de Aguilar-Nascimento JE. The combination of haloperidol, dexamethasone, and ondansetron for prevention of postoperative nausea and vomiting in laparoscopic sleeve gastrectomy: a randomized double-blind trial. *Obes Surg.* (2013) 23:1389–96. doi: 10.1007/s11695-013-0923-1
20. Li Y, Wei X, Zhang S, Zhou L, Zhang J. A meta-analysis of palonosetron for the prevention of postoperative nausea and vomiting in adults. *Journal of Perianesthesia Nurs.* (2015) 30:398–405. doi: 10.1016/j.jopan.2015.05.116
21. Shu C, Yong CY, Chen H, Xiao C, Chao Z, Cheng T, et al. Response of gastric-related neurons in the hypothalamic paraventricular nucleus to acupuncture at Neiguan and Zusanli in a rat model of gastric distension. *Chin J Tissue Eng Res.* (2014) 18:675–80.
22. Cui Y, Wang L, Shi G, Liu L, Pei P, Guo J. Electroacupuncture alleviates cisplatin-induced nausea in rats. *Acupunct Med.* (2016) 34:120–6. doi: 10.1136/acupmed-2015-010833
23. Li Y, Zhu B, Rong P, Ben H, Li YH. Neural mechanism of acupuncture-modulated gastric motility. *World J Gastroenterol.* (2007) 13:709–16. doi: 10.3748/wjg.v13.i5.709
24. Lee A, Chan S, Fan L. Stimulation of the wrist acupuncture point PC6 for preventing postoperative nausea and vomiting. *Cochrane Database Syst Rev.* (2015) 2015:CD003281. doi: 10.1002/14651858.CD003281.pub4
25. Coloma M, White P, Ogunnaike B, Markowitz S, Brown P, Lee A, et al. Comparison of acustimulation and ondansetron for the treatment of established postoperative nausea and vomiting. *Anesthesiology.* (2002) 97:1387–92. doi: 10.1097/00000542-200212000-00009
26. Gu SH, Lang HB, Gan JH, Zheng ZW, Zhao F, Q T. Effect of transcutaneous electrical acupoint stimulation on gastrointestinal function recovery after laparoscopic radical gastrectomy - A randomized controlled trial - ScienceDirect. *Eur J Integr Med.* (2019) 26:11–7. doi: 10.1016/j.eujim.2019.01.001
27. El-Deeb AM, Ahmady MS. Effect of acupuncture on nausea and/or vomiting during and after cesarean section in comparison with ondansetron. *J Anesth.* (2011) 25:698–703. doi: 10.1007/s00540-011-1198-0
28. Wang YJ, Li ZX, Gu HQ, Zhai Y, Jiang Y, Zhao XQ, et al. China stroke statistics 2019: a report from the National Center for Healthcare Quality Management in Neurological Diseases, China National Clinical Research Center for Neurological Diseases, the Chinese Stroke Association, National Center for Chronic and Non-communicable Disease Control and Prevention, Chinese Center for Disease Control and Prevention and Institute for Global Neuroscience and Stroke Collaborations. *Stroke Vasc Neurol.* (2020) 5:211–39. doi: 10.1136/svn-2020-000457
29. Mucci V, Canceri JM, Brown R, Dai M, Yakushin SB, Watson S, et al. Mal de Debarquement syndrome: a retrospective online questionnaire on the influences of gonadal hormones in relation to onset and symptom fluctuation. *Front Neurol.* (2018) 9:362. doi: 10.3389/fneur.2018.00362
30. Canakci E, Catak T, Basar HE, Cebeci Z, Coskun I, Saltali AO, et al. Prevalence study for postoperative nausea vomiting: a training hospital example. *Niger J Clin Pract.* (2021) 24:1633–40. doi: 10.4103/njcp.njcp_399_20
31. Apfel C, Kranke P, Eberhart LJA. Comparison of surgical site and patient's history with a simplified risk score for the prediction of postoperative nausea and vomiting. *Anaesthesia.* (2004) 59:1078–82. doi: 10.1111/j.1365-2044.2004.03875.x
32. Xiong Q, Min S, Wei K, Yang Y, Ma J, Liu D, et al. Transcutaneous electrical acupoint stimulation combined with dexamethasone and tropisetron prevents postoperative nausea and vomiting in female patients undergoing laparoscopic sleeve gastrectomy: a prospective, randomized controlled trial. *Obes Surg.* (2021) 31:1912–20. doi: 10.1007/s11695-020-05205-9

2

Using RNA-Seq to Investigate Immune-Metabolism Features in Immunocompromised Patients with Sepsis

Po-Liang Cheng [1,2], *Hsin-Hua Chen* [3,4,5,6], *Yu-Han Jiang* [1,2], *Tzu-Hung Hsiao* [1,2,7,8], *Chen-Yu Wang* [9,10], *Chieh-Liang Wu* [5,9,11,12], *Tai-Ming Ko* [13,14,15,16] and *Wen-Cheng Chao* [4,9,11,12]*

[1] Department of Medical Research, Taichung Veterans General Hospital, Taichung, Taiwan, [2] Precision Medicine Center, Taichung Veterans General Hospital, Taichung, Taiwan, [3] Division of General Internal Medicine, Department of Internal Medicine, Taichung Veterans General Hospital, Taichung, Taiwan, [4] Big Data Center, Chung Hsing University, Taichung, Taiwan, [5] Department of Industrial Engineering and Enterprise Information, Tunghai University, Taichung, Taiwan, [6] Rong Hsing Research Centre for Translational Medicine, Institute of Biomedical Science, Chung Hsing University, Taichung, Taiwan, [7] Department of Public Health, Fu Jen Catholic University, New Taipei City, Taiwan, [8] Institute of Genomics and Bioinformatics, National Chung Hsing University, Taichung, Taiwan, [9] Department of Critical Care Medicine, Taichung Veterans General Hospital, Taichung, Taiwan, [10] Department of Nursing, Hung Kuang University, Taichung, Taiwan, [11] Department of Computer Science, Tunghai University, Taichung, Taiwan, [12] Department of Automatic Control Engineering, Feng Chia University, Taichung, Taiwan, [13] Department of Biological Science and Technology, National Chiao Tung University, Hsinchu, Taiwan, [14] Department of Biological Science and Technology, National Yang Ming Chiao Tung University, Hsinchu, Taiwan, [15] Institute of Bioinformatics and Systems Biology, National Chiao Tung University, Hsinchu, Taiwan, [16] Institute of Biomedical Sciences, Academia Sinica, Taipei, Taiwan

***Correspondence:**
Wen-Cheng Chao
cwc081@hotmail.com

Objective: Sepsis is life threatening and leads to complex inflammation in patients with immunocompromised conditions, such as cancer, and receiving immunosuppressants for autoimmune diseases and organ transplant recipients. Increasing evidence has shown that RNA-Sequencing (RNA-Seq) can be used to define subendotype in patients with sepsis; therefore, we aim to use RNA-Seq to identify transcriptomic features among immunocompromised patients with sepsis.

Methods: We enrolled patients who were admitted to medical intensive care units (ICUs) for sepsis at a tertiary referral centre in central Taiwan. Whole blood on day-1 and day-8 was obtained for RNA-Seq. We used Gene Set Enrichment Analysis (GSEA) to identify the enriched pathway of day-8/day-1 differentially expressed genes and MiXCR to determine the diversity of T cell repertoire.

Results: A total of 18 immunocompromised subjects with sepsis and 18 sequential organ failure assessment (SOFA) score-matched immunocompetent control subjects were enrolled. The ventilator-day, ICU-stay, and hospital-day were similar between the two groups, whereas the hospital mortality was higher in immunocompromised patients than those in immunocompetent patients (50.0 vs. 5.6%, $p < 0.01$). We found that the top day-8/day-1 upregulated genes in the immunocompetent group were mainly innate immunity and inflammation relevant genes, namely, *PRSS33, HDC, ALOX15, FCER1A*, and *OLR1*, whereas a blunted day-8/day-1 dynamic transcriptome was found among immunocompromised patients with septic. Functional pathway analyses of day-8/day-1 differentially expressed genes identified the upregulated functional biogenesis and T cell-associated pathways in immunocompetent patients recovered from sepsis, whereas merely downregulated metabolism-associated pathways were found in immunocompromised patients with septic. Moreover, we used MiXCR to identify a higher diversity of T cell receptor (TCR) in immunocompetent patients both on day-1 and on day-8 than those in immunocompromised patients.

Conclusions: Using RNA-Seq, we found compromised T cell function, altered metabolic signalling, and decreased T cell diversity among immunocompromised patients with septic, and more mechanistic studies are warranted to elucidate the underlying mechanism.

Keywords: RNA-Seq, sepsis, immunocompromised, immune, metabolism, pathway analyses

BACKGROUND

Sepsis, characterised by a dysregulated host-pathogen inflammation, is a leading cause of death worldwide, and approximately 5.3 million people died from sepsis annually (1). There is a global increase of patients with distinct immunocompromised conditions due to the advance of cancer treatment, increasing biologics, and immunosuppressants for autoimmune diseases and growing organ transplant recipients (2), and it has been estimated that patients with immunocompromised conditions account for approximately 35% of all intensive care unit (ICU) admissions (3). Therefore, there is a crucial need to explore the alternation of immunological responses in sepsis among patients with immunocompromised conditions.

Immunoparalysis, characterised by not only immunologic but also by metabolic dysregulation after sepsis, has been increasingly recognised and attributed to be one of the key biological bases of prolonged impact on long-term mortality in patients with sepsis (4, 5). Recent advances in sequencing technology, such as RNA-Sequencing (RNA-Seq), immune repertoire sequencing, and single-cell RNA-Seq (sc-RNA-Seq), allow for addressing immunological and metabolic features in patients with sepsis and coronavirus disease 2019 (COVID-19) infection (6–8). Several studies have used MicroArray and RNA-Seq to identify the transcriptomic signature, so-called subendotype, in patients with sepsis, and the currently identified sepsis-associated subendotypes included early improvement of organ dysfunction after sepsis and the responsiveness of steroids in patients with a septic shock (6, 9, 10). Additionally, analytic tools, namely, MiXCR, have been recently developed to investigate the diversity of T cell receptor (TCR) using bulk RNA-Seq data (11, 12). Despite increasing studies to explore transcriptomic features of sepsis, the transcriptomic signature of sepsis among immunocompromised patients remains unclear. In the present study, we used RNA-Seq to identify distinct transcriptomic features and MiXCR to explore the diversity of TCR between immunocompromised and severity-matched immunocompetent patients with sepsis.

MATERIALS AND METHODS

Ethical Approval

This study was approved by the Institutional Review Board approval of the Taichung Veterans General Hospital (CE20069B). Informed consent was obtained from all participants prior to the enrolment in the study and collection of blood samples.

Definition of Patients With Immunocompromised Conditions

Patients were defined as immunocompromised if they had at least one of the following conditions, such as patients receiving immunosuppressive therapy due to autoimmune disease, organ transplant recipient, and patients with active malignant disease consisting of active haematological disease, or solid tumour under therapy (13).

Enrolment of Subjects

We enrolled 18 immunocompromised patients and 18 severity-matched (day-1 sequential organ failure assessment (SOFA) score $\pm$ 1) immunocompetent patients who were admitted to the medical ICUs between March 2020 and February 2021 at Taichung Veterans General Hospital, a tertiary referral centre in central Taiwan, for sepsis and extracted blood samples on day-1 and day-8 after the ICU admission. Patients who did not survive until day-8 were not included for analyses; therefore, each enrolled patient for analyses had paired day-1 and day-8 samples in this study. In the present study, we used PAXgene Blood RNA Tube to collect blood samples from enrolled subjects. Clinical variables, such as comorbidities, severity scores (day-1 SOFA score, day-3 SOFA score, day-7 SOFA score, and Acute Physiology and Chronic Health Evaluation (APACHE) II score), laboratory data, and outcomes (ventilator-day, ICU-stay, hospital-stay, and overall mortality) were recorded.

RNA Preparation and Sequencing

We used PAXgene Blood RNA Kit to extract RNA, and the average RNA integrity number (RIN) was 8.31 $\pm$ 0.58 in the present study. The library was constructed in accordance with the manufacturer's instruction, and 800–1,000 ng fragmented RNA was used for further experiments. The RNA-Seq was conducted on the NovaSeq platform (Illumina, San Diego, CA, USA), with at least 50–60 million 150-bp pair-end reads per sample.

Bioinformatics Analyses

The quality of sequencing was good, and Phred scores 30 was applied, and sequence reads were mapped to the human reference genome GRCh38 by HISAT2 (14). Read counts were calculated by featureCounts (15), and the differentially expressed genes were identified by R package DEseq2 (16). The average mapped rate and read counts were 82.3 ± 7.8% and 104.0 ± 43.6 million reads, respectively. Gene Set Enrichment Analysis (GSEA) was used for functional annotation of the whole differentially expressed genes (17), and the visualised enrichment map was performed by using Cytoscape 3.8.2 (18). In brief, we used an enrichment map, which organise gene sets into a similarity network, to visualise GSEA results, and the node, link, and node colour represent gene-set, the overlap of member gene, and enrichment score, respectively (19).

Diversity of TCR Analyses

Raw sequences from RNAseq were conducted into MiXCR v3.0.13 (11, 12) to quantitate the clonotypes of patients with sepsis. After obtaining the quantitated clonotypes, VDJTools v 1.2.1 (20) was used to calculate the sample diversity and counts of complementarity-determining region-3 (CDR3).

Statistical Analyses

Continuous variables were presented as median (interquartile range), and data for categorical variables were shown as numbers (percentages). The differences between the immunocompromised and immunocompetent groups were analysed by the Mann-Whitney U test for continuous variables and Fisher's exact test for categorical variables. Statistical analyses were two-sided, and the level of significance was set at 0.05 for clinical data. Data analyses were conducted using R version 4.0.2.

RESULTS

Patient Characteristics

A total of 36 patients with sepsis were enrolled, consisting of 18 immunocompromised patients and 18 day-1 SOFA score-matched immunocompetent control subjects. Of the 18 immunocompromised patients, the number of subjects with solid tumour receiving therapy, haematological cancer, those with autoimmune disease underwent immunosuppressants, and renal transplant recipients were 3, 6, 7, and 2, respectively. The comorbidities and laboratory data were comparable between the two patient groups. With respect to the outcome, the ventilator-day, ICU-stay, and hospital-day were similar between the two groups, whereas the hospital mortality was much higher in immunocompromised patients compared to those in immunocompetent patients (50.0 vs. 5.6%, $p < 0.01$; **Table 1**; refer to **Supplemental Table 1** for details with regards to pathogens and infection sites).

TABLE 1 | Characteristics of the enrolled immunocompromised and severity-matched immunocompetent critically ill patients with septic.

	Immunocompromised $n = 18$	Immunocompetent $n = 18$	*p*-value
Demographic data			
Age (years)	58.0 (50.3–68.3)	71.0 (57.5–81.5)	0.06
Sex (female)	9 (50.0%)	6 (33.3%)	0.50
Immunocompromised factors			NA
Solid tumour receiving therapy	4 (22.2%)	NA	
Haematological cancer	5 (27.8%)	NA	
Autoimmune disease	7 (38.9%)	NA	
Renal transplant recipient	2 (11.1%)	NA	
Severity scores			
APACHE II score	28.0 (23.0–31.3)	26.0 (22.5–29.5)	0.32
SOFA score, day-1	11.0 (8.5–15.0)	12.0 (8.0–13.3)	1.00
SOFA score, day-3	11.0 (7.0–12.3)	10.0 (5.5–13.0)	0.66
SOFA score, day-7	6.5 (3.8–11.0)	7.0 (3.0–12.0)	0.91
Comorbidities			
Diabetes mellitus	5 (27.8%)	10 (55.6%)	0.18
Congestive heart failure	1 (5.6%)	1 (5.6%)	1.00
COPD	2 (11.1%)	1 (5.6%)	0.50
End-stage renal disease	4 (22.2%)	1 (5.6%)	0.34
Cerebral vascular disease	0 (0%)	4 (22.2%)	0.10
Laboratory data			
White blood cell counts (/ml)	11,445.0 (7640.0–13077.5)	11,175.0 (9342.5–12872.5)	0.89
Platelet count (1000/ml)	41.0 (16.5–145.3)	77.5 (44.5–150.0)	0.12
Creatinine (mg/dl)	1.3 (0.8–4.7)	2.1 (0.8–3.1)	0.91
Albumin (mg/dl)	2.8 (2.5–3.2)	3.1 (2.9–3.4)	0.14
Lactate (mg/dl)	29.0 (19.4–51.0)	39.6 (21.1–73.6)	0.30
C-reactive protein (mg/dl)	11.7 (5.1–26.9)	8.2 (3.4–21.1)	0.56
Outcome			
Ventilator-day, days	12.0 (8.8–25.3)	12.5 (7.8–18.0)	0.54
ICU-stay, days	14.0 (9.5–25.3)	14.5 (11.8–27.5)	0.74
Hospital day	33.5 (14.8–47.8)	28.5 (22.8–41.3)	0.96
Mortality	8 (44.4%)	2 (11.1%)	0.03

Data were presented as median (interquartile range) and number (percentage). APACHE II, acute physiology and chronic health evaluation II; SOFA, sequential organ failure assessment; COPD, chronic obstructive pulmonary disease; ICU, intensive care unit.

Distinct Dynamic Transcriptome in Immunocompetent and Immunocompromised Patients With Sepsis

Principal component analysis was performed on the top 500 variable genes across samples, and we found that the transcriptome was similar on day-1 among immunocompromised and immunocompetent patients (**Figure 1A**). We found that the separation between day-1 and day-8 was apparently better in the immunocompetent group than those in the immunocompromised group, suggesting the regulated recovery from sepsis in the immunocompetent group (**Figures 1B,C**). We then compared gene-expression profiles between day-8 and day-1 in the immunocompromised and immunocompetent groups through using the criteria with $p < 0.01$ and log fold change >0.25 or <-0.25 to define differential expression genes (DEGs). In the immunocompetent group, there were 978 DEGs (362 upregulated and 616 downregulated genes), whereas merely 368 DEGs (200 upregulated and 168 downregulated genes) in the immunocompromised group. We found that the top upregulated genes in the immunocompetent group were mainly innate immunity and inflammation relevant genes, namely, *PRSS33, HDC, ALOX15, FCER1A,* and *OLR1*, whereas a significant downregulation was found in *PCSK9*, which has been implicated with increased clearance of endogenous lipids and bacteria among patients with septic with day-3 functional improvement after resuscitation (6) (**Figure 1D**). In contrast with the highly dynamic transcriptome in immunocompetent patients with septic, we found a relatively blunted dynamic transcriptome among immunocompromised patients with septic (**Figure 1E**).

Enriched Pathway of the Dynamic Transcriptome in Immunocompetent Patients With Sepsis

To illustrate the alteration of biological pathways in the immunocompetent group, we used GSEA and a functional map to illustrate the enriched pathway. In brief, the identified gene ontology (GO) terms were mapped as a network of gene sets (nodes) related by mutual overlap (edges), and the red and blue nodes represent up and downregulated pathways, respectively. We identified a total of 11 clusters with significant over-represented GO terms using normalised $p < 0.005$ (**Figure 2**; **Supplemental Table 2**). We noted that ribosome RNA (rRNA) relevant pathways, such as rRNA biogenesis and metabolic process, were activated, indicating the potential cellular proliferation and tissue repair among immunocompetent patients with septic in the recovery from sepsis. In contrast, autophagy-related pathways, such as macroautophagy, autophagosome organisation, and vesicle budding from the membrane, were downregulated among immunocompetent patients with septic, implicating the resolution of inflammation result from sepsis. Notably, we identified the enriched upregulation of T cell-related pathways, such as T cell selection, positive alpha/beta T cell lineage commitment, and T cell lineage commitment, and the finding indicated the functional T cell immunity in immunocompetent patients was recovered from sepsis. We further used the Reactome to validate our finding in T cell-associated pathway and found an enriched interferon-gamma signalling pathway in which the leading edge genes consisted of *HLA-DRB1, HLA-DPB1, HLA-DPA1, HLA-DRB5, HLA-DQB1,* and *HLA-DRA* (**Supplemental Table 3**). Collectively, the functional pathway analyses identified the upregulated biogenesis and functional T cell signalling in immunocompetent patients recovered from sepsis.

Enriched Pathway of the Dynamic Transcriptome in Immunocompromised Patients With Sepsis

We then explored the alteration of the pathway in immunocompromised patients with septic. Similar to the aforementioned limited differentially expressed genes, we identified merely four downregulated pathways, and no upregulated pathway can be enriched. In contrast with the aforementioned upregulated T cell and metabolic process, we found downregulated antigen processing, antigen presentation, and metabolism-associated pathways in immunocompromised patients clinically recovered from sepsis on day-8 (**Figure 3**; **Supplemental Tables 4, 5**). In detail, the enriched downregulated metabolism-associated pathways included the tricarboxylic acid (TCA) cycle, aerobic respiration, respiratory electron transport chain, and cellular respiration pathway. These results showed an aberrantly blunted immunological pathways and impaired metabolism status among immunocompromised patients clinically recovered from sepsis.

MiXCR to Assess the Diversity of TCR

Given that we found the distinct T cell-associated pathway between immunocompetent and immunocompromised patients recovered from sepsis, we then employed MiXCR to determine the diversity of TCR through using the number of unique CDR3, Shannon's diversity index, and inverse Simpson index (**Figure 4**). We found the day-1 number of unique CDR3 tended to be higher in immunocompetent patients than that in immunocompromised patients. Unlike the mildly increased number of unique CDR3 on day-8 among immunocompetent patients, the number of unique CDR3 in immunocompromised patients remained low (**Figure 4A**). We then used Shannon's diversity index to quantify the diversity of unique CDR3 and found a significantly higher diversity of TCR in immunocompetent patients both on day-1 and on day-8 (**Figure 4B**). We also used the inverse Simpson index, which reflects abundant clonotypes to assess the diversity of unique CDR3 and found a similar trend with a significantly decreased diversity of TCR in immunocompromised, particularly on day-8 (**Figure 4C**).

DISCUSSION

In the present study, we used RNA-Seq, analysed by functional pathway analyses and MiXCR, to identify immunological

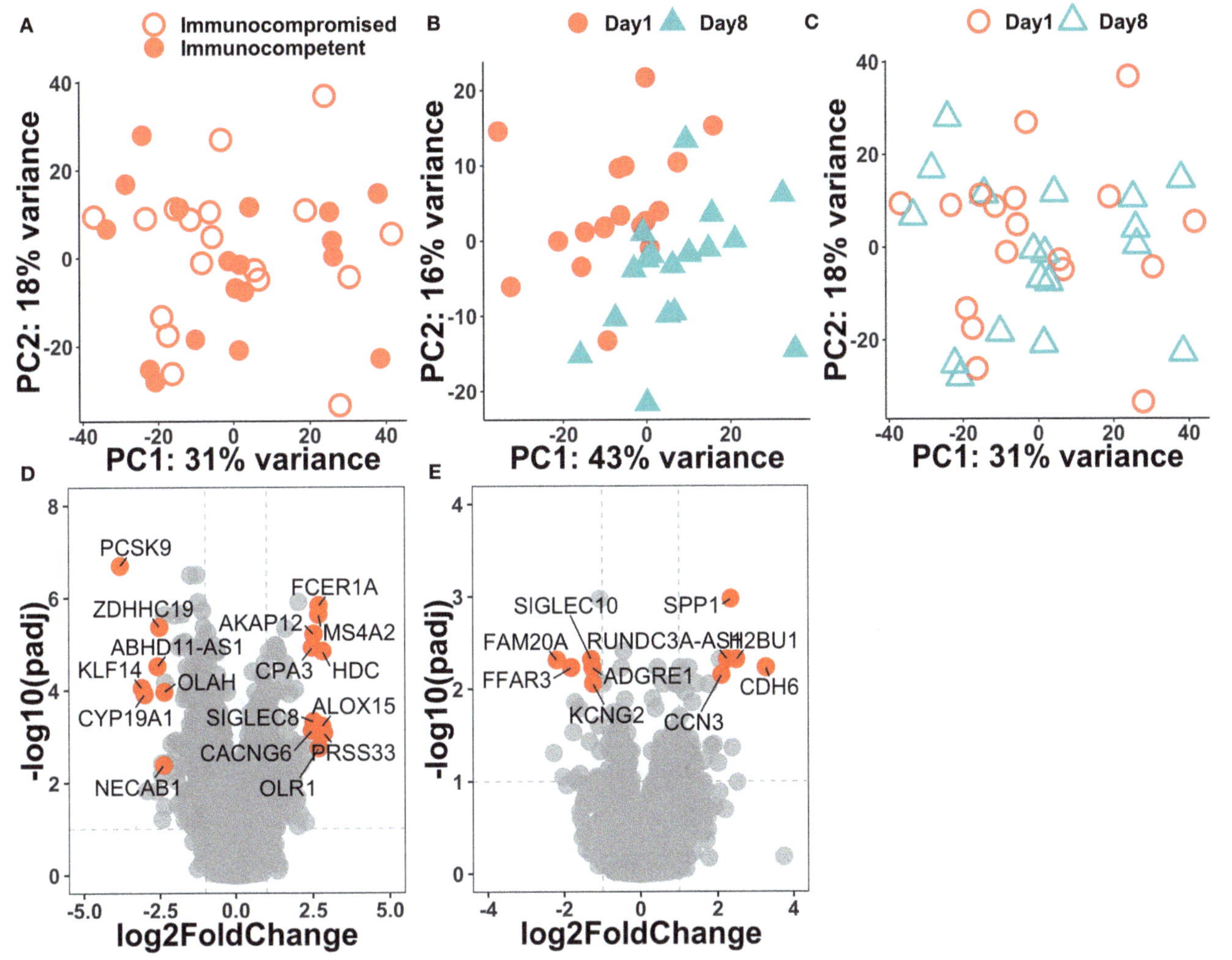

FIGURE 1 | Principal component analysis of day-1 transcriptome among all of the enrolled patients with septic **(A)** and volcano plots of differentially expressed genes between day-1 and day-8 in immunocompetent **(B,D)** and immunocompromised **(C,E)** patients with sepsis.

and metabolic features in immunocompromised patients with sepsis. We found impaired T cell-associated signalling, altered metabolic signalling, and decreased diversity of TCR among immunocompromised patients with septic. The aforementioned immunological and metabolic features indicate a dysregulated recovery in patients with septic with immunocompromised conditions, such as solid cancer underwent therapy, active haematological cancer, and receiving immunosuppressants, due to autoimmune disease or renal transplant recipient. These findings demonstrate the application of RNA-Seq to characterise the subendotype with immunoparalysis in patients with septic, particularly among immunocompromised patients.

The WHO recognises sepsis as a global health priority in 2017 (21), and it is estimated that that sepsis affects 48.9 million patients (38.9–62.9) worldwide and accounts for 19.7% (18.2–21.4) of all global deaths in 2017 (22). Immunocompromised conditions have been found to affect the outcome of sepsis substantially; however, the underlying mechanism remains elusive due to the complexity and high heterogeneity of sepsis (23, 24). The RNA-Seq has been increasingly used to address complex diseases, namely, sepsis, which disrupts the pathophysiological homeostasis result from complex, numerous, intertwined, and subcellular biological events (25). Several studies have used RNA-Seq to identify the subendotype in sepsis, and the identification of subendotype should be essential for individualised medicine in patients with sepsis (26). Antcliffe et al. recently conducted a *post-hoc* transcriptomic analysis among 176 patients in VANISH trial which aimed to explore the mortality impact of vasopressors and corticosteroid in patients with a septic shock and reported two transcriptomic sepsis response signatures (SRSs), such as relatively immunosuppressed signature (SRS-1) and relatively immunocompetent signature (SRS-2) (9). Notably, Antcliffe et al. found that the use of corticosteroids was associated with increased 28-day mortality in patients with septic with SRS-2, whereas the mortality was independent of the use of corticosteroids in patients with septic with SRS-1 (9).

In the present study, the upregulated T cell and Human Leukocyte Antigen (HLA)-associated pathway in immunocompetent patients with septic should be consistent

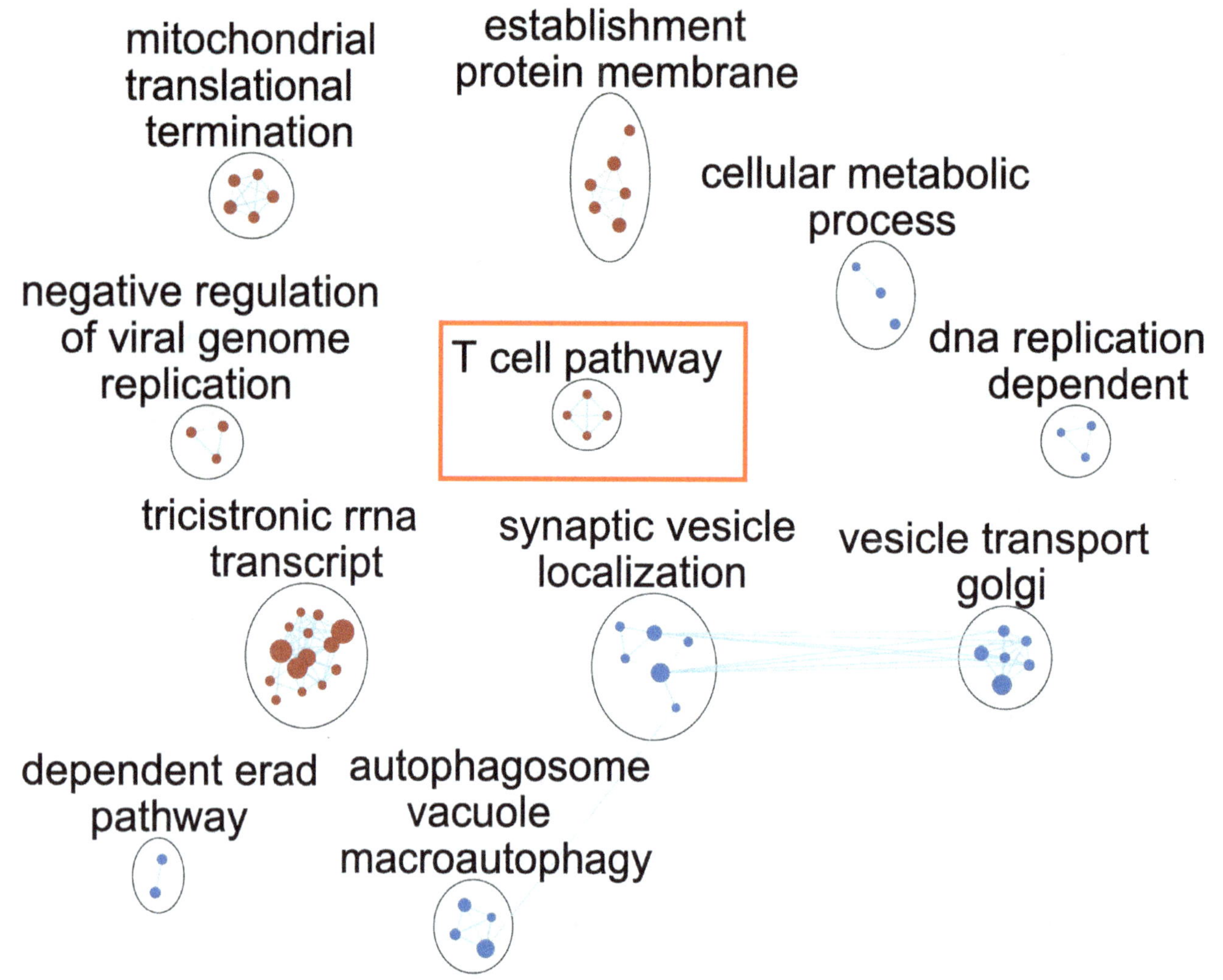

FIGURE 2 | Network of enriched gene ontology term clusters in immunocompetent patients with sepsis. Red circles represent the upregulated pathways, and blue circles represent the downregulated pathways.

with the aforementioned SRS-2 (**Figure 2**). The potentially harmful effect of corticosteroid among patients with septic with specific endotype was recently corroborated using the same dataset by Wong et al., whose team has developed a 100-gene-expression array, which was designed to assess adaptive immunity and glucocorticoid receptor signalling in paediatric septic shock (27). In brief, Wong et al. found that among the 44 patients with endotype A, a phenotype with relatively suppressed adaptive immunity, the mortality tended to be higher among the 26 patients receiving corticosteroid compared with 18 patients without corticosteroid (12/26, 46% vs. 4/18, 22%, $p = 0.105$) (27). Accordingly, the aforementioned evidence and our data demonstrated that the transcriptomic signature should have a crucial role in precision medicine among patients with sepsis.

Sepsis is a complex disease with a robust innate response and dysregulated inflammation, which in turn leads to organ dysfunction (28). In the present study, we used over-representation analysis (ORA) to identify several DEGs in immunocompetent patients, and the identified DEGs, namely, *PRSS33, HDC, ALOX15, FCER1A, OLR1*, and *PCSK9*, were mainly innate immunity and cellular damage-associated genes (7, 29–33). For example, *ALOX15* and *FCER1A* were monocyte-associated genes, which have been found to play a pivotal role in the pathogenesis of bacterial sepsis (7, 31). Moreover, we also used CIBERSORT to estimate cellular types and found the relative abundance of monocyte in enrolled patients, and this finding was in line with the increasing data to show the crucial role of monocyte in the pathogenesis of sepsis (**Supplemental Figure 1**) (7, 31). Notably, the transcriptome was similar on day-1 among immunocompromised and immunocompetent patients (**Figure 1A**), and the findings highlight the crucial need of using paired day-1 and day-8 samples to address the dynamic transcriptome in patients with septic with high heterogeneity as shown in this study and the previous study (6). Furthermore, we employed functional pathway analysis to demonstrate the essential role of T cell

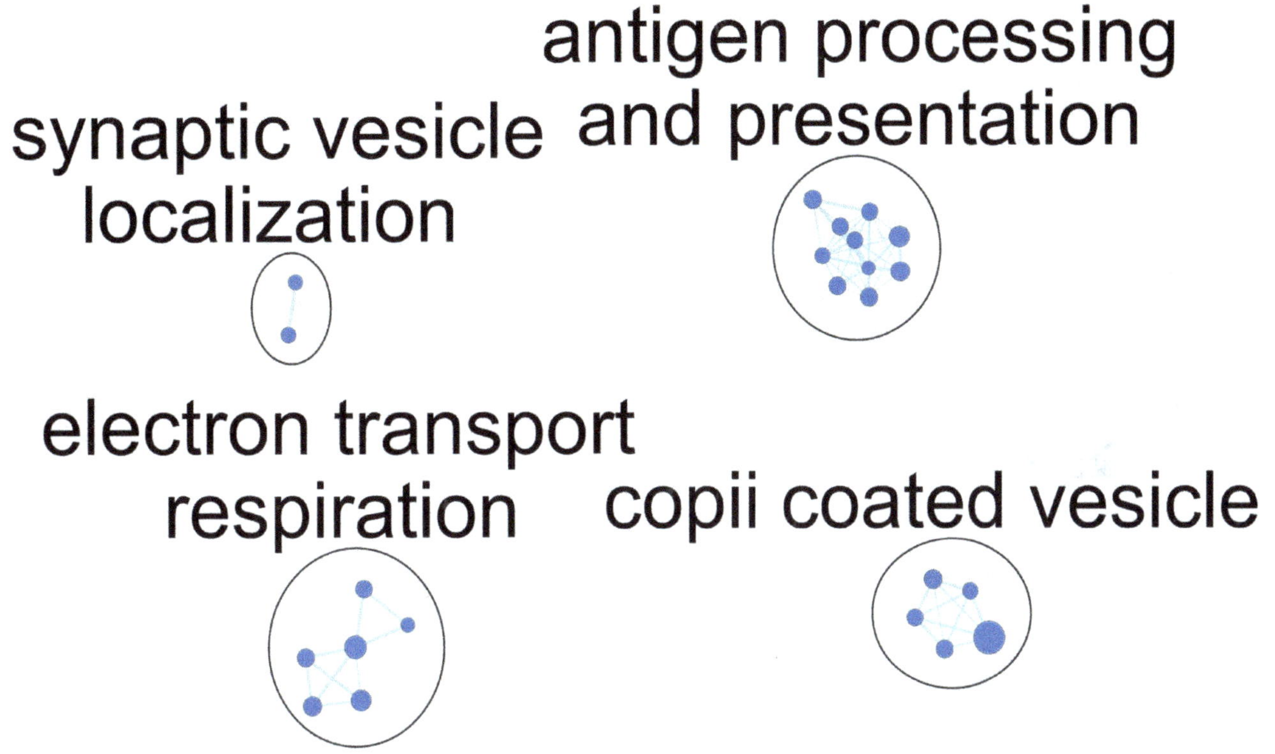

FIGURE 3 | Network of enriched gene ontology term clusters in immunocompromised patients with sepsis. Blue circles represent the downregulated pathways.

immunity-relevant pathways among immunocompromised patients with sepsis. The aforementioned findings highlight that ORA-based analysis alone may not be adequate to address the complex disease with a high number of differentially expressed genes given that the top DEGs may represent the robust dysregulated immunological and cellular function (34). In contrast, functional pathway-based analyses enable us to identify the distinct T cell-associated pathways as we have shown in the present study (**Figure 2**).

Several transcriptomic studies have been used to address the T cell immunity in sepsis, and distinct terms were used, such as T cell exhaustion, immunoparalysis, and immune-suppressive signatures (4, 9, 26). Cheng et al. reported an *in vitro* model of innate immunotolerance/immunoparalysis defined by diminished production of lactate and pro-inflammatory cytokines in lipopolysaccharide (LPS) or *Candida albicans*-treated monocytes isolated from patients with sepsis and found not only compromised innate immunity but also impaired energy metabolism in patients with septic with immunoparalysis (4, 26). Increasing evidence has further validated the key role of metabolic abnormality in sepsis (35, 36), and our data also found impaired metabolic pathways, such as TCA cycle and cellular respiration, in immunocompromised patients with sepsis (**Figure 3**). Additionally, alteration in the metabolic state of T cells has been implicated with the impaired capacity of T cell expansion and effector function of T cells (37, 38). The impaired metabolic signalling as we have shown in this clinical study may hence be associated with the T cell paralysis in the immunocompromised patient with septic, although more mechanistic studies are warranted to elucidate the complex immune-metabolism interaction (4).

Increasing studies have shown the role of T cell exhaustion in patients with sepsis; however, few studies addressed the T cell diversity in patients with septic, particularly immunocompromised patients. Venet et al. conducted a pilot study to explore day-1 and day-7 diversity of TCR in 41 patients with a septic shock through using genomic DNA and multiplex PCR (39). Venet et al. reported that a reduced day-7 TCR β-chain diversity tended to be associated with an increased risk of mortality in the univariable analysis (39). Furthermore, patients who developed a nosocomial infection after the sepsis episode appeared to have a lower day-1 TCR β-chain diversity compared with those without nosocomial infection (39). Recently, there are crucial advances, such as 5′ rapid amplification of cDNA ends (RACE) and measurement of TCR in RNA-level (40). Genomic DNA was widely used to measure the diversity of TCR due to high stability and fixed copy number per cell; however, PCR-associated error result from unused segments and introns remains a major limitation of the DNA-based approach for TCR repertoire (40). In contrast, using RNA with a simplified PCR amplification strategy enables the comprehensive identification of TCR variants and is increasingly applied (41). MiXCR is a framework that allows for analysing raw sequences of RNA-Seq to determine clonotypes of TCR. Therefore, the

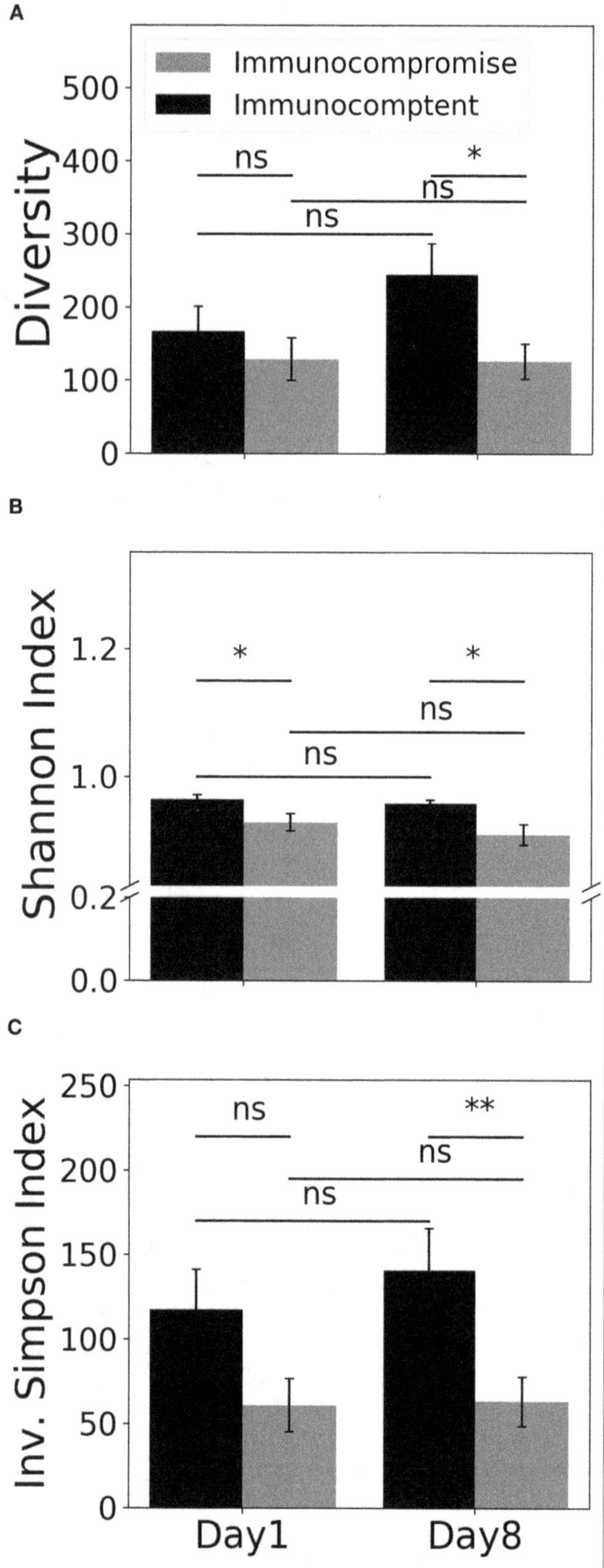

FIGURE 4 | Diversity of the T cell receptor. Counts **(A)**, Shannon's diversity index **(B)**, and inverse Simpson index **(C)** of unique CDR3. (CDR3, complementarity-determining region-3). * < 0.05, ** < 0.005.

approach with MiXCR enables us to simultaneously conduct whole transcriptome and diversity of TCR (11). Similar to our approach, Zhigalova et al. recently demonstrated the utility of using MiXCR and RNA-Seq data to determine the dynamic diversity of TCR among tumour-infiltrating T cells treated with programmed death receptor 1 (PD-1) antibody in mouse melanoma model (42). In the present study, we used RNA-Seq to identify the impaired T cell signalling and MiXCR to reveal the decreased diversity of TCR among immunocompromised patients with septic, and the consistent findings indicate the immunocompromised condition-associated T cell paralysis in sepsis. Similar to our results in immunocompromised patients with septic, Cabrera-Perez et al., conducting qualitative and quantitative analyses of Ag-specific CD4 T cell populations in cecal ligation puncture-treated mice, found a prolonged alteration of Ag-specific T cell repertoire after sepsis despite the recovered number of T cells (43). Collectively, this evidence highlights the feasibility of using data of RNA-Seq and MiXCR to address the diversity of TCR in patients with sepsis and point out the crucial role of reduced diversity of TCR in immunocompromised patients with sepsis.

There are limitations to this study. First, the relatively small number of immunocompromised patients with septic. However, we enrolled severity-matched controls, and the highly comparable controls should allow us the identification of distinct pathways between the two groups. Second, the use of bulk RNA-Seq and future sc-RNA-Seq and functional experiments are warranted for validation at the cellular level. Third, we used RNA-Seq data to assess the diversity of TCR, and future T cell repertoire using 5′RACE should be needed to clarify the issue of TCR in patients with sepsis.

CONCLUSION

The increased number of immunocompromised patients with sepsis is a growing issue worldwide, and the RNA-Seq can be used to address the complex immunologic and metabolic features. In the present study, we enrolled immunocompromised patients with septic with severity-matched controls and conducted RNA-Seq with functional pathway and MiXCR analyses. We found that not only dysregulated innate immunity but also compromised T cell function, altered metabolic signalling, and decreased T cell diversity among immunocompromised patients with septic. These data highlight the feasibility of using RNA-Seq to characterise immunologic and metabolic features in immunocompromised patients with septic, and studies using sc-RNA-Seq and 5′RACE are warranted to elucidate the underlying cellular pathway.

ETHICS STATEMENT

The studies involving human participants were reviewed and approved by Institutional Review Board approval of the Taichung Veterans General Hospital (CE20069B). The patients/participants provided their written informed consent to participate in this study.

AUTHOR CONTRIBUTIONS

P-LC, H-HC, C-YW, C-LW, T-MK, and W-CC: conceived and designed the experiments. P-LC, Y-HJ, and W-CC: acquired data. P-LC, T-HH, and W-CC: contributed materials/analysis tools. P-LC and W-CC: wrote the manuscript. All authors contributed to the article and approved the submitted version.

REFERENCES

1. Fleischmann C, Scherag A, Adhikari NK, Hartog CS, Tsaganos T, Schlattmann P, et al. Current estimates and limitations. *Am J Respir Crit Care Med.* (2016) 193:259–72. doi: 10.1164/rccm.201504-0781OC
2. Harpaz R, Dahl RM, Dooling KL. Prevalence of Immunosuppression Among US Adults, 2013. *JAMA.* (2016) 316:2547–8. doi: 10.1001/jama.2016.16477
3. Azoulay E, Russell L, Van de Louw A, Metaxa V, Bauer P, Povoa P, et al. Diagnosis of severe respiratory infections in immunocompromised patients. *Intensive Care Med.* (2020) 46:298–314. doi: 10.1007/s00134-019-05906-5
4. Cheng SC, Scicluna BP, Arts RJ, Gresnigt MS, Lachmandas E, Giamarellos-Bourboulis EJ, et al. Broad defects in the energy metabolism of leukocytes underlie immunoparalysis in sepsis. *Nat Immunol.* (2016) 17:406–13. doi: 10.1038/ni.3398
5. van Vught LA, Klein Klouwenberg PM, Spitoni C, Scicluna BP, Wiewel MA, Horn J, et al. Incidence, risk factors, and attributable mortality of secondary infections in the intensive care unit after admission for sepsis. *JAMA.* (2016) 315:1469–79. doi: 10.1001/jama.2016.2691
6. Barcella M, Bollen Pinto B, Braga D, D'Avila F, Tagliaferri F, Cazalis MA, et al. Identification of a transcriptome profile associated with improvement of organ function in septic shock patients after early supportive therapy. *Crit Care.* (2018) 22:312. doi: 10.1186/s13054-018-2242-3
7. Reyes M, Filbin MR, Bhattacharyya RP, Billman K, Eisenhaure T, Hung DT, et al. An immune-cell signature of bacterial sepsis. *Nat Med.* (2020) 26:333–40. doi: 10.1038/s41591-020-0752-4
8. Grant RA, Morales-Nebreda L, Markov NS, Swaminathan S, Querrey M, Guzman ER, et al. Circuits between infected macrophages and T cells in SARS-CoV-2 pneumonia. *Nature.* (2021) 590:635–41. doi: 10.1038/s41586-020-03148-w
9. Antcliffe DB, Burnham KL, Al-Beidh F, Santhakumaran S, Brett SJ, Hinds CJ, et al. Transcriptomic signatures in sepsis and a differential response to steroids from the VANISH randomized trial. *Am J Respir Crit Care Med.* (2019) 199:980–6. doi: 10.1164/rccm.201807-1419OC
10. Davenport EE, Burnham KL, Radhakrishnan J, Humburg P, Hutton P, Mills TC, et al. Genomic landscape of the individual host response and outcomes in sepsis: a prospective cohort study. *Lancet Respir Med.* (2016) 4:259–71. doi: 10.1016/S2213-2600(16)00046-1
11. Bolotin DA, Poslavsky S, Mitrophanov I, Shugay M, Mamedov IZ, Putintseva EV, et al. MiXCR: software for comprehensive adaptive immunity profiling. *Nat Methods.* (2015) 12:380–1. doi: 10.1038/nmeth.3364
12. Bolotin DA, Poslavsky S, Davydov AN, Frenkel FE, Fanchi L, Zolotareva OI, et al. Antigen receptor repertoire profiling from RNA-seq data. *Nat Biotechnol.* (2017) 35:908–11. doi: 10.1038/nbt.3979
13. Le Gall JR, Lemeshow S, Saulnier F. A new Simplified Acute Physiology Score (SAPS II) based on a European/North American multicenter study. *JAMA.* (1993) 270:2957–63. doi: 10.1001/jama.270.24.2957
14. Kim D, Langmead B, Salzberg SL. HISAT: a fast spliced aligner with low memory requirements. *Nat Methods.* (2015) 12:357–60. doi: 10.1038/nmeth.3317
15. Liao Y, Smyth GK, Shi W. featureCounts: an efficient general purpose program for assigning sequence reads to genomic features. *Bioinformatics.* (2014) 30:923–30. doi: 10.1093/bioinformatics/btt656
16. Anders S, Huber W. Differential expression analysis for sequence count data. *Genome Biol.* (2010) 11:R106. doi: 10.1186/gb-2010-11-10-r106
17. Subramanian A, Tamayo P, Mootha VK, Mukherjee S, Ebert BL, Gillette MA, et al. Gene set enrichment analysis: a knowledge-based approach for interpreting genome-wide expression profiles. *Proc Natl Acad Sci USA.* (2005) 102:15545–50. doi: 10.1073/pnas.0506580102
18. Shannon P, Markiel A, Ozier O, Baliga NS, Wang JT, Ramage D, et al. Cytoscape: a software environment for integrated models of biomolecular interaction networks. *Genome Res.* (2003) 13:2498–504. doi: 10.1101/gr.1239303
19. Merico D, Isserlin R, Stueker O, Emili A, Bader GD. Enrichment map: a network-based method for gene-set enrichment visualization and interpretation. *PLoS ONE.* (2010) 5:e13984. doi: 10.1371/journal.pone.0013984
20. Andersen ES. Prediction and design of DNA and RNA structures. *N Biotechnol.* (2010) 27:184–93. doi: 10.1016/j.nbt.2010.02.012
21. Reinhart K, Daniels R, Kissoon N, Machado FR, Schachter RD. and S. Finfer recognizing sepsis as a global health priority—a WHO resolution. *N Engl J Med.* (2017) 377:414–7. doi: 10.1056/NEJMp1707170
22. Rudd KE, Johnson SC, Agesa KM, Shackelford KA, Tsoi D, Kievlan DR, et al. Global, regional, and national sepsis incidence and mortality, 1990-2017: analysis for the Global Burden of Disease Study. *Lancet.* (2020) 395:200–11. doi: 10.1016/S0140-6736(19)32989-7
23. Tolsma V, Schwebel C, Azoulay E, Darmon M, Souweine B, Vesin A, et al. Sepsis severe or septic shock: outcome according to immune status and immunodeficiency profile. *Chest.* (2014) 146:1205–13. doi: 10.1378/chest.13-2618
24. Jamme M, Daviaud F, Charpentier J, Marin N, Thy M, Hourmant Y, et al. Time course of septic shock in immunocompromised and nonimmunocompromised patients. *Crit Care Med.* (2017) 45:2031–9. doi: 10.1097/CCM.0000000000002722
25. Evangelatos N, Satyamoorthy K, Levidou G, Bauer P, Brand H, Kouskouti C, et al. Multi-omics research trends in sepsis: a bibliometric, comparative analysis between the United States, the European Union 28 Member States, and China. *OMICS.* (2018) 22:190–97. doi: 10.1089/omi.2017.0192
26. Scicluna BP, van Vught LA, Zwinderman AH, Wiewel MA, Davenport EE, Burnham KL, et al. Classification of patients with sepsis according to blood genomic endotype: a prospective cohort study. *Lancet Respir Med.* (2017) 5:816–26. doi: 10.1016/S2213-2600(17)30294-1
27. Wong HR, Hart KW, Lindsell CJ, Sweeney TE. External corroboration that corticosteroids may be harmful to septic shock endotype a patients. *Crit Care Med.* (2021) 49:e98–101. doi: 10.1097/CCM.0000000000004709
28. Singer M, Deutschman CS, Seymour CW, Shankar-Hari M, Annane D, Bauer M, et al. The third international consensus definitions for sepsis and septic shock (Sepsis-3). *JAMA.* (2016) 315:801–10. doi: 10.1001/jama.2016.0287
29. Juss JK, House D, Amour A, Begg M, Herre J, Storisteanu DM, et al. Acute respiratory distress syndrome neutrophils have a distinct phenotype and are resistant to phosphoinositide 3-kinase inhibition. *Am J Respir Crit Care Med.* (2016) 194:961–73. doi: 10.1164/rccm.201509-1818OC
30. Hattori M, Yamazaki M, Ohashi W, Tanaka S, Hattori K, Todoroki K, et al. Critical role of endogenous histamine in promoting end-organ tissue injury in sepsis. *Intensive Care Med Exp.* (2016) 4:36. doi: 10.1186/s40635-016-0109-y
31. Tang-Huau TL, Gueguen P, Goudot C, Durand M, Bohec M, Baulande S, et al. Human *in vivo*-generated monocyte-derived dendritic cells and macrophages cross-present antigens through a vacuolar pathway. *Nat Commun.* (2018) 9:2570. doi: 10.1038/s41467-018-04985-0

32. Wu Z, Sawamura T, Kurdowska AK, Ji HL, Idell S, Fu J. LOX-1 deletion improves neutrophil responses, enhances bacterial clearance, and reduces lung injury in a murine polymicrobial sepsis model. *Infect Immun.* (2011) 79:2865–70. doi: 10.1128/IAI.01317-10
33. Walley KR, Thain KR, Russell JA, Reilly MP, Meyer NJ, Ferguson JF, et al. PCSK9 is a critical regulator of the innate immune response and septic shock outcome. *Sci Transl Med.* (2014) 6:258ra143. doi: 10.1126/scitranslmed.3008782
34. Khatri P, Sirota M, Butte AJ. Ten years of pathway analysis: current approaches and outstanding challenges. *PLoS Comput Biol.* (2012) 8:e1002375. doi: 10.1371/journal.pcbi.1002375
35. Weiss SL, Zhang D, Bush J, Graham K, Starr J, Murray J, et al. Mitochondrial Dysfunction is Associated With an Immune Paralysis Phenotype in Pediatric Sepsis. *Shock.* (2020) 54:285–93. doi: 10.1097/SHK.0000000000001486
36. McBride MA, Owen AM, Stothers CL, Hernandez A, Luan L, Burelbach KR, et al. The Metabolic Basis of Immune Dysfunction Following Sepsis and Trauma. *Front Immunol.* (2020) 11:1043. doi: 10.3389/fimmu.2020.01043
37. Waickman AT, Powell JD. mTOR, metabolism, and the regulation of T-cell differentiation and function. *Immunol Rev.* (2012) 249:43–58. doi: 10.1111/j.1600-065X.2012.01152.x
38. Jensen IJ, Sjaastad FV, Griffith TS, Badovinac VP. Sepsis-Induced T Cell Immunoparalysis: the ins and outs of impaired T cell immunity. *J Immunol.* (2018) 200:1543–53.
39. Venet F, Filipe-Santos O, Lepape A, Malcus C, Poitevin-Later F, Grives A, et al. Decreased T-cell repertoire diversity in sepsis: a preliminary study. *Crit Care Med.* (2013) 41:111–9. doi: 10.1097/CCM.0b013e3182657948
40. Six A, Mariotti-Ferrandiz ME, Chaara W, Magadan S, Pham HP, Lefranc MP, et al. The past, present, and future of immune repertoire biology—the rise of next-generation repertoire analysis. *Front Immunol.* (2013) 4:413. doi: 10.3389/fimmu.2013.00413
41. Rosati E, Dowds CM, Liaskou E, Henriksen EKK, Karlsen TH, Franke A. Overview of methodologies for T-cell receptor repertoire analysis. *BMC Biotechnol.* (2017) 17:61. doi: 10.1186/s12896-017-0379-9
42. Zhigalova EA, Izosimova AI, Yuzhakova DV, Volchkova LN, Shagina IA, Turchaninova MA, et al. RNA-Seq-based TCR profiling reveals persistently increased intratumoral clonality in responders to anti-PD-1 therapy. *Front Oncol.* (2020) 10:385. doi: 10.3389/fonc.2020.00385
43. Cabrera-Perez J, Condotta SA, James BR, Kashem SW, Brincks EL, Rai D, et al. Alterations in antigen-specific naive CD4 T cell precursors after sepsis impairs their responsiveness to pathogen challenge. *J Immunol.* (2015) 194:1609–20. doi: 10.4049/jimmunol.1401711

3

Association Between Epidural Analgesia and Cancer Recurrence or Survival After Surgery for Renal Cell Carcinoma: A Propensity Weighted Analysis

Fang-Yu Yen [1,2†], Wen-Kuei Chang [1,2†], Shih-Pin Lin [1,2], Tzu-Ping Lin [2,3] and Kuang-Yi Chang [1,2]*

[1] Department of Anesthesiology, Taipei Veterans General Hospital, Taipei, Taiwan, [2] School of Medicine, National Yang Ming Chiao Tung University, Taipei, Taiwan, [3] Department of Urology, Taipei Veterans General Hospital, Taipei, Taiwan

***Correspondence:**
Kuang-Yi Chang
kychang@vghtpe.gov.tw

† These authors have contributed equally to this work

Whether epidural anesthesia and analgesia (EA) is beneficial for postoperative cancer outcomes remains controversial and we conducted this historical cohort study to evaluate the association between EA and long-term outcomes following surgery for renal cell carcinoma (RCC). We collected patients receiving RCC surgery from 2011 to 2017 and followed up them until February 2020. Patient attributes, surgical factors and pathological features were gathered through electronic medical chart review. The association between EA and recurrence-free and overall survival after surgery was evaluated using Cox regression models with inverse probability of treatment weighting (IPTW) to balance the observed covariates. The median follow-up time for the 725 included patients was 50 months (interquartile range: 25.3–66.5) and 145 of them (20%) received perioperative EA. We demonstrated EA use was associated with better recurrence-free survival [IPTW adjusted hazard ratio (HR): 0.64, 95% confidence interval (CI): 0.49–0.83, $p < 0.001$] and overall survival [IPTW adjusted HR: 0.66, 95% CI: 0.49–0.89, $p = 0.006$] in patients receiving surgical resection for RCC. More prospective studies are needed to verify this connection between EA and superior cancer outcomes after RCC surgery.

Keywords: epidural analgesia, inverse probability of treatment weighting, recurrence, renal cell carcinoma, survival

INTRODUCTION

Although life expectancy is increasing along with the progression and improvement of medical care, cancer remains one of the leading causes of death around the world and cancer treatment is still a great challenge in contemporary medicine (1). Surgical intervention is the mainstay treatment for the control and cure of most solid tumors but postoperative local or distant metastasis, which causes 90% of deaths, remains a common reason for morbidity and mortality in cancer patients (2, 3).

It should be noted that the perioperative period is associated with an increased formation of new metastatic foci and accelerated growth of micrometastatic disease (2). Surgical procedures themselves also suppress the host's immunity which is inhibiting pre-existing micro-metastases, and manipulation during surgery can disseminate cancer cells which are shed from the primary tumor to the blood stream or lymphatic system intraoperatively (4). Moreover, surgery can directly activate the hypothalamic-pituitary-adrenal axis and sympathetic nerve system to increase the levels of catecholamine, prostaglandins and acute inflammatory cytokines (interleukin-6, interleukin-8) that further suppress the cytotoxic activity of macrophages and natural killer (NK) cells (5).

Also, accumulating evidence shows that anesthetic intervention and analgesia could affect the pathophysiological processes associated with long-term cancer outcomes (6). Since immunity plays a major role in cancer progression (7), perioperative pain management could be very important for preventing surgery-induced immunosuppression. Perioperative epidural anesthesia and analgesia (EA) effectively attenuate neuroendocrine stress responses related to surgery, they also reduce intraoperative volatile anesthetics and opioid consumption by blocking noxious afferent inputs transmitted to the central nervous system, and further preserve host immunity (4, 7, 8). Previous studies have demonstrated that patients with perioperative EA had better prostate, ovarian, colon, gastro-esophageal and breast cancer outcomes compared with those without (7, 9). Nevertheless, few studies have investigated the association between EA and postoperative outcomes after surgery for renal cell carcinoma (RCC) (8).

To fill this gap, we hypothesized that EA is beneficial to long-term outcomes after curative surgery for RCC and we conducted this retrospective study to evaluate the association between EA and cancer recurrence or overall survival. We used a novel propensity weighted analysis to promote analytical power and to reduce potential confounding effects by incorporating important prognostic factors in the analysis. Sensitivity analysis using the two other regression approaches was also employed to ensure the consistency of the estimated results.

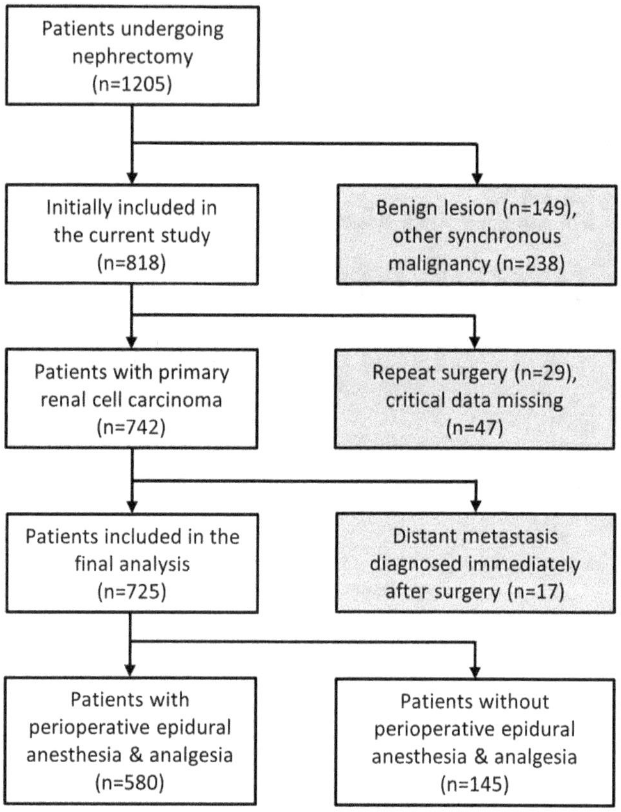

FIGURE 1 | Flow diagram for patient selection.

METHODS

Setting and Patient Selection

The current study was approved by the Institutional Review Board (IRB) of the Taipei Veterans General Hospital, Taipei, Taiwan (IRB-TPEVGH no. 2018-06-009CC, Jul 2018), and written informed consent was waived by the IRB of the Taipei Veterans General Hospital. All methods were performed in accordance with the relevant guidelines and local regulations. Patients who underwent curative surgery for RCC between January 1st 2012 and December 31st 2017, as determined by reviewing the electronic medical records at our hospital, were included in the study. The exclusion criteria were: patients with benign pathological reports, non-RCC, reoperation for metastasis lesions, missing pathological data or perioperative pain management (**Figure 1**). All included patients were further classified into two groups based on whether they received perioperative EA or not. The reasons why patients did not receive EA included contraindications to EA, failed epidurals and the preference of the anesthesiologist, surgeon or patient, etc. For those who did not receive perioperative EA, intravenous patient-controlled analgesia with morphine was used to control postoperative pain.

Anesthetic Management

During general anesthesia, the induction of anesthesia consisted in intravenous fentanyl 1–3 μg/kg, propofol 1–2.5 mg/kg and a neuromuscular blocking drug of either cisatracurium 0.15–0.2 mg/kg or rocuronium 0.6–1.2 mg/kg to facilitate tracheal intubation. Anesthesia was maintained with sevoflurane 2–3 vol% or desflurane 6–8 vol%. All epidural catheters were inserted at the lower thoracic or high lumbar region (T10–L2). Patients scheduled to receive EA had an epidural catheter implanted preoperatively which was tested using 2% lidocaine 2 ml to ensure it functioned properly. A loading dose of 1–1.5% lidocaine with or without fentanyl 50 μg was given before the surgical incision, and then bupivacaine 0.25% was continuous infused at a rate of 5–10 ml/h intraoperatively depending on the hemodynamic stability. EA was administered with bupivacaine 0.0625% for postoperative pain management and typically maintained for 48–72 h. Patients who did not receive EA had intravenous patient-controlled analgesia (PCA) *via* an ambulatory infusion pump (Gemstar Yellow, Hospira, IL, USA) to deliver morphine with an infusion rate of 0.5–1.0 mg/h and a bolus dose of 1 mg with a lockout time of 5–10 mins.

TABLE 1 | Patient demographics.

	Original data			After IPTW		
	Non-EA group (n = 580)	EA group (n = 145)	SDD	Non-EA group (n = 725)	EA group (n = 622)	SDD
Age	59 ± 14	56 ± 14	22.06	58 ± 14	58 ± 12	1.92
BMI	25.65 ± 4.10	25.39 ± 3.84	6.60	25.61 ± 4.10	25.68 ± 3.81	1.86
ASA physical status > 3	162 (27.9%)	38 (26.2%)	3.88	201 (27.7%)	168 (27.0%)	1.52
Charlson comorbidity index	4.08 ± 1.70	3.79 ± 1.76	16.93	4.03 ± 1.69	4.13 ± 1.78	5.84
Anesthesia time*	8.55 ± 0.36	8.57 ± 0.38	3.69	8.56 ± 0.36	8.58 ± 0.39	4.14
Intraoperative blood loss*	7.65 ± 1.89	8.03 ± 1.93	19.82	7.73 ± 1.90	7.65 ± 2.05	3.75
Sex, male	396 (68.3%)	100 (69.0%)	1.49	497 (68.6%)	450 (72.2%)	8.04
Smoking	134 (23.1%)	38 (26.2%)	7.21	172 (23.7%)	151 (24.2%)	1.13
Surgical year			42.61			9.87
< 2015	281 (48.4%)	100 (69.0%)		381 (52.6%)	358 (57.5%)	
Packed RBC transfusion	131 (22.6%)	41 (28.3%)	13.09	173 (23.8%)	148 (23.8%)	0.07
Laparoscopic or robotic surgery	321 (55.3%)	12 (8.3%)	117.12	333 (45.9%)	238 (38.2%)	15.73
Partial nephrectomy	351 (60.5%)	86 (59.3%)	2.46	437 (60.3%)	368 (59.1%)	2.34
Cancer subtype			12.87			7.46
Clear cell	441 (76.0%)	102 (70.3%)		543 (74.9%)	486 (78.1%)	
Others**	139 (24.0%)	43 (29.7%)		182 (25.1%)	136 (21.9%)	
Fuhrman grade > 2	215 (37.1%)	56 (38.6%)	3.20	271 (37.4%)	201 (32.3%)	10.70
Tumor necrosis	190 (32.8%)	54 (37.2%)	9.41	242 (33.4%)	179 (28.7%)	10.17
Capsular invasion	61 (10.5%)	10 (6.9%)	12.87	71 (9.8%)	40 (6.4%)	12.21
Hilar vein invasion	104 (17.9%)	27 (18.6%)	1.78	131 (18.1%)	138 (22.2%)	10.37
Renal sinus invasion	70 (12.1%)	22 (15.2%)	9.06	93 (12.8%)	92 (14.7%)	5.57
Cancer stage			7.18			2.76
I	369 (63.6%)	87 (60.0%)		454 (62.7%)	389 (62.5%)	
II	40 (6.9%)	14 (9.7%)		54 (7.5%)	39 (6.3%)	
III	141 (24.3%)	30 (20.7%)		171 (23.6%)	150 (24.2%)	
IV	30 (5.2%)	14 (9.7%)		45 (6.2%)	43 (7.0%)	

Values were mean ± SD or counts (percent), or median (interquartile range). Standardized difference (SDD) is the difference in mean or proportion divided by the pooled standard error, expressed as percentage; imbalance is defined as absolute value greater than 20 (small effect size).
**On base-2 logarithmic scale. **Other morphological types of RCC include chromophobe, papillary, Xp11.2 translocation, etc.*
BMI, body mass index; EA, epidural anesthesia and analgesia; IPTW, inverse probability treatment weighting; RBC, red blood cell; SDD, standardized difference.

Postoperative Cancer Control

RCC staging was defined according to the American Joint Committee on Cancer 2010 tumor-node-metastasis cancer classification system (10). After the primary tumor resection, additional surgeries for metastatic disease were performed depending on the lesion locations, including hepatectomy, colectomy, IVC thrombectomy, etc. Postoperative surveillance was performed regularly at an outpatient clinic and followed the National Comprehensive Cancer Network guidelines (11).

Data Collection

We reviewed the patient's electronic medical records and collected their demographic characteristics, including age, sex, body mass index (BMI), American Society of Anesthesiologists (ASA) physical status and Charlson comorbidity index (12). We also collected potential risk factors which might affect cancer prognosis, including cancer staging, pathological features (histologic tumor necrosis, capsular invasion, hilar vein invasion, renal sinus invasion), perioperative blood transfusion, minimal invasive or traditional open surgery, partial or radical nephrectomy and smoking. Current disease status and date of death were also obtained from the medical records. Local recurrence or distant metastasis was determined using imaging studies (computed tomography, magnetic resonance imaging, bone scan) or a tissue biopsy. The primary outcome was recurrence-free survival (RFS) which was defined as the time interval between the date of surgery and the discovery date of cancer recurrence or new metastatic foci. The secondary outcomes were overall survival (OS) and cancer-specific survival (CSS). All patients were followed until they were lost to follow-up, death or the 29th February 2020, whichever came first. For those without cancer progression, survival times were defined as the corresponding censored observation. Competing risk events were regarded as censoring in the analysis of cancer-specific survival.

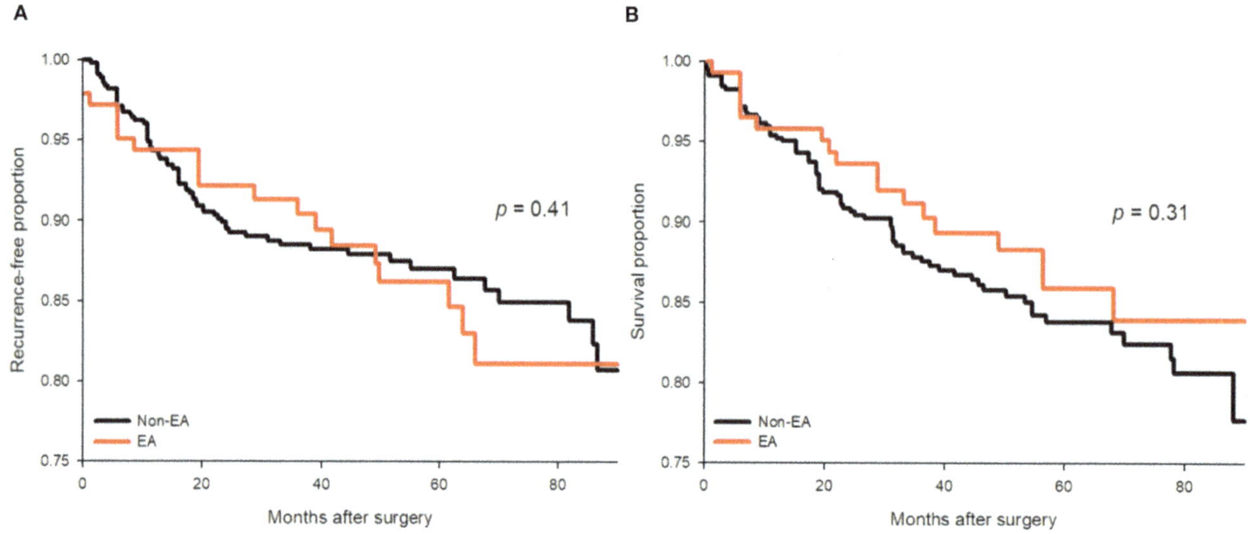

FIGURE 2 | Kaplan-Meier curves for cancer recurrence and all-cause mortality of EA (epidural anesthesia and analgesia) and non-EA groups. No significant difference in cancer recurrence **(A)** or all-cause mortality **(B)** was found after renal cell carcinoma resection between the EA with non-EA groups.

Statistical Analysis

All the patients were classified into the two groups depending on whether they received EA or not. Continuous and categorical variables are presented as the mean with standard deviation and count with the percentage, respectively. Logarithmic transformation was conducted to reduce the skewness of non-normal continuous variables. Standardized differences were used to evaluate balance in the collected variables between the two groups. The Kaplan-Meier method was used to compare the RFS and OS between the two groups. Univariate Cox regression analysis was also performed to assess the effects of EA and other covariates on RFS, OS and CSS. An inverse probability of treatment weighting (IPTW) method based on propensity scores was used to balance the distributions of the collected variables in the EA and non-EA groups and 1% of subjects at the end of weighting distribution were truncated to reduce the impact of large weights on the analytical results (13). Note that the propensity scores were generated from the logistic regression analysis (**Supplementary Table S1**) and reflected the probability of receiving EA given the collected variables. IPTW methodology weighted study subjects by the inverse probability of receiving EA or not to create a pseudo-population where the EA assignment is independent of the collected variables like randomization for unbiased estimation of average EA effects. Accordingly, weighted Cox regression analysis was applied to evaluate the association between EA and RFS, OS or CSS based on IPTW. For sensitivity analysis, all of the patients were further divided into the five equal groups using the quintiles of the generated propensity scores and a stratified Cox regression analysis was conducted to obtain a pooled hazard across the five strata to estimate the association of EA with RFS, OS and CSS. In addition, multivariable Cox regression analysis with a stepwise model selection strategy was used to identify independent predictors of RFS, OS and CSS, and to evaluate the effects of EA on these long-term outcomes. The significance level of all hypothesis testing was set at 0.05 and all the statistical analyses were conducted using SAS software, version 9.4 (SAS Institute Inc., Cary, NC, USA).

RESULTS

Patient Characteristics

A total of 725 patients were included in the study. They had a median follow-up interval of 50 with an interquartile range of 25.3 to 66.5 months and of these patients, 145 (20%) received EA. In the original sample, patients in the EA groups tended to be younger and have a higher chance of receiving open surgery (**Table 1**). Compared with the non-EA group, more cases in the EA group received surgery before 2015. However, after IPTW the imbalances in these covariate distributions between the two groups were removed (**Table 1**).

Recurrence-Free Survival

The 5-year RFS rates were 81.6% [95% confidence interval (CI): 74.5–88.7%] and 78.7% (95% CI: 74.8–82.6%) in the EA and non-EA groups, respectively. No significant difference in RFS distribution was noted between the EA and non-EA groups (p = 0.408 by log rank test, **Figure 2A**). The crude hazard ratio (HR) of the EA group was 0.84 with a 95% CI of 0.55–1.28. However, after IPTW, the weighted Cox regression analysis demonstrated a significant association between the EA and a better RFS (adjusted HR = 0.64, 95% CI: 0.49–0.83; $p < 0.001$). For sensitivity analysis, multivariable regression analysis identified six independent prognostic factors for cancer recurrence, including perioperative transfusion, anesthesia time, tumor necrosis, capsular invasion, cancer staging and EA (adjusted HR = 0.62, 95% CI: 0.40–0.96, **Table 2**). Notice that the association between EA and superior

TABLE 2 | Forward model selection for recurrence-free survival before weighting.

	HR	95% CI	P
Epidural analgesia	0.62	0.40–0.96	0.031
Anesthesia time*	2.12	1.29–3.47	0.003
Packed RBC transfusion	1.65	1.12–2.42	0.010
Tumor necrosis	2.40	1.63–3.54	<0.001
Capsular invasion	1.61	1.05–2.47	0.030
Cancer stage			<0.001
II vs. I	2.69	1.47–4.92	0.001
III vs. I	2.55	1.59–4.08	<0.001
IV vs. I	9.90	5.75–17.05	<0.001

On base-2 logarithmic scale. CI, confidence interval; HR, hazard ratio; RBC, red blood cell.

TABLE 3 | Forward model selection for overall survival before weighting.

	HR	95% CI	p
Epidural analgesia	0.63	0.37–1.07	0.086
BMI	0.93	0.88–0.99	0.025
Charlson comorbidity index	1.17	1.06–1.29	0.003
Anesthesia time*	3.15	1.84–5.39	<0.001
Tumor necrosis	2.83	1.75–4.60	<0.001
Capsular invasion	1.75	1.05–2.91	0.031
Cancer stage			<0.001
II vs. I	2.33	1.09–4.96	0.028
III vs. I	1.78	0.99–3.22	0.054
IV vs. I	11.44	6.26–20.94	0.000

On base-2 logarithmic scale. CI, confidence interval; HR, hazard ratio.

RFS was significant in the quintile-stratified analysis (pooled HR = 0.64, 95% CI: 0.40–1.00; $p = 0.05$).

Overall and Cancer-Specific Survivals

The 5-year OS rates were 86.8% (95% CI: 80.5–93.1%) and 83.8% (95% CI: 80.3–87.3%) in the EA and non-EA groups, respectively. There was no significant association between EA and better OS in the univariate analysis (p = 0.305 by log rank test, **Figure 2B**). The crude HR of EA was 0.76 with a 95% CI of 0.45–1.29. EA was significantly associated with superior OS after IPTW (adjusted HR = 0.66, 95% CI: 0.49–0.89; $p = 0.006$) and in the quintile-stratified analysis (HR = 0.54, 95% CI: 0.31–0.94; $p = 0.03$). The multivariable analysis identified six independent prognostic factors of OS, including BMI, Charlson comorbidity index, anesthesia time, tumor necrosis, capsular invasion and cancer stage (**Table 3**). The association between EA and better OS after RCC surgery was not significant after the adjustment for these significant predictors (HR = 0.63, 95% CI: 0.37–1.07, $p = 0.09$). With respect to the CSS, significant associations between EA and better CSS were noted after IPTW (adjusted HR = 0.68, 95% CI: 0.49–0.94; $p = 0.02$) and in the quintile-stratified analysis (HR = 0.52, 95% CI: 0.28–0.97; $p = 0.04$). Six predictors of CSS were identified after the model selection processes and a significant protective effect of EA on CSS was also noted (HR = 0.49, 95% CI: 0.27–0.89, $p = 0.02$, **Table 4**).

TABLE 4 | Forward model selection for cancer-specific survival before weighting.

	HR	95% CI	P
Epidural analgesia	0.45	0.27–0.89	0.011
Anesthesia time*	2.72	1.46–4.91	0.001
Packed RBC transfusion	1.86	1.12–3.05	0.016
Tumor necrosis	3.48	1.97–5.95	<0.001
Capsular invasion	1.91	1.15–3.32	0.017
Cancer stage			<0.001
II vs. I	2.41	0.87–5.27	0.060
III vs. I	2.56	1.17–4.37	0.007
IV vs. I	13.51	5.68–23.00	<0.001

On base-2 logarithmic scale. CI, confidence interval; HR, hazard ratio; RBC, red blood cell.

DISCUSSION

In recent decades, perioperative management has been identified as a factor that could impact cancer outcomes by altering the microenvironment and it has been receiving more clinical attention (14). All tissue trauma, including the sterile dissection carried out by surgeons, and inflammation have been associated with tumor progression (2). This study demonstrated the hypothetical benefits of perioperative EA for long-term cancer control and survival in patients following RCC resection. To the best of our knowledge, the current study is the largest comparative epidural study to date which has investigated the association between EA and long-term outcomes after RCC surgery. The current study had several strengths, including a relatively large sample size, and the fact that we took more prognostic and pathologic factors into account. We also used sound analytical approaches such as IPTW and other regression-based sensitivity analyses to ensure the consistency of the estimated results (9). Charlson comorbidity index was also used to control for the potential influence of comorbidity severity on the outcomes of interest in the analysis (15). All these efforts were used to try and provide more precise and reliable estimated results to determine the actual association between EA and RFS or OS after curative surgery for RCC.

Although opioids are widely used to control postoperative pain, they are believed to have negative effects on the immune system (8). The evidence from clinical observational studies indicates that opioids suppress cellular and humoral immunity, promote angiogenesis, and enhance progression of metastatic disease (2). Overexpression of μ-opioid receptors on cancer cells is observed and associated with angiogenesis and oncogenic signaling (4). Perioperative EA is administered near the nerve roots to block sensory and sympathetic nerves. It attenuates the neuroendocrine stress responses of the hypothalamic-pituitary-adrenal axis and sympathetic nervous system activation (4) and minimizes volatile agent and opioid consumption (7, 9). Therefore, it has been suggested that EA preserves immune function and prevents cancer recurrence after curative surgery but previous studies have reported inconsistent results (7, 14). Zimmitti et al. reported improved RFS but not OS in patients receiving general anesthesia with EA compared to those without after hepatic resection for colorectal liver metastases (16). However, the study did not take pre-existing medical conditions, perioperative blood transfusion or pathological features into account. Myles et al. (17) found no significant difference in RFS or OS between the EA and non-EA groups following abdominal cancer surgeries in a *post hoc* review of randomized control trials. A systemic review and meta-analysis revealed a lower risk of OS but not cancer recurrence among patients with perioperative regional anesthesia and analgesia (9). A recent study compared perioperative systemic analgesia (SA group) with perioperative EA in addition to systemic analgesia (EA group) following surgical resection of localized RCC, which suggested that EA usage was associated with a significantly improved OS but did not significantly impact cancer-specific survival (8). Accordingly, more prospective studies are needed to elucidate the associations between EA and long-term outcomes after curative cancer surgeries.

During cancer development, circulating tumor cells may leave the primary tumor and form clinically undetectable metastatic foci (2). Micrometastases remain in an immunologic equilibrium between tumor cell proliferation and host immunity (4). However, a cascade of local, systemic cellular and humoral inflammation events may reduce the ability of the host immune system to detect and eradicate cancer cells and could help to disseminated cancer cells which survive the host's defensive mechanisms (2, 14). Clinical evidence shows that tissue trauma caused during surgery can accelerate subsequent neoplastic disease (2, 6). Moreover, an experimental trial reported that the more extensive the surgery is the more potential there is for postoperative inflammation and complications, which further increase the recurrence rate (18). Some studies have suggested that open cancer surgery was associated with shorter disease-free survival compared with minimally invasive surgery, which limited surgical trauma (2, 19), however our investigation did not support the beneficial effects of minimally invasive surgery and partial nephrectomy compared with open surgery and radical nephrectomy, respectively. Notice that similar findings were also noted in another two studies which investigated oncological outcomes in patients undergoing minimally invasive surgery compared with open surgery for clinical T2 RCC and locally advanced RCC, respectively (20, 21). Similar findings were also noted in another study comparing partial or radical nephrectomy for clear cell RCC larger than 7 cm (22).

Interestingly, we also noted that a longer anesthesia time was associated with worse RFS and OS in the stepwise regression analysis. Singh et al. (23) had similar findings in an analysis of minimally-invasive surgeries for endometrial cancer. In their study, longer operative time was also associated with increased medical, surgical and overall complication rates. In fact, longer anesthesia time, as a surrogate for longer surgical time, may reflect the underlying aggressiveness of the disease or the complexity and difficulty of the surgery, or both. Since we have taken miscellaneous surgical and oncological factors into consideration to reduce confounding effects, anesthesia time is highly suspected as an independent risk factor of cancer recurrence and mortality in patients receiving RCC surgery.

Still, there are other factors which may have an effect on long-term cancer outcomes, including the use of steroids (14), non-steroidal anti-inflammatory drugs (4, 18, 19) and systemic lidocaine (4, 14), hypothermia (2, 14, 18), postoperative infections (2), blood transfusions (2, 14), etc. Red blood cells (RBC) are commonly given to cancer patients before, during or after major surgery for a number of different reasons. Although the value of blood transfusions for saving lives is indisputable (24), blood-component therapy can induce negative effects on the recipients' immune system (25), a condition called "transfusion-related immunomodulation" (25, 26). The detrimental effects of immunomodulation are thought to have an association with systemic inflammation (26, 27) and various immunologic changes, including inhibition of cytotoxic cell activity, and immunosuppressive prostaglandin release (26). In the sensitivity analysis, we observed that perioperative packed RBC transfusion was associated with a worse RFS in the multivariable regression analysis. Abu-Ghanem et al. (28) also reported that transfusion reduced RFS, CSS and OS in patients undergoing nephrectomy for RCC. Tsivian et al. (29) found that perioperative blood transfusion was independently associated with worse oncological outcomes for localized RCC after curative surgery and that the recipients were associated with roughly a two-fold increase in metastatic progression, all-cause and RCC-specific mortality. Moreover, negative clinical outcomes were also observed in colon (26, 27) and esophageal (30) cancer patients who received transfusion during curative-intent surgeries. Based on these findings, it has been suggested that blood transfusion can influence the different stages of tumor development including initiation, promotion, malignant conversion, invasion and metastasis (24). To reduce the potential confounding of perioperative blood transfusion on the outcomes of interest, the IPTW methodology was used to balance the exposure of transfusion in both the EA and non-EA groups.

The current study had several limitations. First, patients were not randomized to either group, they instead received EA depending on the preference of the patient, the surgeon or the anesthesiologist. Second, the influence of unmeasured covariates such as dose of opioid, local anesthetics or volatile agents and non-steroidal anti-inflammatory drugs use on cancer outcomes cannot be evaluated due to a lack of available data. Third, the clinical outcomes of loss to follow-up patients are unknown and the last observed censoring time was used in the analysis, which may have affected the results.

In conclusion, we demonstrated an association between perioperative EA use and better RFS and OS in patients undergoing curative surgery for RCC. Future prospective studies and randomized clinical trials with careful design are needed to confirm this relationship between EA and cancer outcomes after curative surgery for RCC and to elucidate the underlying mechanisms.

ETHICS STATEMENT

The studies involving human participants were reviewed and approved by Institutional Review Board (IRB) of the Taipei Veterans General Hospital, Taipei, Taiwan (IRB-TPEVGH No. 2018-06-009CC, Jul 2018). Written informed consent for participation was not required for this study in accordance with the national legislation and the institutional requirements.

AUTHOR CONTRIBUTIONS

F-YY: data collection and manuscript preparation. S-PL: data verification and interpretation. T-PL: data verification and manuscript revision. W-KC: statistical review and manuscript revision. K-YC: study design, data analysis, manuscript preparation, and critical content editing. All authors contributed to the article and approved the submitted version.

REFERENCES

1. Bray F, Ferlay J, Soerjomataram I, Siegel R, Torre L, Jemal A. Global cancer statistics 2018: GLOBOCAN estimates of incidence and mortality worldwide for 36 cancers in 185 countries. *CA Cancer J Clin.* (2018) 68:394–424. doi: 10.3322/caac.21492
2. Tohme S, Simmons RL, Tsung A. Surgery for cancer: a trigger for metastases. *Cancer Res.* (2017) 77:1548–52. doi: 10.1158/0008-5472.Can-16-1536
3. Gupta GP, Massagué J. Cancer metastasis: building a framework. *Cell.* (2006) 127:679–95. doi: 10.1016/j.cell.2006.11.001
4. Kim R. Effects of surgery and anesthetic choice on immunosuppression and cancer recurrence. *J Transl Med.* (2018) 16:8. doi: 10.1186/s12967-018-1389-7
5. Shakhar G, Ben-Eliyahu S. Potential prophylactic measures against postoperative immunosuppression: could they reduce recurrence rates in oncological patients? *Ann Surg Oncol.* (2003) 10:972–92. doi: 10.1245/aso.2003.02.007
6. Tai YH, Chang WK, Wu HL, Chan MY, Chen MY, Chang KY. The effect of epidural analgesia on cancer progression in patients with stage IV colorectal cancer after primary tumor resection: a retrospective cohort study. *PLoS One.* (2018) 13:e0200893. doi: 10.1371/journal.pone.0200893
7. Lennon FE, Moss J, Singleton PA Tsou MY, Chang KY. The μ-opioid receptor in cancer progression: is there a direct effect? *Anesthesiology.* (2012) 116:940–5. doi: 10.1097/ALN.0b013e31824b9512
8. Kovac E, Firoozbakhsh F, Zargar H, Fergany A, Elsharkawy H. Perioperative epidural analgesia is not associated with increased survival from renal cell cancer, but overall survival may be improved: a retrospective chart review. *Can J Anaesth.* (2017) 64:754–62. doi: 10.1007/s12630-017-0875-3
9. Sun Y, Li T, Gan TJ. The effects of perioperative regional anesthesia and analgesia on cancer recurrence and survival after oncology surgery: a systematic review and meta-analysis. *Reg Anesth Pain Med.* (2015) 40:589–98. doi: 10.1097/aap.0000000000000273
10. Edge SB, Compton CC. The American Joint Committee on Cancer: the 7th edition of the AJCC cancer staging manual and the future of TNM. *Ann Surg Oncol.* (2010) 17:1471–4. doi: 10.1245/s10434-010-0985-4
11. Stewart SB, Thompson RH, Psutka SP, Cheville JC, Lohse CM, Boorjian SA, et al. Evaluation of the National Comprehensive Cancer Network and American Urological Association renal cell carcinoma surveillance guidelines. *J Clin Oncol.* (2014) 32:4059–65. doi: 10.1200/jco.2014.56.5416
12. Charlson M, Szatrowski TP, Peterson J, Gold J. Validation of a combined comorbidity index. *J Clin Epidemiol.* (1994) 47:1245–51. doi: 10.1016/0895-4356(94)90129-5
13. Austin PC, Stuart EA. Moving towards best practice when using inverse probability of treatment weighting (IPTW) using the propensity score to estimate causal treatment effects in observational studies. *Stat Med.* (2015) 34:3661–79. doi: 10.1002/sim.6607
14. Wall T, Sherwin A, Ma D, Buggy DJ. Influence of perioperative anaesthetic and analgesic interventions on oncological outcomes: a narrative review. *Br J Anaesth.* (2019) 123:135–50. doi: 10.1016/j.bja.2019.04.062
15. Lin JX, Huang YQ, Xie JW, Wang JB, Lu J, Chen QY, et al. Age-adjusted Charlson Comorbidity Index (ACCI) is a significant factor for predicting survival after radical gastrectomy in patients with gastric cancer. *BMC Surg.* (2019) 19:53. doi: 10.1186/s12893-019-0513-9
16. Zimmitti G, Soliz J, Aloia TA, Gottumukkala V, Cata JP, Tzeng CW, et al. Positive impact of epidural analgesia on oncologic outcomes in patients undergoing resection of colorectal liver metastases. *Ann Surg Oncol.* (2016) 23:1003–11. doi: 10.1245/s10434-015-4933-1
17. Myles PS, Peyton P, Silbert B, Hunt J, Rigg JRA, Sessler DI. Perioperative epidural analgesia for major abdominal surgery for cancer and recurrence-free survival: randomised trial. *BMJ.* (2011) 342:d1491. doi: 10.1136/bmj.d1491
18. Hiller JG, Perry NJ, Poulogiannis G, Riedel B, Sloan EK. Perioperative events influence cancer recurrence risk after surgery. *Nat Rev Clin Oncol.* (2018) 15:205–18. doi: 10.1038/nrclinonc.2017.194
19. Hogan BV, Peter MB, Shenoy HG, Horgan K, Hughes TA. Surgery induced immunosuppression. *Surgeon.* (2011) 9:38–43. doi: 10.1016/j.surge.2010.07.011
20. Lee H, Lee CU, Yoo JH, Sung HH, Jeong BC, Jeon SS, et al. Comparisons of oncological outcomes and perioperative complications between laparoscopic and open radical nephrectomies in patients with clinical T2 renal cell carcinoma (≥7cm). *PLoS ONE.* (2018) 13:e0191786. doi: 10.1371/journal.pone.0191786
21. Bragayrac LA, Abbotoy D, Attwood K, Darwiche F, Hoffmeyer J, Kauffman EC, et al. Outcomes of minimal invasive vs open radical nephrectomy for the treatment of locally advanced renal-cell carcinoma. *J Endourol.* (2016) 30:871–6. doi: 10.1089/end.2016.0082
22. Simone G, Tuderti G, Anceschi U, Papalia R, Ferriero M, Misuraca L, et al. Oncological outcomes of minimally invasive partial versus minimally invasive radical nephrectomy for cT1-2/N0/M0 clear cell renal cell carcinoma: a propensity score-matched analysis. *World J Urol.* (2017) 35:789–94. doi: 10.1007/s00345-016-1923-2
23. Singh S, Swarer K, Resnick K. Longer operative time is associated with increased post-operative complications in patients undergoing minimally-invasive surgery for endometrial cancer. *Gynecol Oncol.* (2017) 147:554–7. doi: 10.1016/j.ygyno.2017.09.024
24. Fischer D, Neb H, Choorapoikayil S, Zacharowski K, Meybohm P. Red blood cell transfusion and its alternatives in oncologic surgery - a critical evaluation. *Crit Rev Oncol Hematol.* (2019) 134:1–9. doi: 10.1016/j.critrevonc.2018.11.011
25. Goubran H, Sheridan D, Radosevic J, Burnouf T, Seghatchian J. Transfusion-related immunomodulation and cancer. *Transfus Apher Sci.* (2017) 56:336–40. doi: 10.1016/j.transci.2017.05.019

26. Aquina CT, Blumberg N, Becerra AZ, Boscoe FP, Schymura MJ, Noyes K, et al. Association among blood transfusion, sepsis, and decreased long-term survival after colon cancer resection. *Ann Surg.* (2017) 266:311–7. doi: 10.1097/sla.0000000000001990
27. McSorley ST, Tham A, Dolan RD, Steele CW, Ramsingh J, Roxburgh C, et al. Perioperative blood transfusion is associated with postoperative systemic inflammatory response and poorer outcomes following surgery for colorectal cancer. *Ann Surg Oncol.* (2020) 27:833–43. doi: 10.1245/s10434-019-07984-7
28. Abu-Ghanem Y, Zilberman DE, Dotan Z, Kaver I, Ramon J. Perioperative blood transfusion adversely affects prognosis after nephrectomy for renal cell carcinoma. *Urol Oncol.* (2018) 36:12.e15–20. doi: 10.1016/j.urolonc.2017.09.006
29. Tsivian M, Abern MR, Tsivian E, Sze C, Jibara G, Rampersaud EN, et al. Effect of blood transfusions on oncological outcomes of surgically treated localized renal cell carcinoma. *Urol Oncol.* (2018) 36:362.e361–7. doi: 10.1016/j.urolonc.2018.04.014
30. Boshier PR, Ziff C, Adam ME, Fehervari M, Markar SR, Hanna GB. Effect of perioperative blood transfusion on the long-term survival of patients undergoing esophagectomy for esophageal cancer: a systematic review and meta-analysis. *Dis Esophagus.* (2018) 31:134. doi: 10.1093/dote/dox134

4

Evaluation of the Time Spent by Anesthetist on Clinical Tasks in the Operating Room

Vincent Compère [1,2], Emmanuel Besnier [1], Thomas Clavier [1,2], Nicolas Byhet [3], Florent Lefranc [4], Frederic Jegou [5], Nicolas Sturzenegger [5], Jean Baptiste Hardy [6], Bertrand Dureuil [1] and Thomas Elie [1]*

[1] Department of Anaesthesiology and Intensive Care, Rouen University Hospital, Rouen, France, [2] Normandie Université, UNIROUEN, INSERM U982, Mont-Saint-Aignan, France, [3] Department of Anaesthesiology, Dieppe General Hospital, Dieppe, France, [4] Department of Anaesthesiology, Hôpital privé de l'estuaire, Le Havre, France, [5] Department of Anaesthesiology, Clinique du Cèdre, Bois-Guillaume, France, [6] Department of Anaesthesiology, Evreux General Hospital, Evreux, France

***Correspondence:**
Vincent Compère
Vincent.Compere@chu-rouen.fr

Background: Changes in the health system in Western countries have increased the scope of the daily tasks assigned to physicians', anesthetists included. As already shown in other specialties, increased non-clinical burden reduces the clinical time spent with patients.

Methods: This was a multicenter, prospective, observational study conducted in 6 public and private hospitals in France. The primary endpoint was the evaluation by an external observer of the time spent per day (in minutes) by anesthetists on clinical tasks in the operating room. Secondary endpoints were the time spent per day (in minutes) on non-clinical organizational tasks and the number of task interruptions per hour of work.

Results: Between October 2017 and April 2018, 54 anesthetists from six hospitals (1 public university hospital, two public general hospitals and three private hospitals) were included. They were followed for 96 days corresponding to 550 hours of work. The proportion of overall clinical time was 62% (58% 95%CI [53; 63] for direct care. The proportion of organizational time was higher in public hospitals (11% in the university hospital ($p < 0.001$) and 4% in general hospitals ($p < 0.01$)) compared to private hospitals (1%). The number of task interruptions (1.5/h ± 1.4 in all hospitals) was 4 times higher in the university hospital (2.2/h ± 1.6) compared to private hospitals (0.5/h ± 0.3) ($p < 0.05$).

Conclusions: Most time in the operating room was spent on clinical care with a significant contrast between public and private hospitals for organizational time.

Keywords: clinical tasks, efficiency, anesthesia organization time, interruption task, anesthesia

HIGHLIGHTS

Most time in the operating room was spent on clinical care 62 % (58 % direct care and 4 % indirect care) with a significant contrast between public and private hospitals for organizational time (11% in the university hospital and 4% in general hospitals compared to 1% in private hospitals).

INTRODUCTION

Changes in the health system in Western countries have increased the scope of the tasks assigned to physicians in their daily lives. The burden of administrative tasks reduces the time spent with the patient. A recent work showed that in four different specialties (general medicine, internal medicine, cardiology and orthopedics), for every hour spent with a patient, a physician spent 2 h on tasks in the patient's absence (1). This result is consistent with that of the study of Wenger *et al.* which found a ratio of 1 to 3 for time spent with the patient vs. administrative tasks in a population of 36 internal medicine residents (2).

Anesthetists are confronted with the same reality as other specialties but no recent work has investigated this topic. A first study published in 1976 showed that anesthetists spent most of their time in contact with their patients: in direct observation (e.g. auscultation) or indirect observation (monitoring of constants) and adapting anesthesia drugs (3). A decade later, McDonald *et al.* reported a clinical time of 61% with 17% directly with the patient (4). In German multicentric study published in 2011, anesthesiologists spent 28.5% of each workday on indirect patient care, 14.7% on direct patient care and 18.8% on administrative work (5). Communication took up 19.9% of anesthesiologists' time, breaks and disruptions 15.2% and other job tasks 2.9%. The time spent on other non-clinical tasks (administrative, organization, etc) appears to be similar than specialties other than anesthesia (20% in the work of Sinsky *et al.*) (1).

A correlation has been shown between the importance of computer tasks in everyday routine and the occurrence of burnout (6). A reduction in clinical time with the patient could be a major source of dissatisfaction for physicians, which can lead to burnout. Anesthetists are more and more confronted with organizational tasks in the operating room that reduce their time spent with patients. No recent work has specifically evaluated the proportion of time spent by anesthetists on clinical and non-clinical tasks in the operating room. The primary objective of this social study was to evaluate the time spent per day by anesthetists on clinical tasks in the operating room. Secondary objectives were the time spent per day on non-clinical organizational tasks and the number of task interruptions per hour of work.

MATERIALS AND METHODS

Study Model

We conducted a multicenter, prospective and observational study in six hospitals in Normandy, France: one university hospital (Rouen University Hospital), two general hospitals (Dieppe General Hospital and Evreux General Hospital) and three private hospitals (Clinique du Cèdre, private hospital in Bois-Guillaume, Hôpital privé de l'estuaire, private hospital in Le Havre and Clinique Pasteur private hospital in Evreux). Fifty-four anesthetists were eligible and volunteered to participate in the study.

Study Protocol

We evaluated the time spent by anesthetists on clinical tasks during 1 day in the operating room. Each day between 8 a.m. and 3 p.m., an anesthetist, who had been selected the day before, was continuously monitored by an external observer, a student nurse anesthetist who was carrying out a research internship. There were 13 external observers, each of whom was followed up over the 3 weeks of the internship. All external observers had a 1-h training session by an anesthetist (TE) to explain the purpose of the study and the use of software for monitoring tasks. The training session consisted in a dedicated program on how to define and categorize clinical tasks and how to use recording devices. At the end of the training session, they were evaluated to assess their good comprehension of the different information. The information was also available on electronic devices. In case of difficulty, the two investigating anesthetists (TE and VC) were available at any time.

Organization of the Operating Rooms of Participating Hospitals

The three public hospitals (Rouen University Hospital, Dieppe General Hospital and Evreux General Hospital), operated with one nurse anesthetist in each operating room. An anesthetist was always in charge of two operating rooms. The organization was different according to the type of public hospital. The university hospital has specialty operating rooms (cardiac surgery, digestive and urological surgery, neurosurgery, pediatric surgery, orthopedic surgery and vascular and thoracic surgery) as well as shared operating rooms for emergency and ambulatory surgery, while the two general hospitals each have shared operating rooms integrating all specialties. The three private hospitals each have shared operating rooms. In the three private hospitals, an anesthetist was in charge of two operating rooms but there was only one nurse anesthetist for two operating rooms.

Data Collection

The data were anonymously collected using a digital tablet with atracker? software. This software was previously configured to monitor 15 items divided into five categories (**Table 1**): clinical time; non-clinical time; time spent on communication media to perform tasks; time spent in different locations; the number of task interruptions.

When the anesthetist started one of the tasks listed in the software, the external observer clicked on the corresponding task, triggering a stopwatch that stopped as soon as the observer clicked on it again. Several tasks could be followed in parallel. At the end of the day, data were automatically classified by the software and then sent in the form of a table on an Excel database.

For each anesthetist, observers recorded: age, the number of patients cared for during 1 day, the hospital, a satisfaction score of 0 to 10 filled by the anesthetist.

Study Outcomes

The primary endpoint was the evaluation by an external observer of the time spent per day (in minutes) by anesthetist on clinical tasks in the operating room.

TABLE 1 | Description of tasks.

Categories and daily tasks	Description
Clinical time	
Direct care (All tasks directly related to patient care)	- Direct communication with patient - Monitoring machines - Performing medical procedures
Indirect care (all tasks indirectly related to patient care)	- Searching for a patient's medical record - Preparing for a procedure
Pedagogical time	Time spent training residents
Non-clinical time	
Personal time	Breaks and lunch
Organizational time	Flow management in the operating room, staff meeting for patient programming
Administrative time	Meetings, scheduling, etc.
Other time	Any time not previously defined
Communication media	
Paper	Time spent writing on paper
Telephone	Time spent on the professional telephone
Computer	Time spent on the computer for professional tasks
Location	
Medical office	Time spent in the office
PACU	Time spent in the PACU
Operating room	Time spent in the operating room
Other	Time spent in the staff room, rest room etc.
Task interruption	
	Number of task interruptions

PACU, post anesthesia care unit.

Secondary endpoints were: the time spent per day (in minutes) on non-clinical organizational tasks; the proportion of time spent in different locations; the proportion of time spent on different communication media; the number of task interruptions per hour of work and stakeholders responsible for task interruptions; and anaesthetists' satisfaction of their working day. The definition used for task interruption was the unexpected cessation of human activity, temporary or permanent. The reason could be specific to the operator or, on the contrary, be external to him.

Ethical Considerations

The protocol was validated by the ethics committee for non-interventional research of Rouen University Hospital (E2017-27) and was registered in clinical trials (NCT03446482). The requirement for written informed consent was waived by the Committee.

TABLE 2 | Characteristics of anesthetists population.

	Anesthetists *n*	Age years	Treated patients *n*/day
Overall	54	39 (±10)	8 (±4.6)
General hospitals	13	44 (±11)[#]	8 (±3)
Private hospitals	14	43 (±8)	10 (±5.6)
University hospital	27	35 (±8.6)*	6.7 (±4.3)*

*Results are presented as means (± standard deviations) or absolute values. *$p < 0.05$ corresponding to a significant difference between the university Hospital and private hospitals. #$p < 0.05$ corresponding to a significant difference between the university hospital and general hospitals.*

Statistical Analysis

As described by Hauschild *et al.*, we wanted to include at least 500 h of anesthesiologist work in a minimum of five different hospitals (5). The values are presented as a mean (± standard deviation) for the characteristics of the study population. The results are presented in proportion, rounded to the nearest unit for the main results. The percentages (IC95%) expressed correspond to the time spent for each item per day and per anesthetist reported on the total observation time per physician. The number of task interruption is expressed as an average of the number of events per hour (± standard deviation). The different parameters were compared using the Kruskall Wallis test and Bonferroni correction. The correlation coefficients were calculated from the Pearson correlation test. We considered an alpha risk of 5%. The data were analyzed using Microsoft Excel ?, XLSTAT? and Prism ? software and the biostaTGV website.

RESULTS

Characteristics of Population

Between October 2017 and April 2018, 54 anesthetists from six hospitals were included. They were followed for 96 days corresponding to 550 h of assessed work hours. The characteristics of anesthetists according to hospitals are summarized in **Table 2**. The sex ratio was 2.6.

Evaluation of the Proportion of Time Spent on the Different Tasks

The proportion of time spent on clinical tasks was 58% 95%CI [53; 63]. The results are summarized in **Table 3**. The different stakeholders responsible for task interruptions are displayed in **Table 4**.

Correlation

There was no correlation between anaesthetists' job satisfaction and the number of patients cared for ($r = 0.19$, 95%CI[−0.03; 0.38], $p = 0.08$). Similarly, the correlation between the satisfaction score and the time spent in the patient's presence was not significant ($r = 0.18$, 95% CI[−0.03; 0.39], $p = 0.09$).

TABLE 3 | Time spent by anesthetists on clinical and non-clinical tasks in the operating room.

	Total	University hospital	General hospitals	Private hospitals
Anesthetists (n)	54	27	13	14
Task % [95%CI]				
Direct care	58% [53; 63]	53%*** [47; 59]	48% [40; 56]	78%+++ [71; 85]
Indirect care	4% [2.7; 5.4]	4% [2.2; 5.8]	2% [0.4; 3.6]	7%+ [3.3; 10.7]
Pedagogical time	4% [2.5; 6.2]	7%** [4.7; 9.3]	4% (2, 10)	<1%
Administrative time	4% [1.2; 5.9]	5% [0.5; 9.5]	1% (1, 3)	2% [0.3; 3.7]
Organizational time	7% [4.8; 9]	11%*** [7.6; 14.4]	4%## [0.3; 7.7]	1% [0; 2]
Personal time	14% [11.9; 5.3]	14% [11.3; 16.7]	15% [12.3; 17.7]	11% [7.5; 14.5]
Other time	9%	6%	26%	0
Communication media % [95%CI]				
Computer	7% [5.2; 9.7]	5%*** [3.2; 6.8]	1%## [0.2; 2.8]	17%+++ [12; 22]
Telephone	2% [1.7; 2.9]	3%* [1.4; 4.6]	1%## [0.4; 1.6]	2% [1.1; 2.9]
Paper	4% [2.7; 4.8]	5%*** [3.7; 6.3]	5% (2, 8)	<1%+
Location % [95%CI]				
Operating room	74% [69; 79]	77% [69; 85]	58%## [49; 57]	83%+++ [73; 93]
Medical office	6% [3.2; 8]	4% [1.2; 6.8]	13%## (6, 20)	2%++ [−0.1; 4.1]
PACU	13% [8.7; 15.6]	12% [4.4; 19.6]	16% [9; 23]	10% [2.7; 15.3]
Other	7% [3.7; 10.2]	7% [1.7; 12.3]	13% [5; 21]	5%+ [−0.1; 6.1]
Task interruption n/hour	1.5 (±1.4)	2.2 (±1.6)*	0.6 (±0.6)#	0.5(±0.3)
Satisfaction	7.2 (±1.6)	6.7(±1.7)**	7.4 (±1.8)	8 (±0.8)

Results are presented as percentages corresponding to the averages of proportions of anaesthetists' follow-up time for tasks, location and support and as an absolute value corresponding to the averages over the total observation time for interruptions and satisfaction.

**Corresponding to a difference between the university hospital and private hospitals.*

#Corresponding to a difference between the university hospital and general hospitals.

+Corresponding to a difference between the general hospitals and private hospitals.

, #, + $p < 0.05$, **, ##, ++ $p < 0.01$, *, ###, +++ $p < 0.001$.*

The correlation between the satisfaction score and the number of task interruptions during the day was significant and inversely proportional (r = −0.28, 95%CI[−0.46; −0.07], p = 0.009). The correlation between the satisfaction score and organizational time was significant and inversely proportional (r = −0.34, 95%CI[−0.52; −0.13], p = 0.002). The correlation between the satisfaction score and computer time was significant and positive (r = 0.26, 95%CI [0.05; 0.45], p = 0.02).

DISCUSSION

In this work based on an evaluation by external observers of the tasks in the operating room of 54 anesthetists corresponding to 550 h of follow-up in six centers, the overall clinical time of anesthetist was 62 % (58 % direct care and 4 % indirect care). This result is the same as that of an older work, published by Kennedy et al. in 1976, which focused on the proportion of time spent on the different tasks of the anesthetists during one day in the operating room. anesthetists spent most of their time in contact with their patients in the operating room to monitor and adapt anesthesia (>50%). These authors reported that anesthetists spent too much time (>30%) on tasks considered secondary (data recording, equipment preparation, etc.) because not related to direct care but which could be included in our definition of clinical time (3). About 10 years later, Mc Donald *et al.* evaluated the division of tasks of anesthetists in the operating room in order to analyze the impact of the modernization of monitoring on time spent in direct care. These authors found that 17% of anaesthetists' time was spent directly observing patients and about 40% on ancillary tasks (data recording, preparation, etc.) or observing the monitoring screens. However, if we add the clinical tasks related to anesthesia, the overall proportion of time spent on care was more than 70%, higher than our results (4). It is difficult to compare the results of our work with these two studies because of major changes in the practice of anesthesia over the past 30 years. Similarly, the definition of the tasks they used were not fully comparable with ours. The most recent wok shows that German anesthesiologists spent 28.5% of each workday on indirect patient care, 14.7% on direct patient care and 18.8% on administrative work (5). The type of hospital could change the ratio between different tasks. Indeed, Dexter *et al.* found 53.2% for direct clinical care, 11.5% for indirect clinical care, 10.3% for education and 12.9% for management (7).

Nevertheless, these results relative to ours suggest a continuous decrease in clinical time over the years. Our results are also consistent with those of different studies that focused on other specialties. In the study by Sinsky et al., the clinical time in the presence of patients was 33% in ambulatory practice (family medicine, internal medicine etc.) (1). Wenger et al. found similar results in a population of medical residents The authors attributed the decrease in clinical time to the increasing importance of computer tools (2). In an intensive care unit, the proportion of direct care ranged from 16 to 19% (8). Our results show that, on average, anesthetists spend 2–3 times longer on direct care than other medical specialties. One of the reasons is that in the French model, anesthetists are in charge of two operating rooms and are therefore responsible for two patients at the same time.

In our work, we found a significant difference in the time spent on direct care between public (48 and 53% for general hospitals and the university hospital, respectively) and private hospitals (78%). There are several explanations for this result. First, in the private hospitals observed, the anesthetist worked with only one nurse anesthetist for two rooms, which required the anesthetist to be present continuously in one of the two operating rooms and therefore the time in the presence of the

TABLE 4 | Stakeholders responsible for task interruptions.

Anesthetist	Nurse	Nurse anesthetist	Medical doctor	Resident	Surgeon	Surgical nurse	Unknown
3%	22%	15%	14%	4%	3%	7%	32%

patient was higher. In addition, in public hospitals, particularly in university hospitals, time is spent training residents (7%), which is not the case in private hospitals. Finally, this work highlights the higher organizational constraints in public hospitals (11% in the university hospital and 4% in general hospitals) compared to private hospitals (1%). This organizational time, which is at the expense of clinical time, is correlated with anaesthetists' satisfaction. This result suggests that in public hospitals, and more particularly in university hospitals, there is a difficulty in anticipating the organizational constraints of the operating room and that these latter regulate the work flow in real time. This organizational aspect, through a shift in tasks, is largely the responsibility of the anesthetist who may not be trained to assume this responsibility. Finally, organizational constraints could be a source of conflict between the many different medical professionals working alongside each other in the operating room (surgeons, surgical nurses, nurse anesthetists, nurse assistants).

The time spent on computer media was relatively low (7% of total observation time) compared to other specialties studied in the literature. Indeed, several studies showed that nearly a half of physicians' time was spent on computer tasks (1, 2). In our work, computer media were mainly used in private hospitals compared to public hospitals. In the private hospitals studied, intraoperative processes, including intraoperative monitoring, intra- and post-operative prescriptions and anesthesia consultation, were computerized, while in public hospitals, only post-operative prescriptions were computerized. Unlike other studies, we found a positive correlation between the use of computer media and anaesthetists' job satisfaction (6, 9). This result seems to be in discrepancy with that of another study which showed that the progressive use of electronic devices was rather a source of dissatisfaction for physicians in the U.S (10).

The number of task interruptions in our work was 1.5/h. Savoldelli et al. observed a frequency of distracting events of 5 per induction out of 37 inductions in the context of emergency surgery, the duration of which occupied 35% of the total induction time (11). In another work in the perioperative period, Campbell et al. followed 30 procedures during which they observed 13.8 distracting events per hour (17.4/h during induction, 9/h during maintenance of anesthesia and 30/h during the recovery phase) (12). Finally, out of 32 procedures, Jothiraj *et al.* observed 60 distractor events per hour of which 19.2 scored 2 on the Heavey scale (13). The difference observed between our study and these different works is the definition of task interruption. These other studies evaluated all the events likely to interfere with the physician's vigilance (distraction, disruption and interruption) whereas we only considered those that were responsible for cessation of activity, which reduced the number of our observations. In the context of critical care, several studies have focused on the quantification of interruption with a similar definition to ours. A work by Berg *et al.*, published in 2016, found a rate of 5/h in a population of physicians and nurses in an Emergency Department (14). A recent work by Li et al. evaluated task distribution and associated interruptions in an intensive care unit. The time spent in contact with the patient was only 16%, and 4.2/h of task interruptions were recorded In comparison, in a population of specialists not involved in critical care, Westbrook et al. found a 15% rate of patient contact time and a number of task interruptions of 2.9/h (8, 15). These task interruptions had consequences on the satisfaction of anesthetists since we found a correlation between their dissatisfaction and the number of task interruptions per day. Similarly, the work of Berg et al. found this result between dissatisfaction and task interruption (14).

Borrowed from aviation, some authors have put forward the concept of a sterile cockpit, particularly for the induction and recovery phases, to limit task interruptions by staying focused on clinical tasks (16). The International Civil Aviation Organization defines this concept as "the entire period during which the crew should not be disturbed except for matters essential to the safety of the aircraft" and in fact implies the restriction of crew members' activities to those that are operationally essential during particularly complex flight phases (take-off, landing,....). Apart from the exclusion of all non-management discussions, this concept also introduces the use of checklists and also a standardization of communication between the different professionals. This concept has not been specifically studied in anesthesia but other disciplines have shown interest in it. In a before/after study in cardiac surgery, the authors showed that formalizing the elements of communication made it possible to reduce the number of task interruptions (7.3 compared to 11.5 per case) (17). Without necessarily seeking total silence in the operating theater, simple measures such as banning unnecessary movement of people, reducing background noise, temporarily diverting telephone calls can create a more serene, professional and safe atmosphere. The physician (surgeon or anaesthesist) can also ask team members to refocus by warning them that a risky phase of a procedure is about to begin (18). Finally, training physicians to perform or manage multiple tasks simultaneously appears to be an interesting way (19, 20).

Our study presents a number of limitations that need to be included in discussion. We conducted a briefing session with external observers before their observation days to standardize the evaluation, but inter-observer variability between the 13 different external observers cannot be excluded. In addition, the choice of anesthetist to be followed during the day was defined by the study investigator a few days earlier without drawing lots from a population of volunteer physicians to be followed. Since the evaluation took place over 7 consecutive hours and because of the multitude of tasks observed, the observers' attention may have fluctuated, the evaluation and the number of task interruptions were probably underestimated compared to reality especially since as described by Hauschild et al., we didn't perform a multitasking analysis (5). Although the anesthetists volunteered to participate in the study, there is a potential bias that there might not be happy with the working environment.

CONCLUSION

In this study, most time in the operating room was spent on clinical tasks with a significant contrast between public and private hospitals for organizational time. The enlargement of the scope of the anesthetists could in part lead to anaesthetists' dissatisfaction.

AUTHOR CONTRIBUTIONS

VC helped in the study conception and design, in resident recruitment, in study coordination, in interpretation of data, and in manuscript draft and revision. EB helped in the study conception and design, in acquisition of data, in analysis and interpretation of data and in manuscript draft. TC, NB, FL, FJ, NS, JH, and BD helped in interpretation of data and manuscript revision. TE helped in the study conception and design, in acquisition of data, in statistical analysis, in analysis and interpretation of data and in manuscript draft. All authors read and approved the final manuscript.

ACKNOWLEDGMENTS

The authors are grateful to Nikki Sabourin-Gibbs, Rouen University Hospital, for her help in editing the manuscript and to student nurse anesthetists, Rouen University Hospital, for their participation as external observers.

REFERENCES

1. Sinsky C, Colligan L, Li L. Allocation of physician time in ambulatory practice: a time and motion study in 4 specialties. *Ann Intern Med.* (2016) 165:753–60. doi: 10.7326/M16-0961
2. Wenger N, Méan M, Castioni J, Marques-Vidal P, Waeber G, Garnier A. Allocation of internal medicine resident time in a swiss hospital: a time and motion study of day and evening shifts. *Ann Intern Med.* (2017) 166:579–86. doi: 10.7326/M16-2238
3. Kennedy PJ, Feingold A, Wiener EL, Hosek RS. Analysis of tasks and human factors in anesthesia for coronary-artery bypass. Anesth Analg. (1976) 55:374–7. doi: 10.1213/00000539-197605000-00020
4. McDonald JS, Dzwonczyk RR. A time and motion study of the anaesthetist's intraoperative time. *Br J Anaesth.* (1988) 61:738–42. doi: 10.1093/bja/61.6.738
5. Hauschild I, Vitzthum K, Klapp BF, Groneberg DA, Mache S. Time and motion study of anesthesiologists' workflow in German hospitals. *Wien Med Wochenschr.* (2011) 161:433–40. doi: 10.1007/s10354-011-0028-1
6. Shanafelt TD, Dyrbye LN, Sinsky C, Hasan O, Satele D, Sloan J, et al. Relationship between clerical burden and characteristics of the electronic environment with physician burnout and professional satisfaction. *Mayo Clin Proc.* (2016) 91:836–48. doi: 10.1016/j.mayocp.2016.05.007
7. Dexter F, Wachtel RE, Todd MM, Hindman BJ. The "Fourth Mission": the time commitment of anesthesiology faculty for management is comparable to their time commitments to education, research, and indirect patient care. *A A Case Rep.* 2015 5:206–11. doi: 10.1213/XAA.0000000000000149
8. Li, Ling; Hains, Isla; Hordern, Toni; Milliss, David; Raper, Ray and Westbrook, Johanna. What do ICU doctors do? a multisite time and motion study of the clinical work patterns of registrars. *Crit Care Resusc.* (2015) 17:159–66.
9. Friedberg MW, Chen PG, Van Busum KR, Aunon F, Pham C, Caloyeras J, et al. Factors affecting physician professional satisfaction and their implications for patient care, health systems, and health policy. *Rand Health Quarterly.* (2014) 3:1. doi: 10.7249/RB9740
10. Shanafelt TD, Hasan O, Dyrbye LN, Sinsky C, Satele D, Sloan J, et al. Changes in burnout and satisfaction with work-life balance in physicians and the general US working population between 2011 and 2014. *Mayo Clin Proc.* (2015) 90:1600–13. doi: 10.1016/j.mayocp.2015.08.023
11. Savoldelli GL, Thieblemont J, Clergue F, Waeber JL, Forster A, Garnerin P. Incidence and impact of distracting events during induction of general anaesthesia for urgent surgical cases. *Eur J Anaesthesiol.* (2010) 27:683–9. doi: 10.1097/EJA.0b013e328333de09
12. Campbell G, Arfanis K, Smith AF. Distraction and interruption in anaesthetic practice. *Br J Anaesth.* (2012) 109:707–15. doi: 10.1093/bja/aes219
13. Jothiraj H, Howland-Harris J, Evley R, Moppett IK. Distractions and the anaesthetist: a qualitative study of context and direction of distraction. *Br J Anaesth.* (2013) 111:477–82. doi: 10.1093/bja/aet108
14. Berg LM, Källberg AS, Göransson KE, Östergren J, Florin J, Ehrenberg A. Interruptions in emergency department work: an observational and interview study. *BMJ Qual Saf.* (2013) 22:656. doi: 10.1136/bmjqs-2013-001967
15. Westbrook JI, Woods A, Rob MI, Dunsmuir WM, Day RO. Association of interruptions with an increased risk and severity of medication administration errors. *Arch Intern Med.* (2010) 170:683–90. doi: 10.1001/archinternmed.2010.65
16. Broom MA, Capek AL, Carachi P, Akeroyd MA, Hilditch G. Critical phase distractions in anaesthesia and the sterile cockpit concept. *Anaesthesia.* (2011) 66:175–9. doi: 10.1111/j.1365-2044.2011.06623.x
17. Wadhera RK, Parker SH, Burkhart HM, Greason KL, Neal JR, Levenick KM, et al. Is the ≪ sterile cockpit ≫ concept applicable to cardiovascular surgery critical intervals or critical events? The impact of protocol-driven communication during cardiopulmonary bypass. *J Thorac Cardiovasc Surg.* (2010) 139:312–9. doi: 10.1016/j.jtcvs.2009.10.048
18. Aerden D, Smets D, Poelaert J, Oste J, Van den Brande P. Fighting human error : what surgeons can learn from aviators. *Acta Chir Belg.* (2014) 114:228–32. doi: 10.1080/00015458.2014.11681017
19. Rasmussen SR, Konge L, Mikkelsen PT, Sørensen MS, Andersen SAW. Notes from the field: secondary task precision for cognitive load estimation during virtual reality surgical simulation training. *Eval Health Prof.* (2016) 39:114–20. doi: 10.1177/0163278715597962
20. Schneider W, Detweiler M. The role of practice in dual-task performance: toward workload modeling in a connectionist/control architecture. *Hum Factors.* (1988) 30:539–66. doi: 10.1177/001872088803000502

5

Sequential Organ Failure Assessment Score for Prediction of Mortality of Patients with Rhabdomyolysis Following Exertional Heatstroke: A Longitudinal Cohort Study in Southern China

Ming Wu [1,2†], *Conglin Wang* [2†], *Zheyeng Liu* [2] *and Zhifeng Liu* [2,3*]

[1] *Department of Critical Care Medicine and Hospital Infection Prevention and Control, Health Science Center, The Second People's Hospital of Shenzhen, First Affiliated Hospital of Shenzhen University, Shenzhen, China,* [2] *Department of Critical Care Medicine, General Hospital of Southern Theatre Command of Peoples Liberation Army, Guangzhou, China,* [3] *Key Laboratory of Hot Zone Trauma Care and Tissue Repair of Peoples Liberation Army, General Hospital of Southern Theatre Command of Peoples Liberation Army, Guangzhou, China*

Correspondence:
Zhifeng Liu
Zhifengliu7797@163.com

† These authors have contributed equally to this study

Background: Heatstroke is a medical emergency that causes multi-organ injury and death without intervention, but limited data are available on the illness scores in predicting the outcomes of exertional heat stroke (EHS) with rhabdomyolysis (RM). The aim of our study was to investigate the Sequential Organ Failure Assessment (SOFA) score in predicting mortality of patients with RM after EHS.

Methods: A retrospective cohort study was performed, which included all patients with EHS admitted into the intensive care unit (ICU) of General Hospital of Southern Theater Command of Peoples Liberation Army from January 2008 to June 2019. RM was defined as creatine kinase (CK) > 1,000 U/L. Data, including the baseline data at admission, vital organ function indicators, and 90-day mortality, were reviewed.

Results: A total of 176 patients were enrolled; among them, 85 (48.3%) had RM. Patients with RM had a significantly higher SOFA score (4.0 vs. 3.0, $p = 0.021$), higher occurrence rates of disseminated intravascular coagulation (DIC) (53.1 vs. 18.3%, $p < 0.001$) and acute liver injury (ALI) (21.4 vs. 5.5%, $p = 0.002$) than patients with non-RM. RM was positively correlated with ALI and DIC, and the correlation coefficients were 0.236 and 0.365, respectively (both p-values <0.01). Multivariate logistics analysis showed that the SOFA score [odds ratio (OR) 1.7, 95% CI 1.1–2.6, $p = 0.024$] was the risk factor for 90-day mortality in patients with RM after EHS, with the area under the curve (AUC) 0.958 (95% CI 0.908–1.000, $p < 0.001$) and the optimal cutoff 7.5 points.

Conclusions: Patients with RM after EHS have severe clinical conditions, which are often accompanied by DIC or ALI. The SOFA score could predict the prognosis of patients with RM with EHS. Early treatment strategies based on decreasing the SOFA score at admission may be pivotal to reduce the 90-day mortality of patients with EHS.

Keywords: exertional heatstroke, rhabdomyolysis, mortality, risk factors, SOFA score

INTRODUCTION

Heatstroke is an acute medical emergency characterized by the central nervous system (CNS) dysfunction, multi-organ failure, and extreme hyperthermia (usually >40.5°C) with a mortality rate of 40 to 70% and a disability rate of 30%. It is typically classified as exertional heat stroke (EHS) and classical heatstroke (CHS) (1). Rhabdomyolysis (RM) is one of the complications in patients with EHS, which ranges from an asymptomatic illness with an elevated creatine kinase (CK) level to a life-threatening condition associated with extreme elevations in CK, electrolyte imbalances, acute kidney injury (AKI), or disseminated intravascular coagulation (DIC). However, the relationships between RM and organ function and prognosis are poorly documented.

Some studies have also shown that RM caused by heatstroke may be an important factor in initiating sepsis (2–6) and will further cause the disturbance of blood coagulation, which can easily lead to the occurrence of DIC (7) and AKI (8, 9). Research showed that the Sequential Organ Failure Assessment (SOFA) score was an independent risk factor affecting the survival of patients (10); therefore, treatments based on reducing the SOFA score may be pivotal for reducing the mortality of EHS complicated with AKI (11). However, so far there are few clinical studies on the clinical characteristics and prognosis of EHS complicated with RM, and there is no scoring system that can predict prognosis in patients with RM with EHS. To provide a reference for timely and effective treatment, a retrospective cohort study was designed in a tertiary-care teaching hospital in southern China over 10 years, in which the clinical characteristics, the relationships between RM and organ function, and risk factors and 90-day mortality were analyzed.

METHODS

Study Design and Participants

This retrospective cohort study was performed in the intensive care unit (ICU) of General Hospital of Southern Theater Command of Peoples Liberation Army from January 2008 to June 2019. The inclusion criteria of EHS are as follows (1): patients exposed to high temperature, high humidity, and history of strenuous exercise, with an excessively high body temperature (central temperature higher than 40°C) or/and nervous system dysfunction (including delirium, cognitive impairment, coma, etc.). The exclusion criteria were as follows: (1) death or discharged within 24 h after admission, (2) incomplete data regarding key indicators, (3) incomplete outcome evaluation data obtained *via* telephone follow-up, and (4) a previous history of organ dysfunction, such as skeletal muscle disease and chronic kidney disease.

Comprehensive treatments were provided to all patients, such as body cooling, the volume of infusion, and anti-inflammation drugs. Meanwhile, organ function supports were provided for patients with RM under clinical guidelines if necessary, including appropriate hydration, alkalization of urine, blood purifications with polymer interception, and so on.

Research Procedures

The basic characteristics of patients were reviewed, including the Acute Physiology and Chronic Health Evaluation II (APACHE II) score, SOFA score, Glasgow Coma Score (GCS), and inflammatory and organ function indicators at admission. The indicators included blood count (lymphocyte and platelets), kidney function markers [blood urea nitrogen (BUN) and serum creatinine (Scr)], liver function markers [total bilirubin, alanine aminotransferase (ALT), and aspartate aminotransferase (AST)], C-reactive protein (CRP), procalcitonin (PCT), cardiac markers [CK, MB isoenzyme of creatine kinase (CK-MB), MB, and cardiac troponin I (cTNI)], clotting factors [prothrombin time (PT), international normalized ratio (INR), activated partial thromboplastin time (APTT), thrombin time (TT), fibrinogen (FIB), and D-dimer], and blood transfusion during treatment. All patients were assigned to the RM group and the non-RM group according to the presence of RM. Survival time was defined as the duration from onset to death; when the survival time was longer than 90 days, it was recorded as 90 days. The main results, including the 90-day mortality, ICU time, and the total cost during hospitalization, were analyzed. The survival curve analysis was performed.

Definitions

(1) RM (12): General fatigue, muscle soreness, and soy sauce-like urine; elevated laboratory CK; and elevated non-cardiogenic MB. This study adopted the current consensus opinion that CK > 1,000 U/L or increased more than five times the normal level was considered as elevated CK, whereas an increase in CK due to cardiogenic shock (CK-MB/CK < 5%) was excluded.
(2) DIC (13): International Society for Thrombosis and Haemostasis (ISTH) standard: An ISTH score ≥5 points.
(3) AKI (14): The Kidney Disease: Improving Global Outcomes (KDIGO) standard: Scr increased to ≥26.5 μmol/L (≥0.3 mg/dl) within 48 h, Scr increased to ≥1.5 times the baseline within 7 days, or urine output <0.5 ml/(kg h) for 6 h.
(4) Acute liver injury (ALI) (15): Plasma TBIL ≥ 34.2 μmol/L and INR ≥ 1.5, or with any grade of hepatic encephalopathy.
(5) Lymphocytopenia (16): Absolute lymphocytes less than 0.8 $\times 10^9$/L.

Statistical Analysis

The continuous variables conformed to a normal distribution are expressed as $\bar{x} \pm s$. For continuous variables that did not conform to a normal distribution are presented as medians and interquartile ranges (IQRs), and the categorical data were summarized as numbers and percentages. Continuous variables were compared using the independent two-sample t test or Mann–Whitney U tests. Categorical variables were compared using the Chi-Square test or Fisher's exact test. Significant indicators were analyzed using single factor analysis. Indicators with a P value < 0.1 were included in the multivariate logistic regression (LR) model: OR (odds ratio) and 95% confidence interval levels (95% CI), and forward stepwise regression was

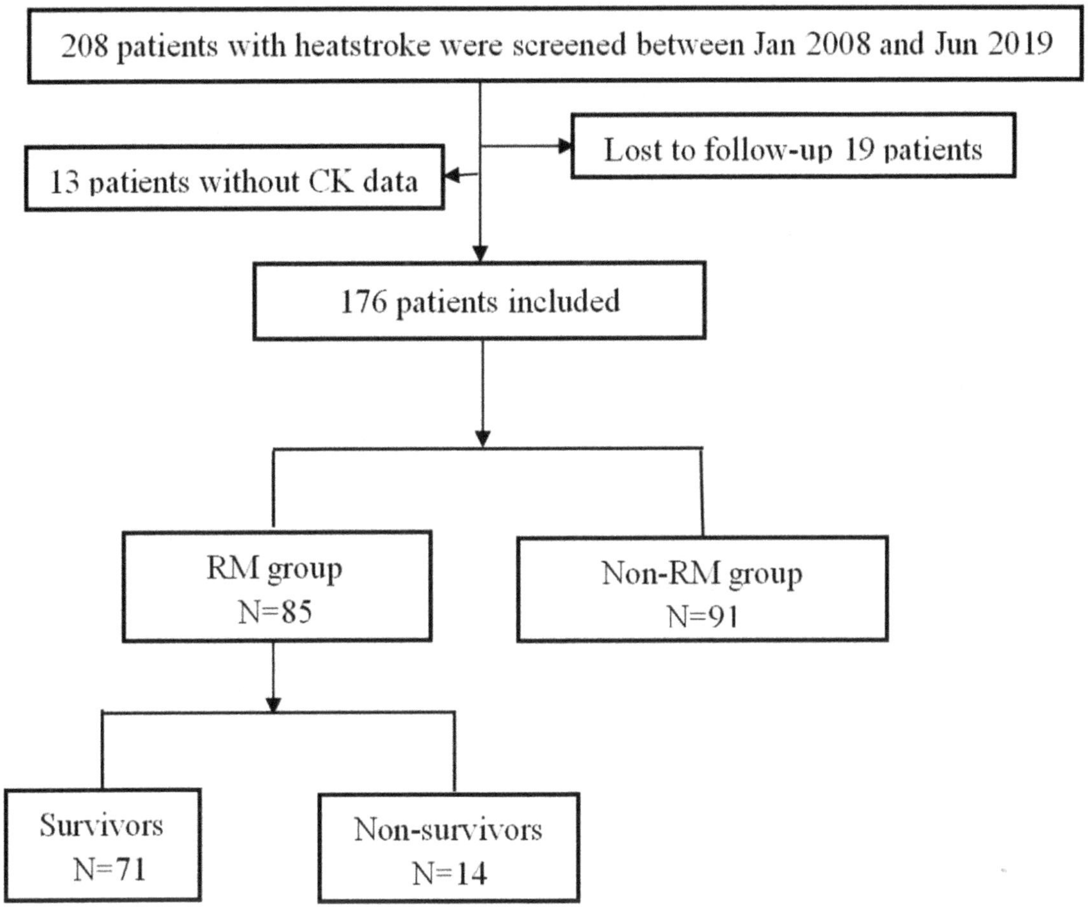

FIGURE 1 | Flowchart of all excluded and included patients.

used to gradually eliminate each variable. The predictive ability of SOFA score for 90-day mortality was assessed using the area under the receiver operating characteristic (AU-ROC) curve, and the optimal cutoff value was determined by Youden's index. We analyzed the 90-day mortality in the RM and non-RM groups using the Kaplan–Meier's method and assessed the differences by the log-rank test. The relationship between RM and organ injury was performed using the Pearson correlation analysis. Statistical analyses were performed using the IBM SPSS Windows version 23.0 (IBM Corp., Armonk, NY, USA), Empower (R) (http://www.empowerstats.com, X&Y solutions, Inc., Boston, MA, USA), and R (http://www.R-project.org) software. The p-values (two-tailed) less than 0.05 were considered statistically significant.

RESULTS

Clinical Characteristics of the Patients With EHS

A total of 208 patients fulfilled the inclusion criteria; among them, 32 patients were excluded because of loss to follow-up or missing CK data. Finally, 176 patients were included, who were all men; among them, there were 91 patients (51.7%) without RM, and 85 patients (48.3%) with RM (**Figure 1**). There was no statistical difference in age between the two groups [20.0 vs. 22.0 (years), $p = 0.472$]. Compared with the patients with non-RM, the patients with RM had a significantly higher SOFA score (4.0 vs. 3.0, $p = 0.021$), higher incidence of DIC (53.1 vs. 18.3%, $p < 0.001$) and ALI (21.4% vs. 5.5%, $p = 0.002$). These patients also had lower lymphocyte and platelet, significantly increased CK, MB, PCT, PT, APTT, D-dimer, ALT, and AST, and higher blood transfusion proportion than patients with non-RM (all $p < 0.05$). However, there were no statistically significant differences in APACHE II (12.0 vs. 10.0, $p = 0.285$) and GCS scores (10.0 vs. 12.0, $p = 0.429$) and also in the incidence of lymphocytopenia (44.6 vs. 33.0%, $p = 0.116$) and AKI (48.8 vs. 39.6%, $p = 0.218$). Interestingly, the 90-day mortality of patients with RM was not significantly increased (16.5% vs. 8.8%, $p = 0.124$), whereas the total cost of hospitalization was particularly higher [51,986.3 vs. 31,810.5 (RMB), $p = 0.036$] than that of patients with non-RM (**Table 1**).

Comparisons of Survivors and Non-survivors With EHS Complicated With RM

Among the patients with RM induced by EHS, 71 survived (83.5%) and 14 died (16.5%). Non-survivors had higher APACHE

TABLE 1 | Comparisons of clinical characteristics between patients with rhabdomyolysis (RM) and non-RM with exertional heat stroke (EHS).

Variables	Non-RM ($n = 91$)	RM ($n = 85$)	*p*-value
APACHE II score, median (IQR)	10.0 (8.0–15.0)	12.0 (8.0–17.8)	0.285
SOFA score, median (IQR)	3.0 (2.0–5.0)	4.0 (2.0–9.0)	0.021
GCS score, median (IQR)	12.0 (7.0–14.0)	10.0 (7.0–13.0)	0.429
Age (years), median (IQR)	20.0 (19.0–26.5)	22.0 (19.0–27.0)	0.472
Lymphocyte (1×10^9/L), median (IQR)	1.3 (0.7–2.3)	0.9 (0.5–1.7)	0.044
Platelets (1×10^9/L), median (IQR)	186.0 (139.0–230.5)	106.0 (59.0–177.5)	<0.001
TBIL (μmol/L), median (IQR)	12.2 (8.6–21.5)	19.9 (13.3–37.6)	<0.001
ALT (U/L), median (IQR)	22.0 (15.0–41.5)	91.0 (33.0–868.0)	<0.001
AST (U/L), median (IQR)	36.0 (26.0–62.0)	173.0 (88.0–837.0)	<0.001
BUN (mmol/L), median (IQR)	5.5 (4.4–6.6)	6.2 (4.9–8.1)	0.022
Scr (μmol/L), median (IQR)	127.0 (94.0–150.5)	131.0 (93.0–186.0)	0.164
Cystatin C (mg/L), median (IQR)	1.0 (0.8–1.2)	1.0 (0.8–1.2)	0.838
CK (U/L), median (IQR)	372.0 (212.0–636.0)	2,918.0 (1,536.0–5,568.0)	<0.001
CK-MB (ng/ml), median (IQR)	26.0 (19.5–34.5)	72.0 (45.0–128.5)	<0.001
MB (ng/ml), median (IQR)	239.1 (73.3–646.5)	954.0 (317.8–1000.0)	<0.001
cTNI (pg/ml), median (IQR)	90.0 (26.4–281.1)	200.0 (30.0–699.9)	0.481
PT (s), median (IQR)	14.7 (13.7–16.4)	18.1 (15.8–26.2)	<0.001
INR, median (IQR)	1.2 (1.0–1.3)	1.5 (1.2–2.1)	0.003
APTT (s), median (IQR)	35.0 (31.6–40.9)	43.3 (37.4–76.5)	0.001
TT (s), median (IQR)	17.3 (16.3–18.5)	18.1 (16.8–29.8)	0.003
FIB (g/L), median (IQR)	2.5 (2.1–3.0)	2.4 (1.9–2.8)	0.111
D-Dimer (mg/L), median (IQR)	0.9 (0.4–3.7)	3.7 (0.9–10.1)	<0.001
CRP (mg/dl), median (IQR)	2.0 (0.4–3.7)	3.4 (3.2–7.2)	<0.001
PCT (ng/ml), median (IQR)	1.2 (0.6–2.4)	3.1 (1.4–5.3)	0.008
Transfusion, *N* (%)	14/90 (15.6%)	34/80 (42.5%)	<0.001
Lymphocytopenia, *N* (%)	30/91 (33.0%)	37/83 (44.6%)	0.116
DIC, *N* (%)	13/71 (18.3%)	34/64 (53.1%)	<0.001
AKI, *N* (%)	36/91 (39.6%)	41/84 (48.8%)	0.218
ALI, *N* (%)	5/91 (5.5%)	18/84 (21.4%)	0.002
90-day mortality, *N* (%)	8/91 (8.8%)	14/85 (16.5%)	0.124
ICU time (days), median (IQR)	4.0 (3.0–8.5)	6.0 (4.0–10.0)	0.024
Survival time (days), median (IQR)	90.0 (90.0–90.0)	90.0 (90.0–90.0)	0.118
Hospitalization costs (RMB), median (IQR)	31,810.5 (20,639.3–56,200.3)	51,986.3 (33,642.8–132,146.6)	0.036

AKI, acute kidney injury; ALI, acute liver injury; APTT, activated partial thromboplastin time; APACHE II, Acute Physiology and Chronic Health Evaluation II; BUN, blood urea nitrogen; CK, creatine kinase; CK-MB, MB isoenzyme of creatine kinase; CRP, C-reactive protein; cTNI, cardiac troponin I; DIC, disseminated intravascular coagulation; FIB, fibrinogen; ICU, intensive care unit; INR, international normalized ratio; IQR, interquartile range; PCT, procalcitonin; PT, prothrombin time; Scr, serum creatinine; SOFA, Sequential Organ Failure Assessment; TT, thrombin time.

II score [23.0 (21.0–23.5) vs. 11.0 (8.0–14.5), $p < 0.001$] and SOFA score at admission [12.0 (10.5–14.5) vs. 3.0 (2.0–6.0), $p < 0.001$], and lower GCS scores [6.0 (4.5–7.5) vs. 12.0 (8.0–13.5), $p = 0.005$]. In the non-survivor group, the organ function was worse than that in the survivor group, illustrated by the significantly increased total bilirubin, ALT, AST, Scr, Cystatin C, cTNI, and MB values (all $p < 0.05$), the worse blood coagulation (PT, INR, APTT, and D-dimer, all $p < 0.001$), and higher blood transfusion proportion (90 vs. 35.7%, $p < 0.001$). Furthermore, the non-survivors were easily complicated with DIC (100 vs. 42.3%, $p < 0.001$), AKI (100 vs. 38.6%, $p < 0.001$) and ALI (42.9 vs. 17.1%, $p = 0.032$) but there were no significant differences in the incidence of lymphocytopenia (61.5 vs. 41.4%, $p = 0.180$), inflammation index (PCT/CRP) ($p > 0.05$), and the length of ICU time [5.5 vs. 6.0 (days), $p = 0.381$] between survivors and non-survivors group. However, the total hospitalization costs in the non-survivor group were increased [156,820.3 vs. 45,182.6 (RMB), $p < 0.001$] (**Table 2**).

The Relationship Between RM and Another Organ Injury in EHS

It was found by the Pearson correlation that RM was positively correlated with ALI and DIC, with the correlation coefficients of 0.236 and 0.365, respectively (both $p < 0.01$). However, it was not associated with AKI ($p = 0.220$) and lymphocytopenia ($p = 0.117$) when CK > 1,000 U/L was used as the serological diagnostic standard of RM (**Table 3**).

TABLE 2 | Comparisons of clinical characteristics between survivors and non-survivors with RM induced by EHS.

Variables	Survivor(n = 71)	Non-survivor(n = 14)	p-value
APACHE II score, median (IQR)	11.0 (8.0–14.5)	23.0 (21.0–23.5)	<0.001
SOFA score, median (IQR)	3.0 (2.0–6.0)	12.0 (10.5–14.5)	<0.001
GCS score, median (IQR)	12.0 (8.0–13.5)	6.0 (4.5–7.5)	0.005
Age (years), median (IQR)	22.0 (19.0–27.5)	21.5 (20.2–23.0)	0.311
Lymphocyte (1 × 10^9/L), median (IQR)	1.0 (0.5–1.7)	0.5 (0.3–2.1)	0.368
Platelets (1 × 10^9/L), median (IQR)	127.0 (72.8–186.2)	65.0 (29.0–84.0)	0.004
TBIL (μmol/L), median (IQR)	17.6 (12.9–33.5)	37.4 (21.2–103.6)	<0.001
ALT (U/L), median (IQR)	64.0 (31.0–648.2)	546.5 (95.0–1,648.2)	0.028
AST (U/L), median (IQR)	133.0 (77.5–708.0)	408.5 (306.5–1,849.2)	0.020
BUN (mmol/L), median (IQR)	5.8 (4.5–7.7)	7.9 (6.2–9.0)	0.597
Scr (μmol/L), median (IQR)	114.0 (88.5–149.0)	245.5 (210.0–283.0)	<0.001
Cystatin C (mg/L), median (IQR)	1.0 (0.8–1.2)	1.5 (1.1–2.8)	<0.001
CK (U/L), median (IQR)	2,486.0 (1,462.5–4,927.0)	6,196.0 (2,231.8–8,251.5)	0.583
CK–MB (ng/ml), median (IQR)	71.0 (44.0–105.0)	298.0 (98.0–374.0)	0.332
MB (ng/ml), median (IQR)	658.0 (228.0–1,000.0)	1,000.0 (1,000.0–1,000.0)	0.019
cTNI (pg/ml), median (IQR)	110.0 (20.0–343.1)	1,530.0 (1,019.0–3,860.0)	<0.001
PT (s), median (IQR)	17.1 (15.4–21.9)	38.6 (24.8–45.3)	<0.001
INR, median (IQR)	1.4 (1.2–1.9)	4.2 (2.8–5.0)	<0.001
APTT (s), median (IQR)	41.2 (36.4–49.8)	93.8 (68.5–123.8)	<0.001
TT (s), median (IQR)	17.7 (16.6–22.2)	40.7 (28.9–58.7)	<0.001
FIB (g/L), median (IQR)	2.5 (2.1–2.8)	1.3 (0.9–1.8)	0.002
D–Dimer (mg/L), median (IQR)	2.9 (0.7–6.6)	10.1 (10.0–20.0)	<0.001
CRP (mg/dl), median (IQR)	3.6 (3.2–7.7)	3.3 (3.3–3.3)	0.454
PCT (ng/ml), median (IQR)	3.0 (1.3–4.8)	4.6 (1.7–8.1)	0.433
Transfusion, N (%)	25/70 (35.7%)	9/10 (90%)	<0.001
Lymphocytopenia, N (%)	29/70 (41.4%)	8/13 (61.5%)	0.180
DIC, N (%)	22/52 (42.3%)	12/12 (100.0%)	<0.001
AKI, N (%)	27/70 (38.6%)	14/14(100.0%)	<0.001
ALI, N (%)	12/70 (17.1%)	6/14 (42.9%)	0.032
ICU time (days), median (IQR)	6.0 (4.0–10.8)	5.5 (5.0–8.8)	0.381
Survival time (days), median (IQR)	90.0 (90.0–90.0)	5.5 (5.0–8.8)	<0.001
Hospitalization costs (RMB), median (IQR)	45,182.6 (29,738.0–93,106.3)	156,820.3 (133,525.5–214,730.5)	<0.001

AKI, acute kidney injury; ALI, acute liver injury; APTT, activated partial thromboplastin time; APACHE II, Acute Physiology and Chronic Health Evaluation II; BUN, blood urea nitrogen; CK, creatine kinase; CK-MB, MB isoenzyme of creatine kinase; CRP, C-reactive protein; cTNI, cardiac troponin I; DIC, disseminated intravascular coagulation; FIB, fibrinogen; ICU, intensive care unit; INR, international normalized ratio; IQR, interquartile range; PCT, procalcitonin; PT, prothrombin time; Scr, serum creatinine; SOFA, Sequential Organ Failure Assessment; TT, thrombin time.

Risk Factors of 90-Day Mortality for EHS Complicated With RM

The univariate analysis showed that APACHE II, SOFA, GCS, Cystatin C, MB ≥ 1,000 ng/ml, INR, FIB, and D-dimer were closely related to the 90-day mortality of patients with RM (all $p < 0.001$). The multivariate logistic regression showed that the SOFA score [OR 1.7 (1.1, 2.6), $p = 0.024$] was an independent risk factor affecting 90-day mortality in patients with EHS complicated with RM (**Table 4**). The area under the ROC curve for prediction of mortality based on the SOFA score was 0.958 (95% CI 0.908–1.000, $p < 0.001$), the optimal cutoff was 7.5 points, with SEN 100% and SPE 83.7% (**Figure 2**). However, there was no significant difference in the 90-day mortality between patients with RM and non-RM ($p = 0.11$) (**Figure 3**).

DISCUSSION

In this study, we observed clinical characteristics and risk factors in critically ill patients with RM induced by EHS in southern China. When CK ≥ 1,000 U/L was used as the serological diagnostic standard of RM, the results showed that the SOFA score of patients with RM was higher than that of patients with non-RM, which were mainly involving ALI and DIC. While non-survivors with EHS complicated with RM had a higher incidence of DIC and AKI at admission. The SOFA score at admission was an independent risk factor for 90-day mortality in patients with RM following EHS.

There are many causes leading to RM. Patients with RM caused by EHS were often doing strenuous exercise under high temperature and humidity, which are different from crush

TABLE 3 | The relationship between RM and another organ injury in EHS.

Variables	RM		
	Correlation	95%CI	*p*-value
AKI	0.093	0.056, 0.238	0.220
ALI	0.236	0.090, 0.371	0.002
Lymphocytopenia	0.119	−0.030, 0.263	0.117
DIC	0.365	0.209, 0.503	<0.001

AKI, acute kidney injury; ALI, acute liver injury; DIC, disseminated intravascular coagulation.

TABLE 4 | Risk factors for 90-day mortality with RM induced by EHS.

Variables	Univariate OR (95%CI) *p*-value	Multivariate OR (95%CI) *p*-value
APACHE II score	1.5 (1.3, 1.9) < 0.001	1.3 (0.8, 1.9) 0.272
SOFA score	2.2 (1.5, 3.1) < 0.001	1.7 (1.1, 2.6) 0.024
GCS score	0.6 (0.4, 0.8) < 0.001	1.2 (0.7, 2.2) 0.497
DIC	18.4 (5.0, 67.2) < 0.001	9.1 (0.2, 489.7) 0.277
AKI	19.7 (4.4, 87.5) < 0.001	9.5 (0.1, 748.2) 0.312
Cystatin C	2.7 (1.6, 4.5) < 0.001	NA
MB ≥ 1,000 ng/ml	7.4 (2.7, 20.4) < 0.001	NA
INR	2.1 (1.4, 3.0) < 0.001	NA
FIB	0.2 (0.1, 0.5) < 0.001	NA
D-dimer	1.1 (1.0, 1.2) < 0.001	NA
ALI	1,486,691.7 (0.0, Inf) 0.992	NA

Adjust model adjust for: Age. AKI, acute kidney injury; ALI, acute liver injury; APACHE II, Acute Physiology and Chronic Health Evaluation II; DIC, disseminated intravascular coagulation; FIB, fibrinogen; GCS, Glasgow Coma Score; OR, odds ratio; SOFA, Sequential Organ Failure Assessment.

syndrome. Vascular endothelial cells are more severely damaged due to the high temperature, which leads to a higher incidence of DIC. On the other hand, heatstroke could induce ALI *via* IL-1β and HMGB1-induced pyroptosis (17). It may be related to the pathogenesis as followed. RM releases myoglobin that can be decomposed into myosin, which plays an important role in the coagulation cascades, including both coagulation factors and fibrinolysis (18). In addition, some nuclear proteins are released by muscle cell injuries, such as histone 3 (19, 20) and HMGB1 (21), which can activate platelets and then lead to the occurrence and development of DIC and ALI. Previous studies have found that the renal tubular injury in RM caused by crush syndrome is mainly caused by apoptosis (22), which shows that RM is prone to AKI. The mechanism of its occurrence may include the following two aspects or the result of a combination: the deficiency of effective circulating blood volume caused by fluid loss and dehydration (23), and the mechanical obstruction of renal tubules caused by MB released RM (24). It has even been reported that myoglobin oxidative stress directly leads to renal tubular epithelial injury, but the specific mechanism of this injury is not completely clear yet (25). Furthermore, our study also showed that non-survived patients with RM were more likely complicated with AKI and DIC ($p < 0.001$). The reasons may be caused by the direct damage to vascular endothelial cells due to heat shock (26) and significantly reduced renal perfusion due to DIC, which are different from crush syndrome. Therefore, it is necessary to further explore the mechanism of RM on renal tubules under heatstroke.

Due to the imbalance between production and dissipation of heat, the occurrence of EHS is high when doing strenuous exercise under high temperature conditions. It often damages from CNS, striated muscle, kidney, and the coagulation system. The mechanism may be related to vascular endothelial cell damage, and the activation of inflammatory cells and platelets (21). A single-center retrospective study of 140 critical patients with severe heatstroke found that RM at admission was an independent risk factor for mortality (27). However, there was no further study on the effects of RM and other key organ functions and mortality. Therefore, we analyzed the effect of RM on the indicators of key organ functions and 90-day mortality by using RM as an exposure factor. The results showed that patients with EHS complicated with RM had more severe organ injuries. RM was positively correlated with ALI and DIC (all $p < 0.01$) whereas not associated with AKI ($p = 0.220$) and lymphocytopenia ($p = 0.117$), but there was no difference in 90-day mortality ($p = 0.11$) between patients with RM and non-RM. We speculated that the underlying reason is the inaccuracy of CK ≥ 1,000 U/L as the serological diagnostic criteria for RM in evaluating RM and organ function. In addition, there were other factors leading to AKI, such as glomerular perfusion pressure decreased because of the lower cardiac output, renal tubular apoptosis, renal interstitial edema, inflammatory exudation, and so on (25, 28). Multicenter prospective studies are needed to confirm CK thresholds at different organ injuries.

Multivariate logistic regression showed that only the SOFA score was an independent risk factor for 90-day mortality in patients with EHS complicated with RM, but not the APACHE II score. The APACHE II score is an important scoring system for evaluating the prognosis of critically ill patients, which involves age and chronic health. However, our patients were previously healthy and had a median age of 21 years. In addition, because the APACHE II score excluded some vital acute organ functions including coagulation function and liver function, it is not as comprehensive as that of the SOFA score. Therefore, the APACHE II score is not appropriate to evaluate prognosis in young patients with EHS. The optimal cutoff for the prediction of 90-day mortality based on the SOFA score was 7.5 points, with SEN 100% and SPE 83.7%. Moreover, SOFA scores in survivors and non-survivors with RM induced by EHS were 3.0 and 12.0, respectively. This indicates that the SOFA score can accurately predict the 90-day mortality of patients with RM induced by EHS. Survival curves showed there was no significant difference in the 90-day mortality between patients with RM (CK ≥ 1,000 U/L) and non-RM. Because the serologic diagnostic standard of RM with CK ≥ 1,000 U/L is too lenient, it does not reflect the true organ function status and predict the prognosis of patients. Multicenter prospective studies are needed to confirm CK thresholds for 90-day mortality in different disease states.

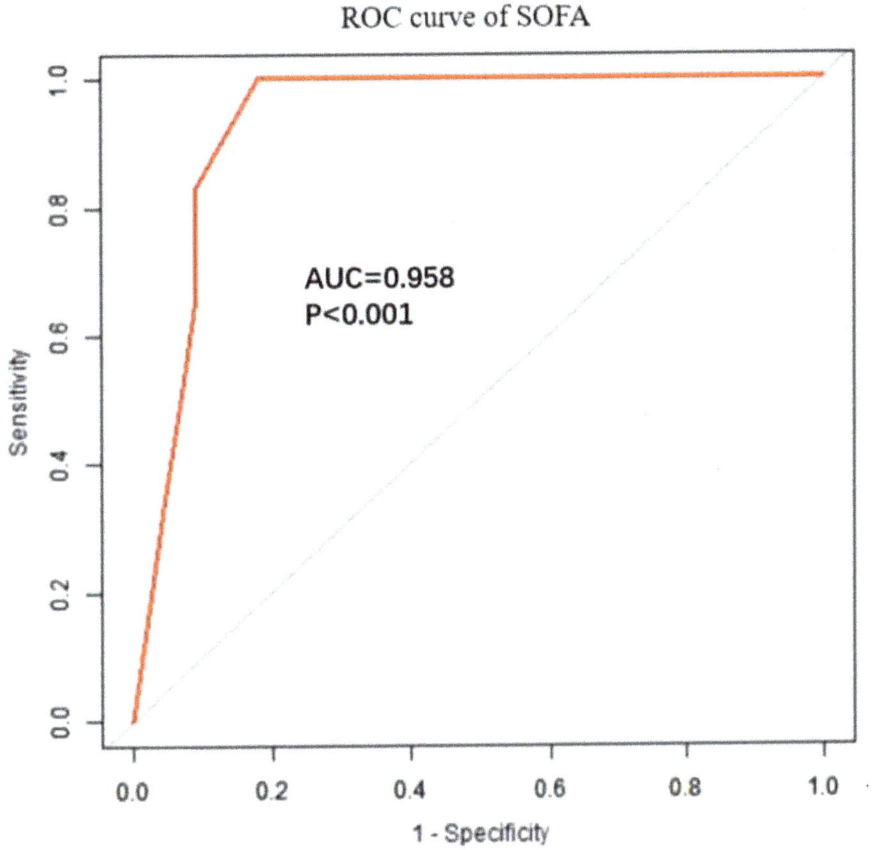

FIGURE 2 | The ROC curve of SOFA in predicting 90-day mortality with patients with RM induced by EHS. EHS, exertional heat stroke; RM, rhabdomyolysis; ROC, receiver operating characteristic; SOFA, Sequential Organ Failure Assessment.

There are many measures that can be used to treat RM in ICU, including removal of MB by blood purification (29), antioxidation (30), anti-inflammation (31), and so on. Only the SOFA score was an independent risk factor for mortality, suggesting that the follow-up treatment with the primary aim of protecting key organ function is an important way to reduce mortality.

This study has some limitations. It was a single-center retrospective cohort study with a comparatively small number of cases. In addition, this study excluded 32 patients, which may cause selective bias in the results. Because all the patients were male and the average age was relatively young, though the type of heatstroke was restricted to EHS, the results do not fully reflect the overall conditions of the heatstroke population. Expanding the sample size and employing a prospective cohort study should be designed to achieve higher-level clinical results in the subsequent studies.

CONCLUSIONS

Patients with RM after EHS have severe clinical conditions, which are often accompanied by DIC or ALI. The SOFA score was an important independent risk factor for 90-day mortality in patients with EHS complicated with RM. Early treatment strategies based on decreasing the SOFA score at admission may be pivotal to reduce the 90-day mortality rate of patients with EHS.

ETHICS STATEMENT

The studies involving human participants were reviewed and approved by the Research Ethics Committee of the General Hospital of Southern Theatre Command of Peoples Liberation Army (HE-2020-09). Written informed consent for participation was not required for this study in accordance with the national legislation and the institutional requirements.

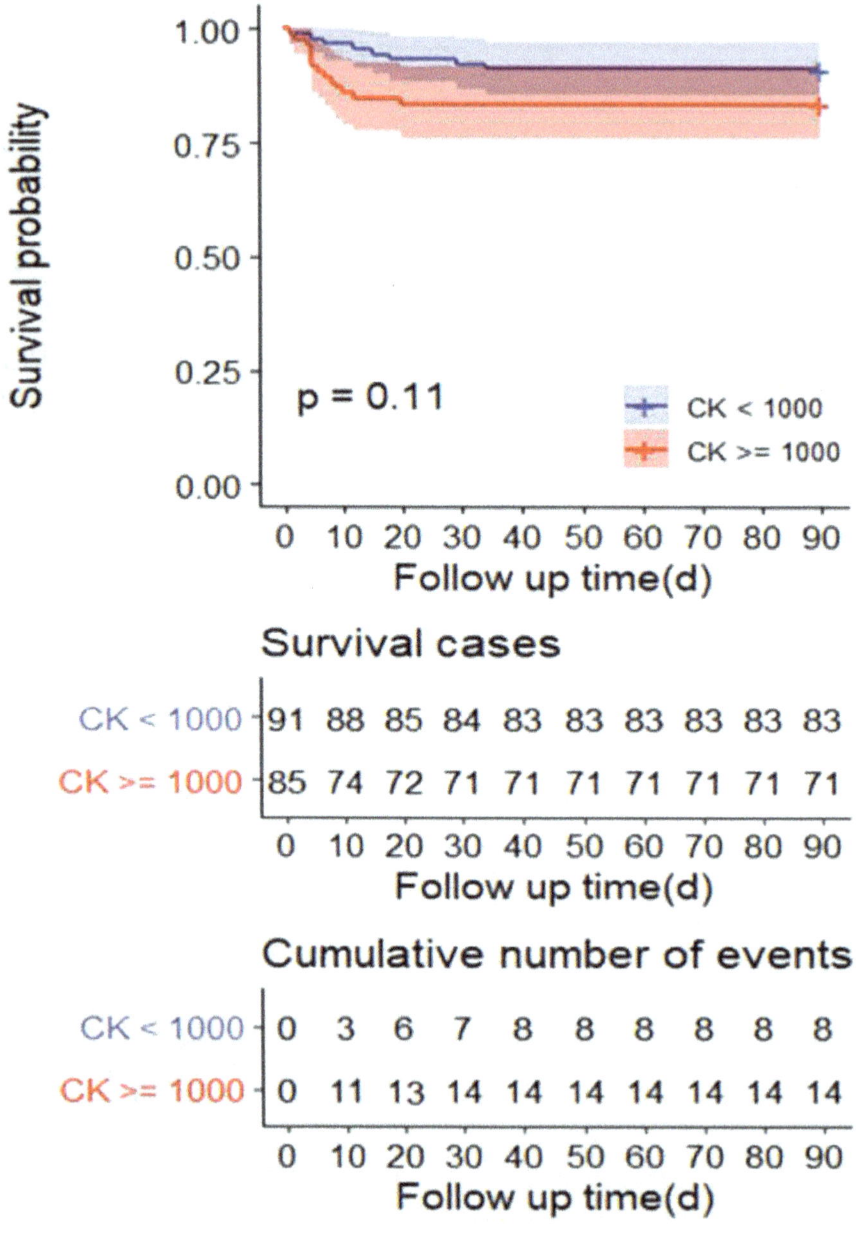

FIGURE 3 | Survival curves of 90-day mortality rate in the R) group (CK ≥ 1,000 U/L) and non-RM group (CK < 1,000 U/L). CK, creatine kinase; RM, rhabdomyolysis.

AUTHOR CONTRIBUTIONS

ZFL and MW contributed to the study concept and design. MW, CW, and ZYL collected the data. MW and CW performed the statistical analysis. ZFL, MW, and CW drafted the manuscript. All the authors had full access to all the data in the study and take responsibility for the integrity of the data and the accuracy of the data analysis.

FUNDING

This study was supported by grants from the National Natural Science Foundation of China (No. 82072143), Natural Science Foundation of Guangdong Province of China (No. 2021A1515010170), the Peoples Liberation Army Logistics Research Project of China (18CXZ030 and BLJ20J006), Sanming Project of Medicine in Shenzhen (SZSM20162011), Shenzhen Science and Technology Innovation Commission (JCYJ20170306091335008 and JCYJ20190806163603504), and Clinical Research Project of Shenzhen Municipal Health Commission (SZLY2017007).

REFERENCES

1. Epstein Y, Yanovich R. Heatstroke. *N Engl J Med.* (2019) 380:2449–59. doi: 10.1056/NEJMra1810762
2. Moreno JA, Martín-Cleary C, Gutiérrez E, Toldos O, Blanco-Colio LM, Praga M, et al. AKI associated with macroscopic glomerular hematuria: clinical and pathophysiologic consequences. *Clin J Am Soc Nephrol.* (2012) 7:175–84. doi: 10.2215/CJN.01970211
3. Jang HR, Rabb H. The innate immune response in ischemic acute kidney injury. *Clin Immunol.* (2009) 130:41–50. doi: 10.1016/j.clim.2008.08.016
4. Gonzalez-Michaca L, Farrugia G, Croatt AJ, Alam J, Nath KA. Heme: a determinant of life and death in renal tubular epithelial cells. *Am J Physiol Renal Physiol.* (2004) 286:F370–7. doi: 10.1152/ajprenal.00300.2003
5. Moreno JA, Martín-Cleary C, Gutiérrez E, Rubio-Navarro A, Ortiz A, Praga M, et al. Haematuria: the forgotten CKD factor? *Nephrol Dial Transplant.* (2012) 27:28–34. doi: 10.1093/ndt/gfr749
6. Wagener FA, Feldman E, de Witte T, Abraham NG. Heme induces the expression of adhesion molecules ICAM-1, VCAM-1, and E selectin in vascular endothelial cells. *Proc Soc Exp Biol Med.* (1997) 216:456–63. doi: 10.3181/00379727-216-44197
7. Guis S, Mattei JP, Cozzone PJ, Bendahan D. Pathophysiology and clinical presentations of rhabdomyolysis. *Joint Bone Spine.* (2005) 72:382–91. doi: 10.1016/j.jbspin.2004.04.010
8. Komada T, Usui F, Kawashima A, Kimura H, Karasawa T, Inoue Y, et al. Role of NLRP3 inflammasomes for rhabdomyolysis-induced acute kidney injury. *Sci Rep.* (2015) 5:10901. doi: 10.1038/srep10901
9. Wu M, Su L. Current research situation of ferroptosis in rhabdomyolysis-induced acute kidney injury. *Chin J Crit Care Intensive Care Med.* (2017) 3:231–7. doi: 10.3877/j.issn.2096-1537.2017.03.015
10. Zhong L, Wu M, Liu Z, Liu Y, Ren G, Su L, et al. Risk factors for the 90-day prognosis of severe heat stroke: a case-control study. *Shock.* (2021) 55:61–6. doi: 10.1097/SHK.0000000000001589
11. Wu M, Wang C, Liu Z, Zhong L, Yu B, Cheng B, et al. Clinical characteristics and risk factors associated with acute kidney injury inpatient with exertional heatstroke: an over 10-year intensive care survey. *Front Med.* (2021) 8:678434. doi: 10.3389/fmed.2021.678434
12. Cervellin G, Comelli I, Lippi G. Rhabdomyolysis: historical background, clinical, diagnostic and therapeutic features. *Clin Chem Lab Med.* (2010) 48:749–56. doi: 10.1515/CCLM.2010.151
13. Taylor FJ, Toh CH, Hoots WK, Wada H, Levi M. Towards definition, clinical and laboratory criteria, and a scoring system for disseminated intravascular coagulation. *Thromb Haemost.* (2001) 86:1327–30. doi: 10.1055/s-0037-1616068
14. Stevens PE, Levin A. Evaluation and management of chronic kidney disease: synopsis of the kidney disease: improving global outcomes 2012 clinical practice guideline. *Ann Intern Med.* (2013) 158:825–30. doi: 10.7326/0003-4819-158-11-201306040-00007
15. Ji J, Gao J, Wang C, Ouyang L, Liu Z, Liu Z. Characteristics and outcome of exertional heatstroke patients complicated by acute hepatic injury: a cohort study. *J Clin Transl Hepatol.* (2021). doi: 10.14218/JCTH.2021.00084. [Epub ahead of print].
16. Mira JC, Gentile LF, Mathias BJ, Efron PA, Brakenridge SC, Mohr AM, et al. Sepsis pathophysiology, chronic critical illness, and persistent inflammation-immunosuppression and catabolism syndrome. *Crit Care Med.* (2017) 45:253–62. doi: 10.1097/CCM.0000000000002074
17. Geng Y, Ma Q, Liu YN, Peng N, Yuan FF Li XG, et al. Heatstroke induces liver injury via IL-1β and HMGB1-induced pyroptosis. *J Hepatol.* (2015) 63:622–33. doi: 10.1016/j.jhep.2015.04.010
18. Deguchi H, Morla S, Griffin JH. Novel blood coagulation molecules: skeletal muscle myosin and cardiac myosin. *J Thromb Haemost.* (2021) 19:7–19. doi: 10.1111/jth.15097
19. Bruchim Y, Ginsburg I, Segev G, Mreisat A, Avital Y, Aroch I, et al. Serum histones as biomarkers of the severity of heatstroke in dogs. *Cell Stress Chaperones.* (2017) 22:903–10. doi: 10.1007/s12192-017-0817-6
20. Ito T, Totoki T, Yokoyama Y, Yasuda T, Furubeppu H, Yamada S, et al. Serum histone H3 levels and platelet counts are potential markers for coagulopathy with high risk of death in septic patients: a single-center observational study. *J Intensive Care.* (2019) 7:63. doi: 10.1186/s40560-019-0420-2
21. Leon LR, Bouchama A. Heat stroke. *Compr Physiol.* (2015) 5:611–47. doi: 10.1002/cphy.c140017
22. Li O, Geng X, Ma Q, Wang W, Liu R, Yin Z, et al. Gene microarray integrated with high-throughput proteomics for the discovery of transthyretin in rhabdomyolysis-induced acute kidney injury. *Cell Physiol Biochem.* (2017) 43:1673–88. doi: 10.1159/000484028
23. Nose H, Kamijo YI, Masuki S. Interactions between body fluid homeostasis and thermoregulation in humans. *Handb Clin Neurol.* (2018) 156:417–29. doi: 10.1016/B978-0-444-63912-7.00025-4
24. Holt S, Moore K. Pathogenesis of renal failure in rhabdomyolysis: the role of myoglobin. *Exp Nephrol.* (2000) 8:72–6. doi: 10.1159/000020651
25. Plotnikov EY, Chupyrkina AA, Pevzner IB, Isaev NK, Zorov DB. Myoglobin causes oxidative stress, increase of NO production and dysfunction of kidney's mitochondria. *Biochim Biophys Acta.* (2009) 1792:796–803. doi: 10.1016/j.bbadis.2009.06.005
26. Pei Y, Geng Y, Su L. Pyroptosis of HUVECs can be induced by heat stroke. *Biochem Biophys Res Commun.* (2018) 506:626–31. doi: 10.1016/j.bbrc.2018.10.051
27. Zhiguo P. *Study on incidence and mechanisms of sever heatstroke and rhabdomyolysis.* Guangzhou University of Chinese Medicine (2012).
28. Panizo N, Rubio-Navarro A, Amaro-Villalobos JM, Egido J, Moreno JA. Molecular mechanisms and novel therapeutic approaches to rhabdomyolysis-induced acute kidney injury. *Kidney Blood Press Res.* (2015) 40:520–32. doi: 10.1159/000368528
29. Scharf C, Liebchen U, Paal M, Irlbeck M, Zoller M, Schroeder I. Blood purification with a cytokine adsorber for the elimination of myoglobin in critically ill patients with severe rhabdomyolysis. *Crit Care.* (2021) 25:41. doi: 10.1186/s13054-021-03468-x
30. Gois P, Canale D, Volpini RA, Ferreira D, Veras MM, Andrade-Oliveira V, et al. Allopurinol attenuates rhabdomyolysis-associated acute kidney injury: renal and muscular protection. *Free Radic Biol Med.* (2016) 101:176–89. doi: 10.1016/j.freeradbiomed.2016.10.012
31. Sun G, Wang J, Wang P, Ren H, Yue Y, Song Z, et al. Donepezil protects glycerol-induced acute renal failure through the cholinergic anti-inflammatory and nitric oxide pathway in rats. *Immunopharmacol Immunotoxicol.* (2020) 42:625–31. doi: 10.1080/08923973.2020.1835950

6

The Effect of Dexmedetomidine as a Sedative Agent for Mechanically Ventilated Patients with Sepsis

Caimu Wang, Qijiang Chen, Ping Wang, Weisheng Jin, Chao Zhong, Zisheng Ge and Kangmin Xu*

General Intensive Care Unit, Ninghai First Hospital, Ningbo, China

Correspondence:
Caimu Wang
caimuwang001@gmail.com

Purpose: Dexmedetomidine has been shown to improve clinical outcomes in critically ill patients. However, its effect on septic patients remains controversial. Therefore, the purpose of this meta-analysis was to assess the effect of dexmedetomidine as a sedative agent for mechanically ventilated patients with sepsis.

Methods: We searched PubMed, Embase, Scopus, and Cochrane Library from inception through May 2021 for randomized controlled trials that enrolled mechanically ventilated, adult septic patients comparing dexmedetomidine with other sedatives or placebo.

Results: A total of nine studies involving 1,134 patients were included in our meta-analysis. The overall mortality (RR 0.97, 95%CI 0.82 to 1.13, $P = 0.67$, $I^2 = 25\%$), length of intensive care unit stay (MD −1.12, 95%CI −2.89 to 0.64, $P = 0.21$, $I^2 = 71\%$), incidence of delirium (RR 0.95, 95%CI 0.72 to 1.25, $P = 0.70$, $I^2 = 0\%$), and delirium free days (MD 1.76, 95%CI −0.94 to 4.47, $P = 0.20$, $I^2 = 80\%$) were not significantly different between dexmedetomidine and other sedative agents. Alternatively, the use of dexmedetomidine was associated with a significant reduction in the duration of mechanical ventilation (MD −0.53, 95%CI −0.85 to −0.21, $P = 0.001$, $I^2 = 0\%$) and inflammatory response (TNF-α: MD −5.27, 95%CI −7.99 to −2.54, $P < 0.001$, $I^2 = 0\%$; IL-1β: MD −1.25, 95%CI −1.91 to −0.59, $P < 0.001$, $I^2 = 0\%$).

Conclusions: For patients with sepsis, the use of dexmedetomidine as compared with other sedative agents does not affect all-cause mortality, length of intensive care unit stay, the incidence of delirium, and delirium-free days. But the dexmedetomidine was associated with the reduced duration of mechanical ventilation and inflammatory response.

Keywords: sepsis, anesthesiology, meta-analysis, dexmedetomidine, mechanical ventilation, sedation

INTRODUCTION

Sepsis, defined as a life-threatening organ dysfunction due to a dysregulated immune response to infection, affects millions of patients per year and carries a high risk of mortality, becoming a major global health problem (1, 2). According to the Global Burden of Diseases Study, in 2017, an estimated 48.9 million incident cases of sepsis were reported worldwide with nearly 11.0 million patients dying, accounting for 19.7% of all global deaths (3).On the other hand, sepsis is often complicated with acute respiratory distress syndrome that requires mechanical ventilatory support (4, 5), research showed that more than 20% of septic patients needed invasive ventilation in the USA (6).

Sedation is an integral component of care for mechanically ventilated patients to reduce the anxiety and stress associated with tracheal intubation and other invasive interventions (7, 8). However, the appropriate choice of a preferred sedative agent for patients with sepsis remains controversial. For decades, γ-aminobutyric acid (GABA) receptor agonists (such as propofol and midazolam) were widely used as sedative drugs in the intensive care units (ICU) (9–11). Recently, dexmedetomidine, a highly selective α-2 adrenergic receptor agonist, is a unique alternative sedative compared with GABA receptor agonists considering its analgesic properties with wider safety margin due to the lack of suppressive effects on respiration (12). Using dexmedetomidine to induce sedation while preserving a degree of arousability for critically ill patients. Limited but increasing evidence suggests that dexmedetomidine has a promising future as a sedative agent in the ICU, its use resulted in a shorter duration of mechanical ventilation (MV) or ICU length of stay (13–17), a reduced incidence of coma or delirium (15, 17–19).

Recently, Hughes and coworkers conducted the MENDS II trial concerning the effect of dexmedetomidine vs. propofol on the short-term and long-term outcomes of mechanically ventilated adults with sepsis. In this pragmatic randomized controlled trial (RCT) involving more than 400 patients, there was no significant difference in the delirium or ventilator-free days, ICU length of stay, and 90-day mortality between the patients receiving dexmedetomidine or propofol. Therefore, the effects of dexmedetomidine in septic patients receiving MV remains controversial. We aimed to assess the effects of dexmedetomidine on clinical outcomes in mechanically ventilated patients with sepsis.

METHODS

Our study was conducted following the Preferred Reporting Items for Systematic Reviews and Meta-Analyses (PRISMA) statement (20) (**Supplementary Material 1**). The study protocol was registered in PROSPERO (CRD42019145061). A literature search was performed in PubMed, Embase, Scopus, and Cochrane Library for eligible RCTs in English from inception through May 2021. The search used broad search terms containing "sepsis," "ventilation," "dexmedetomidine," and "randomized." In addition, full details on our search terms and strategy detailed were recorded in **Supplementary Material 2**.

Eligibility Criteria

Study inclusion criteria were as follows: (1). Population: adult ($\geq$18 years old) patients with sepsis receiving mechanical ventilation and intravenous sedation; (2). Intervention: the use of IV dexmedetomidine regardless of dose, start time, and duration; (3). Comparison: the use of other IV sedative drugs or placebo regardless of dose, start time, and duration; (4). Outcomes: the primary outcome was overall mortality (including ICU, hospital, 28/30-day mortality). The secondary outcomes were duration of mechanical ventilation, ICU length of stay, and inflammatory responses (serum levels of inflammatory markers after 24 h). (5). Design: RCT.

The following studies would be excluded: (1). If the study evaluated obstetrical patients because sedation practices and mechanical ventilation strategies are different in the patient population (21); (2). Patients did not receive IV sedatives or mechanical ventilation; (3). Studies published only in abstract form.

Data Extraction and Quality Assessment

Two authors independently retrieved relevant studies and extracted data from included studies. The characteristics of studies (first author, years of publication, study design, population, sedation goal, intervention, and control sedative agents, outcomes) were recorded in **Table 1**. Further information (study design, number of participants, sex ratio, mean age, inclusion, and exclusion criteria) was recorded in **Supplementary Material 3.**

Two authors independently assessed the methodological quality of the included studies by using the Cochrane risk of bias tool (22).

Statistical Synthesis and Analysis

We combined the data from the included studies to estimate the pooled relative ratio (RR) with a 95% CI for the primary outcome, and the secondary outcomes were pooled as mean difference (MD) with 95%CI.

The heterogeneity between studies was tested by the Chi-squared test with significance set at a *P*-value of 0.1, and quantitatively by inconsistency (I^2) statistics (23). Substantial heterogeneity was identified when $I^2 > 30\%$ and we employed a random-effects model to perform the analysis, otherwise, a fixed-effects model would be used. In addition, we used the funnel plot and Egger's regression test to assess the publication bias (24).

A predefined subgroup analysis was stratified by population (sepsis or septic shock) and control drug (propofol or others) to investigate the potential source of heterogeneity. Furthermore, we performed a sensitivity analysis to explore the effect of individual studies by omitting each one at a time.

RESULTS

Study Identification and Characteristics

A total of nine studies (25–33) involving 1,134 patients were included (search process in **Figure 1**). Among the nine included studies, two studies were subgroup analyses of patients with

TABLE 1 | Characteristics of the included studies.

First author, year	Design	Patients	Interventions	Sedation goals	Outcomes
Hughes et al. (33)	Multicenter, double-blind	422 patients with sepsis	Intervention group: DEX for 0.15 to 1.5 μg/kg·h; Control group: propofol for 5 to 50 μg/kg·h	RASS score of −2 to 0	30-day mortality, 90-day mortality, delirium free days
Cioccari et al. (31)	Multicenter, open-label	83 patients with septic shock	Intervention group: DEX start at 1 μg/kg·h, followed at adjusted dose (maximunm at 1.5 μg/kg·h); Control group: propofol directed by the treating physician	RASS score of −2 to +1	ICU mortality, in-hospital mortality, 90-day mortality, duration of mechanical ventilation, ICU length of stay, incidence of delirium
Liu et al. (32)	Single-center, open-label	200 patients with septic shock	Intervention group: DEX start at a loading dose of 1 μg/kg·h, followed at 0.2 to 0.3 μg/kg·h; Control group: propofol start at a loading dose of 1 mg/kg, followed at 1 to 3 mg/kg·h	RASS score of −2 to 0	28-day mortality, duration of mechanical ventilation, ICU length of stay
Kawazoe et al. (30)	Multicenter, open-label	201 patients with sepsis	Intervention group: DEX start at start at 0.1 μg/kg·h then at 0.1–0.7 μg/kg·h; Control group: propofol at 0–3 mg/kg/h or midazolam at 0–0.15 mg/kg/h	RASS score of −2 to 0	28-day mortality, duration of mechanical ventilation, ICU length of stay, incidence of delirium
Guo et al. (29)	Single-center, open-label	45 patients with septic shock	Intervention group: DEX for 0.2 to 0.7 μg/kg·h; Control group 1: propofol; Control group 2: midazolam;	RASS score of −2 to −1	In-hospital mortality, duration of mechanical ventilation, ICU length of stay
Pandharipande et al. (28)	Multicenter, double-blind	63 patients with sepsis	Intervention group: DEX at a median rate of 0.74 μg/kg·h, max does at 1.5 μg/kg·h; Control group: lorazepam at a median rate of 3 mg/h, max does at 10 mg/h	RASS score of −2 to +1	28-day mortality, ICU length of stay, delirium free days
Tasdogan et al. (27)	Single-center, open-label	40 patients with sepsis	Intervention group: DEX at a loading does of 1 μg/kg for 10 min, followed by 0.2–2.5 μg/kg·h; Control group: propofpl at a loading does of 1 mg/kg·h for 15 min, followed by 1–3 mg/kg·h	RSS≤2	28-day mortality, duration of mechanical ventilation, ICU length of stay, levels of TNF-α and IL-1β
Memis et al. (27)	Single-center, open-label	40 patients with septic shock	Intervention group: DEX at a loading does of 1 μg/kg for 10min, followed by 0.2–2.5 μg/kg·h; Control group: propofpl at a loading does of 1 mg/kg·h for 15 min, followed by 1–3 mg/kg·h	RSS≤2	ICU mortality, ICU length of stay
Memis et al. (27)	Single-center, open-label	40 patients with sepsis	Intervention group: DEX at a loading does of 1 μg/kg for 10 min, followed by 0.2–2.5 μg/kg·h; Control group: midazolam at a loading does of 0.2 mg/kg·h for 10 min, followed by 0.1–0.5 mg/kg·h	RSS < 2	ICU mortality, levels of TNF-α and IL-1β

DEX, dexmedetomidine; RASS, Richmond agitation sedation scale; RSS, Ramsay sedation score.

sepsis from previous RCTs [Cioccari et al. (31) performed a subgroup analysis of the SPICE III trial (34), Pandharipande et al. (28) performed a subgroup analysis of the MENDS trial (35)]. **Table 1** shows the characteristics of the included studies. Five trials used dexmedetomidine in patients with sepsis (25, 27, 28, 30, 33), and four in patients with septic shock (26, 29, 31, 32). Different control drugs were also identified: propofol in six arms (26, 27, 29, 31–33), midazolam in two arms (25, 29), lorazepam in

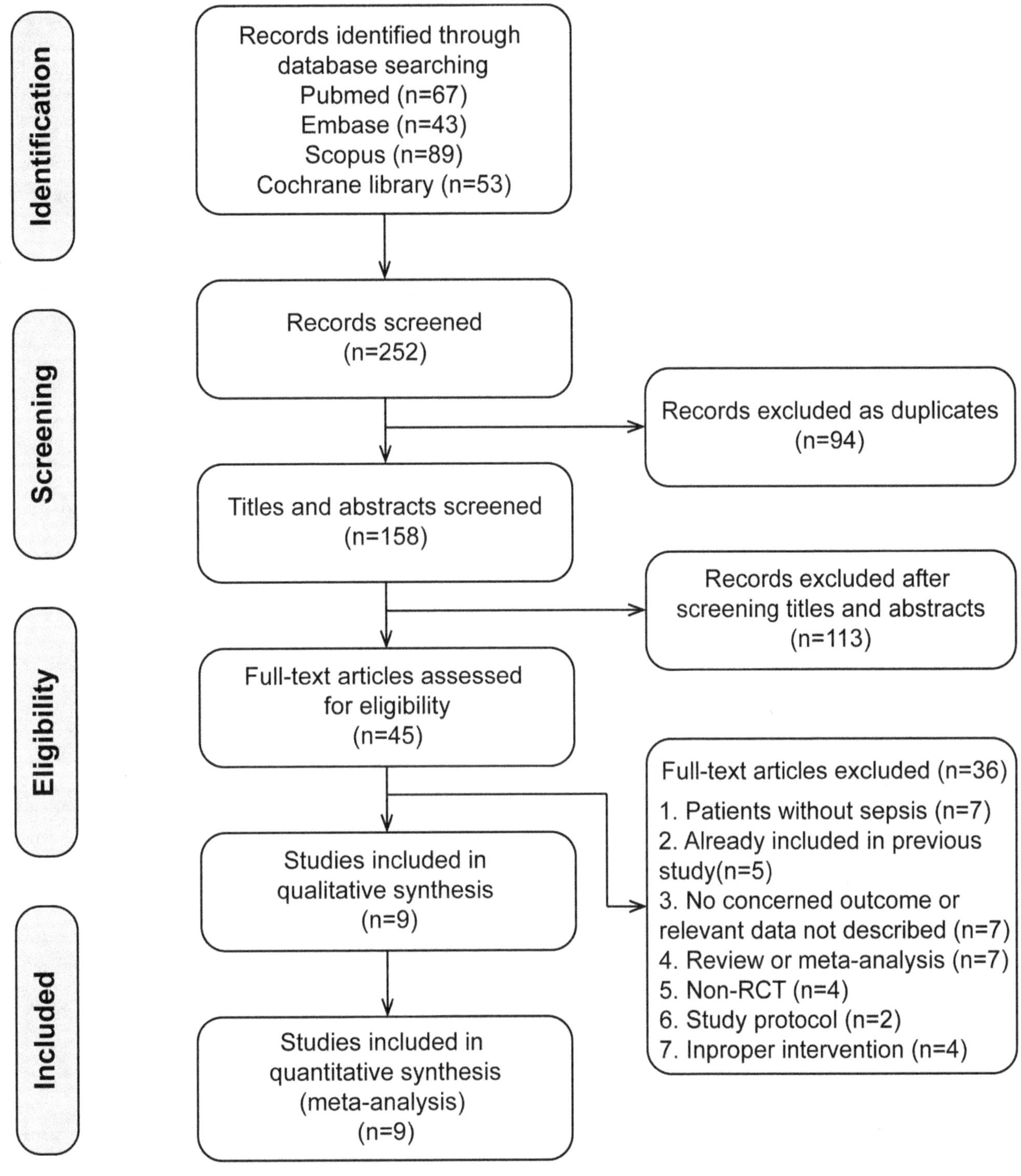

FIGURE 1 | Flow chart of database search and study selection.

one arm (28), and propofol plus midazolam in one arm (30). Five studies (25–27, 31, 32) used a loading dose of dexmedetomidine at 1 μg/kg·h, the other four studies (28–30, 33) used infusion dose of dexmedetomidine between 0.1 to 1.5 μg/kg·h. The target sedation goals were Richmond Agitation Sedation Scale of −2 to 0 in three trials (30, 32, 33), −2 to 1 in two trials (28, 31), −2 to −1 in one trial (29), and Ramsay Sedation Score <2 in three trials (25–27).

Other detailed information of included studies (e.g., study design, sex ratio, age, APACHE II and SOFA score at trial enrollment, definitions of sepsis or septic shock) were reported in **Supplementary Material 3**.

Quality Assessment

The quality assessment by the Cochrane risk of bias tool was summarized in **Figure 2**. Seven studies (25–27, 29–32) had a high risk of bias because they were open-label trials. Three studies (25, 29, 32) did not report the details of random sequence generation and allocation concealment. The blinding method for outcome assessment was not reported in five studies (25, 26, 29, 31, 32), which would either underestimate or overestimate the size of the effect. Moreover, in the trial by Guo et al. (29), the doses of control sedative drugs were not reported. The details for quality assessment and reason for judgment were recorded in **Supplementary Material 3**.

We used the funnel plot and Egger's test to assess the publication bias (**Supplementary Material 4**), the results showed there was a potential risk of publication bias for the overall mortality and length of ICU stay (Egger's test, $P < 0.01$). Thus, we performed an additional analysis by using the trim and fill method. The imputed studies produced a symmetrical funnel plot and the analysis after imputing continued to show no association between the use of dexmedetomidine and overall mortality (RR 1.05, 95%CI 0.91 to 1.22 $P = 0.67$, $I^2 = 32\%$), but a shortened length of ICU stay was observed (MD −2.42, 95%CI −4.15 to -0.68, $P < 0.01$, $I^2 = 75\%$).

Primary Outcome

All studies involving 1,134 patients reported mortality (two studies reported the ICU mortality, four studies reported the 28/30-day mortality, one study reported the in-hospital mortality, one study reported the 30-day and 90-day mortality, one study reported the ICU, in-hospital, and 90-day mortality). The risk for overall mortality was similar between dexmedetomidine and control regimens without significant heterogeneity (RR 0.97; 95%CI 0.82 to 1.13, $P = 0.67$, $I^2 = 25\%$; **Table 2**, **Figure 3**). Similarly, the use of dexmedetomidine had no significant effect on the ICU mortality, 28/30-day mortality, in-hospital mortality, and 90-day mortality (**Table 2**, **Supplementary Material 5**).

We performed predefined subgroup analyses stratified by population (sepsis or septic shock) and control drug (propofol or others). Compared with propofol, the use of dexmedetomidine does not affect the overall mortality (RR 1.01, 95%CI 0.86 to 1.20, $P = 0.87$, $I^2 = 4\%$; **Figure 4A**). However, a trend toward the reduction of all-cause mortality by dexmedetomidine when compared with other sedations (RR 052, 95%CI 0.25 to 1.06, $P = 0.07$, $I^2 = 0\%$; **Figure 4A**) was observed, although it was not statistically significant. The use of dexmedetomidine had no different effect on mortality for patients with sepsis or septic shock (**Figure 4B**). Moreover, the sensitivity analysis by removing each trial showed similar results to the overall analysis, indicating good robustness (**Supplementary Material 5**).

Secondary Outcomes

A total of seven studies with eight cohorts reported the length of ICU stay and there was no significant difference between patients who received dexmedetomidine and other sedative drugs (MD −1.12, 95%CI −2.89 to 0.64, $P = 0.21$, $I^2 = 71\%$; **Table 2**, **Figure 5A**). The overall analysis from five studies (six cohorts) showed that the use of dexmedetomidine was associated with a slight reduction in the duration of MV (MD −0.53, 95%CI −0.85 to −0.21, $P = 0.001$, $I^2 = 0\%$; **Table 2**, **Figure 5B**). However, since the significant heterogeneity, this result should be interpreted prudently.

In the subgroup analysis, compared with propofol, the use of dexmedetomidine was associated with the shortened duration of MV, but no significant difference in the length of ICU stay. Furthermore, the population (sepsis or septic shock) has no significant effect on the length of ICU stay. The positive effect of dexmedetomidine in reducing the duration of MV became not significant in the sepsis subgroup (**Table 2**, **Supplementary Material 5**). The sensitivity analysis by removing each trial showed no significant difference in the length of ICU stay, indicating good robustness. The positive effect of dexmedetomidine in reducing the duration of MV became not significant after omitting the study by Liu et al. (32) (**Supplementary Material 5**).

Two studies reported the serum levels of inflammatory markers including the tumor necrosis factor α (TNF-α) and interleukin 1β (IL-1β) after 24 h of treatment. In the group of patients receiving dexmedetomidine, the serum levels of TNF-α and IL-1β after 24 h of treatment were significantly lower than that in the control group (TNF-α: MD −5.27, 95%CI −7.99 to −2.54, $P < 0.001$, $I^2 = 0\%$; IL-1β: MD −1.25, 95%CI −1.91 to −0.59, $P < 0.001$, $I^2 = 0\%$; **Table 2**, **Figure 5C**).

In addition, four studies reported the incidence of delirium or the delirium-free days. The results indicated that the use of dexmedetomidine had no significant effect on the incidence of delirium (RR 0.95, 95%CI 0.72 to 1.25, $P = 0.70$, $I^2 = 0\%$; **Table 2**, **Figure 6A**) and delirium free days (MD 1.76, 95%CI −0.94 to 4.47, $P = 0.20$, $I^2 = 80\%$; **Table 2**, **Figure 6B**).

Furthermore, there were no differences in the use of vasopressor, the incidence of hypotensive, and mean arterial pressure during the study period between the dexmedetomidine and control groups (**Supplementary Material 6**).

DISCUSSION

In this meta-analysis, we systematically and comprehensively reviewed nine studies with 1,134 patients to evaluate the effect of dexmedetomidine for mechanically ventilated patients with sepsis. Overall, compared with other sedation, the use of dexmedetomidine does not affect the overall mortality, length of ICU stay, incidence of delirium, or the delirium-free days. We found that patients with sepsis receiving dexmedetomidine had a shortened duration of MV, limited evidence suggested that the use of dexmedetomidine was associated with a lower level of TNF-α and IL-1β.

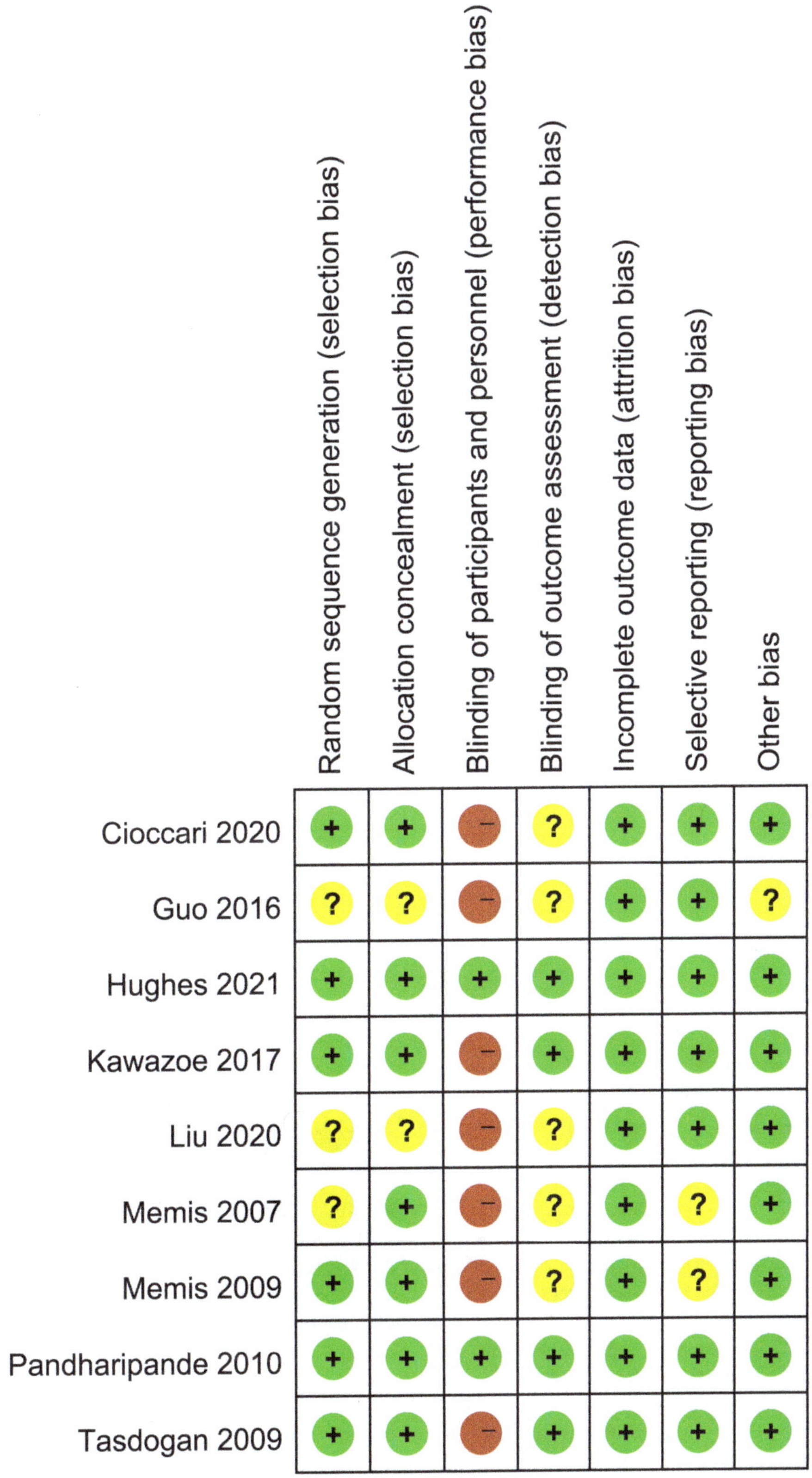

FIGURE 2 | Assessment of quality by the Cochrane risk of bias tool. Red denotes high risk, yellow unclear risk and green low risk.

TABLE 2 | Primary and secondary outcomes of this meta-analysis.

Outcome	N	Result
Overall mortality	9	RR 0.97, 95%CI 0.82 to 1.13, $P = 0.67$, $I^2 = 25\%$
ICU mortality	3	RR 0.60, 95%CI 0.30 to 1.21, $P = 0.15$, $I^2 = 0\%$
28/30-day mortality	5	RR 1.00, 95%CI 0.84 to 1.18, $P = 0.98$, $I^2 = 56\%$
In-hospital mortality	2	RR 0.74, 95%CI 0.38 to 1.45, $P = 0.37$, $I^2 = 0\%$
90-day mortality	2	RR 0.94, 95%CI 0.75 to 1.18, $P = 0.67$, $I^2 = 29\%$
Length of ICU stay	8	MD −1.12, 95%CI −2.89 to 0.64, $P = 0.21$, $I^2 = 71\%$
Duration of MV	6	MD −0.53, 95%CI −0.85 to −0.21, $P = 0.001$, $I^2 = 0\%$
Inflammatory response		
TNF-α	2	MD −5.27, 95%CI −7.99 to −2.54, $P < 0.001$, $I^2 = 0\%$
IL-1β	2	MD −1.25, 95%CI −1.91 to −0.59, $P < 0.001$, $I^2 = 0\%$
Incidence of delirium	2	RR 0.95, 95%CI 0.72 to 1.25, $P = 0.70$, $I^2 = 0\%$
Delirium free days	2	MD 1.76, 95%CI −0.94 to 4.47, $P = 0.20$, $I^2 = 80\%$

N, number of studies; ICU, intensive care unit; RR, risk ratio; CI, confidence interval; MV, mechanical ventilation; MD, mean difference; TNF-α, tumor necrosis factor-α; IL-1β, interleukin-1β.

Study or Subgroup	Experimental Events	Experimental Total	Control Events	Control Total	Weight	Risk Ratio M-H, Fixed, 95% CI
Cioccari 2020	9	44	12	39	6.9%	0.66 [0.31, 1.41]
Guo 2016	2	14	4	31	1.3%	1.11 [0.23, 5.35]
Hughes 2021	74	214	57	208	31.3%	1.26 [0.95, 1.68]
Kawazoe 2017	19	100	28	101	15.1%	0.69 [0.41, 1.14]
Liu 2020	64	100	62	100	33.6%	1.03 [0.83, 1.28]
Memis 2007	2	20	3	20	1.6%	0.67 [0.12, 3.57]
Memis 2009	3	20	4	20	2.2%	0.75 [0.19, 2.93]
Pandharipande 2010	5	31	13	32	6.9%	0.40 [0.16, 0.98]
Tasdogan 2009	1	20	2	20	1.1%	0.50 [0.05, 5.08]
Total (95% CI)		**563**		**571**	**100.0%**	**0.97 [0.82, 1.13]**
Total events	179		185			

Heterogeneity: Chi² = 10.73, df = 8 (P = 0.22); I² = 25%
Test for overall effect: Z = 0.43 (P = 0.67)

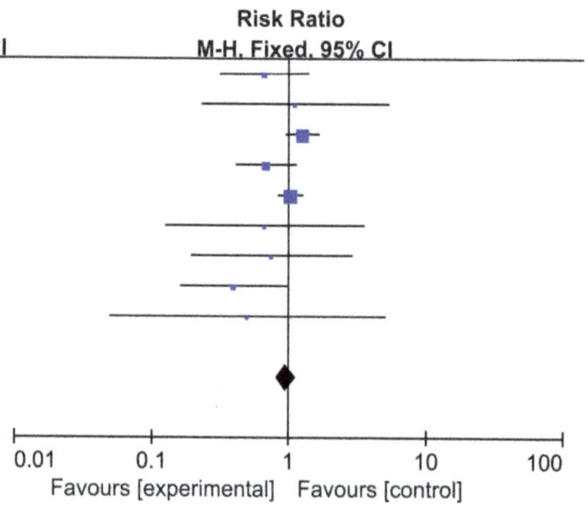

FIGURE 3 | Forest plot comparing the effect of DEX on mortality.

Moreover, we found survival benefits in comparison with other sedations including lorazepam and midazolam, but not with propofol.

There are three previous systematic reviews and meta-analyses (36–38) comparing the effect of dexmedetomidine vs. other sedative agents on clinical outcomes of patients with sepsis. The results of previous studies showed that compared with other sedatives, the use of dexmedetomidine had beneficial effects on 28-day mortality, but there were no significant differences in the length of ICU stay and duration of MV (36–38). Our meta-analysis indicated that the use of dexmedetomidine was associated with the shortened duration of MV for mechanically ventilated patients with sepsis, but no significant differences in the overall mortality. These differences may result from several newly published RCTs. In contrast to previous meta-analyses, our research updated the findings by including recently published RCTs (31–33), especially the MENDS II trial. In this pragmatic RCT involving 400 patients from 13 medical centers, there are many important methodologic advances including a higher degree of trial drug allocation concealment and blinding, better separation between groups concerning sedative exposure, and stricter adherence to light sedation approaches (33). The increased trials and number of patients could provide more robust results. Moreover, in the subgroup analyses, we found survival benefits in comparison with lorazepam, not with propofol.

Dexmedetomidine could promote macrophage phagocytosis and bactericidal killing further enhancing the mucosal immunity and bacterial clearance, which are of great importance for patients with sepsis and septic shock. Previous research has shown that dexmedetomidine had potential anti-inflammatory effects in both animal and human studies (39). Results of our meta-analysis also suggest that after 24 h of receiving dexmedetomidine, the levels of TNF-α and IL-1β were significantly lower than the control group. This anti-inflammatory effect of dexmedetomidine can suppress the exaggerated production of inflammatory cytokines in septic shock (4, 40, 41).

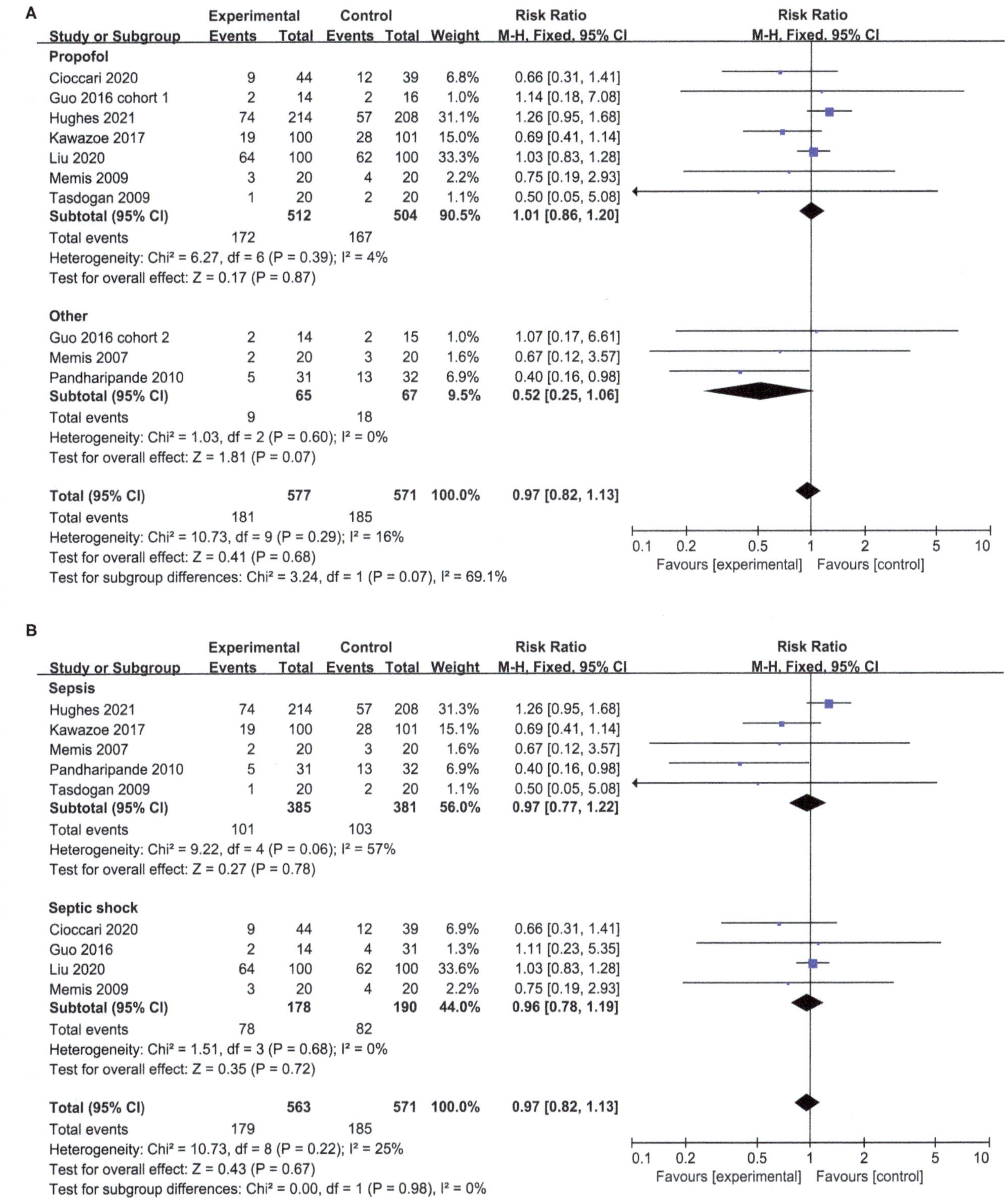

FIGURE 4 | Subgroup analysis for mortality **(A)** propofol vs. other sedation, **(B)** sepsis vs. septic shock.

A

Study or Subgroup	Experimental Mean	Experimental SD	Experimental Total	Control Mean	Control SD	Control Total	Weight	Mean Difference IV, Random, 95% CI
Cioccari 2020	5.7	5.75	44	5.33	6.39	39	14.3%	0.37 [-2.26, 3.00]
Guo 2016 cohort 1	15.2	5.6	14	19.7	5.7	15	9.8%	-4.50 [-8.61, -0.39]
Guo 2016 cohort 2	15.2	5.6	14	17.8	5.7	16	10.0%	-2.60 [-6.65, 1.45]
Kawazoe 2017	7.67	6.02	100	8.67	7.52	101	17.0%	-1.00 [-2.88, 0.88]
Liu 2020	13.5	2.8	100	17	4	100	19.8%	-3.50 [-4.46, -2.54]
Memis 2009	14	8	20	12	7	20	8.5%	2.00 [-2.66, 6.66]
Pandharipande 2010	13.4	15.1	31	12.2	9.8	32	5.7%	1.20 [-5.11, 7.51]
Tasdogan 2009	7.33	3.99	20	6.33	3.99	20	14.9%	1.00 [-1.47, 3.47]
Total (95% CI)			**343**			**343**	**100.0%**	**-1.12 [-2.89, 0.64]**

Heterogeneity: $Tau^2 = 3.85$; $Chi^2 = 24.22$, df = 7 (P = 0.001); $I^2 = 71\%$
Test for overall effect: Z = 1.25 (P = 0.21)

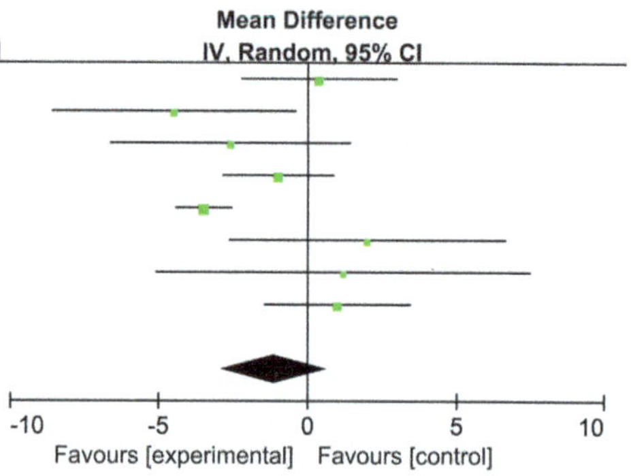

B

Study or Subgroup	Experimental Mean	Experimental SD	Experimental Total	Control Mean	Control SD	Control Total	Weight	Mean Difference IV, Fixed, 95% CI
Cioccari 2020	3.07	3.68	44	4.53	6.47	39	2.0%	-1.46 [-3.76, 0.84]
Guo 2016 cohort 1	14.2	5.7	14	17.7	5.7	15	0.6%	-3.50 [-7.65, 0.65]
Guo 2016 cohort 2	14.2	5.7	14	16.9	5.7	16	0.6%	-2.70 [-6.79, 1.39]
Kawazoe 2017	6.67	6.02	100	6.67	6.02	101	3.8%	0.00 [-1.66, 1.66]
Liu 2020	4.75	1	100	5.25	1.4	100	92.6%	-0.50 [-0.84, -0.16]
Tasdogan 2009	9.67	7.18	20	9.67	9.57	20	0.4%	0.00 [-5.24, 5.24]
Total (95% CI)			**292**			**291**	**100.0%**	**-0.53 [-0.85, -0.21]**

Heterogeneity: $Chi^2 = 4.13$, df = 5 (P = 0.53); $I^2 = 0\%$
Test for overall effect: Z = 3.20 (P = 0.001)

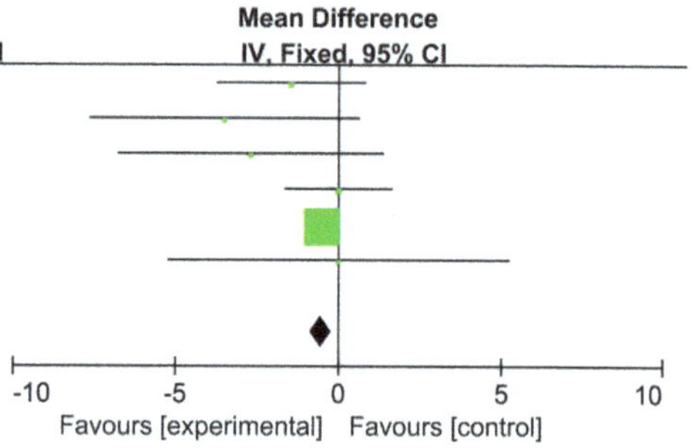

C

Study or Subgroup	Experimental Mean	Experimental SD	Experimental Total	Control Mean	Control SD	Control Total	Weight	Mean Difference IV, Fixed, 95% CI
TNF-α								
Memis 2007	14.6	4	20	19.5	5.8	20	4.3%	-4.90 [-7.99, -1.81]
Tasdogan 2009	14.66	4.4	18	21.21	11.37	17	1.2%	-6.55 [-12.32, -0.78]
Total (95% CI)			**38**			**37**	**5.6%**	**-5.27 [-7.99, -2.54]**
Heterogeneity: $Chi^2 = 0.24$, df = 1 (P = 0.62); $I^2 = 0\%$								
Test for overall effect: Z = 3.79 (P = 0.0001)								
IL-1								
Memis 2007	5	0.3	20	6.29	2	20	52.7%	-1.29 [-2.18, -0.40]
Tasdogan 2009	5.03	0.15	18	6.23	2.09	17	41.7%	-1.20 [-2.20, -0.20]
Total (95% CI)			**38**			**37**	**94.4%**	**-1.25 [-1.91, -0.59]**
Heterogeneity: $Chi^2 = 0.02$, df = 1 (P = 0.89); $I^2 = 0\%$								
Test for overall effect: Z = 3.70 (P = 0.0002)								

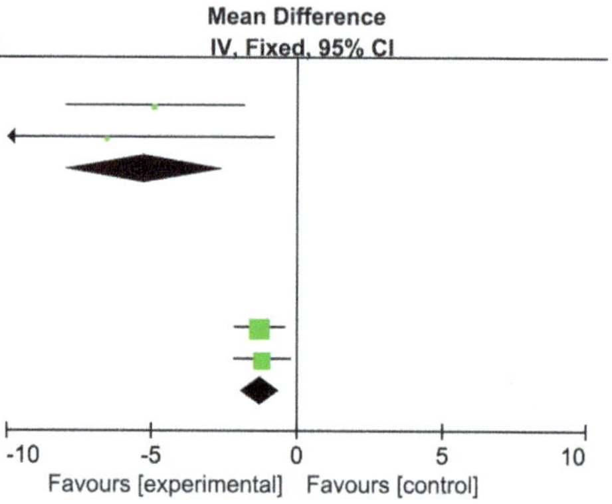

FIGURE 5 | Forest plot comparing the effect of DEX on **(A)** length of ICU stay, **(B)** duration of MV, **(C)** inflammatory response.

The strengths of our study include the comprehensive and up-to-date search strategies, specific and targeted inclusion criteria, comprehensive and rigorous analytical methods. Three studies included in our meta-analysis are recently published RCTs (31–33) with large populations. The predefined subgroup analysis found survival benefits of dexmedetomidine in comparison with other sedations including lorazepam and midazolam.

However, our meta-analysis also had several limitations. First of all, the main limitation is the limited number of included studies and the small sample size. Six of the included trials are typically characterized as small studies because the sample size was smaller than 100 patients, which may lead to small study effect bias (42). Second, the diagnostic criteria for sepsis or septic shock, the dose of the sedative drug, and target sedation goals were varied among included studies. These factors may cause clinical heterogeneity. Third, the follow-up duration in most included studies was relatively short, only two studies reported 90-day mortality as the long-term outcome. More RCTs with long follow-ups were necessary to demonstrate the effects of dexmedetomidine on long-term outcomes. Last but not the least, in some included studies, the dexmedetomidine was combined with other sedative agents including opioids or benzodiazepines in the intervention

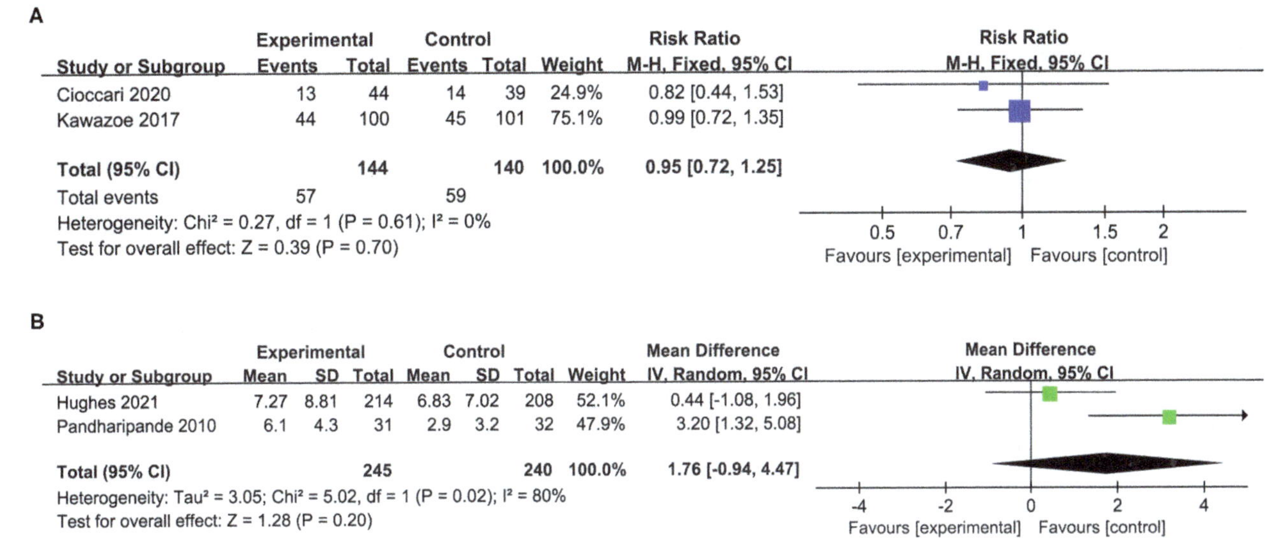

FIGURE 6 | Forest plot comparing the effect of DEX on **(A)** incidence of delirium, **(B)** delirium free days.

group for sedation. Therefore, the actual efficacy of single administration with dexmedetomidine for patients with sepsis requires further validation.

CONCLUSION

In conclusion, our meta-analysis suggests that for patients with sepsis or septic shock, the use of dexmedetomidine has no effect on all-cause mortality and length of ICU stay, but may offer advantages in terms of reducing the duration of mechanical ventilation and inflammatory response. However, considering the significant heterogeneity and the limited number of included studies with small sample sizes. Well-designed, multicenter RCTs with a large sample size are needed to further evaluate the effect of dexmedetomidine on short-term and long-term clinical outcomes for patients with sepsis and to compare its effects with other sedative agents.

AUTHOR CONTRIBUTIONS

CW contributed to the acquisition and analysis of the data, the initial draft writing of this paper, and the final approval of the version to be published. QC, PW, and WJ contributed to the collection and interpretation of data. CZ, ZG, and KX contributed to the concept of the review and the revision of this paper. All authors contributed to the article and approved the submitted version.

REFERENCES

1. Singer M, Deutschman CS, Seymour CW, Shankar-Hari M, Annane D, Bauer M, et al. The Third International Consensus Definitions for Sepsis and Septic Shock (Sepsis-3). *JAMA.* (2016) 315:801–10. doi: 10.1001/jama.2016.0287
2. Fleischmann C, Scherag A, Adhikari NK, Hartog CS, Tsaganos T, Schlattmann P, et al. Assessment of Global Incidence and Mortality of Hospital-treated Sepsis. Current Estimates and Limitations. *Am J Respir Crit Care Med.* (2016) 193:259–72. doi: 10.1164/rccm.201504-0781OC
3. Rudd KE, Johnson SC, Agesa KM, Shackelford KA, Tsoi D, Kievlan DR, et al. Global, regional, and national sepsis incidence and mortality, 1990–2017: analysis for the Global Burden of Disease Study. *Lancet.* (2020) 395:200–11. doi: 10.1016/S0140-6736(19)32989-7
4. Angus DC, van der Poll T. Severe sepsis and septic shock. *N Engl J Med.* (2013) 369:840–51. doi: 10.1056/NEJMra1208623
5. Auriemma CL, Zhuo H, Delucchi K, Deiss T, Liu T, Jauregui A, et al. Acute respiratory distress syndrome-attributable mortality in critically ill patients with sepsis. *Intensive Care Med.* (2020) 46:1222–31. doi: 10.1007/s00134-020-06010-9
6. Dhital R, Basnet S, Poudel DR. Predictors and outcome of invasive mechanical ventilation in hospitalized patients with sepsis: data from National Inpatient Sample. *J Community Hosp Intern Med Perspect.* (2018) 8:49–52. doi: 10.1080/20009666.2018.1450592
7. Patel SB, Kress JP. Sedation and analgesia in the mechanically ventilated patient. *Am J Respir Crit Care Med.* (2012) 185:486–97. doi: 10.1164/rccm.201102-0273CI
8. Reade MC, Finfer S. Sedation and delirium in the intensive care unit. *N Engl J Med.* (2014) 370:444–54. doi: 10.1056/NEJMra1208705
9. Wunsch H, Kahn JM, Kramer AA, Rubenfeld GD. Use of intravenous infusion sedation among mechanically ventilated patients in the United States. *Crit Care Med.* (2009) 37:3031–9. doi: 10.1097/CCM.0b013e3181b02eff

10. Jacobi J, Fraser GL, Coursin DB, Riker RR, Fontaine D, Wittbrodt ET, et al. Clinical practice guidelines for the sustained use of sedatives and analgesics in the critically ill adult. *Crit Care Med.* (2002) 30:119–41. doi: 10.1097/00003246-200201000-00020
11. Martin J, Franck M, Fischer M, Spies C. Sedation and analgesia in German intensive care units: how is it done in reality? Results of a patient-based survey of analgesia and sedation. *Intensive Care Med.* (2006) 32:1137–42. doi: 10.1007/s00134-006-0214-6
12. Keating GM. Dexmedetomidine: a Review of Its Use for Sedation in the Intensive Care Setting. *Drugs.* (2015) 75:1119–30. doi: 10.1007/s40265-015-0419-5
13. Tan JA, Ho KM. Use of dexmedetomidine as a sedative and analgesic agent in critically ill adult patients: a meta-analysis. *Intensive Care Med.* (2010) 36:926–39. doi: 10.1007/s00134-010-1877-6
14. Fraser GL, Devlin JW, Worby CP, Alhazzani W, Barr J, Dasta JF, et al. Benzodiazepine versus nonbenzodiazepine-based sedation for mechanically ventilated, critically ill adults: a systematic review and meta-analysis of randomized trials. *Crit Care Med.* (2013) 41(9 Suppl 1):S30–8. doi: 10.1097/CCM.0b013e3182a16898
15. Constantin JM, Momon A, Mantz J, Payen JF, De Jonghe B, Perbet S, et al. Efficacy and safety of sedation with dexmedetomidine in critical care patients: a meta-analysis of randomized controlled trials. *Anaesth Crit Care Pain Med.* (2016) 35:7–15. doi: 10.1016/j.accpm.2015.06.012
16. Pasin L, Greco T, Feltracco P, Vittorio A, Neto CN, Cabrini L, et al. Dexmedetomidine as a sedative agent in critically ill patients: a meta-analysis of randomized controlled trials. *PLoS ONE.* (2013) 8:e82913. doi: 10.1371/journal.pone.0082913
17. Xia ZQ, Chen SQ, Yao X, Xie CB, Wen SH, Liu KX. Clinical benefits of dexmedetomidine versus propofol in adult intensive care unit patients: a meta-analysis of randomized clinical trials. *J Surg Res.* (2013) 185:833–43. doi: 10.1016/j.jss.2013.06.062
18. Nelson S, Muzyk AJ, Bucklin MH, Brudney S, Gagliardi JP. Defining the role of dexmedetomidine in the prevention of delirium in the intensive care unit. *Biomed Res Int.* (2015) 2015:635737. doi: 10.1155/2015/635737
19. Pasin L, Landoni G, Nardelli P, Belletti A, Di Prima AL, Taddeo D, et al. Dexmedetomidine reduces the risk of delirium, agitation and confusion in critically Ill patients: a meta-analysis of randomized controlled trials. *J Cardiothorac Vasc Anesth.* (2014) 28:1459–66. doi: 10.1053/j.jvca.2014.03.010
20. Liberati A, Altman DG, Tetzlaff J, Mulrow C, Gøtzsche PC, Ioannidis JP, et al. The PRISMA statement for reporting systematic reviews and meta-analyses of studies that evaluate healthcare interventions: explanation and elaboration. *BMJ.* (2009) 339:b2700. doi: 10.1136/bmj.b2700
21. Plaat F, Naik M. Critical care in pregnancy. *Critical Care.* (2011) 15:1014. doi: 10.1186/cc10479
22. Higgins JP, Altman DG, Gøtzsche PC, Jüni P, Moher D, Oxman AD, et al. The Cochrane Collaboration's tool for assessing risk of bias in randomised trials. *BMJ.* (2011) 343:d5928. doi: 10.1136/bmj.d5928
23. Higgins JP, Thompson SG, Deeks JJ, Altman DG. Measuring inconsistency in meta-analyses. *BMJ.* (2003) 327:557–60. doi: 10.1136/bmj.327.7414.557
24. Egger M, Davey Smith G, Schneider M, Minder C. Bias in meta-analysis detected by a simple, graphical test. *BMJ.* (1997) 315:629–34. doi: 10.1136/bmj.315.7109.629
25. Memiş D, Hekimoglu S, Vatan I, Yandim T, Yüksel M, Süt N. Effects of midazolam and dexmedetomidine on inflammatory responses and gastric intramucosal pH to sepsis, in critically ill patients. *Br J Anaesth.* (2007) 98:550–2. doi: 10.1093/bja/aem017
26. Memiş D, Kargi M, Sut N. Effects of propofol and dexmedetomidine on indocyanine green elimination assessed with LIMON to patients with early septic shock: a pilot study. *J Crit Care.* (2009) 24:603–8. doi: 10.1016/j.jcrc.2008.10.005
27. Tasdogan M, Memis D, Sut N, Yuksel M. Results of a pilot study on the effects of propofol and dexmedetomidine on inflammatory responses and intraabdominal pressure in severe sepsis. *J Clin Anesth.* (2009) 21:394–400. doi: 10.1016/j.jclinane.2008.10.010
28. Pandharipande PP, Sanders RD, Girard TD, McGrane S, Thompson JL, Shintani AK, et al. Effect of dexmedetomidine versus lorazepam on outcome in patients with sepsis: an a priori-designed analysis of the MENDS randomized controlled trial. *Crit Care.* (2010) 14:R38. doi: 10.1186/cc8916
29. Guo F, Wang Q, Yan CY, Huang HY, Yu X, Tu LY. Clinical application of different sedation regimen in patients with septic shock. *Zhonghua Yi Xue Za Zhi.* (2016) 96:1758–61. doi: 10.3760/cma.j.issn.0376-2491.2016.22.010
30. Kawazoe Y, Miyamoto K, Morimoto T, Yamamoto T, Fuke A, Hashimoto A, et al. Effect of dexmedetomidine on mortality and ventilator-free days in patients requiring mechanical ventilation with sepsis: a randomized clinical trial. *JAMA.* (2017) 317:1321–8. doi: 10.1001/jama.2017.2088
31. Cioccari L, Luethi N, Bailey M, Shehabi Y, Howe B, Messmer AS, et al. The effect of dexmedetomidine on vasopressor requirements in patients with septic shock: a subgroup analysis of the Sedation Practice in Intensive Care Evaluation [SPICE III] Trial. *Crit Care.* (2020) 24:441. doi: 10.1186/s13054-020-03115-x
32. Liu J, Shi K, Hong J, Gong F, Mo S, Chen M, et al. Dexmedetomidine protects against acute kidney injury in patients with septic shock. *Ann Palliat Med.* (2020) 9:224–30. doi: 10.21037/apm.2020.02.08
33. Hughes CG, Mailloux PT, Devlin JW, Swan JT, Sanders RD, Anzueto A, et al. Dexmedetomidine or propofol for sedation in mechanically ventilated adults with sepsis. *N Engl J Med.* (2021) 384:1424–36. doi: 10.1056/NEJMoa2024922
34. Shehabi Y, Howe BD, Bellomo R, Arabi YM, Bailey M, Bass FE, et al. Early sedation with dexmedetomidine in critically Ill patients. *N Engl J Med.* (2019) 380:2506–17. doi: 10.1056/NEJMoa1904710
35. Pandharipande PP, Pun BT, Herr DL, Maze M, Girard TD, Miller RR, et al. Effect of sedation with dexmedetomidine vs lorazepam on acute brain dysfunction in mechanically ventilated patients: the MENDS randomized controlled trial. *JAMA.* (2007) 298:2644–53. doi: 10.1001/jama.298.22.2644
36. Zamani MM, Keshavarz-Fathi M, Fakhri-Bafghi MS, Hirbod-Mobarakeh A, Rezaei N, Bahrami A, et al. Survival benefits of dexmedetomidine used for sedating septic patients in intensive care setting: a systematic review. *J Crit Care.* (2016) 32:93–100. doi: 10.1016/j.jcrc.2015.11.013
37. Zhang WQ, Xu P, Zhan XH, Zheng P, Yang W. Efficacy of dexmedetomidine for treatment of patients with sepsis: a meta-analysis of randomized controlled trials. *Medicine (Baltimore).* (2019) 98:e15469. doi: 10.1097/MD.0000000000015469
38. Chen P, Jiang J, Zhang Y, Li G, Qiu Z, Levy MM, et al. Effect of dexmedetomidine on duration of mechanical ventilation in septic patients: a systematic review and meta-analysis. *BMC Pulm Med.* (2020) 20:42. doi: 10.1186/s12890-020-1065-6
39. Flanders CA, Rocke AS, Edwardson SA, Baillie JK, Walsh TS. The effect of dexmedetomidine and clonidine on the inflammatory response in critical illness: a systematic review of animal and human studies. *Crit Care.* (2019) 23:402. doi: 10.1186/s13054-019-2690-4
40. MacLaren R. Immunosedation: a consideration for sepsis. *Crit Care.* (2009) 13:191. doi: 10.1186/cc8034
41. Xiang H, Hu B, Li Z, Li J. Dexmedetomidine controls systemic cytokine levels through the cholinergic anti-inflammatory pathway. *Inflammation.* (2014) 37:1763–70. doi: 10.1007/s10753-014-9906-1
42. Zhang Z, Xu X, Ni H. Small studies may overestimate the effect sizes in critical care meta-analyses: a meta-epidemiological study. *Crit Care.* (2013) 17:R2.doi: 10.1186/cc11919

7

PPV May be a Starting Point to Achieve Circulatory Protective Mechanical Ventilation

Longxiang Su[1†], Pan Pan[2†], Huaiwu He[1], Dawei Liu[1] and Yun Long[1]*

[1] Department of Critical Care Medicine, State Key Laboratory of Complex Severe and Rare Diseases, Peking Union Medical College Hospital, Chinese Academy of Medical Science and Peking Union Medical College, Beijing, China, [2] College of Pulmonary and Critical Care Medicine, Chinese PLA General Hospital, Beijing, China

***Correspondence:**
Yun Long
ly_icu@aliyun.com

† These authors have contributed equally to this work

Pulse pressure variation (PPV) is a mandatory index for hemodynamic monitoring during mechanical ventilation. The changes in pleural pressure (P_{pl}) and transpulmonary pressure (P_L) caused by mechanical ventilation are the basis for PPV and lead to the effect of blood flow. If the state of hypovolemia exists, the effect of the increased P_{pl} during mechanical ventilation on the right ventricular preload will mainly affect the cardiac output, resulting in a positive PPV. However, P_L is more influenced by the change in alveolar pressure, which produces an increase in right heart overload, resulting in high PPV. In particular, if spontaneous breathing is strong, the transvascular pressure will be extremely high, which may lead to the promotion of alveolar flooding and increased RV flow. Asynchronous breathing and mediastinal swing may damage the pulmonary circulation and right heart function. Therefore, according to the principle of PPV, a high PPV can be incorporated into the whole respiratory treatment process to monitor the mechanical ventilation cycle damage/protection regardless of the controlled ventilation or spontaneous breathing. Through the monitoring of PPV, the circulation-protective ventilation can be guided at bedside in real time by PPV.

Keywords: pulse pressure variation, mechanical ventilation, cardiopulmonary interactions, circulatory-protection, blood flow

HIGHLIGHTS

- Pulse pressure variation (PPV) is a mandatory index for hemodynamic monitoring during mechanical ventilation.
- PPV originates from increased pleural pressure (P_{pl}) and transpulmonary pressure (PL).
- P_{pl} mainly affects the right ventricular preload, while PL is more influenced by right heart overload.
- The role of PPV in right heart overload should be emphasized in lung and circulatory protection during mechanical ventilation, reducing the occurrence of ventilator-induced lung injury (VILI), and patient self-inflicted lung injury (P-SILI).
- PPV is a real-time monitoring index for the mechanical ventilation that can promptly alert for abnormal breathing and circulation at the bedside.

Hemodynamic monitoring is essential to improve gas exchange, optimize organ and tissue perfusion, and avoid ventilation-related lung injury (VILI) in the mechanical ventilation patients. Therefore, the low-tidal volume lung protection strategies are widely used in clinical practice. However, in the process of mechanical ventilation for the patients with acute respiratory distress syndrome (ARDS) or even coronavirus disease 2019 (COVID-19), we have increasingly realized that only low-tidal volume lung protective ventilation is far from sufficient. Many patients still die from acute circulatory failure caused by ventilation-related lung injury (VILI) or patient self-inflicted lung injury (P-SILI) (1, 2). In clinical work, we are always thinking about whether we can use a direct indicator to reflect the mechanical ventilation management to achieve circulatory protection on the basis of lung protection at the same time. The cardiopulmonary interaction produced by positive pressure ventilation leads to the changes in pleural pressure (P_{pl}) and transpulmonary pressure (P_L), and the accompanying hemodynamic effects provide clues for us, which make it possible to monitor the hemodynamic changes under mechanical ventilation (3–5). Specific indicators can prompt the hemodynamic situation of a patient to the doctor at the bedside and provide precise treatment directions. In the intensive care unit (ICU), it is necessary to establish the central venous catheters and peripheral arterial catheters for critically ill patients. The analysis of the central venous pressure, arterial blood pressure, pressure waveform, and blood gas of arteries and veins can enable doctors to perform more precise and individualized strategies in circulation and respiratory management for the patients (6). When the peripheral arterial catheter is indwelled for arterial blood pressure measurement, the arterial pressure waveform has a periodic change with the respiratory cycle that can be displayed in the monitor, which we call pulse pressure variation (PPV). The previous studies have shown that during strictly controlled mechanical ventilation, a PPV value >13% indicates that the patients have fluid responsiveness when high tidal volume or lung compliance exists (7, 8). However, sometimes we find that the PPV value is more than 13%, but the mechanical ventilation patients have no fluid responsiveness. At this time, the decline in patient cardiac output is often due to high right ventricle afterload. Therefore, expanding the usage of PPV can identify and evaluate the hemodynamic dysfunction of a patient early during mechanical ventilation and better implement circulatory and lung protection ventilation therapy.

MECHANISM OF PPV

Positive-pressure ventilation changes the normal respiratory physiology of a patient, leading to the changes in P_{pl} and P_L. The changed cardiopulmonary interaction produced by P_{pl} and P_L can result in the changes in preload and afterload of the two ventricles, which in turn causes the blood flow changes (3, 5). In controlled ventilation mode, inhalation can increase P_{pl} and reduce venous return, reducing the preload of the right ventricle. After the gas is inhaled, the lung tissue stress during tidal inhalation is the pressure distending the lung, called P_L, the difference between airway pressure and P_{pl}. P_L causes an increase in afterload to the right ventricle due to the increased pulmonary vascular resistance during inhalation (9). The result is that the output of the right ventricle is the lowest at the end of inspiration (4, 9). For the left ventricle, the increase in P_{pl} during inhalation can lead to a decrease in the afterload of the left ventricle due

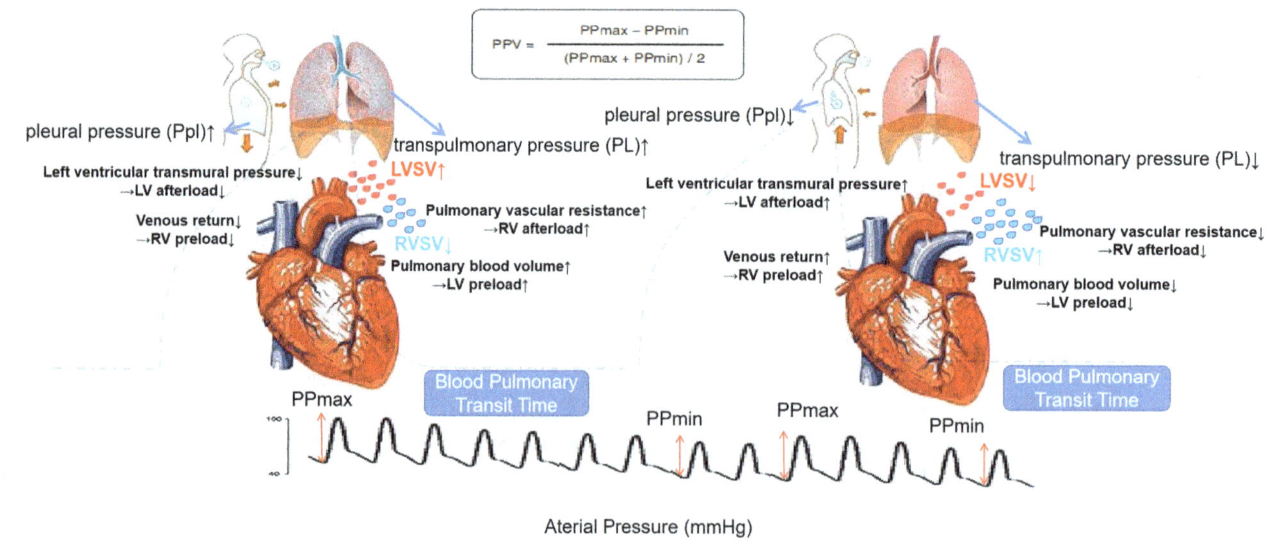

FIGURE 1 | Schematic effects of high transpulmonary pressure (P_L) and pleural pressure (P_{pl}) on the right ventricle (RV) vs. left ventricle (LV) to explain the mechanisms of pulse pressure variation (PPV). Blood pulmonary transit time means 2–4 heartbeat cycles for this blood flow effect conducting from the right heart to left heart. When exhaling, the effect of the drop in the stroke volume (SV) of the right heart during inhalation will affect the left heart. Top: calculation formula of PPV; background dotted line: airway pressure tracing; bottom: arterial pressure tracing. The left side is the inspiratory phase, and the right side is the expiratory phase.

to the decrease in left ventricular transmural pressure. At the same time, the P_L causes an increase in the preload of the left ventricle. Therefore, the result for left ventricle output can be the largest at the end of inhalation (10). However, as the left and right hearts are connected, the influence of inhalation on the reduction of right ventricle output will result in the reduction of left ventricle preload. There are 2–4 heartbeat cycles for this blood flow effect conducting from the right heart to the left heart, which is called the blood pulmonary transit time. At this time, the inhalation changes to exhalation, and eventually, the left ventricle output decreases during exhalation. The different cardiac outputs of inhalation and exhalation create the basis for the existence of PPV. The maximum pulse pressure difference appears during inhalation, and the minimum pulse pressure difference appears during exhalation. The ratio of the difference between the two values to the average of the two values is defined as PPV. **Figure 1** shows the schematic effects of the mechanisms of pulse pressure variation.

PPV AND BLOOD FLOW DURING MECHANICAL VENTILATION

P_{pl} and P_L can affect the pulmonary blood flow during mechanical ventilation. The P_{pl} causes a change in the right ventricle inflow and the left ventricle outflow. P_L causes the changes in right ventricle outflow and left ventricle inflow. From the above, we know that the P_{pl} during mechanical ventilation causes a decrease in the right ventricle preload, and the P_L causes an increase in the right ventricle afterload, both of which are responsible for the decrease in global cardiac output. However, we need to determine which pressure constitutes the bulk of decreased cardiac output so that we can better determine whether fluid resuscitation or P_L should be reduced. The wrong judgments will lead to the wrong treatments and ultimately cause patient injury.

In general, we focused on the hemodynamic effect of capacity status on right ventricle preload. When both the left and right ventricles have fluid responsiveness, the global cardiac output will increase as the capacity increases. At this time, the increased PPV can represent whether the patients have fluid responsiveness. If any one of the ventricles has no fluid responsiveness, the global cardiac output will ultimately not increase due to fluid resuscitation (10). When pulmonary compliance is normal or slightly decreased, a high tidal volume can cause P_{pl} to affect the change in alveolar pressure by 50% or more. At this time, if combined with a hypovolemic state, the influence of increased P_{pl} on right ventricle preload will constitute the bulk of cardiac output, resulting in a positive PPV (11). Therefore, when using PPV to predict the fluid responsiveness during mechanical ventilation, the doctors need to consider pulmonary compliance and tidal volume (7, 12).

In addition, PPV can be used to predict the hemodynamic effect of positive end-expiratory pressure (PEEP) on the right ventricle (13). High PEEP can cause decreased cardiac output, resulting in increased PPV, but not all the patients have fluid responsiveness. Research has suggested that the higher the PPV before using mechanical ventilation, the more obvious the decrease in cardiac output caused by PEEP (13). However, for the patients without fluid responsiveness, if the high PPV does not represent reduced right ventricle preload, we need to consider whether it is due to the increased right ventricle afterload that causes the decrease in cardiac output. This suggests that the high PPV in the patients with ARDS may not mean hypovolemia but a significant increase in P_L, which causes an increase in right ventricle afterload and a decreased left ventricle inflow. At this time, we should not only take note of cardiac output decreases but also be alerted of the incidence of acute cor pulmonale (ACP).

PPV AND RIGHT VENTRICLE AFTERLOAD

Positive pressure ventilation affects the right ventricle afterload, which in turn affects pulmonary blood flow, resulting in a decrease in cardiac output and an increase in PPV. At this time, the patients usually have no fluid responsiveness. P_L rises during mechanical ventilation, which can compress the alveolar capillaries. Since right heart failure is more sensitive to afterload than preload, the decrease in right ventricular outflow during inhalation has a greater relationship with right ventricle afterload. Two clinical studies have reported that in the case of right heart failure, the patients with high PPV have no fluid responsiveness. Moritz et al. found that in the early stage after cardiac surgery or during septic shock, the patients with increased pulmonary artery pressure had a poor response to fluid resuscitation, and PPV could not be used to predict the fluid responsiveness (14). Yazine Mahjoub et al. (15) found that right heart failure can lead to false-positive PPV. Such patients can be combined with the tricuspid annular systolic velocity (Sta) to identify whether the patients have increased right ventricular afterload. Therefore, we emphasize that when the capacity of a patient is sufficient but lung compliance is significantly reduced or when the ventilator support conditions are high, P_L can significantly increase the right ventricular afterload or cause ACP, resulting in a decrease in cardiac output (3). As mentioned before, the effects of mechanical ventilation on preload and afterload of the right ventricle can cause cardiac output and blood pressure to decrease, leading to an increase in PPV, but different effects will have completely different treatments. When decreased right ventricular preload contributes to the bulk of decreased cardiac output, it indicates the need for fluid resuscitation; when the right ventricular afterload effect is dominant, fluid resuscitation is not recommended or may even be harmful. In this case, limiting P_L is the first choice, that is, the essence and connotation of circulation-protective ventilation.

PPV AND SPONTANEOUS BREATHING

Many studies have recommended reducing the dose of sedatives during mechanical ventilation and allowing the patients to maintain spontaneous breathing. However, the abnormal spontaneous breathing of the mechanically ventilated patients, defined here as excessive spontaneous breathing, can cause hemodynamic disturbances. Excessive spontaneous breathing causes negative changes in the Ppl and increases the P_L, resulting in excessive alveolar expansion, increased functional residual capacity (FRC), increased pulmonary vascular resistance (PVR), decreased pulmonary blood flow, increased V/Q ratio, and increased dead space ventilation (16). The injury caused by spontaneous breathing not only affects the alveoli but also affects pulmonary blood flow. Transvascular pressure is the difference between intravascular pressure and pressure outside the vessels. The more negative P_{pl} generated during spontaneous breathing will increase transvascular pressure and aggravate pulmonary edema due to promoting alveolar flooding and increased RV flow (17). In the healthy lung, the changes in local P_{pl} are evenly transmitted across the lung surface; this phenomenon is called "fluid-like" behavior. However, the injured lungs exhibit "solid-like" behavior, where a non-aerated lung region impedes the rapid generalization of a local change in P_L. In such cases, the lung expansion is heterogeneous. Therefore, there will be different regional P_{Ls} and different degrees of lung inflation. At this time, if spontaneous breathing is superimposed, it will undoubtedly cause more changes in P_{pl} and uneven conduction, resulting in uneven lung expansion or even excessive expansion (18, 19). Eventually, lack of synchronization between the reserved spontaneous breathing and mechanical ventilation of a patient as well as mediastinal swing may impair pulmonary circulation and right heart function (20, 21). The hemodynamic effects caused by the above conditions can also be predicted by PPV.

PPV AND COVID-19 AND ARDS

In COVID-19 pneumonia, a large proportion of the patients have L-type ARDS. Their lung gas volume is usually high, lung recruitability is minimal, and hypoxemia likely results from the loss of hypoxic pulmonary vasoconstriction and impaired regulation of pulmonary blood flow (22). During hypoxia, the patients are usually forced to increase their tidal volume and thus increase minute ventilation volume (23). At this time, if the patients maintain spontaneous breathing, there will be an increase in the work of spontaneous breathing, which will cause the P_{pl} negative changes and increase the transvascular pressure. In the case of increased pulmonary vessel permeability caused by inflammation, increased transvascular pressure will extremely increase the risk of pulmonary edema resulting from vascular leakage (24), which will progress L-type ARDS toward H-type ARDS. Manifestation of H-type is similar to typical ARDS. The lung lesions are distributed in a dependent area. The movement of the diaphragm during spontaneous breathing is mainly in the dependent area, which is conducive to the recruitment maneuvers and increased pulmonary blood flow in the dependent area (25–27). When mild and moderate ARDS occurs, the patients have a relatively low P_L, and spontaneous breathing can increase transpulmonary vascular pressure, reduce pulmonary vascular resistance, increase pulmonary blood flow, and improve ventilation while improving oxygenation. However, in severe ARDS, the patients have higher P_L, spontaneous breathing can cause uneven blood flow and airflow distribution, alveoli easily expand excessively, pulmonary vascular resistance increases and decreases pulmonary blood flow in normal ventilation areas, and transpulmonary vascular pressure increases and exacerbates pulmonary edema in dependent areas. Unfortunately, we have not yet seen the publication of studies on the treatment or prognosis of PPV in the patients with COVID-19 until now. However, according to the principle of PPV, a high PPV plays an important role in the monitoring of circulation damage/protection during mechanical ventilation. We hypothesize that the PPV abnormalities in the patients with COVID-19 may be a common phenomenon. Through PPV monitoring, the circulation management of mechanical ventilation can be incorporated into the entire mechanical ventilation and weaning process.

LIMITATIONS OF PPV

When PPV is used as an index to predict fluid responsiveness, we need to clarify whether PPV is positive. We must also be

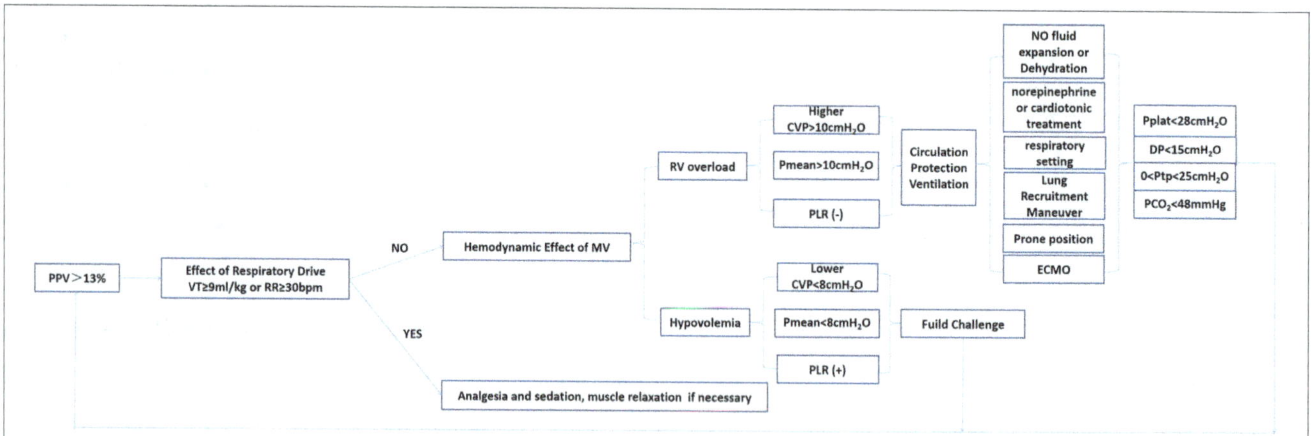

FIGURE 2 | Management and intervention process based on PPV monitoring. PPV, pulse pressure variation; MV, mechanical ventilation; RV, right ventricle; CVP, central venous pressure; P_{mean}, mean airway pressure; PLR, passive leg raising test; ECMO, extracorporeal membrane oxygenation; DP, driving pressure; Ptp, transpulmonary pressure.

alert to the possibility of false negatives and positives and the corresponding reasons. Multiple studies have shown that the threshold index for PPV to assess fluid responsiveness is 13% (8, 28). In the clinical applications, it should be noted that when the tidal volume is >8 ml/kg tidal volume (VT) mechanical ventilation, the PPV fluctuates at "9% < PPV ≤ 13%" and may also prompt the possibility of fluid responsiveness (29). Myatra et al. proposed that PPV is poor in predicting fluid responsiveness at 6 ml/kg VT (AUROC curve, 0.69). When VT increased to 8 ml/kg, PPV more reliably predicted fluid responsiveness (AUROC curve, 0.91). The study also found that during the increase in VT, if the absolute value of PPV increases by ≥3.5%, the fluid responsiveness can be predicted quite accurately (AUROC curve, 0.99) (30). Messina et al. (31) conducted a tidal volume challenge (TVC) in the prone position patients, that is, increasing the tidal volume from 6 to 8 ml/kg in a short period of time, and attempting to use pulse pressure variability and stroke volume variability to assess the fluid responsiveness of a patient. In addition, the studies have pointed out that when the PPV of a patient is >13%, the passive leg raising tests are performed. If the PPV decreases, it indicates that the patient has fluid responsiveness. If the PPV is unchanged, it indicates that the right ventricle afterload of a patient increases (32). Therefore, we must pay attention to the premise of ensuring tidal volume (8 ml/kg PBW) when we use PPV to judge potential fluid responsiveness. Additionally, we can combine or use more indicators for judging fluid responsiveness, for example, transmural central vascular pressure, to further improve the accuracy of PPV (33, 34). However, we may not need to emphasize whether the patient is in a fully controlled ventilation state or whether the tidal volume needs to be increased to 8 ml/kg when we use PPV as an indicator of right ventricle afterload. What we need to pay attention to is whether P_L affects the pulmonary circulation and right heart function. However, the only concern is to identify whether the patient has arrhythmia. Arrhythmia has become the most important obstacle that affects the accurate determination of PPV. In addition, we should also notice the effect of increased intra-abdominal pressure on P_{pl} and P_L. In general, the clinical significance of positive PPV has a new extension and significance than before.

CIRCULATION-PROTECTIVE VENTILATION STRATEGY

At present, the lung-protection ventilation strategies have been affirmed and widely used, such as low tidal volume, limiting plateau pressure (<27 cmH_2O), and driving pressure (<15 cmH_2O), to reduce lung stress injury caused by mechanical ventilation. Recruitment maneuver and perform reasonable PEEP titration can also be considered. Applying P_L monitoring achieves the end-expiratory P_L > 0 cmH_2O and end-inspiratory P_L < 25 cmH_2O. As high $PaCO_2$ can aggravate pulmonary vasoconstriction, treatment should be used to limit hypercapnia ($PaCO_2$ < 48 mmHg). Prone position ventilation is used to reduce pulmonary circulation resistance, improve ventilation and blood flow matching, and improve right heart function. Therefore, based on the above treatment to prevent secondary injury (35), what else can we do? A new understanding of PPV will help us to protect the circulation during mechanical ventilation. After the relevant circulation-protective ventilation treatment, the criterion for whether we successfully protect circulation is whether the PPV returns to normal. Therefore, in the process of related lung protection ventilation, the following circulation-protective procedures can be considered to guide our mechanical ventilation to achieve lower PPV, such as evaluating and treating the spontaneous breathing effort and respiratory support conditions and monitoring and optimizing the flow status and volume status of a patient. Combined with our previous studies (36, 37), we propose a possible processing procedure for the PPV abnormalities, as shown in **Figure 2**.

In summary, we should pay attention to the role of P_{pl} and P_L in the cardiopulmonary interaction and their effect on blood flow. We should be sufficiently aware of the universality of increased right ventricle afterload caused by mechanical ventilation. PPV is an indicator that can help us distinguish the causes of decreased cardiac output and has become a necessary indicator for monitoring circulatory damage in ARDS during mechanical ventilation. At the bedside, we can adjust our mechanical ventilation parameter by monitoring the PPV to achieve circulation-protective mechanical ventilation. Therefore, we believe that PPV is the starting point to achieve circulation-protective mechanical ventilation. During mechanical ventilation, PPV should be continuously monitored, and its abnormalities should be treated clinically and dealt with immediately instead of shelving.

AUTHOR CONTRIBUTIONS

PP, LS, and HH wrote the manuscript. DL and YL responsible to this manuscript. All authors contributed to the article and approved the submitted version.

REFERENCES

1. Grieco DL, Menga LS, Eleuteri D, Antonelli M. Patient self-inflicted lung injury: implications for acute hypoxemic respiratory failure and ARDS patients on non-invasive support. *Minerva Anestesiol.* (2019) 85:1014–23. doi: 10.23736/S0375-9393.19.13418-9

2. Yoshida T, Grieco DL, Brochard L, Fujino Y. Patient self-inflicted lung injury and positive end-expiratory pressure for safe spontaneous breathing. *Curr Opin Crit Care.* (2020) 26:59–65. doi: 10.1097/MCC.0000000000000691

3. Jardin F, Farcot JC, Gueret P, Prost JF, Ozier Y, Bourdarias JP. Cyclic changes in arterial pulse during respiratory support. *Circulation.* (1983) 68:266–74. doi: 10.1161/01.cir.68.2.266
4. Robotham JL, Cherry D, Mitzner W, Rabson JL, Lixfeld W, Bromberger-Barnea B. A re-evaluation of the hemodynamic consequences of intermittent positive pressure ventilation. *Crit Care Med.* (1983) 11:783–93. doi: 10.1097/00003246-198310000-00005
5. Pinsky MR. The influence of positive-pressure ventilation on cardiovascular function in the critically ill. *Crit Care Clin.* (1985) 1:699–717
6. Su LX, Liu DW. Personalized critical hemodynamic therapy concept for shock resuscitation. *Chin Med J.* (2018) 131:1240–3. doi: 10.4103/0366-6999.231511
7. Michard F, Boussat S, Chemla D, Anguel N, Mercat A, Lecarpentier Y, et al. Relation between respiratory changes in arterial pulse pressure and fluid responsiveness in septic patients with acute circulatory failure. *Am J Respir Crit Care Med.* (2000) 162:134–8. doi: 10.1164/ajrccm.162.1.9903035
8. Yang X, Du B. Does pulse pressure variation predict fluid responsiveness in critically ill patients? A systematic review and meta-analysis. *Crit Care.* (2014) 18:650. doi: 10.1186/s13054-014-0650-6
9. Vieillard-Baron A, Loubieres Y, Schmitt JM, Page B, Dubourg O, Jardin F. Cyclic changes in right ventricular output impedance during mechanical ventilation. *J Appl Physiol.* (1999) 87:1644–50. doi: 10.1152/jappl.1999.87.5.1644
10. Michard F, Teboul JL. Using heart-lung interactions to assess fluid responsiveness during mechanical ventilation. *Crit Care.* (2000) 4:282–9. doi: 10.1186/cc710
11. Jardin F, Genevray B, Brun-Ney D, Bourdarias JP. Influence of lung and chest wall compliances on transmission of airway pressure to the pleural space in critically ill patients. *Chest.* (1985) 88:653–8. doi: 10.1378/chest.88.5.653
12. Freitas FG, Bafi AT, Nascente AP, Assuncao M, Mazza B, Azevedo LC, et al. Predictive value of pulse pressure variation for fluid responsiveness in septic patients using lung-protective ventilation strategies. *Br J Anaesth.* (2013) 110:402–8. doi: 10.1093/bja/aes398
13. Michard F, Chemla D, Richard C, Wysocki M, Pinsky MR, Lecarpentier Y, et al. Clinical use of respiratory changes in arterial pulse pressure to monitor the hemodynamic effects of PEEP. *Am J Respir Crit Care Med.* (1999) 159:935–9. doi: 10.1164/ajrccm.159.3.9805077
14. Wyler von Ballmoos M, Takala J, Roeck M, Porta F, Tueller D, Ganter CC, et al. Pulse-pressure variation and hemodynamic response in patients with elevated pulmonary artery pressure: a clinical study. *Crit Care.* (2010) 14:R111. doi: 10.1186/cc9060
15. Mahjoub Y, Pila C, Friggeri A, Zogheib E, Lobjoie E, Tinturier F, et al. Assessing fluid responsiveness in critically ill patients: false-positive pulse pressure variation is detected by Doppler echocardiographic evaluation of the right ventricle. *Crit Care Med.* (2009) 37:2570–5. doi: 10.1097/CCM.0b013e3181a380a3
16. Cortes-Puentes GA, Oeckler RA, Marini JJ. Physiology-guided management of hemodynamics in acute respiratory distress syndrome. *Ann Transl Med.* (2018) 6:353. doi: 10.21037/atm.2018.04.40
17. Dreyfuss D, Soler P, Basset G, Saumon G. High inflation pressure pulmonary edema. Respective effects of high airway pressure, high tidal volume, and positive end-expiratory pressure. *Am Rev Respir Dis.* (1988) 137:1159–64. doi: 10.1164/ajrccm/137.5.1159
18. Raj JU, Bland RD, Lai-Fook SJ. Microvascular pressures measured by micropipettes in isolated edematous rabbit lungs. *J Appl Physiol.* (1986) 60:539–45. doi: 10.1152/jappl.1986.60.2.539
19. Yoshida T, Torsani V, Gomes S, De Santis RR, Beraldo MA, Costa EL, et al. Spontaneous effort causes occult pendelluft during mechanical ventilation. *Am J Respir Crit Care Med.* (2013) 188:1420–7. doi: 10.1164/rccm.201303-0539OC
20. Vieillard-Baron A, Prin S, Schmitt JM, Augarde R, Page B, Beauchet A, et al. Pressure-volume curves in acute respiratory distress syndrome: clinical demonstration of the influence of expiratory flow limitation on the initial slope. *Am J Respir Crit Care Med.* (2002) 165:1107–12. doi: 10.1164/ajrccm.165.8.2106104
21. Tabuchi A, Nickles HT, Kim M, Semple JW, Koch E, Brochard L, et al. Acute lung injury causes asynchronous alveolar ventilation that can be corrected by individual sighs. *Am J Respir Crit Care Med.* (2016) 193:396–406. doi: 10.1164/rccm.201505-0901OC
22. Gattinoni L, Chiumello D, Rossi S. COVID-19 pneumonia: ARDS or not? *Crit Care.* (2020) 24:154. doi: 10.1186/s13054-020-02880-z
23. Vaporidi K, Akoumianaki E, Telias I, Goligher EC, Brochard L, Georgopoulos D. Respiratory drive in critically ill patients. Pathophysiology and clinical implications. *Am J Respir Crit Care Med.* (2020) 201:20–32. doi: 10.1164/rccm.201903-0596SO
24. Brochard L, Slutsky A, Pesenti A. Mechanical ventilation to minimize progression of lung injury in acute respiratory failure. *Am J Respir Crit Care Med.* (2017) 195:438–42. doi: 10.1164/rccm.201605-1081CP
25. Neumann P, Wrigge H, Zinserling J, Hinz J, Maripuu E, Andersson LG, et al. Spontaneous breathing affects the spatial ventilation and perfusion distribution during mechanical ventilatory support. *Crit Care Med.* (2005) 33:1090–5. doi: 10.1097/01.ccm.0000163226.34868.0a
26. Glenny RW. Determinants of regional ventilation and blood flow in the lung. *Intensive Care Med.* (2009) 35:1833–42. doi: 10.1007/s00134-009-1649-3
27. Gattinoni L, Chiumello D, Caironi P, Busana M, Romitti F, Brazzi L, et al. COVID-19 pneumonia: different respiratory treatments for different phenotypes? *Intensive Care Med.* (2020) 46:1099–102. doi: 10.1007/s00134-020-06033-2
28. Bentzer P, Griesdale DE, Boyd J, MacLean K, Sirounis D, Ayas NT. Will this hemodynamically unstable patient respond to a bolus of intravenous fluids? *JAMA.* (2016) 316:1298–309. doi: 10.1001/jama.2016.12310
29. Min JJ, Gil NS, Lee JH, Ryu DK, Kim CS, Lee SM. Predictor of fluid responsiveness in the 'grey zone': augmented pulse pressure variation through a temporary increase in tidal volume. *Br J Anaesth.* (2017) 119:50–6. doi: 10.1093/bja/aex074
30. Myatra SN, Prabu NR, Divatia JV, Monnet X, Kulkarni AP, Teboul JL. The changes in pulse pressure variation or stroke volume variation after a "tidal volume challenge" reliably predict fluid responsiveness during low tidal volume ventilation. *Crit Care Med.* (2017) 45:415–21. doi: 10.1097/CCM.0000000000002183
31. Messina A, Montagnini C, Cammarota G, Giuliani F, Muratore L, Baggiani M, et al. Assessment of fluid responsiveness in prone neurosurgical patients undergoing protective ventilation: role of dynamic indices, tidal volume challenge, and end-expiratory occlusion test. *Anesth Analg.* (2020) 130:752–61. doi: 10.1213/ANE.0000000000004494
32. Teboul JL, Monnet X, Chemla D, Michard F. Arterial pulse pressure variation with mechanical ventilation. *Am J Respir Crit Care Med.* (2019) 199:22–31. doi: 10.1164/rccm.201801-0088CI
33. Westphal GA, Silva E, Caldeira Filho M, Roman Goncalves AR, Poli-de-Figueiredo LF. Variation in amplitude of central venous pressure curve induced by respiration is a useful tool to reveal fluid responsiveness in postcardiac surgery patients. *Shock.* (2006) 26:140–145. doi: 10.1097/01.shk.0000227439.76418.7d
34. Magder S. Understanding central venous pressure: not a preload index? *Curr Opin Crit Care.* (2015) 21:369–75. doi: 10.1097/MCC.0000000000000238
35. Pan P, Su LX, Liu DW, Wang XT, Chinese Critical Ultrasound Study Group. (2021). Acute respiratory distress syndrome: focusing on secondary injury. *Chin Med J.* (2021) 134:2017. doi: 10.1097/CM9.0000000000001694
36. Pan P, Su L, Zhang Q, Long Y, Wang X, Liu D. Effects of quality control targets (SpO_2 not equal 100%, $PaCO_2$ $\leq$40 mmHg, Pmean $\geq$ 10 cmH_2O) on outcomes in patients in the ICU. *Front Med.* (2020) 7:111. doi: 10.3389/fmed.2020.00111
37. Su L, Pan P, Liu D, Long Y. Mean airway pressure has the potential to become the core pressure indicator of mechanical ventilation: raising to the front from behind the clinical scenes. *J Inten Med.* (2021). doi: 10.1016/j.jointm.2021.04.002

8

Association of Time–Varying Intensity of Ventilation with Mortality in Patients with COVID–19 ARDS: Secondary Analysis of the PRoVENT–COVID Study

Michiel T. U. Schuijt[1], David M. P. van Meenen[1], Ignacio Martin–Loeches[2], Guido Mazzinari[3], Marcus J. Schultz[1,4,5], Frederique Paulus[1,6] and Ary Serpa Neto[1,7,8,9,10,11] for the 'PRactice of VENTilation in COVID-19' (PRoVENT-COVID) Collaborative Group*

[1] Department of Intensive Care, Amsterdam UMC, Location AMC, Amsterdam, Netherlands, [2] Department of Clinical Medicine, Trinity Centre for Health Sciences, Multidisciplinary Intensive Care Research Organization (MICRO), St James's Hospital, Dublin, Ireland, [3] Department of Anaesthesiology, Hospital Universitario y Politécnico la Fe, Valencia, Spain, [4] Mahidol Oxford Tropical Medicine Research Unit (MORU), Mahidol University, Bangkok, Thailand, [5] Nuffield Department of Medicine, University of Oxford, Oxford, United Kingdom, [6] ACHIEVE, Centre of Applied Research, Amsterdam University of Applied Sciences, Faculty of Health, Amsterdam, Netherlands, [7] Australian and New Zealand Intensive Care Research Centre (ANZIC–RC), Monash University, Melbourne, VIC, Australia, [8] Department of Intensive Care, Austin Hospital, Melbourne, VIC, Australia, [9] Data Analytics Research and Evaluation (DARE) Centre, Austin Hospital, Melbourne, VIC, Australia, [10] Department of Critical Care, Melbourne Medical School, University of Melbourne, Melbourne, VIC, Australia, [11] Department of Critical Care Medicine, Hospital Israelita Albert Einstein, São Pãulo, Brazil

***Correspondence:**
Ary Serpa Neto
ary.serpaneto@monash.edu

Background: High intensity of ventilation has an association with mortality in patients with acute respiratory failure. It is uncertain whether similar associations exist in patients with acute respiratory distress syndrome (ARDS) patients due to coronavirus disease 2019 (COVID–19). We investigated the association of exposure to different levels of driving pressure (ΔP) and mechanical power (MP) with mortality in these patients.

Methods: PRoVENT–COVID is a national, retrospective observational study, performed at 22 ICUs in the Netherlands, including COVID–19 patients under invasive ventilation for ARDS. Dynamic ΔP and MP were calculated at fixed time points during the first 4 calendar days of ventilation. The primary endpoint was 28–day mortality. To assess the effects of time–varying exposure, Bayesian joint models adjusted for confounders were used.

Results: Of 1,122 patients included in the PRoVENT–COVID study, 734 were eligible for this analysis. In the first 28 days, 29.2% of patients died. A significant increase in the hazard of death was found to be associated with each increment in ΔP (HR 1.04, 95% CrI 1.01–1.07) and in MP (HR 1.12, 95% CrI 1.01–1.36). In sensitivity analyses, cumulative exposure to higher levels of ΔP or MP resulted in increased risks for 28–day mortality.

Conclusion: Cumulative exposure to higher intensities of ventilation in COVID–19 patients with ARDS have an association with increased risk of 28–day mortality. Limiting exposure to high ΔP or MP has the potential to improve survival in these patients.

Clinical Trial Registration: www.ClinicalTrials.gov, identifier: NCT04346342.

Keywords: coronavirus disease 2019, acute respiratory distress syndrome, driving pressure, mechanical power, mortality

INTRODUCTION

The coronavirus disease 2019 (COVID−19) is an infection caused by the highly contagious Severe Acute Respiratory Coronavirus−2 (SARS-CoV−2), of which the first outbreak was reported in Wuhan, China in the beginning of December, 2019 (1). Worldwide, healthcare workers are faced with surges of infected patients who need hospitalization and eventually admission to an intensive care unit (ICU) because of need for invasive ventilation. The care of coronavirus disease 2019 (COVID−19) patients receiving ventilation is challenging and the outcomes are poor (2). Mortality rates as high as 50% have been reported in invasively ventilated COVID−19 patients that develop acute respiratory distress syndrome (ARDS) (2).

Different ventilation strategies have been studied in the setting of acute respiratory failure, and evidence from randomized clinical trials supports the use of ventilation with a low tidal volume (V_T) and a low plateau pressure to decrease the risk of ventilator-induced lung injury (VILI) in patients with acute respiratory distress syndrome (ARDS) (3-5). There is increasing interest in limiting exposure to driving pressure (ΔP) and mechanical power (MP) in invasively ventilated patients (6-8). ΔP, the pressure applied by the ventilator to support the delivery of tidal volume, (7) is a surrogate for cyclic lung strain (9). MP, a parameter that combines several ventilatory variables, including respiratory rate (RR), V_T, flow and ΔP, represents the amount of energy transferred from the ventilator to the respiratory system (8, 10). Associations of ΔP and MP with outcomes in patients receiving mechanical ventilation is well described (7, 8, 11-19).

A potential limitation of earlier studies is the inclusion of patients with spontaneous efforts during ventilation (18, 20). Even if appropriately adjusted for resistance, flow, and chest wall elastance, any estimate of these variables during spontaneous efforts would reflect both the ventilator's contribution and respiratory muscle activity, and thus would not represent the total energy imparted during inflation (20). Also, mechanical ventilation is a dynamic process, and thus far only one investigation studied the cumulative effect of ΔP and MP beyond baseline (12). To date, there have been no studies that assessed the impact of intensity of ventilation on outcome of COVID−19 patients with ARDS. To ascertain the effect of time-varying exposure to different levels of ΔP and MP on 28-day mortality in COVID−19 patients with ARDS, we conducted a secondary analysis of a national multicenter investigation, named the "PRactive of VENTilation in COVID−19" (PRoVENT-COVID) study. Our objectives were to estimate the effects of different levels of ΔP and MP over the first 4 days of ventilation on 28-day mortality in COVID−19 patients with ARDS, and whether there was a cumulative effect of exposure over time. We hypothesized that intensity of ventilation has an association with mortality in patients with COVID−19 ARDS, in a similar way as has been described in patients with ARDS from another cause.

METHODS

Study Design and Participants

This is a preplanned secondary analysis of the "Practice of VENTilation in COVID−19" (PRoVENT-COVID) study, an investigator-initiated, multicenter, observational cohort study in patients with COVID−19 ARDS undertaken at 22 ICUs during the first 3 months of the pandemic in the Netherlands (21-23). The protocol of the PRoVENT-COVID study was prepublished, (21) and the statistical analysis plan for the current analysis, finalized before assessing the database, is available online (22). The institutional review boards of each participating center approved the study protocol, and need for individual patient informed consent was waived based on the observational nature of the study. Study sites were recruited through direct contact by members of the steering committee of the PRoVENT-COVID study. Study coordinators contacted the local doctors, trained and helped the data collectors, and monitored the study according to the International Conference on Harmonization Good Clinical Practice-guidelines. Integrity and timely completion of data collection was ensured by the study coordinators.

Consecutive patients aged 18 yr or older were eligible for participation if they were admitted to one of the participating ICUs and had received invasive mechanical ventilation for COVID−19 ARDS. The PRoVENT-COVID study itself had no exclusion criteria—for the current analysis we excluded patients if they had spontaneous breathing activity in more than half the observations, or when life status was unknown at day 28.

Procedures and Outcome

Demographics and data regarding premorbid diseases and home medication were collected at baseline. In the first hour of invasive ventilation, and every 8 h thereafter at fixed time points ventilator settings and parameters were collected up to day 4. Since plateau pressure was not recorded in the current study, all measurements of dynamic ΔP were calculated as peak inspiratory pressure (P_{peak}) minus positive end-expiratory pressure. Dynamic MP was calculated as $0.098 * RR * VT * [P_{peak} - (0.5 \times \text{dynamic } \Delta P)]$. Both variables were calculated only considering moments without evidence of spontaneous breathing (additional information in **eMethods** in **Supplementary Information**). The Berlin definition for ARDS was used for classification of severity as mild, moderate and severe (24).

The primary outcome was 28-day mortality. In secondary analyses, we investigated whether the strength of association between intensity of ventilation and 28-day mortality changed over time. In addition, we quantified the effect of cumulative response, and we examined whether ARDS severity class changed the effects of time-varying ΔP and MP on 28-day mortality.

Analysis Plan

For the final assessment, patients receiving ventilation without evidence of spontaneous breathing at less than 50% of the available timepoints were identified and deselected

TABLE 1 | Baseline patient characteristics and outcomes.

	Participants (*n* = 734)
Age, years	65 (57–72)
Male gender–no (%)	540 (73.6)
Body mass index, kg/m^2	27.8 (25.4–31.1)
Transferred under invasive ventilation	109 (14.9)
Days between intubation and admission	0.0 (0.0–0.0)
Use of non-invasive ventilation prior to intubation–no (%)	66/661 (10.0)
Duration of non-invasive ventilation, hours	6 (2–14)
Chest CT scan performed–no (%)	254/715 (35.5)
Lung parenchyma affected–no (%)	
0%	9/254 (3.5)
25%	77/254 (30.3)
50%	80/254 (31.5)
75%	71/254 (28.0)
100%	17/254 (6.7)
Chest X-ray performed–no (%)	397/455 (87.3)
Quadrants affected–no (%)	
1	28/395 (7.1)
2	97/395 (24.6)
3	117/395 (29.6)
4	153/395 (38.7)
Severity of ARDS–no (%)	
Mild	65 (8.9)
Moderate	424 (57.8)
Severe	245 (33.4)
Co-existing disorders–no (%)	
Hypertension	247 (33.7)
Heart failure	27 (3.7)
Diabetes	163 (22.2)
Chronic kidney disease	29 (4.0)
Baseline creatinine, μmol/L*	78 (62–100)
Liver cirrhosis	2 (0.3)
Chronic obstructive pulmonary disease	62 (8.4)
Active hematological neoplasia	9 (1.2)
Active solid neoplasia	21 (2.9)
Neuromuscular disease	3 (0.4)
Immunosuppression	15 (2.0)
Previous medication–no (%)	
Systemic steroids	28 (3.8)
Inhalation steroids	83 (11.3)
Angiotensin converting enzyme inhibitor	126 (17.2)
Angiotensin II receptor blocker	81 (11.0)
Beta-blockers	131 (17.8)
Insulin	46 (6.3)
Metformin	116 (15.8)
Statins	217 (29.6)
Calcium channel blockers	137 (18.7)
Vital signs at day 01	
Heart rate, bpm**	84 (74–98)
Mean arterial pressure, mmHg**	80 (73–88)
Laboratory tests at day 01	
pH**	7.36 (7.30–7.41)
Worst PaO_2/FiO_2, mmHg***	117 (91–154)
$PaCO_2$, mmHg**	45 (39–51)
Lactate mmol/L**	1.2 (0.9–1.5)
Organ support at day 01–no (%)	
Continuous sedation	703/732 (96.0)
Inotropic or vasopressor	574/732 (78.4)
Vasopressor	573/732 (78.3)
Inotropic	37/732 (5.1)
Fluid balance, mL****	637 (77–1445)
Urine output, mL****	675 (360–1116)
Ventilation support at day 01	
Assisted ventilation–no (%)[a]	185/731 (25.3)
Volume controlled	125/731 (17.1)
Pressure controlled	421/731 (57.6)
Pressure support	12/731 (1.6)
Synchronized intermittent mandatory ventilation	68/731 (9.3)
Airway pressure release ventilation	3/731 (0.4)
INTELLiVENT-ASV	12/731 (1.6)
Other	90/731 (12.3)
Tidal volume, mL/kg PBW**[b]	6.3 (5.9–7.0)
Tidal volume ≤ 8 mL/kg PBW	609 (95.9)
PEEP, cmH_2O**[b]	13 (12–15)
Peak pressure, cmH_2O**[b]	27 (24–30)
Driving pressure, cmH_2O**[b]	14 (12–16)
Driving pressure > 15 cmH_2O	206/640 (32.2)
Mechanical power, J/min**[b]	18.9 (15.7–22.8)
Mechanical power > 17 J/min	381/640 (59.5)
Dynamic compliance, mL/cmH_2O**[b]	32 (27–40)
Total respiratory rate, mpm**[b]	22 (20–24)
Set respiratory rate, mpm**[b]	22 (20–24)
Minute ventilation, L/min**[b]	9.5 (8.4–11.0)
FiO_2**	0.60 (0.50–0.70)
$etCO_2$, mmHg**	37 (32–42)
Rescue therapy at day 01–no (%)	
Prone positioning	225/719 (31.3)
Duration, hours	8 (4–12)
Recruitment maneuver	15/590 (2.5)
ECMO	
Use of NMBA	212/731 (29.0)
Hours of use of use	0 (0–8)
Clinical outcome	
28-day mortality	214 (29.2)

Data are median (quartile 25%–quartile 75%) or No (%). Percentages may not total 100 because of rounding. CT, computed tomography; PEEP positive end expiratory pressure; ECMO, extracorporeal membrane oxygenation; FiO_2, inspired fraction of oxygen; PEEP, positive end-expiratory pressure; NMBA, neuromuscular blocking agent.

**Most recent measurement in 24 h before intubation, or at ICU admission under invasive ventilation.*

***Aggregate as the mean of a maximum of four values.*

****Worst value of four available.*

*****Collected in the period after intubation or ICU admission with ventilation until 24:00.*

[a]Assisted ventilation defined as any mode other than pressure or volume controlled. The mode of ventilation reported is the mode used 1 h after intubation.

[b]Only assessed in moments without spontaneous breathing activity.

(**Supplementary Information eMethods**). Continuous variables were reported as median (25th - 75th percentile) and compared with Wilcoxon rank–sum tests, and categorical variables as number and percentage, and compared with Fisher exact tests. The following variables were considered for adjustment in all models described below: age, gender, body mass index, PaO_2 to FiO_2 ratio, plasma creatinine, medical history of hypertension, heart failure, diabetes, chronic kidney disease, chronic obstructive pulmonary disease, active hematological neoplasia and/or active solid tumor, use of angiotensin converting enzyme inhibitors, use of angiotensin II receptor blockers, use of a vasopressor or inotropes, fluid balance, arterial pH, mean arterial pressure, and heart rate. These baseline covariates were selected according to clinical relevànce and as used in previous study (23). Finally, all continuous variables were standardized to interpret their effect on outcome in standard deviation units.

To estimate the association of subject-specific longitudinal profiles of either ΔP and MP with 28–day mortality, we used Bayesian joint models with shared random effects and adjusted for the covariates described above (25, 26). The repeated values of ΔP and MP (a maximum of 13 measurements) were included as time–varying exposure variables. Natural cubic splines were used in both the fixed–effects and random–effects models to account for the non-linearity of the longitudinal exposure profiles. To investigate whether the association between ΔP and MP and 28–day mortality changed over time, p–splines were included in an interaction term and presented in time–varying plots. Estimation of Bayesian joint model was done considering 28,000 iterations, 3,000 adapt, 3,000 burn–in, and 50 of thinning. Model diagnostics were done by visual inspection of the diagnostic plots. These results were presented as hazard ratios with corresponding 95% credible intervals (CrI).

To further expand the findings of the original model, 3 additional analyses were performed. First, the model described above was expanded to a multivariate joint model. In addition to the baseline covariates, the following time–varying covariates were included: daily use of prone positioning and daily use of inotropes or vasopressors. Second, the calculation of dynamic ΔP and MP were further restricted to moments when a neuromuscular blocking agent was administered, thereby decreasing the chance of including moments at which a patient was having spontaneous breathing activity. Third, patients with missing data in their 28–day vital status were not excluded but assessed in 2 different scenarios: i. best–case scenario (these patients were all considered alive at day 28); and ii. worst–case scenario (these patients were all considered to have died before or at day 28).

Three sensitivity analyses were added. First, to quantify the effect of cumulative exposure, we estimate the association between the percentage of moments with high ΔP and MP and 28–day mortality. The cut–off used to determine high ΔP was 15 cm H_2O; the cut–off used for high MP was 17 J/min (7, 8, 12, 27). Second, we investigated the relationship between cumulative dose and 28–day mortality using the area under the ΔP and MP time curve above the thresholds described above divided by the number of hours of exposure, as a measure of dose. Using this definition, 1 cm H_2O or 1 J/min of dose describes that a patient's average ΔP and MP were 1 cmH_2O or 1 J/min per mL/cm H_2O above the thresholds described for the duration of the exposure window. Third, we investigated the impact of time–weighted average ΔP and MP calculated as the area under the ΔP and MP time curve divided by the number of hours of exposure. For these 3 exposures, the impact on outcome was assessed using (shared–frailty) Cox proportional hazard models adjusted by the covariates described above.

The models were reassessed in a subgroup analysis according to ARDS severity at baseline (24). The models were repeated, considering an interaction between ΔP and MP and ARDS severity at baseline. The amount of missing data is < 3% for the variables of interest, as shown in the **Appendix** (**Supplementary Information Table 1**). For the final models, missing data in covariates were imputed by the median due to the low number of missing, and in the repeated measurements of ΔP and MP over the days a linear imputation was used (**Supplementary Information Figure 1**). All analyses were performed using R version 4.0.2 (R Foundation for Statistical Computing), and a $p < 0.05$ was considered significant. *P* values for the Bayesian models were calculated as the tail probabilities using the formula $2 \times \min\{P(\theta > 0), P(\theta < 0)\}$, with θ denoting the corresponding regression coefficient from the survival submodel.

RESULTS

From March 1, 2020, through June 1, 2020, 31 ICUs were invited for participation in the PRoVENT–COVID study, and 22 met inclusion criteria. A total of 1,340 individuals were screened. Of the 1,122 invasively ventilated COVID−19 patients, 734 (66.6%) were included in the current analysis (**Supplementary Information Figure 2**). Reasons for exclusion were evidence for presence of spontaneous breathing activity in more than 50% of available timepoints of data collection (n = 368), and unknown life status at day 28 (n = 20). Demographic characteristics and ventilation characteristics are presented in **Table 1**. The patients had a median age of 65 yr [IQR 57–72] and 194 (26%) of them were women. 8.9% of the patients had mild ARDS, and 57.8% and 33.4% moderate or severe ARDS, respectively. The most prevalent premorbid conditions were hypertension and diabetes. 29.2% of the patients died within the first 28 days of follow–up. Additional clinical outcomes and use of rescue therapies are presented in the **Appendix** (**Supplementary Information Table 2**).

In the first calendar day of ventilation, median ΔP was 14 (13–17) cm H_2O, and median MP was 18.9 (15.7-22.8) J/min (**Table 1**). ΔP was > 15 cm H_2O in 32.2% of the patients, and MP was > 17 J/min in 59.5% in 66.1% of the patients. ΔP and MP over the first 4 calendar days of ventilation are shown in **Figure 1**.

In the first 4 calendar days of ventilation, and after adjusting for confounders, both a high time–varying ΔP (HR, 1.04 [95% CrI, 1.01–1.07]) and a high time–varying MP (HR, 1.12 [95% CrI, 1.01–1.36]) had an association with increased risk of 28–day mortality (**Table 2**). The strength of the association of ΔP as well as of MP with 28–day

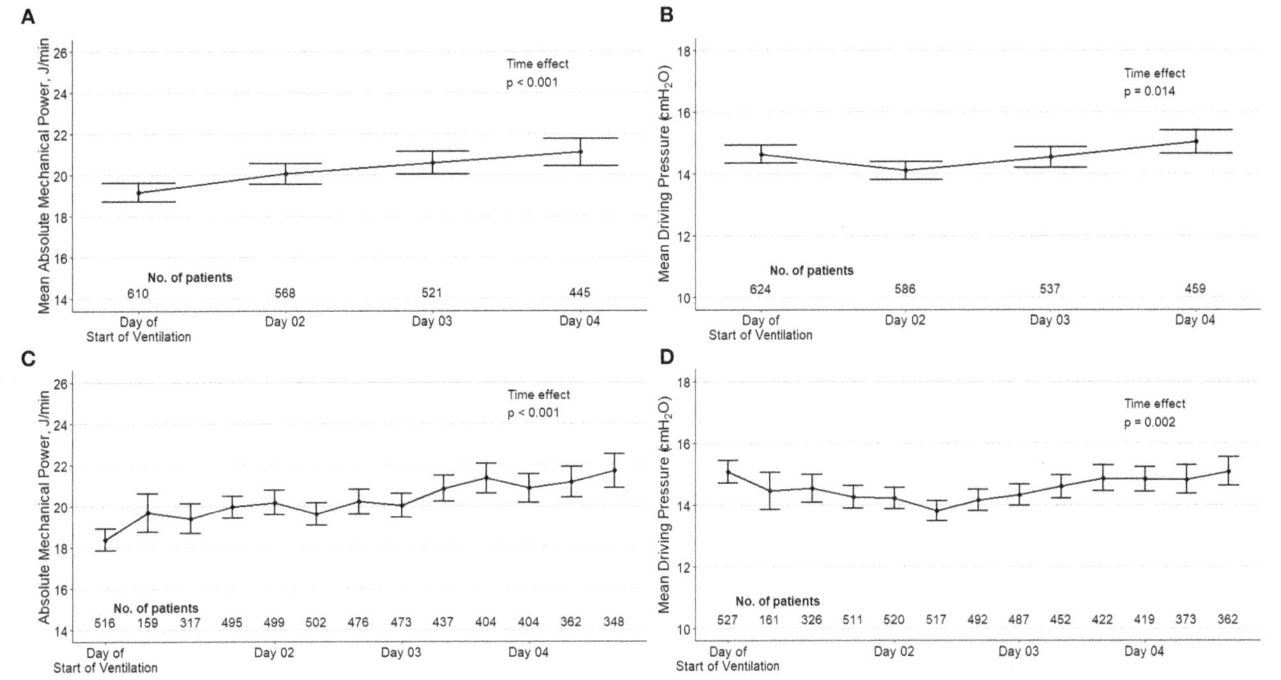

FIGURE 1 | Driving pressure and mechanical power over the first four days of ventilation in the included patients. Top panels **(A, B)**: mean daily values of ΔP and MP according to a maximum of four measurements in the day of start of ventilation and three measurements in the next days. Bottom panels **(C, D)**: ΔP and MP per time point of assessment. Circles are means and error bars are 95% confidence intervals. Both variables were calculated using only measurements without spontaneous breathing activity. *P* values from a mixed-effect model with time as fixed effect (as continuous variable) and patients as random effect to account for repeated measurements.

mortality decreased slightly over the first 4 days (**Figure 2**). As shown in the **Appendix**, the effect of time-varying ΔP was more pronounced in patients with ARDS classified as severe (**Supplementary Information Figure 3**). The full multivariable model is reported in **Supplementary Information Table 3.** After adjustment for the daily use of prone positioning and inotropes or vasopressors, both higher ΔP (HR, 1.04 [95% CrI, 1.00–1.09]) and higher MP (HR, 1.06 [95% CrI, 1.00–1.15]) had an association with increased risk of 28-day mortality (**Table 2**). When restricting the measurements to moment at which neuromuscular blocking agents were administered, both ΔP (HR, 1.38 [95% CrI, 1.14–1.61]) and MP (HR, 1.35 [95% CrI, 1.06–1.73]) had an association with 28-day mortality (**Table 2**). The findings of the best- and worst-case scenario confirmed the findings of the primary analysis (**Table 2**).

The number and percentage of measurements per patient with ΔP > 15 cm H_2O and MP > 17 J/min in the first 4 days of ventilation are shown in the **Appendix** (**Supplementary Information Figure 4**). A higher percentage of measurements with ΔP > 15 cm H_2O (HR, 1.61 [95% CI, 1.03–2.51] $p = 0.037$) or with MP > 17 J/min (HR, 2.42 [95% CI, 1.44–4.07] $p < 0.001$) had an association with increased risk of 28-day mortality (**Figure 3**). Comparison of baseline characteristics and outcomes according to the median ΔP and MP in the first 4 calendar days is shown in **Supplementary Information Table 4.**

Time-weighted average and cumulative dose of ΔP and MP are shown in the **Appendix** (**Supplementary Information Figure 5**). Cumulative dose of ΔP > 15 cm H_2O (HR, 1.09 [95% CI, 1.05–1.14]; $p < 0.001$) and MP > 17 J/min (HR, 1.06 [1.03–1.09]; $p < 0.001$) had an association with increased risk of 28-day mortality (**Figure 3**). In accordance, time-weighted average ΔP (HR, 1.06 [95% CI, 1.03–1.09]; $p < 0.001$) and time-weighted average MP (HR, 1.04 [95% CI, 1.02–1.06]; $p < 0.001$) also had an association with an increased risk on 28-day mortality.

DISCUSSION

The findings of this observational study assessing the impact of time-varying ΔP and MP on 28-day mortality in invasively ventilated COVID–19 patients with ARDS, can be summarized as follows: (1) exposure to both higher ΔP and higher MP during the first 4 calendar days of ventilation had associations with increased risk of 28-day mortality in joint models; and (2) a higher cumulative exposure to ΔP > 15 cm H_2O or MP > 17 J/min over the first 4 days of ventilation had associations with increased risk for 28-day mortality. These findings support the suggestion that limiting the intensity of ventilation in COVID–19 patients with ARDS by using strategies that result in a lower ΔP or MP could improve patient outcome, alike what has been suggested in patients with ARDS from another origin.

TABLE 2 | Multivariable model assessing the association of time-varying driving pressure and mechanical power over the first four days of ventilation with 28-day mortality.

	Time-varying models		Models of cumulative exposure	
	Hazard ratio (95% CrI)	***p* value***	**Hazard ratio (95% CI)**	***p* value**
Time-varying models (main models)				
Driving pressure	1.04 (1.01 to 1.07)	0.010	–	–
Mechanical power	1.12 (1.01 to 1.36)	0.018	–	–
Sensitivity time-varying models				
Multivariate joint model**				
Driving pressure	1.04 (1.00 to 1.09)	0.030	–	–
Mechanical power	1.06 (1.00 to 1.15)	0.049	–	–
Restricted to moments when NMBA was used				
Driving pressure	1.38 (1.14 to 1.61)	<0.001	–	–
Mechanical power	1.35 (1.06 to 1.73)	<0.001	–	–
Best-case scenario***				
Driving pressure	1.03 (1.01 to 1.07)	0.007		
Mechanical power	1.13 (1.02 to 1.32)	0.014		
Worst-case scenario***				
Driving pressure	1.03 (1.00 to 1.07)	0.018		
Mechanical power	1.09 (1.01 to 1.22)	0.014		
Models of cumulative exposure				
Percentage of moments with $\Delta P > 15$ cmH_2O	–	–	1.61 (1.03 to 2.51)	0.037
Percentage of moments with $MP > 17$ J/min	–	–	2.42 (1.44 to 4.07)	< 0.001
Cumulative dose of $\Delta P > 15$ cmH_2O	–	–	1.09 (1.05 to 1.14)	< 0.001
Cumulative dose of $MP > 17$ J/min	–	–	1.06 (1.03 to 1.09)	< 0.001
Time-weighted average ΔP	–	–	1.06 (1.03 to 1.09)	< 0.001
Time-weighted average MP	–	–	1.04 (1.02 to 1.06)	< 0.001

CrI, credible interval; CI, confidence interval; NMBA, neuromuscular blocking agents. Hazard ratios were the adjusted hazard ratios associated with a 1-standard deviation increment. Values higher than 1 indicate increased mortality.

**P values calculated as the tail probabilities using the formula 2 x min {P(θ > 0), P(θ < 0)}, with θ denoting the corresponding regression coefficient from the survival submodel.*

***Expansion of the original joint models further adjusted by the following time-varying covariates: daily use of prone positioning and daily use of inotropes or vasopressor.*

****In the best-case scenario, 20 patients with missing in 28-day mortality were considered alive at day 28. In the worst-case scenario, 20 patients with missing in 28-day mortality were considered dead at day 28.*

The findings of our study are in line with previous investigations of ΔP and MP in patients with ARDS from another cause than COVID−19. Indeed, in patients with ARDS from another origin, a higher ΔP and higher MP at baseline have been shown to have an association with increased mortality (7–10, 12–16). A recent study showed the adverse effect of exposure to higher cumulative doses of ΔP and MP over the duration of ventilation in critically ill patients receiving ventilation due to respiratory failure (12). We also found that a high time-varying ΔP and MP, and a higher cumulative exposure to harmful levels of ΔP and MP have an association with increased 28-day mortality, and as in the previous study these effects were more pronounced in patients with more severe forms of ARDS at baseline.

Considering all the available evidence, monitoring intensity of ventilation seems an attractive approach, both in patients with ARDS due to COVID−19 and in patients with ARDS from another origin. Yet, it remains uncertain whether the found association only reflects the relationship between respiratory system compliance and patient outcome. It is also uncertain whether measures to lower the intensity will result in better outcomes. Nevertheless, our results, corrected for baseline covariates and time-varying confounding, could represent a causal effect. Thus, ventilation strategies aiming to lower the intensity of ventilation need to be studied, preferably in randomized clinical trials.

The present cohort of COVID−19 patients with ARDS is comparable to other COVID−19 cohorts in relation to baseline characteristics and clinical outcomes (28–31). Key variables of ventilation management, like V_T, RR and ΔP were comparable to what was described in previous studies in patients with COVID−19, and in line with recommendations for lung-protective ventilation in patients with ARDS (28–31). MP in our cohort was lower than what was reported in one study in COVID−19 patients, (30) suggesting a better adoption of lung-protective ventilation in our study.

Our study has strengths. We restricted the analysis to patients who were without spontaneous breathing activity for the majority of time, and ΔP and MP was only calculated for the moments a patient was passive. Calculation ΔP and MP in the presence of spontaneous breathing is not yet validated. For the main analyses we used joint models, which allows the examination of the effect of

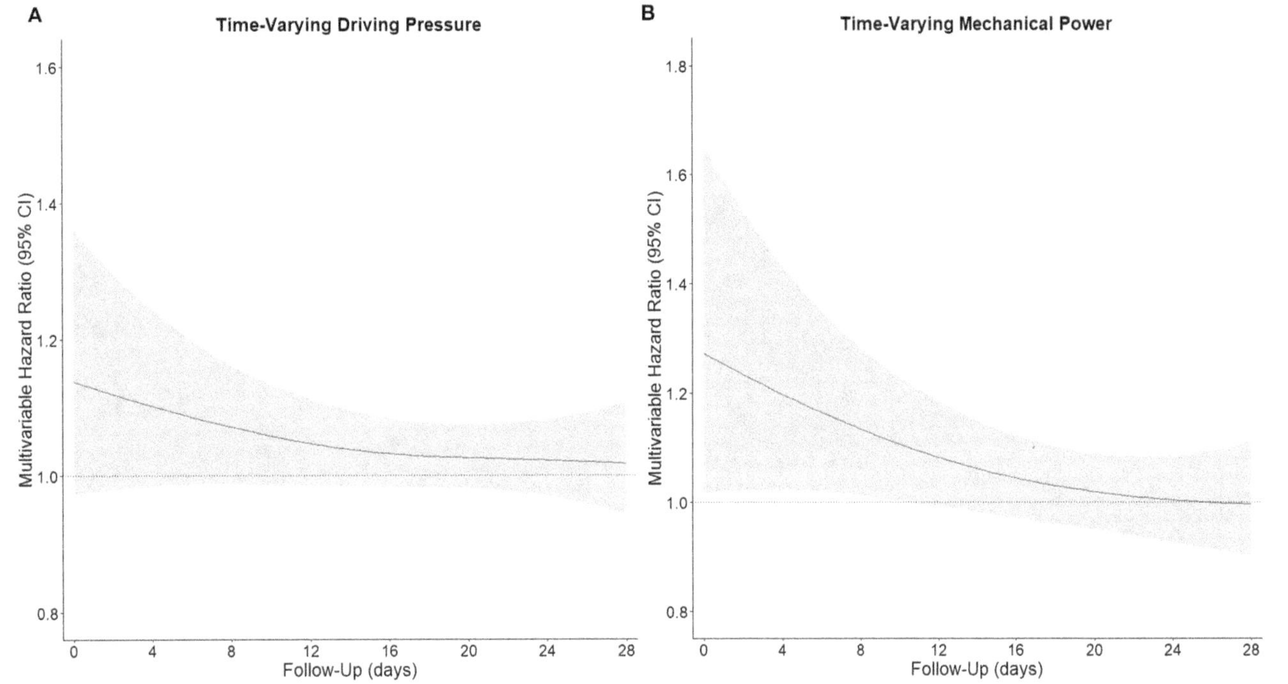

FIGURE 2 | Time-varying hazard ratio of driving pressure and mechanical power for 28-day mortality. **(A)**, Time-varying ΔP, and **(B)** time-varying MP. Time-varying hazard ratio obtained from a Bayesian joint model estimating the association between ΔP and MP and 28-day mortality, including p-splines in an interaction term. The strength of the association decreased over time. All models were adjusted for age, gender, body mass index, PaO_2 to FiO_2 ratio, plasma creatinine, medical history of hypertension, heart failure, diabetes, chronic kidney disease, chronic obstructive pulmonary disease, active hematological neoplasia and/or active solid tumor, use of angiotensin converting enzyme inhibitors, use of angiotensin II receptor blockers, use of a vasopressor or inotropes, fluid balance, arterial pH, mean arterial pressure, and heart rate. Natural cubic splines were used in both the fixed-effects and random-effects models to account for the nonlinearity of the longitudinal exposure profiles.

a time–varying, endogenous covariate on a time–to–event outcome, accounting for non–random dropouts due to death during follow–up.

Our study also has limitations. First, our study was conducted very early in the local outbreak, and anti–inflammatory strategies, like steroids and other treatments such as anti–IL–6, were not yet extensively used. We did not collect data regarding the use of steroids or other anti–inflammatory drugs. Also, we did not collect D–dimer levels and other laboratory tests that may have predictive value, as these were not yet routinely performed so early in the local outbreak. However, the variables used for adjustment are in line with previous studies assessing the impact of ΔP and MP in patients receiving ventilation (12, 14, 15). Our models used several important clinical variables. Of note, we only had measurements of dynamic airway ΔP as plateau or transpulmonary pressures were not routinely connected. Airway ΔP does correlate with transpulmonary ΔP, but it represents a surrogate, which might be affected by other factors. However, recent data suggested that this calculation is reliable (32). Also, we could not adjust for all possible yet unmeasured confounders and due to the observational nature, no causal relationship can be inferred or determined. A high incidence of thromboembolic complications has been found in the present study, which is in line with other reports on COVID–19 patients (33). Pulmonary embolism could cause an increase in dead space, as such affecting the intensity of ventilation. Another limitation is that participating centers did not all use the same disease severity score. Indeed, some centers reported either APACHE II or APACHE IV scores, others used the SAPS II, and some only SOFA scores. These scores cannot be used interchangeably. However, several baseline covariates were used in our models, representing all organ systems, several supportive treatments and pre–existing comorbidities. The mortality rate in our study is lower than that reported in one recent cohort of COVID–19 patients, (2) but higher than in other reports (34, 35). It remains to be determined whether the associations found here are also present in cohorts with other mortality rates. In addition, the models used had some limitations. All baseline covariates were assumed to be measured without error. The joint models assume the correct specification of random effect structure, and all interdependencies between longitudinal and time–to–event outcomes should be explained by the latent, subject–specific random effects structure. Also, there is a risk of residual confounding.

CONCLUSIONS

In conclusion, in this cohort of COVID–19 patients with ARDS, exposure to higher ΔP or MP, or to a higher cumulative exposure

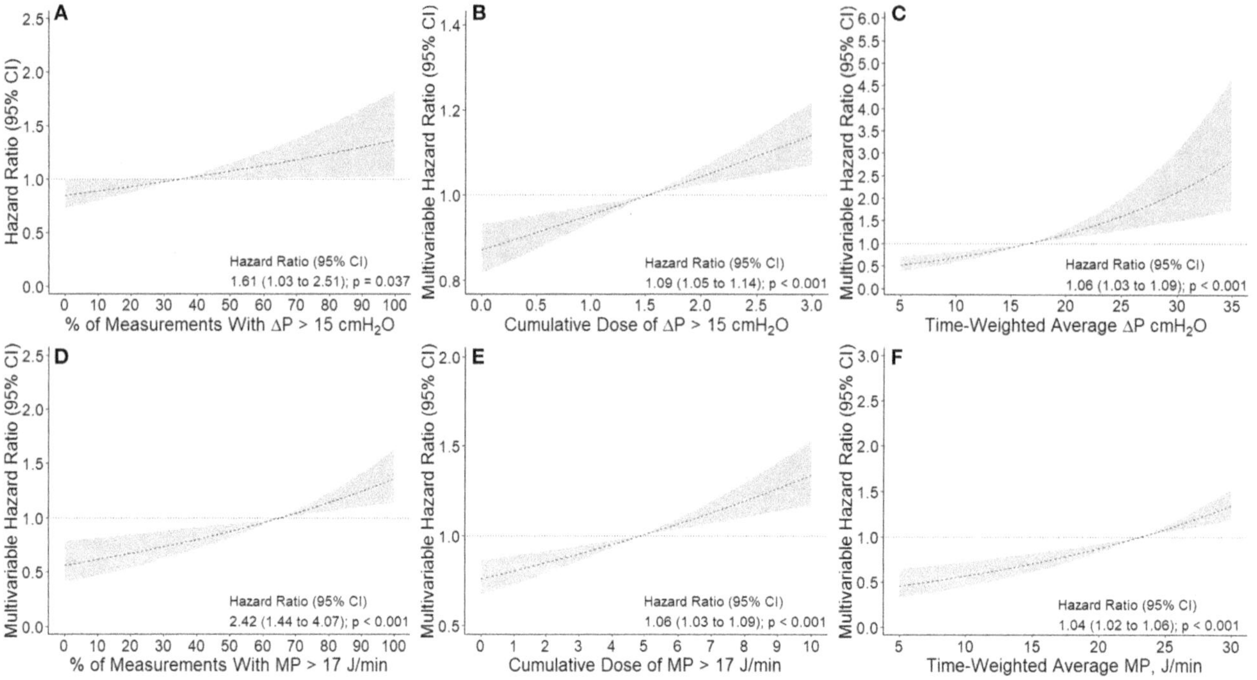

FIGURE 3 | Association between intensity of exposure to higher driving pressure and mechanical power and 28-day mortality. **(A, D):** Association between percentage of measurements with $\Delta P > 15$ cmH_2O and $MP > 17$ J/min and 28-day mortality. Percentage calculated from a maximum of 13 measurements extracted every 8 h. **(B, E):** Association between cumulative dose of $\Delta P > 15$ cmH_2O and $MP > 17$ J/min and 28-day mortality. Cumulative dose calculated as area under the ΔP and MP time curve above the thresholds described above divided by the number of hours of exposure, as a measure of dose. Using this definition, 1 cmH_2O or 1 J/min of dose describes that a patient's average ΔP or MP was 1 cmH_2O or 1 J/min above the thresholds described for the duration of the exposure window, respectively. **(C,F)** Association between time-weighted average ΔP and MP and 28-day mortality. Time-weighted average calculated as the area under the ΔP and MP time curve divided by the number of hours of exposure. All models were adjusted for age, gender, body mass index, PaO_2 to FiO_2 ratio, plasma creatinine, medical history of hypertension, heart failure, diabetes, chronic kidney disease, chronic obstructive pulmonary disease, active hematological neoplasia and/or active solid tumor, use of angiotensin converting enzyme inhibitors, use of angiotensin II receptor blockers, use of a vasopressor or inotropes, fluid balance, arterial pH, mean arterial pressure, and heart rate. Dashed lines and gray areas represent hazard ratio and 95% confidence interval for increasing values the variable analyzed as a continuous variable and centralized in the mean of each variable. *ΔP is driving pressure and MP is mechanical power.*

to a $\Delta P > 15$ cm H_2O or a $MP > 17$ J/min over the first 4 calendar days of ventilation had associations with increased risk for 28-day mortality. To ascertain a causal relationship between ΔP and MP with mortality, randomized clinical trials are needed.

ETHICS STATEMENT

The studies involving human participants were reviewed and approved by the institutional review boards of each participating center. Written informed consent for participation was not required for this study in accordance with the national legislation and the institutional requirements.

PROVENT-COVID COLLABORATIVE GROUP

Monitored email address: provent-covid@amsterdamumc.nl.
Investigators: J.P. van Akkeren; A.G. Algera; C.K. Algoe; R.B. van Amstel; O.L. Baur; P. van de Berg; D.C.J.J. Bergmans; D.I. van den Bersselaar; F.A. Bertens; A.J.G.H. Bindels; M.M. de Boer; S. den Boer; L.S. Boers; M. Bogerd; L.D.J. Bos; M. Botta; J.S. Breel; H. de Bruin; S. de Bruin; C.L. Bruna; L.A. Buiteman-Kruizinga; O. Cremer; R.M. Determann; W. Dieperink; D.A. Dongelmans; H.S. Franke; M.S. Galek Aldridge; M.J. de Graaff; L.A. Hagens; J.J. Haringman; N.F.L. Heijnen; S.Hiel; S.T. van der Heide; P.L.J. van der Heiden; L.L. Hoeijmakers; L. Hol; M. W. Hollmann; M.E. Hoogendoorn; J. Horn; R. van der Horst; E.L.K. Ie; D. Ivanov; N.P. Juffermans; E. Kho; E.S. de Klerk; A.W.M. Koopman; M. Koopmans; S. Kucukcelebi; M.A. Kuiper; D.W. de Lange; D.M.P. van Meenen; I. Martin-Loeches, G. Mazzinari; N. van Mourik; S.G. Nijbroek; M. Onrust; E.A.N. Oostdijk; F. Paulus; C.J. Pennartz; J. Pillay; L. Pisani; I.M. Purmer; T.C.D. Rettig; J.P Roozeman; M.T.U. Schuijt; M.J. Schultz; A. Serpa Neto; M.E. Sleeswijk; M.R. Smit; P.E. Spronk; W. Stilma; A.C. Strang; A.M. Tsonas; P.R Tuinman; C.M.A. Valk; F.L. Veen; A.P.J. Vlaar; L.I. Veldhuis; P. van Velzen; W.H. van der Ven; P. van Vliet; P. van der Voort; H.H. van der Wier; L. van Welie; H.J.F.T. Wesselink; B. van Wijk; T. Winters; W.Y. Wong; A.R.H. van Zanten.

AUTHOR CONTRIBUTIONS

MiS and AS had full access to all data in the study and take responsibility for the integrity of the data and the accuracy of the data analysis. MiS, MaS, GM, FP, and AS concept and design. All authors contributed to acquisition, analysis or interpretation of data, drafting the manuscript, and critical revision of the manuscript for important intellectual content. MiS and AS statistical analysis. FP and MaS obtained funding. MaS, FP, and AS supervision. All authors contributed to acquisition, analysis or interpretation of data, drafting the manuscript, and critical revision of the manuscript for important intellectual content. All authors contributed to the article and approved the submitted version.

REFERENCES

1. Guan W, Ni Z, Hu Y, Liang W, Ou C, He J, et al. Clinical characteristics of coronavirus disease 2019 in China. *N Engl J Med.* (2020) 382:1708–20. doi: 10.1056/NEJMoa2002032
2. Domecq JP, Lal A, Sheldrick CR, Kumar VK, Boman K, Bolesta S, et al. Outcomes of patients with coronavirus disease 2019 receiving organ support therapies: the international viral infection and respiratory illness universal study registry. *Crit Care Med.* (2021) 49:437–48. doi: 10.1097/CCM.0000000000005007
3. Slutsky A, Ranieri V. Ventilator-induced lung injury. *N Engl J Med.* (2013) 369:2126–36. doi: 10.1056/NEJMra1208707
4. Fan E, Del Sorbo L, Goligher EC, Hodgson CL, Munshi L, Walkey AJ, et al. An official American Thoracic Society/European Society of intensive care medicine/society of critical care medicine clinical practice guideline: Mechanical ventilation in adult patients with acute respiratory distress syndrome. *Am J Respir Crit Care Med.* (2017) 195:1253–63. doi: 10.1164/rccm.19511erratum
5. The ARDS. Network. Ventilation with lower tidal volumes as compared with traditional tidal volumes for acute lung injury and the acute respiratory distress syndrome. *N Engl J Med.* (2000) 342:1301–8. doi: 10.1056/NEJM200005043421801
6. Goligher EC, Ferguson ND, Brochard LJ. Clinical challenges in mechanical ventilation. *The Lancet.* (2016) 387:1856–66. doi: 10.1016/S0140-6736(16)30176-3
7. Amato MBP, Meade MO, Slutsky AS, Brochard L, Costa ELV, Schoenfeld DA, et al. Driving pressure and survival in the acute respiratory distress syndrome. *N Engl J Med.* (2015) 372:747–55. doi: 10.1056/NEJMsa1410639
8. Serpa Neto A, Deliberato RO, Johnson AEW, Bos LD, Amorim P, Pereira SM, et al. Mechanical power of ventilation is associated with mortality in critically ill patients: an analysis of patients in two observational cohorts. *Intensive Care Med.* (2018) 44:1914–22. doi: 10.1007/s00134-018-5375-6
9. Protti A, Andreis DT, Monti M, Santini A, Sparacino CC, Langer T, et al. Lung stress and strain during mechanical ventilation: any difference between statics and dynamics? *Crit Care Med.* (2013) 41:1046–55. doi: 10.1097/CCM.0b013e31827417a6
10. Gattinoni L, Tonetti T, Cressoni M, Cadringher P, Herrmann P, Moerer O, et al. Ventilator-related causes of lung injury: the mechanical power. *Intensive Care Med.* (2016) 42:1567–75. doi: 10.1007/s00134-016-4505-2
11. Marini JJ, Jaber S. Dynamic predictors of VILI risk: beyond the driving pressure. *Intensive Care Medicine.* (2016) 32:1597–600. doi: 10.1007/s00134-016-4534-x
12. Urner M, Jüni P, Hansen B, Wettstein MS, Ferguson ND, Fan E. Time-varying intensity of mechanical ventilation and mortality in patients with acute respiratory failure: a registry-based, prospective cohort study. *Lancet Respir Med.* (2020) 8:905–13. doi: 10.1016/S2213-2600(20)30325-8
13. Zhang Z, Zheng B, Liu N, Ge H, Hong Y. Mechanical power normalized to predicted body weight as a predictor of mortality in patients with acute respiratory distress syndrome. *Intensive Care Med.* (2019) 45:856–64. doi: 10.1007/s00134-019-05627-9
14. Tonna JE, Peltan I, Brown SM, Herrick JS, Keenan HT, Grissom CK, et al. Mechanical power and driving pressure as predictors of mortality among patients with ARDS. *Intensive Care Med.* (2020) 46:1941–3. doi: 10.1007/s00134-020-06130-2
15. Coppola S, Caccioppola A, Froio S, Formenti P, De Giorgis V, Galanti V, et al. Effect of mechanical power on intensive care mortality in ARDS patients. *Crit Care.* (2020) 24:1–10. doi: 10.1186/s13054-020-02963-x
16. Parhar KKS, Zjadewicz K, Soo A, Sutton A, Zjadewicz M, Doig L, et al. Epidemiology, mechanical power, and 3-year outcomes in acute respiratory distress syndrome patients using standardized screening: An observational cohort study. *Ann Am Thorac Soc.* (2019) 16:1263–72. doi: 10.1513/AnnalsATS.201812-910OC
17. Gattinoni L, Marini JJ, Collino F, Maiolo G, Rapetti F, Tonetti T, et al. The future of mechanical ventilation: Lessons from the present and the past. *Crit Care.* (2017) 21:1–11. doi: 10.1186/s13054-017-1750-x
18. Huhle R, Serpa Neto A, Schultz MJ, Gama de. Abreu M. Is mechanical power the final word on ventilator-induced lung injury?—no. *Ann Transl Med.* (2018) 6:394. doi: 10.21037/atm.2018.09.65
19. Vasques F, Duscio E, Pasticci I, Romitti F, Vassalli F, Quintel M, et al. Is the mechanical power the final word on ventilator-induced lung injury?—we are not sure. *Ann Transl Med.* (2018) 6:395–395. doi: 10.21037/atm.2018.08.17
20. Cressoni M, Cadringher P, Chiurazzi C, Amini M, Gallazzi E, Marino A, et al. Lung inhomogeneity in patients with acute respiratory distress syndrome. *Am J Respir Crit Care Med.* (2014) 189:149–58. doi: 10.1164/rccm.201308-1567OC
21. Boers NS, Botta M, Tsonas AM, Algera AG, Pillay J, Dongelmans DA, et al. PRactice of VENTilation in Patients with Novel Coronavirus Disease (PRoVENT-COVID): rationale and protocol for a national multicenter observational study in The Netherlands. *Ann Transl Med.* (2020) 8:1251. doi: 10.21037/atm-20-5107
22. PROVENT-COVID. Available online at: https://sites.google.com/view/provent-covid/. (accessed Mar 10, 2021)
23. Botta M, Tsonas AM, Pillay J, Boers LS, Algera AG, Bos LDJ, et al. Ventilation management and clinical outcomes in invasively ventilated patients with COVID-19 (PRoVENT-COVID): a national, multicentre, observational cohort study. *Lancet Respir Med.* (2021) 9:139–48. doi: 10.1016/S2213-2600(20)30459-8
24. Ranieri VM, Rubenfeld GD, Thompson BT, Ferguson ND, Caldwell E, Fan E, et al. Acute respiratory distress syndrome: the Berlin definition. *JAMA - J Am Med Assoc.* (2012) 307:2526–33. doi: 10.1001/jama.2012.5669
25. Rizopoulos D. The R package jmbayes for fitting joint models for longitudinal and time-to-event data using MCMC. *J Stat Softw.* (2016) 72:46. doi: 10.18637/jss.v072.i07
26. Rizopoulos D, Ghosh P. A bayesian semiparametric multivariate joint model for multiple longitudinal outcomes and a time-to-event. *Stat Med.* (2011) 30:1366–80. doi: 10.1002/sim.4205
27. Giosa L, Busana M, Pasticci I, Bonifazi M, Macrì MM, Romitti F, et al. Mechanical power at a glance: a simple surrogate for volume-controlled ventilation. *Intensive Care Med Exp.* (2019) 7:61. doi: 10.1186/s40635-019-0276-8
28. Ferrando C, Suarez-Sipmann F, Mellado-Artigas R, Hernández M, Gea A, Arruti E, et al. Clinical features, ventilatory management, and outcome of ARDS caused by COVID-19 are similar to other causes of ARDS. *Intensive Care Med.* (2020) 46:2200–11. doi: 10.1007/s00134-020-06251-8

29. Gupta S, Hayek SS, Wang W, Chan L, Mathews KS, Melamed ML, et al. Factors associated with death in critically ill patients with coronavirus disease 2019 in the US. *JAMA Intern Med.* (2020) 180:1–12. doi: 10.1001/jamainternmed.2020.3596
30. COVID-ICU Group on behalf of the REVA Network and the COVID-ICU Investigators. Clinical characteristics and day-90 outcomes of 4244 critically ill adults with COVID-19: a prospective cohort study. *Intensive Care Med.* (2021) 47:60–73. doi: 10.1007/s00134-020-06294-x
31. Cummings MJ, Baldwin MR, Abrams D, Jacobson SD, Meyer BJ, Balough EM, et al. Epidemiology, clinical course, and outcomes of critically ill adults with COVID-19 in New York City: a prospective cohort study. *Lancet.* (2020) 395:1763–70. doi: 10.1016/S0140-6736(20)31189-2
32. Chiumello D, Gotti M, Guanziroli M, Formenti P, Umbrello M, Pasticci I, et al. Bedside calculation of mechanical power during volume- and pressure-controlled mechanical ventilation. *Crit Care.* (2020) 24:417–23. doi: 10.1186/s13054-020-03116-w
33. Bompard F, Monnier H, Saab I, Tordjman M, Abdoul H, Fournier L, et al. Pulmonary embolism in patients with COVID-19 pneumonia. *Eur Respir J.* (2020) 56:17–20. doi: 10.1183/13993003.01365-2020
34. Grasselli G, Zangrillo A, Zanella A, Antonelli M, Cabrini L, Castelli A, et al. Baseline Characteristics and Outcomes of 1591 Patients Infected with SARS-CoV-2 Admitted to ICUs of the Lombardy Region, Italy. *JAMA - J Am Med Assoc.* (2020) 323:1574–81.
35. Grasselli G, Tonetti T, Protti A, Langer T, Girardis M, Bellani G, et al. Pathophysiology of COVID-19-associated acute respiratory distress syndrome: a multicentre prospective observational study. *Lancet Respir Med.* (2020) 8:1201–08. doi: 10.1016/S2213-2600(20)30370-2

9

Effects of Dexmedetomidine on Postoperative Nausea and Vomiting in Adult Patients Undergoing Ambulatory Thyroidectomy

*Cuiyu Xie[1], Caihui Zhang[1], Hao Sun[1] and Yao Lu[1,2]**

[1] Department of Anesthesiology, The First Affiliated Hospital of Anhui Medical University, Hefei, China, [2] Ambulatory Surgery Center, The First Affiliated Hospital of Anhui Medical University, Hefei, China

***Correspondence:**
Yao Lu
luyao@ahmu.edu.cn

Background: Postoperative nausea and vomiting (PONV) is a common and disturbing problem in patients undergoing ambulatory thyroidectomy. This prospective trial aimed to explore whether dexmedetomidine (DEX) combined with azasetron (AZA) can further drop the incidence of PONV in patients undergoing ambulatory thyroidectomy compared with AZA.

Methods: This single-center, randomized, double-blind trial involved 172 adult patients undergoing ambulatory thyroidectomy. The individuals were randomized to DEX + AZA group and AZA group. In the DEX + AZA group, patients received dexmedetomidine 0.5 $\mu g\ kg^{-1}$ for 10 min and then the infusion rate was held at 0.1 $\mu g\ kg^{-1}\ h^{-1}$ until the completion of the operation, while the same amount of 0.9% saline in the AZA group. At the completion of the surgery, 10 mg azasetron was administered to every patient in both groups. The primary outcome was the incidence of 24 h PONV after ambulatory thyroidectomy. The secondary outcomes included residence time in recovery room, pain scores, severity of nausea, and adverse events.

Results: No significant difference was found in the incidence of 24-h PONV between the DEX + AZA group and the AZA group [36% (30 of 84) vs. 38% (32 of 84); relative risk, 0.94; 95% confidence interval (CI), 0.63–1.40; $P = 0.749$]. The incidence of severe nausea was similar between the DEX + AZA group and the AZA group [57% (12 of 21) vs. 43% (9 of 21); relative risk, 1.33; 95% CI, 0.72–2.50; $P = 0.355$].

Conclusions: Intraoperative dexmedetomidine combined with azasetron failed to drop the incidence of 24-h PONV compared with azasetron alone in patients undergoing ambulatory thyroidectomy.

Keywords: dexmedetomidine, postoperative nausea and vomiting, ambulatory, thyroidectomy, anesthesia

INTRODUCTION

At present, thyroid tumors and thyroid disease are on the rise worldwide. In China, people with thyroid tumors are increasing rapidly, and the incidence rate is 3 times more common in women than in men (1, 2). Surgery is the main treatment for thyroid cancer. Guided by the concept of enhanced recovery after surgery, ambulatory thyroidectomy has become a new trend, and more and more thyroidectomies have been performed in the ambulatory operating room (3, 4).

Postoperative nausea and vomiting (PONV) refer to any nausea, retching, and vomiting that happen after the anesthesia and operation (5). Studies have reported that, if not treated, ~35% of patients will develop nausea, vomiting, or both symptoms after surgery, which is a very painful experience, even more serious than postoperative pain (6). However, ~60–80% of patients develop nausea and vomiting after thyroidectomy without antiemetic prophylaxis, which may result in severe complications, such as aspiration pneumonia caused by accidental inhalation of vomitus or postoperative neck hematoma and even airway obstruction caused by hematoma (7). PONV often prolongs the patient's stay in the recovery room or even the discharge time, which is the main reason for accidental readmission after elective surgery (8). However, prophylactic antiemetic agents can improve the condition.

The latest guidelines for the management of PONV advised that the combination of different prophylactic drugs can drop the rate of PONV (9). Dexmedetomidine (DEX) is a novel α2-adrenoreceptor agonist that has good sedative, analgesic, and sympatholytic effects. Because of its advantages of reducing intraoperative opioid dose and accelerating postoperative recovery, dexmedetomidine is increasingly used during anesthesia. Recently, several researches have suggested that intraoperative DEX may have an antiemetic effect and can decrease the incidence of PONV (10, 11). Azasetron (AZA) as a selective serotonin receptor antagonist that is recommended by the guidelines as a first-line antiemetic agent in high-risk patients. However, there have been no studies of dexmedetomidine in combination with azasetron for the prevention of PONV after ambulatory thyroidectomy.

We designed this trial to explore the effect of dexmedetomidine on nausea and vomiting after ambulatory thyroidectomy. We hypothesized that dexmedetomidine combined with azasetron can further decrease the incidence of nausea and vomiting 24 h after ambulatory thyroidectomy compared with azasetron.

METHODS

Ethics

Ethical approval for this study (PJ2020-13-21) was provided by the Ethics Committee of The First Affiliated Hospital of Anhui Medical University, Hefei China (Chairperson Prof Heng Wang) on 29 October 2020. This randomized, double-blind trial was registered at the Chinese Clinical Trial Registry (ChiCTR2000039603, Principal Investigator: Yao Lu, MD, PhD, November 03, 2020). Individuals scheduled to undergo ambulatory thyroidectomy were enrolled. An informed consent was obtained from each patient.

Study Design

Eligible patients were 18–60 years old of any sex with American Society of Anaesthesiologists classification I–II and body mass index of 18–30 kg/m^2. The exclusion criteria included allergy to dexmedetomidine, antiemetic or analgesic medication intake within 24 h before surgery, use of antipsychotic drugs or corticosteroids, previous heart failure or arrhythmia and diabetes mellitus with poor glycemia control, uncontrolled hypertension, liver and kidney dysfunction, gastric dynamic disorder, and vestibular disease.

Randomization and Masking

The investigators, independent of the blind study, prepared the randomized schedule and study drugs. During the study, patients, investigators, anaesthesiologists, nurses in the post-anesthesia care unit (PACU) or ward, and the recorders of each observation index were all unaware of the group assignment. The SPSS version 23.0 generated random numbers, which were delivered in sealed, opaque envelopes. And the envelopes were opened after consent was obtained. The study drugs included dexmedetomidine (100 μg ml^{-1}, diluted with 0.9% saline to 4 μg ml^{-1}), azasetron, and 0.9% saline, all prepared according to random numbers. Patients were randomly allocated into the DEX + AZA group or the AZA group in a 1:1 ratio.

Study Treatments

The patient received routine pre-operative preparation, and no premedication was administered. Standard monitoring was done after arriving at the operating room. Before anesthesia induction, 0.5 μg kg^{-1} for 10 min of dexmedetomidine was administered intravenously and then the infusion rate reduced to 0.1 μg kg^{-1} h^{-1} until the end of surgery in the DEX + AZA group or the same amount of 0.9% saline in the AZA group. General anesthesia was induced i.v. with propofol (2 mg kg^{-1}) and sufentanil (0.4 μg kg^{-1}). To facilitate endotracheal intubation, cisatracurium (0.2 mg kg^{-1}) was administered. Anesthesia was maintained with remifentanil (0.1–0.2 μg kg^{-1} min^{-1}) and propofol (4–6 mg kg^{-1} h^{-1}), with their infusion rate adjusted to keep the bispectral index from 40 to 60. Sufentanil (5–10 μg) was administered to keep the heart rate and blood pressure fluctuations within 20% of baseline. In addition, to maintain adequate muscle relaxation, intermittent doses of cisatracurium were administered. At the end of surgery, every patient in each group was treated with 10 mg azasetron and 50 mg flurbiprofen axetil. Hypotension (mean arterial pressure of $<$60 mmHg or $<$80% of the baseline) was treated with 6 mg ephedrine and bradycardia (heart rate of $<$45 beats min^{-1}) with atropine 0.5 mg. After the operation, when autonomous breathing was regular, tidal volume was $>$6 mL kg^{-1}, SpO2 could be maintained at more than 95% during air intake, the trachea catheter was withdrawn, patients were transported to PACU. No analgesia was routinely applied.

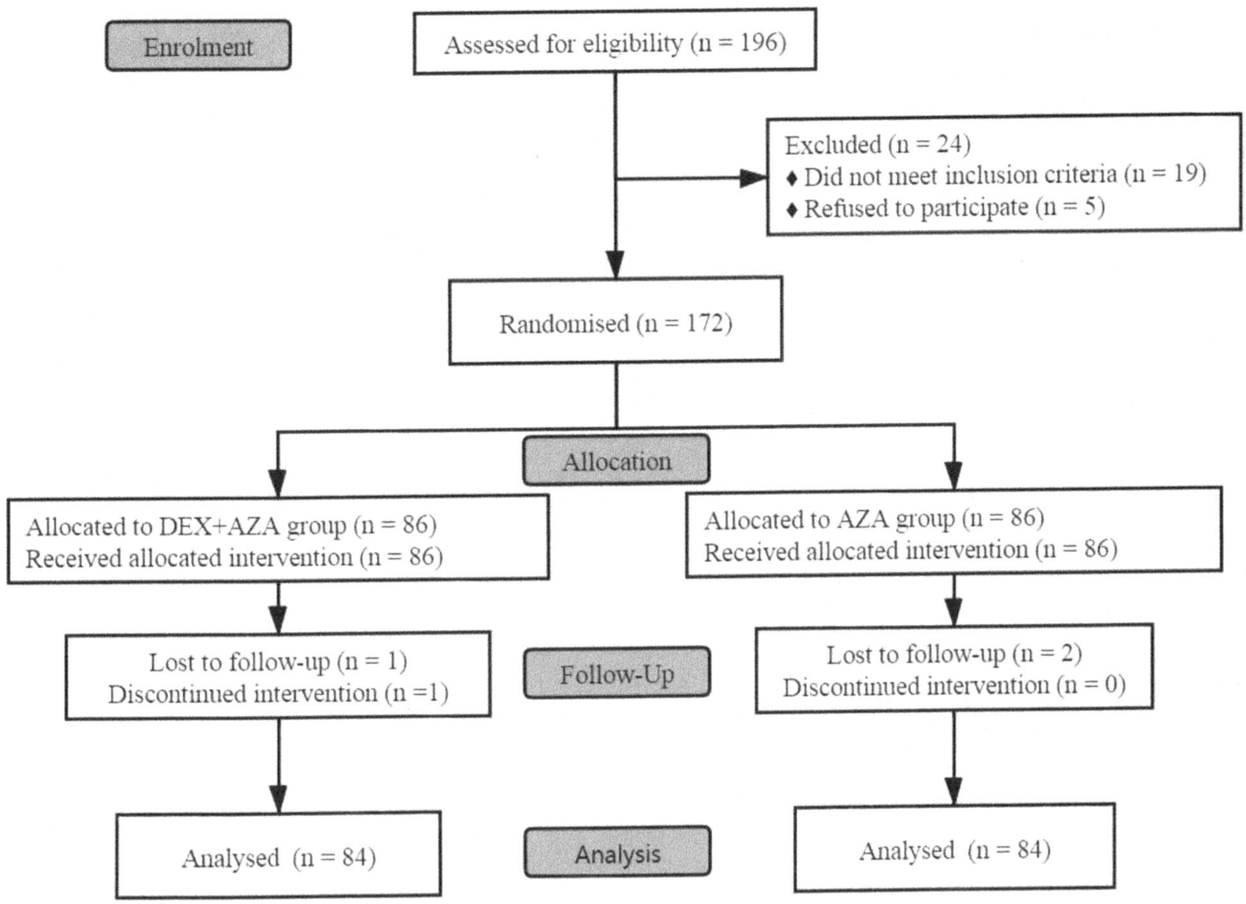

FIGURE 1 | CONSORT flow diagram for this study. This flow diagram shows this single-center, double-blind, randomized trial conducted on adult patients undergoing ambulatory thyroidectomy from November 2020 to January 2021. In the DEX + AZA group, patients received dexmedetomidine 0.5 $\mu g\ kg^{-1}$ for 10 min before anesthesia, and then the infusion rate was held at 0.1 $\mu g\ kg^{-1}\ h^{-1}$ until the completion of operation. In the AZA group, patients received an equal volume of saline with same pattern as the DEX + AZA group. Patients in both groups were given 10 mg azasetron before the end of surgery. DEX + AZA, dexmedetomidine + azasetron; AZA, azasetron.

Outcomes

Data were collected by investigators who were unaware of randomization and did not participate in the whole procedure. Relevant baseline characteristics and perioperative data of patients were carefully recorded.

The primary outcome was the incidence of 24 h PONV after ambulatory thyroidectomy. PONV was defined as at least 1 incident of nausea, vomiting, or retching or a combination of these symptoms. The investigators assessed the incidence of PONV at the time of leaving PACU, 6 and 24 h postoperatively in the ambulatory surgical ward by asking patients if they had experienced nausea and vomiting. Only a "YES" or "NO" answer can be accepted.

The secondary outcomes included severity of nausea, residence time in PACU, visual analog scale (VAS) pain scores at the time of leaving PACU, 6 and 24 h postoperatively, and adverse events.

Moreover, 11-point numerical rating scale (NRS) was used to assess nausea severity (0, no nausea; 10, worst nausea imaginable). Mild nausea is defined as NRS score from 1 to 3, whereas severe nausea is >3 (12). Rescue antiemetic agents will be administered if patients have experienced severe nausea or 2 or more times of vomiting or retching or patients request an antiemetic agent at any time. Intramuscular injection of 10 mg metoclopramide hydrochloride was used as the rescue antiemetic agent. Morphine is not allowed to be used after surgery. Parecoxib sodium 40 mg will be administered for VAS pain score of >3. In the PACU, Ramsay sedation scale (RSS) was used to assess sedation levels (1, agitated; 2, cooperative and oriented; 3, can respond to simple questions; 4, asleep, but with a quick reaction to stimulus; 5, asleep, arousable; 6, asleep, unarousable) (13). Oversedation was defined as RSS value of >4.

Statistical Analysis

Based on our unpublished pilot trial, we observed that, despite 10 mg azasetron being given intraoperatively, ~40% of patients develop PONV after thyroidectomy. A 20% decline in the occurrence of PONV is considered clinically significant; hence,

TABLE 1 | Patient baseline characteristics and intraoperative variables.

Characteristics/intraoperative variables	DEX + AZA (n = 84)	AZA (n = 84)	P-value
Mean age ± SD, yr	44 ± 11	41 ± 10	0.157[a]
Sex, no. (%)			0.717[b]
Female	63 (75)	65 (77)	
Male	21 (25)	19 (23)	
Mean BMI ± SD, kg/m^2	23.5 ± 2.6	23.2 ± 2.7	0.432[a]
ASA classification, no. (%)			0.070[b]
I	25 (30)	15 (18)	
II	59 (70)	69 (82)	
Smoking, no. (%)	7 (8)	5 (6)	0.549[b]
Hypertension, no. (%)	16 (19)	9 (11)	0.129[b]
History of motion sickness, no. (%)	34 (40)	23 (27)	0.073[b]
Median duration of anesthesia (IQR), min	97 (84, 117)	105 (85, 128)	0.059[c]
Median duration of surgery (IQR), min	79 (67, 98)	89 (72, 110)	0.100[c]
Medication administered during surgery			
Median propofol (IQR), mg	595 (500, 675)	558 (482, 656)	0.553
Median remifentanil (IQR), μg	580 (466, 700)	768 (600, 1,019)	<0.001
Median sufentanil (IQR), μg	35 (30, 35)	35 (30, 35)	0.497

DEX, dexmedetomidine; AZA, azasetron; IQR, interquartile range; ASA, American Society of Anesthesiologists; BMI, body mass index.
[a]*Analyzed using Independent-sample t test.*
[b]*Analyzed using χ^2 test.*
[c]*Analyzed using Mann–Whitney U-test.*

TABLE 2 | Nausea and vomiting outcomes and postoperative characteristics.

Outcomes/postoperative characteristics	DEX + AZA (n = 84)	AZA (n = 84)	P-value
PONV, no. (%)			
PACU	0	0	–
PACU-6 h	15 (18)	16 (19)	0.842[a]
6–24 h	20 (24)	24 (29)	0.483[a]
0–24 h	30 (36)	32 (38)	0.749[a]
Nausea, no. (%)			
PACU	0	0	–
PACU-6 h	9 (11)	12 (14)	0.484[a]
6–24 h	13 (15)	12 (14)	0.828[a]
Vomiting, no. (%)			
PACU	0	0	–
PACU-6 h	9 (11)	5 (6)	0.264[a]
6–24 h	12 (14)	18 (21)	0.227[a]
Use of rescue antiemetics, no. (%)	19 (23)	23 (27)	0.476[a]
Use of rescue analgesics, no. (%)	5 (6)	4 (5)	0.732[a]
Median residence time in PACU (IQR), min	45 (40, 55)	45 (40, 55)	0.391[b]

DEX, dexmedetomidine; AZA, azasetron; IQR, interquartile range; PONV, postoperative nausea and/or vomiting; PACU, Post-anesthesia Care Unit.
[a]*Analyzed using χ^2 test.*
[b]*Analyzed using Mann–Whitney U test.*

80 patients are required per group with an alpha level of 0.05 and power of 80%. Finally, we planned to enroll 196 patients to allow for a 20% dropout. Categorical data are presented as number (percentage) and were analyzed by χ^2 test or Fisher's exact test. Independent t-test or Mann-Whitney U-test was applied for analyzing continuous variables, which are presented as mean ± standard deviation or medians (interquartile range). χ^2 test or Fisher's exact test was used to analyze the incidences of PONV, nausea severity, and adverse events presented as number (percentage). Postoperative pain scores are presented as median (interquartile range) and were analyzed with the linear mixed model. Two-tailed $P < 0.05$ was considered statistically significant. SPSS 23.0 was used for data analysis.

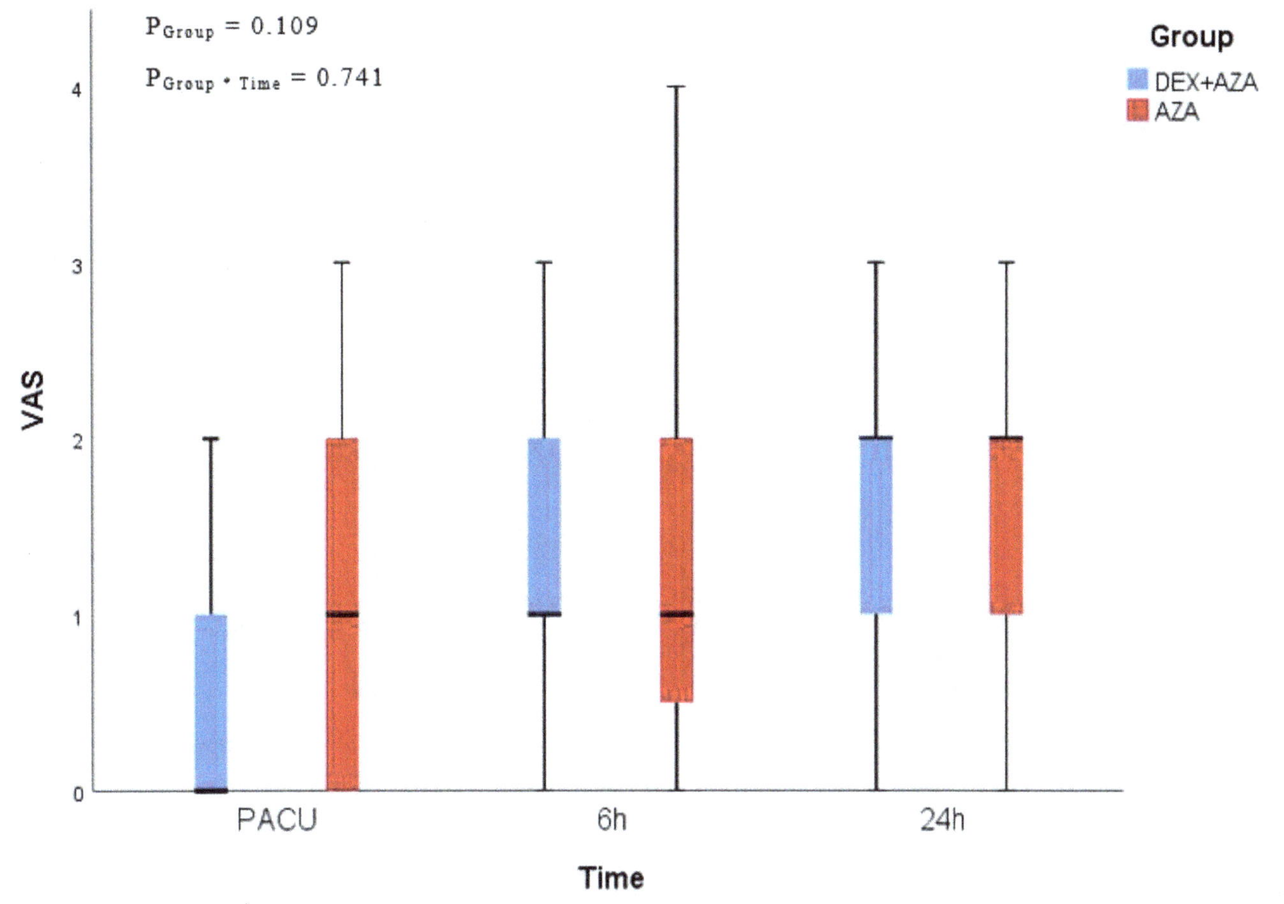

FIGURE 2 | Postoperative pain assessment. We adopted 11-point visual analog scale (VAS) for pain assessment at the time of leaving PACU, 6 and 24 hours after thyroidectomy. VAS presented as median (interquartile range). In the DEX + AZA group (*n* = 84), patients received dexmedetomidine 0.5 μg kg^{-1} for 10 min before anesthesia, and then the infusion rate was held at 0.1 μg kg^{-1} h^{-1} until the completion of operation. In the AZA group (*n* = 84), patients received an equal volume of saline with same pattern as the DEX + AZA group. Patients in both groups were given 10 mg azasetron before the end of surgery. $P_{Group*Time}$ = *P*-value of the group and time interaction obtained by the linear mixed model. DEX + AZA, dexmedetomidine + azasetron; AZA, azasetron.

RESULTS

Before the study began, 24 patients were excluded because they did not meet the inclusion criteria or withdrew their consent, so we enrolled a total of 172 patients between November 2020 to January 2021 (**Figure 1**). In the DEX+AZA group, 1 patient was excluded from the analysis because of failure to pump dexmedetomidine at the beginning of surgery. Because of missing data, 2 patients in each group were excluded from the analysis after being treated with study drugs. In total, 168 patients finished the study and were evaluated for all study outcomes: 84 in the DEX + AZA group and 84 in the AZA group.

No significant differences were found in baseline characteristics, smoking status, or history of motion sickness between two the groups. No significant differences were found in intraoperative variables between groups except the consumption of remifentanil (**Table 1**).

Outcomes

The incidence of 24-h PONV was not significantly different between the two groups (**Table 2**). In the DEX+AZA group, 30 of 84 patients (36%) experienced at least 1 episode of retching, vomiting, or both during the first 24-h postoperative period compared with 32 of 84 patients (38%) in the AZA group (relative risk, 0.94; 95% CI, 0.63–1.40; $P = 0.749$). The postoperative characteristics such as the residence time in PACU and the use of analgesic and antiemetic drugs were not significantly different in the two groups.

Throughout the study period, the VAS scores were not significantly different at any time points between the two groups (**Figure 2**). Postoperative nausea occurred in 21 patients in each group. The severity of nausea was similar in both groups 24 h after surgery; severe nausea (NRS score, >3) occurred in 9 patients (43%) in the AZA group and 12 patients (57%) in the DEX+AZA group (relative risk, 1.33; 95% CI, 0.72–2.50; $P = 0.355$) (**Figure 3**). No serious adverse events were observed during the study. The main intraoperative adverse events were

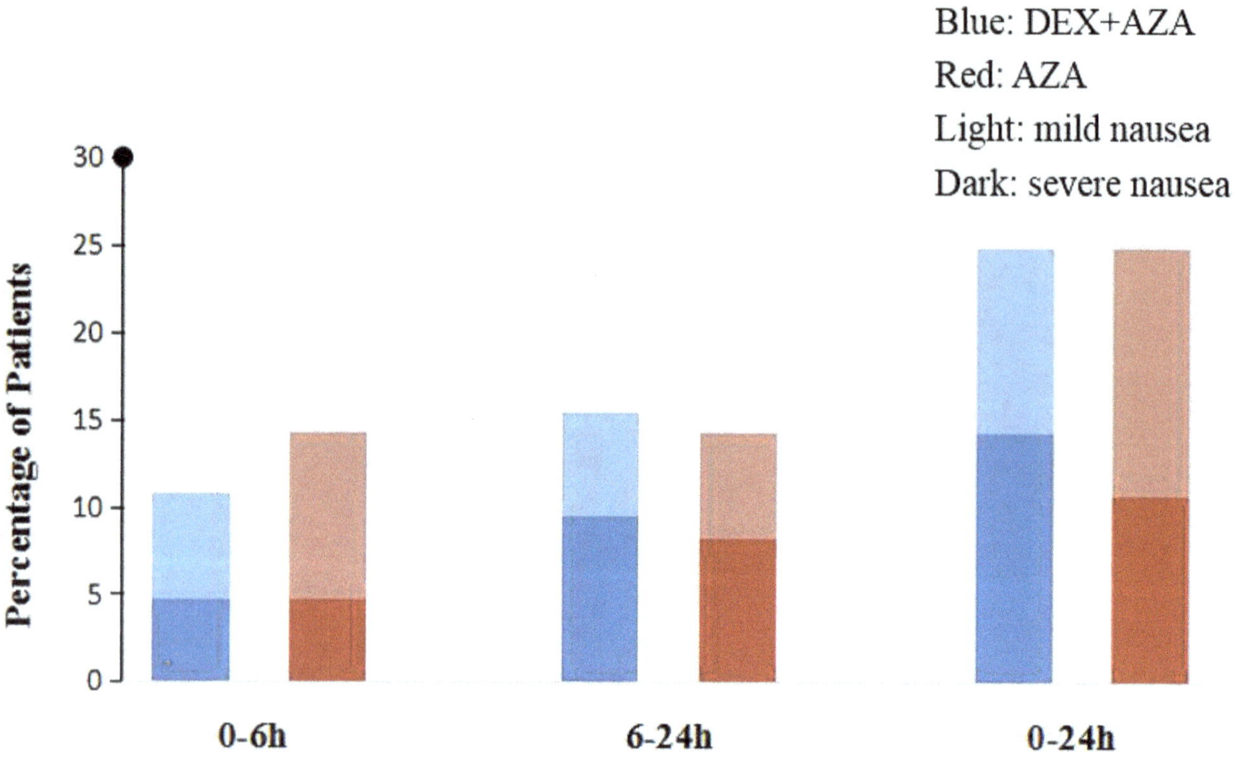

FIGURE 3 | Postoperative nausea intensity assessment. We adopted 11-point numerical rating scale (NRS) to assess nausea severity (0, no nausea; 10, worst nausea imaginable). Mild nausea is defined as NRS score from 1 to 3, whereas severe nausea is >3. In the DEX + AZA group (n = 84), patients received dexmedetomidine 0.5 μg kg^{-1} for 10 min before anesthesia, and then the infusion rate was held at 0.1 μg kg^{-1} h^{-1} until the completion of operation. In the AZA group (n = 84), patients received an equal volume of saline with same pattern as the DEX + AZA group. Patients in both groups were given 10 mg azasetron before the end of surgery. DEX + AZA, dexmedetomidine+ azasetron; AZA, azasetron; Light, mild nausea; Dark, severe nausea.

hypotension and bradycardia, and the rate did not differ between the two groups (**Table 3**).

DISCUSSION

The results in this randomized, double-blind trial suggest that intra-operative dexmedetomidine combined with azasetron did not significantly decrease the rate of 24-h PONV compared with azasetron alone.

The mechanism of PONV is very complex, and the trauma caused by surgery, inflammation, visceral stimulation, pain, hypoxia, and hypotension are the main stimulating factors (14). When the stimulus reaches the vomiting center *via* the afferent nerve, dopamine, histamine, serotonin type 3 (5-HT3), tachykinin 1 (NK1), or muscarinic receptors are activated to trigger the vomiting response (15). Moreover, relevant studies have reported that female sex, non-smoker, history of PONV, and use of postoperative opioids are high-risk factors for PONV, and the occurrence of PONV is also related to the type of surgery and intraoperative anesthesia management (16). The incidence of PONV varies greatly among different types of surgery, such as otolaryngology, gynecological, and endoscopic surgeries with relatively high incidence of PONV. In the maintenance of intraoperative anesthesia, inhalation of anesthetic drugs can easily cause PONV compared with total intravenous anesthesia (TIVA) (17, 18).

Geng et al. (13) conducted a study to investigate the effect of adjuvant dexmedetomidine on PONV during gynecological laparoscopic surgery. The results indicate that intraoperative dexmedetomidine (0.5 μg kg^{-1} loading dose followed by 0.1 μg kg^{-1} h^{-1} infusion until the end of surgery) can reduce the incidence of postoperative nausea 2 h after surgery. Song et al. (19) found that, in orthopedic surgery, adding 10 μg kg^{-1} dexmedetomidine to a fentanyl-based PCA drug mixture improved the frequency and intensity of severe postoperative nausea in patients with high-risk factors of PONV. However, the mechanism of the antiemetic function of dexmedetomidine is still unknown. Possible mechanisms to reduce PONV by dexmedetomidine include the following: dexmedetomidine has sedative and analgesic effects and can reduce the dose of narcotic drugs and opioids. It can also inhibit the excitability of the sympathetic nerve and reduce the release of catecholamine, because catecholamine may be a contributing factor of PONV (5).

This trial aimed to clarify the effect of dexmedetomidine combined with azasetron on PONV. Unfortunately, it fails to

TABLE 3 | Comparison of perioperative adverse events.

Variables	DEX + AZA (n = 84)	AZA (n = 84)	P-value
Adverse events during operation			
Hypotension, no. (%)	2 (2)	2 (2)	–
Bradycardia, no. (%)	6 (7)	8 (10)	0.577[a]
Adverse events in the PACU			
Agitation, no. (%)	1 (1)	3 (4)	0.613[b]
Over sedation, no. (%)	6 (7)	3 (4)	0.493[b]

DEX, dexmedetomidine; AZA, azasetron; PACU, Post-anesthesia Care Unit.
[a]Analyzed using χ^2 test.
[b]Analyzed using continuity correction χ^2 test.

further drop the occurrence of PONV, but the gross incidence of PONV in the 2 groups was not as high as reported in previous articles. This may be caused by the fact that we have adopted a multimodal prophylactic approach to prevent PONV, including TIVA with propofol, no inhalation anesthesia was used and no postoperative opioid used, which reduces the baseline risk of PONV.

There may be several reasons for the differences in the outcomes between the present study and the previous articles. First, a multimodal prophylactic treatment was used to accelerate the patient's recovery after surgery, but too many antiemetic factors may have masked the effect of dexmedetomidine on PONV. Second, due to the sedative and analgesic properties of dexmedetomidine, the amount of intraoperative remifentanil in the experimental group was significantly reduced compared with the control group. However, many studies have reported that remifentanil has a short half-life and quick elimination, and there is no effect on PONV (20–22). Therefore, although dexmedetomidine reduced the dose of intraoperative remifentanil, it fails to drop the occurrence of PONV. Third, Aouad et al. reported that 1, 0.5, and 0.25 μg kg^{-1} dose of dexmedetomidine had no significant difference in the occurrence of PONV, but they cause dose-dependent hypotension (23). For decreasing the incidence of perioperative adverse events and promoting postoperative recovery, the selected dose of dexmedetomidine (0.5 μg kg^{-1} loading dose followed by 0.1 μg kg^{-1} h^{-1} infusion) may be relatively small, which may affect the antiemetic effect of dexmedetomidine. Finally, dexmedetomidine may not decrease the incidence of PONV.

There are several limitations in this study. First, our trial did not adopt a multicenter study method, which may make our results not universal. Second, only one dose of dexmedetomidine was adopted in this trial, and this dose of dexmedetomidine combined with azasetron did not produce significant effects in patients undergoing ambulatory thyroidectomy. Third, we included patients with ambulatory thyroidectomy in our study, and traditional procedures such as cholecystectomy and endoscopic surgery with a high incidence of PONV were not selected. In future studies, we can choose different types of surgery to compare the incidence of PONV.

In summary, we find that intraoperative dexmedetomidine combined with azasetron did not significantly decrease the incidence of 24-h PONV compared with azasetron alone in adult patients undergoing ambulatory thyroidectomy.

ETHICS STATEMENT

The studies involving human participants were reviewed and approved by Ethics Committee of The First Affiliated Hospital of Anhui Medical University. The patients/participants provided their written informed consent to participate in this study.

AUTHOR CONTRIBUTIONS

CX and YL: study design. CX: ethics approval and registration. CX, CZ, and HS: patient recruitment. CX and CZ: data collection. CX and HS: data analysis. CX, CZ, and YL: drafting. All authors contributed to the article and approved the submitted version.

ACKNOWLEDGMENTS

Assistance with the study: The authors thank Dr. Chengyang Hu (Department of Epidemiology and Biostatistics, School of Public Health, Anhui Medical University, Hefei, China) for his help in data analysis and Xiandao Li, MD (Department of Anesthesiology, Changfeng Hospital of Traditional Chinese Medicine, Hefei, China), for his great assistance.

REFERENCES

1. Wang J, Yu F, Shang Y, Ping Z, Liu L. Thyroid cancer: incidenc and mortality trends in China, 2005–2015. *Endocrine.* (2020) 68:163–73. doi: 10.1007/s12020-020-02207-6
2. Du L, Zhao Z, Zheng R, Li H, Zhang S, Li R, et al. Epidemiology of thyroid cancer: incidence and mortality in China, 2015. *Front Oncol.* (2020) 10:1702. doi: 10.3389/fonc.2020.01702
3. Hu QL, Livhits MJ, Ko CY, Yeh MW. Same-day discharge is not associated with increased readmissions or complications after thyroid operations. *Surgery.* (2020) 167:117–23. doi: 10.1016/j.surg.2019.06.054
4. Cozzaglio L, Zuccarelli A, Quagliuolo V. Financial benefit in outpatient thyroid surgery. *J Endocrinol Invest.* (2019) 42:867–8. doi: 10.1007/s40618-019-01043-4
5. Watcha MF, White PF. Postoperative nausea and vomiting. Its etiology, treatment, and prevention. *Anesthesiology.* (1992) 77:162–84. doi: 10.1097/00000542-199207000-00023

6. Apfel CC, Korttila K, Abdalla M, Kerger H, Turan A, Vedder I, et al. A factorial trial of six interventions for the prevention of postoperative nausea and vomiting. *N Engl J Med.* (2004) 350:2441–51. doi: 10.1056/NEJMoa032196
7. Cho YJ, Choi GJ, Kang H. Pharmacologic interventions for postoperative nausea and vomiting after thyroidectomy. *Medicine.* (2019) 98:e14542. doi: 10.1097/MD.0000000000014542
8. Tarantino I, Warschkow R, Beutner U, Kolb W, Lüthi A, Lüthi C, et al. Efficacy of a single preoperative dexamethasone dose to prevent nausea and vomiting after thyroidectomy (the tPONV Study). *Ann Surg.* (2015) 262:934–40. doi: 10.1097/SLA.0000000000001112
9. Gan TJ, Belani KG, Bergese S, Chung F, Diemunsch P, Habib AS, et al. Fourth consensus guidelines for the management of postoperative nausea and vomiting. *Anesth Anal.* (2020) 131:411–48. doi: 10.1213/ANE.0000000000004833
10. Grape S, Kirkham KR, Frauenknecht J, Albrecht E. Intra-operative analgesia with remifentanil vs. dexmedetomidine: a systematic review and meta-analysis with trial sequential analysis. *Anaesthesia.* (2019) 74:793–800. doi: 10.1111/anae.14657
11. Kwak H, Chang YJ, Lee KC, Jung WS, Kwon S, Jo YY. Antiemetic efficacy of dexmedetomidine versus dexmedetomidine-dexamethasone combination in patients undergoing breast surgery. *J Int Med Res.* (2019) 47:5060–9. doi: 10.1177/0300060519872031
12. Hyman JB, Park C, Lin HM, Cole B, Rosen L, Fenske SS, et al. Olanzapine for the prevention of postdischarge nausea and vomiting after ambulatory surgery. *Anesthesiology.* (2020) 132:1419–28. doi: 10.1097/ALN.0000000000003286
13. Geng Z, Liu Y, Wang S, Wang D. Intra-operative dexmedetomidine reduces early postoperative nausea but not vomiting in adult patients after gynaecological laparoscopic surgery. *Eur J Anaesth.* (2016) 33:761–6. doi: 10.1097/EJA.0000000000000491
14. Horn CC, Wallisch WJ, Homanics GE, Williams JP. Pathophysiological and neurochemical mechanisms of postoperative nausea and vomiting. *Eur J Pharmacol.* (2014) 722:55–66. doi: 10.1016/j.ejphar.2013.10.037
15. Gan TJ. Mechanisms underlying postoperative nausea and vomiting and neurotransmitter receptor antagonist-based pharmacotherapy. *Cns Drugs.* (2007) 21:813–33. doi: 10.2165/00023210-200721100-00003
16. Gan TJ, Gan MFF. Risk factors for postoperative nausea and vomiting. *Anesth Anal.* (2006) 102:1884–98. doi: 10.1213/01.ANE.0000219597.16143.4D
17. Yang L, Xu Y, Shen J, Lou F, Zhang J, Wu J. Propofol-based total intravenous anesthesia decreases the incidence of postoperative nausea and vomiting without affecting flap survival in free flap breast reconstruction. *Gland Surg.* (2020) 9:1406–14. doi: 10.21037/gs-20-225
18. Apfel CC, Heidrich FM, Jukar-Rao S, Jalota L, Hornuss C, Whelan RP, et al. Evidence-based analysis of risk factors for postoperative nausea and vomiting [†]. *Br J Anaesth.* (2012) 109:742–53. doi: 10.1093/bja/aes276
19. Song Y, Shim J, Song J, Kim E, Kwak Y. Dexmedetomidine added to an opioid-based analgesic regimen for the prevention of postoperative nausea and vomiting in highly susceptible patients. *Eur J Anaesth.* (2016) 33:75–83. doi: 10.1097/EJA.0000000000000327
20. Oh AY, Kim JH, Hwang JW, Do SH, Jeon YT. Incidence of postoperative nausea and vomiting after paediatric strabismus surgery with sevoflurane or remifentanil–sevoflurane. *Br J Anaesth.* (2010) 104:756–60. doi: 10.1093/bja/aeq091
21. Dershwitz M, Michalowski P, Chang Y, Rosow CE, Conlay LA. Postoperative nausea and vomiting after total intravenous anesthesia with propofol and remifentanil or alfentanil: how important is the opioid? *J Clin Anesth.* (2002) 14:275–8. doi: 10.1016/S0952-8180(02)00353-7
22. Fujimoto D, Egi M, Makino S, Mizobuchi S. The association of intraoperative end-tidal carbon dioxide with the risk of postoperative nausea and vomiting. *J Anesth.* (2020) 34:195–201. doi: 10.1007/s00540-019-02715-4
23. Aoud MT, Zeeni C, Al Nawwar R, Siddik-Sayyid SM, Barakat HB, Yazbeck Karam VG, et al. Dexmedetomidine for improved quality of emergence from general anesthesia. *Anesth Anal.* (2019) 129:1504–11. doi: 10.1213/ANE.0000000000002763

10

Lidocaine and Bupivacaine Downregulate MYB and *DANCR* lncRNA by Upregulating *miR-187-5p* in MCF-7 Cells

Chiao-Yi Lin[1,2], *Wen-Ting Tseng*[1], *Yao-Yin Chang*[3], *Mong-Hsun Tsai*[4,5], *Eric Y. Chuang*[5,6,7], *Tzu-Pin Lu*[5,8] *and Liang-Chuan Lai*[1,5*]

[1] Graduate Institute of Physiology, College of Medicine, National Taiwan University, Taipei, Taiwan, [2] Department of Anesthesiology, Hsinchu MacKay Memorial Hospital, Hsinchu, Taiwan, [3] Department of Electrical Engineering, Graduate Institute of Biomedical Electronics and Bioinformatics, National Taiwan University, Taipei, Taiwan, [4] Graduate Institute of Biotechnology, College of Bioresources and Agriculture, National Taiwan University, Taipei, Taiwan, [5] Bioinformatics and Biostatistics Core, Center of Genomic and Precision Medicine, National Taiwan University, Taipei, Taiwan, [6] Graduate Institute of Biomedical Electronics and Bioinformatics, College of Electrical Engineering and Computer Science, National Taiwan University, Taipei, Taiwan, [7] College of Biomedical Engineering, China Medical University, Taichung, Taiwan, [8] Graduate Institute of Epidemiology and Preventive Medicine, College of Public Health, National Taiwan University, Taipei, Taiwan

***Correspondence:**
Liang-Chuan Lai
llai@ntu.edu.tw

Background: Breast cancer is the most common malignancy and a leading cause of death among women. The majority of patients require surgery, and retrospective studies have revealed an association between anaesthetic techniques during surgery and clinical outcomes. Local anaesthetics (LAs) influence carcinogenesis by interacting with non-coding RNAs (ncRNAs). However, the detailed mechanisms underlying the association between LAs and ncRNAs remain unclear.

Methods: In this study, the effects of two commonly used LAs, lidocaine and bupivacaine, on the malignancy of MCF-7 breast cancer cells were investigated. The expression profiles of the microRNAs (miRNAs) that responded to treatment with LAs were determined through next-generation sequencing.

Results: Data from the functional assay revealed that the LAs suppressed the proliferation of MCF-7 cells. The result of next-generation sequencing revealed that 131 miRNAs were upregulated, following treatment with the LAs. Validation using polymerase chain reaction (PCR) identified *miR-187-5p* as a potential biomarker, and it was selected for further analyses. Prediction with bioinformatics tools and luciferase reporter assays revealed that *MYB* is a direct target gene of *miR-187-5p*. Based on the hypothesis that lncRNAs acts as miRNA sponges, the target lncRNA, *DANCR,* of *miR-187-5p* was predicted using DIANA-LncBase v2 and validated using luciferase reporter assays. In addition, the reciprocal suppressive effect between *DANCR* and *miR-187-5p* was determined.

Conclusions: This study suggests that one of the anti-tumour mechanisms of lidocaine and bupivacaine is mediated through the *DANCR-miR-187-5p-MYB* axis. This may provide a novel molecular mechanism of tumour suppression in breast cancer.

Keywords: ***miR-187-5p*, *MYB*, *DANCR*, bupivacaine, lidocaine**

INTRODUCTION

Breast cancer is one of the most common malignancies and a leading cause of death among women (https://gco.iarc.fr/). Most patients require surgery; however, residual disease from scattered micro-metastases and tumour cells related to surgery is usually inevitable (1). Experimental and clinical retrospective studies indicate an association between the types of anaesthetic techniques used during the cancer resection surgery and outcomes (1, 2). There are conflicting results on the administration of volatile anaesthetics and opioids and cancer development, metastasis, and recurrence (3, 4). Regional anaesthesia is hypothesised to attenuate immunosuppression and surgical stress by minimising the requirement for opioids and volatile anaesthetics, therefore improving the long-term postoperative outcomes (2). The overall survival for different local anaesthetics (LAs) varies among the clinical studies; however, laboratory studies suggest that LAs have direct inhibitory effects on tumour cells (5, 6).

Lidocaine and bupivacaine are commonly used amide-type LAs for regional anaesthesia and peripheral nerve blockade, providing excellent perioperative pain relief, especially in breast cancer surgery (7). The mechanisms underlying the inhibitory effect of LAs on cancer cell proliferation, migration, and metastasis, are elucidated (5, 8, 9). However, the precise mechanism remains unclear; it could involve sodium channel blockade, DNA demethylation (10, 11), or interactions between LAs and non-coding RNAs (ncRNAs). Lidocaine inhibits the growth and invasion of gastric carcinoma cells by upregulating miR-145 (12). It inhibits proliferation and induces apoptosis in colorectal cancer cells by upregulating miR-520a-3p and targeting EGFR (13).

Dysregulated gene expression is a major hallmark of cancer. ncRNAs play a critical role in tumourigenesis, growth, and progression (14–16). NcRNAs are categorised as small ncRNAs (sncRNAs) and long ncRNAs (lncRNAs) with a cut-off length of 200 bp; they are directly or indirectly involved in diverse biological processes through epigenetic, transcriptional, and post-transcriptional mechanisms (17). MicroRNAs (miRNAs) are a type of short ncRNAs that regulate cellular proliferation, differentiation, apoptosis, adhesion, epithelial-mesenchymal transition (EMT), and metastasis in various cancers (18). The competing endogenous RNA (ceRNA) theory (19) states that miRNAs recognise miRNA response elements (MREs) in different RNA molecules, and induce target repression through miRNA-RNA-induced silencing complex (RISC)-mediated degradation. Therefore, the transcriptional regulation of diverse RNAs, including mRNAs and ncRNAs, can regulate biological processes through a novel MRE-mediated mechanism (19).

Abbreviations: LA, local anaesthetic; ncRNA, non-coding RNA; miRNA, microRNA; PCR, polymerase chain reaction; sncRNA, small ncRNA; lncRNA, long ncRNA; EMT, epithelial-mesenchymal transition; ceRNA, competing endogenous RNA; MRE, miRNA response element; RISC, RNA-induced silencing complex; MYB, MYB proto-oncogene, transcription factor; *DANCR*, Differentiation Antagonising Non-Protein Coding RNA; qRT-PCR, quantitative real time polymerase chain reaction; PCA, principal component analysis.

The tumour-suppressive effects of lidocaine and bupivacaine were studied in MCF-7 cells. The effects of these LAs on the function of *miR-187-5p*, Differentiation Antagonising Non-Protein Coding RNA (*DANCR*), and *MYB* were investigated for elucidating the underlying mechanism. Our findings provide novel insights into the process of tumour suppression for future breast cancer therapy.

METHODS

Cell Culture

MCF-7 cells were purchased from Bioresource Collection and Research Center (Hsinchu, Taiwan), and HEK-293T cells were provided by Dr. Shau-Ping Lin (Institute of Biotechnology, National Taiwan University, Taiwan). All cells were cultured in Dulbecco's Modified Eagle Medium (DMEM) (Gibco, Thermo Fisher, CA, USA) containing 1% penicillin-streptomycin (Gibco) and 10% foetal bovine serum (FBS) (HyClone, Logan, UT, USA). The culture plates were maintained at 37°C in a humidified atmosphere of 5% CO_2 and were routinely tested for Mycoplasma sp. using Mycoplasma polymerase chain reaction (PCR) Detection Kit (ABM Inc., Vancouver, BC, Canada).

Cell Viability Assay

MCF-7 cells were seeded at 5×10^3 cell into 96-well plates 1 day before lidocaine or bupivacaine (Sigma, St. Louis, MO, USA) treatment at the indicated concentrations. LAs and the controls were diluted in 200 μL DMEM for each well. For the thiazolyl blue tetrazolium bromide (MTT) colorimetric assay, 5 mg/mL of MTT (Sigma) were added to each well and incubated at 37°C for 4 h. The supernatants were removed and replaced with dimethyl sulfoxide (DMSO) (Sigma). The absorbance was measured using a microtiter plate reader (BioTek, Winooski, VT, USA) at 570 nm.

Wound Healing Assays

MCF-7 cells were seeded at a density of 2.5×10^4 cells/well in a medium containing 10% FBS and incubated overnight. The culture inserts were removed and an image of the gap area at 0 h was captured. The cells were further incubated at 37°C in a 5% CO_2 incubator, and the images were captured at 12, 24, and 36 h, respectively. The cell migration ability in the gap area was quantified using ImageJ v1.8.0 (National Institutes of Health, USA).

Cell Migration

Migration assays were performed using SPLInsert™ Hanging plate (SPL Life Sciences, Pocheon, South Korea). The upper chamber of the transwell unit was seeded at 4×10^4 cells/well in 0.2 mL serum-free DMEM. The lower chambers were loaded with 0.6 mL DMEM containing 10% FBS as chemo-attractant. The MCF-7 cells were incubated at 37°C for 36 h. A methanol: acetic acid (3:1) mixture was added to the lower chamber for fixing the cells by incubating at 25°C for 10 min. The non-migrating cells on the inner transwell membrane were removed carefully, and the membranes were stained with 1 mL of 0.5% crystal violet. The stained cells were solubilized with 10% acetic acid, imaged, and analysed using ImageJ v1.8.0.

Western Blotting

The proteins were extracted from the cells lysed with radioimmunoprecipitation assay buffer (RIPA) Lysis Buffer (EMD Millipore, Billerica, MA, USA) and the concentration was determined using Coomassie Protein Assay Reagent (Thermo Fisher, Waltham, MA, USA). The extracted protein samples (20 µg) were separated using 10% sodium dodecyl sulphate–polyacrylamide gel electrophoresis (SDS-PAGE) and transferred to polyvinylidene fluoride (PVDF) membranes (GE healthcare, Chicago, IL, USA). The membranes were incubated with primary rabbit polyclonal antibodies against c-MYB (Proteintech, Rosemont, IL, USA) and β-actin (GeneTex, Irvine, CA, USA), at 4°C overnight; the samples were hybridised with horseradish peroxidase (HRP) conjugated anti-rabbit IgG (GeneTex) at 25°C for 1 h. The blotted proteins were detected using an enhanced chemiluminescence (ECL) system (Millipore, Billerica, MA, USA) equipped with a BioSpectrum Imaging System (UVP, Upland, CA, USA). The images were analysed using ImageJ v1.8.0.

RNA Extraction, Reverse Transcription, and Quantitative Real Time Polymerase Chain Reaction

The RNA was extracted using TRIZOL (Invitrogen, Carlsbad, CA, USA) and reverse-transcribed using High-Capacity cDNA Reverse Transcription Kit (Applied Biosystems, Carlsbad, CA, USA). The RNA quality was detected by a spectrophotometer (NanoDrop; Thermo Scientific) with the A260/A280 ratio between 1.8~2.0. Samples were kept in RNase free water buffer at neutral pH. All RNA samples were stored at −80°C. One µg of total RNA was reverse-transcribed by High-Capacity cDNA Reverse Transcription Kit (Applied Biosystems, Carlsbad, CA, USA). SuperScript IV Reverse Transcriptase (Invitrogen) was used for reverse transcription of the miRNAs in accordance with the manufacturer's instructions. Two point five percent of each reaction was used as template for quantitative PCR with OmicsGreen qPCR MasterMix (OmicsBio, New Taipei City, Taiwan) and the reactions were performed on StepOnePlus Real-Time PCR System (Thermo Fisher, Waltham, MA, USA). The primers were checked for only generating a single melting curve peak and detailed information are provided in **Supplementary Table 1**. The relative expression was normalised to that of 18S rRNA or U6 snRNA, using the $2^{-\Delta\Delta Ct}$ method.

Library Preparation and Sequencing

The total RNA was extracted using TRIZOL reagent (Invitrogen). The small RNA library was constructed from total RNA (2 µg) using the TruSeq Small RNA Library Prep Kit (Illumina Inc., San Diego, CA, USA), according to the manufacturer's instructions. A total of 75 single-read nucleotides were obtained from each miRNA library using NextSeq500 (Illumina Inc., CIC bioGUNE, Bilbao, Spain). The sequencing data were submitted to the Gene Expression Omnibus (GEO) (accession number: GSE171282).

Sequencing Data Analyses

The raw Illumina FASTQ sequencing reads were mapped to the miRBase mature miRNA reference (http://www.mirbase.org/) using Partek Flow™ v5.0 (Partek Inc., St. Louis, MO, USA) with Bowtie alignment algorithm. The Bowtie alignment method was generally thought to be optimal for sequences less than 50 bp. The adapter sequences were first removed from each FASTQ reads, and the remaining bases were trimmed from the 3′ end with a minimum Phred quality score of 20. A minimum read-length philtre of 15-bases in length was used in this work. A minimum seed length of 10 that was consistent with the standard setting provided by the Partek Flow pipeline was chosen for the Bowtie aligner. The remaining reads were aligned to the human genome reference (RefSeq Hg19). Raw miRNA expression reads were normalised by scale normalisation and then processed by $\log_2$ transformation. Then, miRNAs with extremely low expression ($\log_2$ <5 in all samples) were removed from further analysis. Then, differentially expressed miRNA profiles between groups were identified by $\log_2$ fold-change value ≧2X or <-1X and P-value < 0.05 using a two-sided Student's t-test. Principal component analysis using the expression values of total miRNAs was used to visualise the similarity of different groups.

Transfection

MCF-7 cells were cultured in an antibiotic-free medium to 70–80% confluence in 6-well plates (2.5 × 10^5 cells/well) and transfected with the 0.025 nmol of *miR-187-5p* mimic (GenePharma, Shanghai, China) or negative control (GenePharma), using Lipofectamine 2000 as the transfection reagent (Invitrogen), following the manufacturer's instructions.

The MCF-7 cells were transfected with 0.5 nmol of pcDNA-*DANCR* or the empty vector (Dharmacon, New Taipei city, Taiwan) using jetPRIME (Polyplus-transfection, New York, NY, USA) reagent, following the manufacturer's instructions. After 4 h, the medium was replaced with fresh medium containing serum. The cellular RNA expression after 48 h was determined using qRT-PCR.

Plasmid Construct and Site-Directed Mutagenesis

To determine promoter activity by luciferase assay, the luciferase expression plasmid pMIR-REPORT-*c-MYB 3′UTR* and pMIR-REPORT-*DANCR* was purchased from the BioMed Resource Core of the 1st Core Facility Lab, National Taiwan University College of Medicine (Taipei, Taiwan). Briefly, *c-MYB 3′UTR* region encompassing 2,493–3,684 bp relative to the transcription start site was amplified from the human genomic DNA by PCR. The *c-MYB 3′UTR* was subcloned into pMIR-REPORT vector, and the final construct was called pMIR-REPORT-*c-MYB 3′UTR*. *DANCR* encompassing 1–915 bp relative to the transcription start site was amplified from the human genomic DNA by PCR and the final construct was called pMIR-REPORT-*DANCR*.

miR-187-5p binding sites of *c-MYB 3′UTR* were located at 2,710–2,734 and 3,634–3,656 bp. Besides, *miR-187-5p* binding sites of *DANCR* were located at 134–157 and 380–408 bp. To determine binding activity of *miR-187-5p* by luciferase assay, the luciferase expression plasmid pMIR-REPORT-*c-MYB 3′UTR* S1, pMIR-REPORT-*c-MYB 3′UTR* S2, pMIR-REPORT-c-MYB 3′UTR S12, pMIR-REPORT-*DANCR* S1, pMIR-REPORT-*DANCR* S2, and pMIR-REPORT-DANCR S12 was purchased from the BioMed Resource Core of the 1st Core Facility Lab,

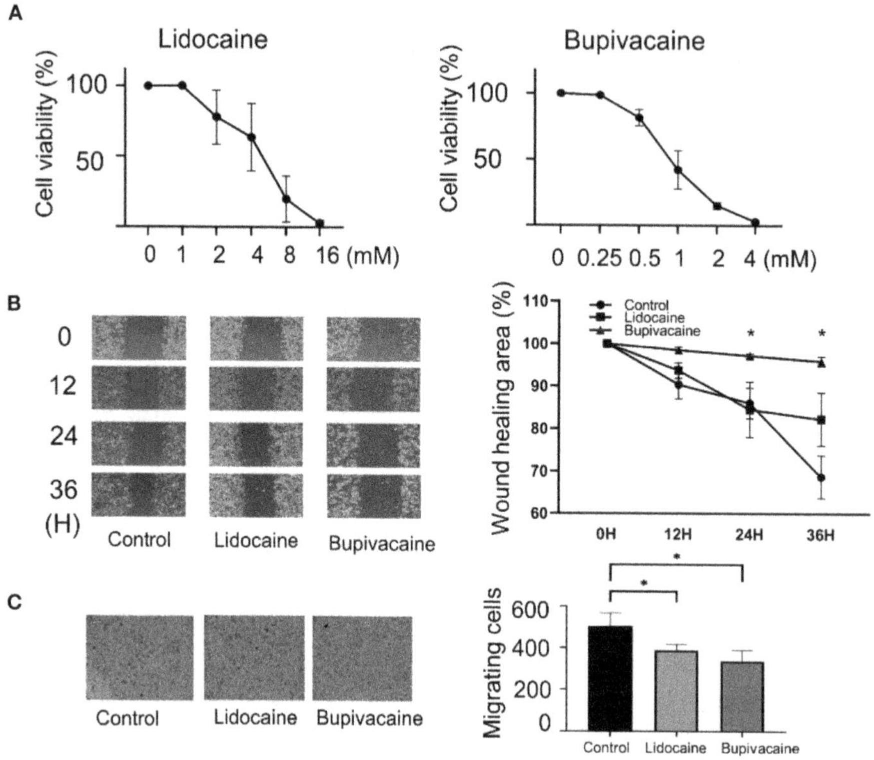

FIGURE 1 | Lidocaine and bupivacaine inhibited the proliferation and migration of MCF-7 cells. **(A)** Cell proliferation determined using the MTT assay. The growth of MCF-7 cells measured after 6 h of treatment with serially diluted concentrations of lidocaine or bupivacaine. The proliferation rate was normalised to that at 0 h. **(B)** Wound healing assay. Left: Images after 0, 12, 24, and 36 h of treatment with lidocaine (4 mM) or bupivacaine (1 mM). Right: The migratory ability quantified using the reduction in wound size over time by ImageJ software v1.8.0. **(C)** Transwell migration assay. Right: The cells were seeded after 24 h of treatment with lidocaine (4 mM) or bupivacaine (1 mM). Left: Cell migration measured after 36 h of seeding. All data are presented as mean ± SD ($n = 3$). $^*p < 0.05$.

NTU-CM (Taipei, Taiwan). In addition, the mutated sequences were validated by sequencing.

Luciferase Reporter Assay

Luciferase assays were performed with HEK-293T cells using the Dual-Glo® luciferase reporter assay system (Promega, Fitchburg, WI, USA). Cells (5×10^4/well) were transfected with 100 ng reporter constructs containing the wild-type or mutant-type of *MYB*, the wild-type or mutant-type of *DANCR* and 2 ng Ranilla luciferase plasmid (BioMed Resource Core of the 1st Core Facility Lab, National Taiwan University College of Medicine, Taiwan), using the jetPRIME (Polyplus-transfection) reagent. The cells were additionally transfected with 0.025 nmol of *miR-187-5p* (GenePharma). After 24 h, the cells were lysed and the Renilla luciferase signals were used for normalisation, according to manufacturer's protocol.

Statistical Analyses

The experimental data are presented as the mean ± standard deviation (SD) of at least three independent experiments. The genes with statistically significant expression patterns in the different samples were determined by a two-tailed Student's t-test using GraphPad Prism v5 (GraphPad Software, Inc., La Jolla, CA, USA). p-values <0.05 were considered statistically significant.

RESULTS

LAs Significantly Suppressed Cell Viability and Migration

To determine the effects of lidocaine and bupivacaine on MCF-7 cells, the cell viability following treatment with different concentrations of lidocaine or bupivacaine for 6 h was determined. Lidocaine and bupivacaine inhibited the growth of MCF-7 cells in a dose-dependent manner (**Figure 1A**). The median lethal dose (LD_{50}) of lidocaine (4 mM) and bupivacaine (1 mM) were used as the concentrations for the following experiments, respectively. Wound healing and transwell invasion assays were performed using MCF-7 cells treated with lidocaine or bupivacaine for 12, 24, and 36 h. Both the LAs significantly reduced the migration and invasive ability of MCF-7 cells (**Figures 1B,C**), suggesting suppression of malignancy in the MCF-7 cells.

Differential miRNA Expression Profiles Following LA Treatment

To identify the miRNAs that mediated the effects of the LAs on MCF-7 cells, next-generation sequencing was used for identifying the differentially expressed miRNAs, following lidocaine or bupivacaine treatment. Principal component analysis (PCA) was

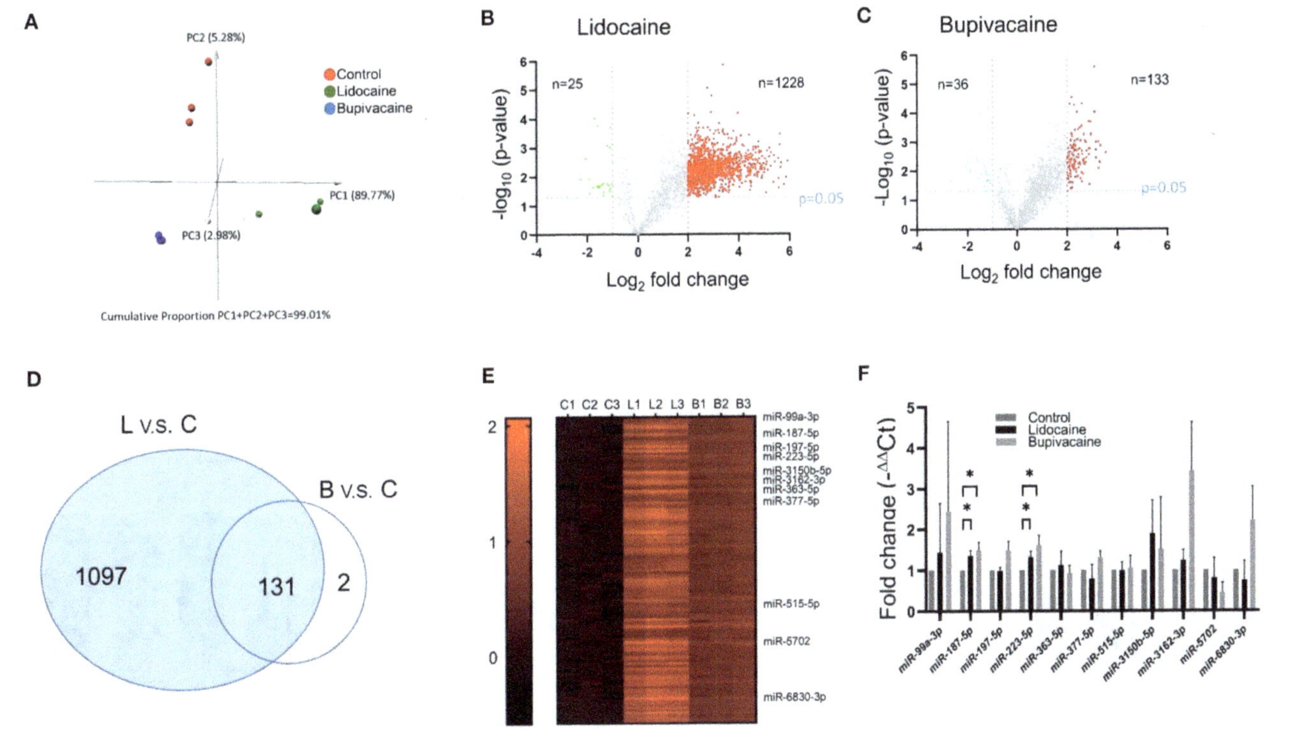

FIGURE 2 | Identification of miRNAs in MCF-7 cells that responded to treatment with lidocaine or bupivacaine. **(A)** PCA of differentially expressed miRNAs in response to treatment with lidocaine (4 mM) or bupivacaine (1 mM). **(B,C)** Volcano plot of the differentially expressed miRNAs in response to treatment with lidocaine **(B)** or bupivacaine **(C)** determined by next-generation sequencing. **(D)** Venn diagram of the differentially expressed miRNAs. The expression of 131 miRNAs was upregulated following treatment with lidocaine or bupivacaine. **(E)** Heat map of the upregulated miRNAs ($n = 131$) that responded to treatment with both lidocaine and bupivacaine. **(F)** PCR validation of the selective differentially expressed miRNAs in MCF-7 cells, following treatment with lidocaine and bupivacaine. The expression levels measured using qRT-PCR and normalised to that of U6 snRNA. L, lidocaine; B, bupivacaine; C, control. All data are presented as mean ± SD ($n = 3$). $^*p < 0.05$.

performed for the samples (lidocaine, bupivacaine, and control groups, nine dots in total) using the data for 2,522 differentially expressed miRNAs in the three groups (**Figure 2A**). The miRNAs in the same group showed similar expression profiles, while the expression profiles in the lidocaine- and bupivacaine-treated groups were distinct from those of the control.

The miRNAs that were differentially expressed in the lidocaine- and bupivacaine-treated groups were filtered using the criteria: fold change ≥ 2.0X and *p*-value ≤0.05. The expression of 1,228 and 133 miRNAs was significantly upregulated in the lidocaine (**Figure 2B**) and bupivacaine groups (**Figure 2C**), respectively (red dots). The expression of 25 and 36 miRNAs was significantly downregulated (fold change <-1X and *p*-value ≤ 0.05) in the lidocaine (**Figure 2B**) and bupivacaine groups (**Figure 2C**), respectively (green dots). The genes that were not differentially expressed are depicted in grey. Among the upregulated miRNAs, 131 were common to both the lidocaine and bupivacaine groups (**Figure 2D**). The number of downregulated miRNAs common to both the groups was low; therefore, only the upregulated miRNAs were selected for subsequent studies. The expression of the selected miRNAs is depicted using a heatmap (**Figure 2E**).

The data from next-generation sequencing was validated by selecting the miRNAs whose expression was significantly higher and for which experimentally validated data were available. The expression of only *miR-187-5p* and *miR-223-5p* was significantly ($p < 0.05$) higher than that of the control. The expression of the other miRNAs examined using qRT-PCR was not statistically different between the lidocaine and bupivacaine groups (**Figure 2F**).

LAs Downregulated MYB Expression via *miR-187-5p*

To identify the genes regulated by *miR-187-5p* and ascertain their functional relevance, we used the TargetScan tool (http://www.targetscan.org/vert_72/) for identifying the downstream target genes. The *MYB* transcription factor, a proto-oncogene, was a predicted target gene of *miR-187-5p. In vitro* and *in vivo* studies indicated that *MYB* plays an important role in different cancers. *MYB* overexpression and dysregulation is observed in almost all breast tumours, and is associated with poor prognosis (20, 21). *MYB* also regulates cell proliferation, differentiation, and angiogenesis (22), and therefore, was selected for further studies.

qRT-PCR and western blotting were used to investigate the mechanism underlying the influence of *miR-187-5p* on cellular function. The mRNA and protein levels of MYB were significantly downregulated in the LA-treated groups (**Figures 3A,B**). The levels of *MYB* mRNA were significantly

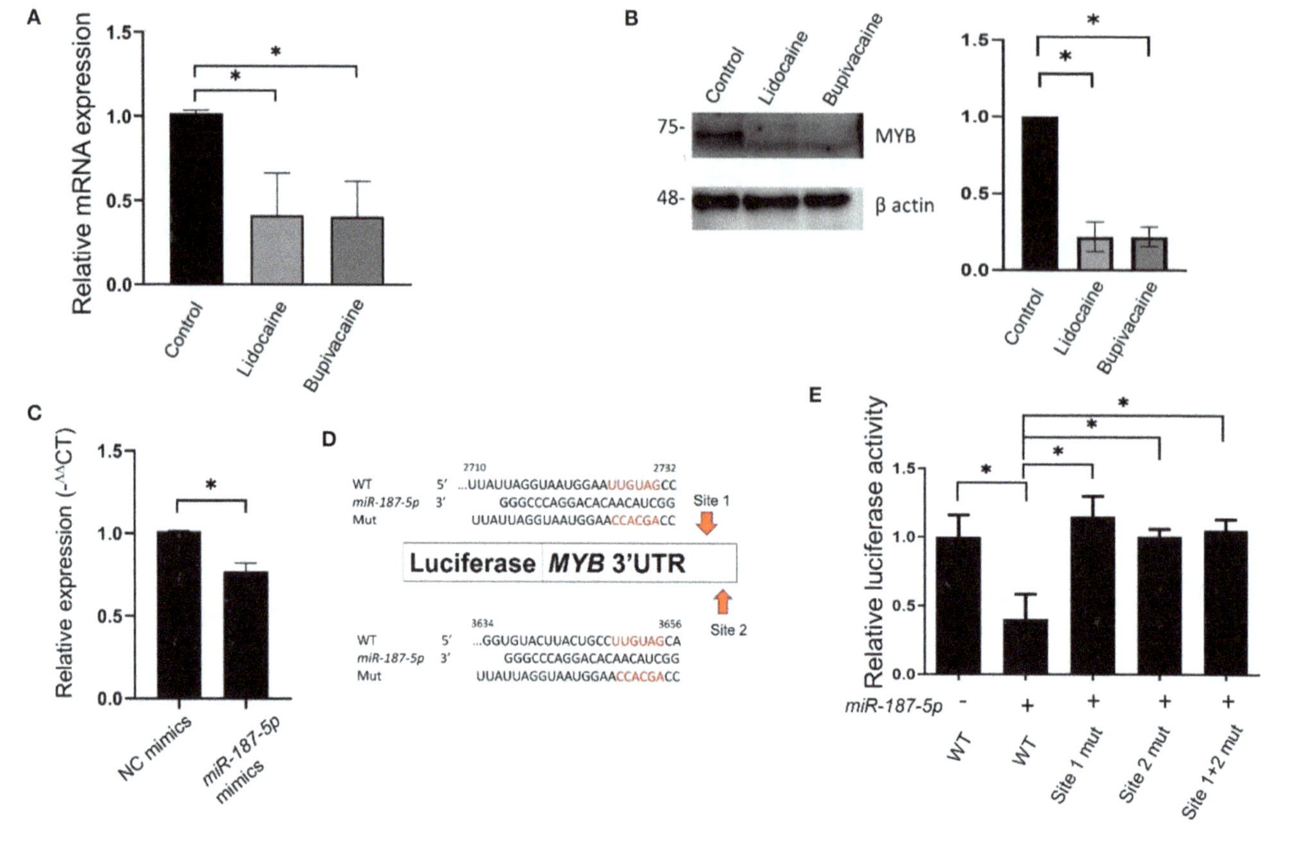

FIGURE 3 | Downregulation of *MYB* in MCF-7 cells following lidocaine and bupivacaine treatment. **(A)** The relative mRNA levels of *MYB* in MCF-7 cells following treatment with lidocaine (4 mM) or bupivacaine (1 mM). The expression levels of *MYB* were measured using qRT-PCR and normalised to that of 18S rRNA. **(B)** Western blots of MYB in MCF-7 cells following treatment with the LAs. Right: graphical representation of the results of western blotting. Left: quantification of the western blots. β actin was used as the loading control. **(C)** Relative expression levels of *MYB* in MCF-7 cells overexpressing *miR-187-5p*. The cells were transfected with 2 μg of *miR-187-5p* or control mimics. The expression levels were detected using qRT-PCR and normalised to that of 18S rRNA. **(D)** Schematic diagram of the putative binding site of *miR-187-5p* in the 3′-UTR region (2,493 ~ 3,684 bp) of *MYB*. **(E)** Luciferase reporter assays of *MYB* 3′-UTR in HEK-293T cells overexpressing *miR-187-5p*. The HEK-293T cells were transfected with *miR-187-5p* mimics, firefly luciferase plasmids, and Renilla luciferase vectors. The relative activity of firefly luciferase was measured and normalised to that of Renilla luciferase. The data are presented as mean ± SD ($n = 3$). $^{*}p < 0.05$.

reduced when *miR-187-5p* was overexpressed (**Figure 3C**). Using bioinformatics analysis, we validated *MYB* as a target gene of *miR-187-5p*; two binding sites (2,710–2,732 nt and 3,634–3,656 nt) were predicted in the 3′-UTR of *MYB*, which were complementary to the seed sequence of *miR-187-5p* (**Figure 3D**). The direct interactions between *miR-187-5p* and *MYB* were examined using luciferase reporter plasmids containing the wild-type *MYB* (*MYB*-wt) and binding site mutants (*MYB*-site1-mut, *MYB*-site2-mut, and *MYB*-site1+2-mut). The luciferase activity of *MYB*-wt decreased significantly, with the transfection of *miR-187-5p* mimics; however, they had no influence on *MYB*-site1, *MYB*-site2, and *MYB*-site1+2 (**Figure 3E**), indicating that *MYB* is a direct target gene of *miR-187-5p*. The LAs, lidocaine and bupivacaine, upregulated the expression of *miR-187-5p*, directly downregulating the expression of *MYB*.

DANCR Decoys *miR-187-5p* by Reciprocal Suppression

LncRNAs act as ceRNAs and influence mRNA levels by sequestering miRNAs that target both lncRNA and mRNAs. To identify the ceRNAs of *miR-187-5p*, we used DIANA-LncBase v2 (23) for predicting the lncRNAs that bind to *miR-187-5p*. Five possible lncRNAs were predicted and validated using qRT-PCR (**Figure 4A**). The expression of *DANCR* was downregulated by the LAs, while that of the *HIF1A-AS2* and *SNHG1* lncRNAs was upregulated; however, these lncRNAs did not function as ceRNAs of *miR-187-5p*. In addition, the expression of *DANCR* significantly decreased when the expression of *miR-187-5p* increased (**Figure 4B**).

Luciferase reporter assays were performed for validating the association between *DANCR* and *miR-187-5p*. Prediction revealed two potential binding sites of *miR-187-5p* at 134–157 nt and 380–408 nt of *DANCR*, which were individually positioned upstream of the luciferase reporter genes (**Figure 4C**). The binding site mutants (sites 1-mut, 2-mut, and 1+2-mut) were constructed and transfected into HEK-293T cells. The luciferase activity of *DANCR*-wt was significantly reduced by the *miR-187-5p* mimics; however, they had no effect on sites 1-mut, 2-mut, and 1+2-mut (**Figure 4D**), indicating that the *DANCR* lncRNA sponges *miR-187-5p* by direct binding.

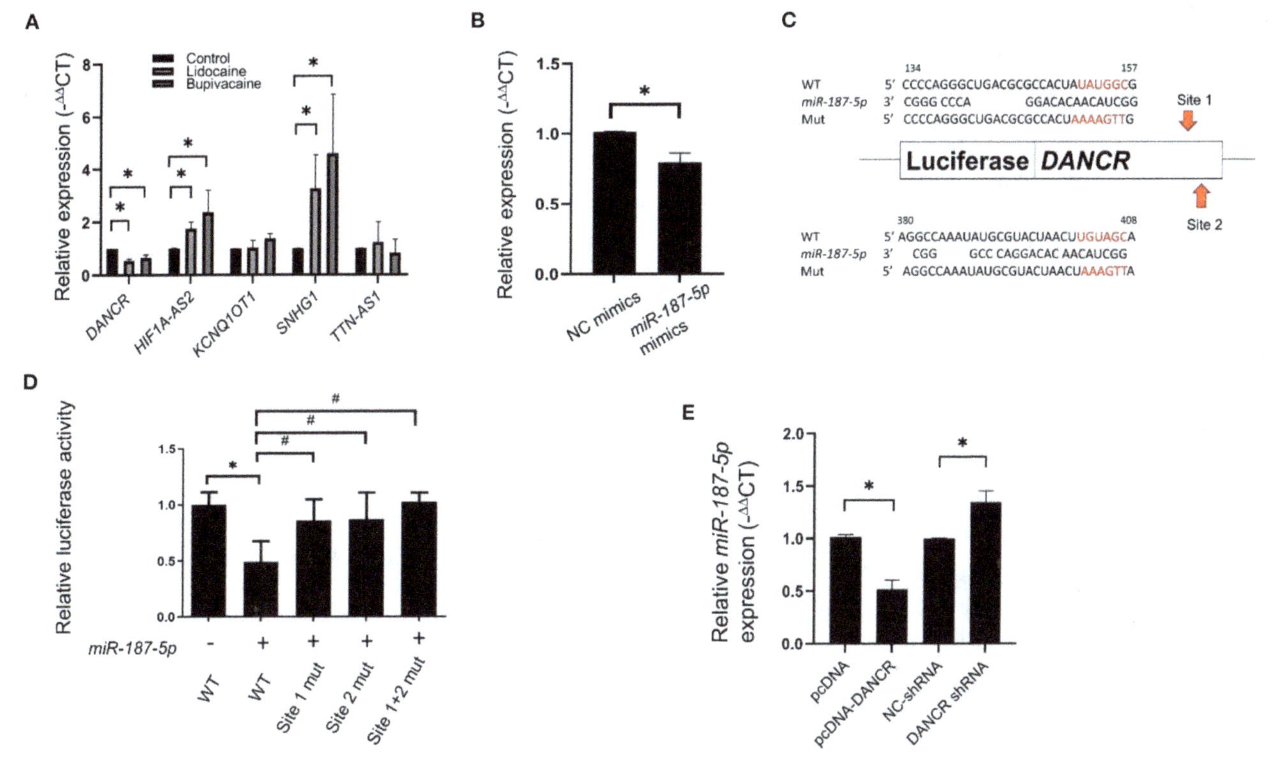

FIGURE 4 | Expression of *DANCR* lncRNA was downregulated in MCF-7 cells following treatment with lidocaine or bupivacaine. **(A)** The relative expression levels of selective lncRNAs in MCF-7 cells following treatment with lidocaine (4 mM) or bupivacaine (1 mM). The expression levels were measured using qRT-PCR and normalised to that of 18S rRNA. **(B)** Relative expression levels of *DANCR* in MCF-7 cells overexpressing *miR-187-5p*. The cells were transfected with 2 μg of *miR-187-5p* or control mimics. The expression levels were detected using qRT-PCR and normalised to that of 18S rRNA. **(C)** Schematic diagram of the putative binding site of *miR-187-5p* in the binding region of *DANCR*. **(D)** Luciferase reporter assays of *DANCR* in HEK-293T cells overexpressing *miR-187-5p*. The HEK-293T cells were transfected with *miR-187-5p* mimics, firefly luciferase plasmids, and Renilla luciferase vectors. The relative activity of firefly luciferase was measured and normalised to that of Renilla luciferase. **(E)** The relative expression levels of *miR-187-5p* in MCF-7 cells overexpressing *DANCR* or shRNAs against *DANCR*. The expression levels were detected using qRT-PCR and normalised to that of U6 snRNA. The data are presented as mean ± SD ($n = 3$). $^*p < 0.05$.

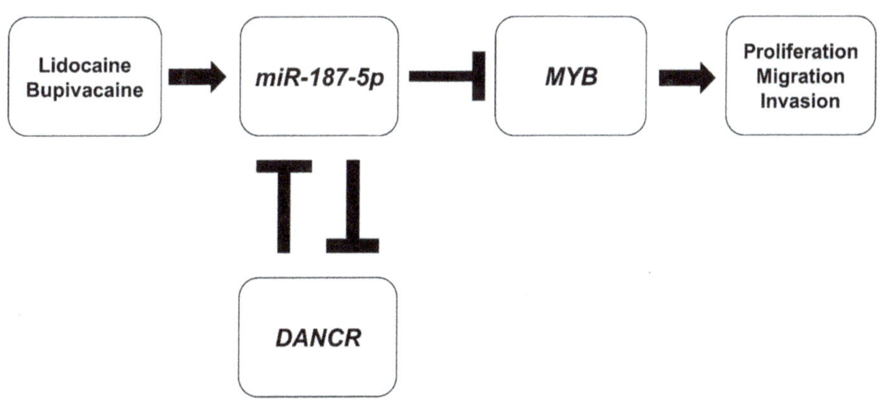

FIGURE 5 | Schematic diagram of the proposed mechanism underlying the inhibitory effect of LAs. Lidocaine and bupivacaine suppress the malignancy of MCF-7 breast cancer cells by upregulating *miR-187-5p*, which in turn downregulates the expression of MYB (MYB proto-oncogene, transcription factor) proteins and the DANCR (Differentiation Antagonising Non-Protein Coding RNA) lncRNA.

The overexpression of *DANCR* suppressed *miR-187-5p* expression, while the downregulation of *DANCR* increased *miR-187-5p* expression (**Figure 4E**). These results demonstrated a reciprocal inhibitory relationship between *DANCR* and *miR-187-5p*, and that *miR-187-5p* could mediate the inhibitory effect of the LAs on MCF-7 cell viability and migration.

DISCUSSION

The LAs, lidocaine and bupivacaine, inhibited MCF-7 cell proliferation and migration. Genomic studies and validation experiments revealed that the LAs promoted *miR-187-5p* expression, which downregulated *MYB* expression. Additionally, the LAs reduced the expression of *DANCR* lncRNA, which could be a ceRNA of *miR-187-5p*. Our study demonstrated a novel mechanism underlying the inhibitory effect of LAs on cancer cell proliferation, migration, and invasion, mediated via the *DANCR-miR-187-5p-MYB* regulatory axis.

LAs inhibit cancer cell proliferation, migration, and invasion by regulating miRNA expression (12, 13). Lidocaine inhibits proliferation and induces apoptosis in retinoblastoma cells by modulating the *miR-520a-3p*/EGFR axis (24). Bupivacaine inhibits gastric cancer progression by regulating the *circ_0000376*/*miR-145-5p* axis (25). Using NGS and qRT-PCR, we demonstrated that lidocaine and bupivacaine upregulated *miR-187-5p* expression. *MiR-187-5p* regulates cellular proliferation and apoptosis in lung cancer (26), hepatocellular carcinoma (27), bladder cancer (28), and acute lymphoblastic leukaemia (29), and is a possible indicator of drug sensitivity in breast cancer (30). This study is the first to identify that *miR-187-5p* regulates the inhibitory effect of LAs on the proliferation, migration, and invasion of MCF-7 cells.

Bioinformatics-based prediction revealed that *MYB* is a target gene of *miR-187-5p*, consistent with the reports that *MYB* functions as an oncogene in different tumours, including breast cancer (21, 31–33). *MYB* could be inhibited in MCF-7 cells through the upregulation of *miR-187-5p* by lidocaine or bupivacaine. These LAs reduced the mRNA and protein levels of MYB, and the *miR-187-5p* mimics significantly reduced *MYB* expression in MCF-7 cells. The luciferase reporter assay confirmed that *miR-187-5p* directly targets the 3′-UTR of *MYB*.

LncRNAs interact with various molecules and have key roles in regulating signalling processes at the epigenetic, transcriptional, and post-transcriptional levels (34, 35). A novel regulatory mechanism elucidates that all types of transcripts, including mRNAs, lncRNAs, and circular RNAs, can act as ceRNAs, forming a complex RNA interactome involving different RNA species, for regulating gene expression (35). The lncRNA-miRNA-mRNA crosstalk could have a prominent role in the anti-tumour effects of LAs. Among the lncRNAs, *DANCR*, encoded by a gene located in human chromosome 4q12, plays an important role in different cancers (36). The *DANCR*-SOCS3-EZH2 axis regulates the inflammatory phenotype and breast cancer cell metastasis (37). *DANCR* promotes progressive osteosarcoma by functioning as a ceRNA and sponging *miR-335-5p* and *miR-1972*, regulating ROCK1 expression (38). In this study, the expression of *DANCR* was inhibited by the LAs, and a reciprocal suppressive effect was observed between *DANCR* and *miR-187-5p*. The luciferase reporter assay confirmed that *DANCR* was the target of *miR-187-5p*. Therefore, the upregulation of *miR-187-5p* and downregulation of *DANCR* could mediate the inhibitory effect of LAs on the proliferation, migration, and invasion of MCF-7 cells. Together, we concluded that the DANCR-miR-187-5p-MYB axis is activated by lidocaine and bupivacaine; the proposed schematic diagram is presented in **Figure 5**.

This study has certain limitations. First, LAs are chemically categorised into amide-ester and amide-amide groups, and the new generation LAs, including ropivacaine and levobupivacaine, are used clinically. Only the older generation LAs, lidocaine and bupivacaine, were considered. LAs have variable anti-tumour effects and mechanisms of action in different cancers (39). Further studies are necessary for confirming whether the *DANCR-miR-187-5p-MYB* axis mediates the inhibitory effects of other LAs. Second, there are several breast cancer types; and therefore, further studies are necessary for confirming the effects of lidocaine and bupivacaine in other breast cancer cell lines and in an animal model, which may improve upon the present findings. Third, although luciferase studies proved the interaction between *DANCR-miR-187-5p-MYB* axis, whether the anti-tumour properties of LAs can be reversed requires more experiments to prove, such as using antagomir to inhibit *miR-187-5p* or overexpressing *MYB* in MCF-7 cells treated with LAs.

This study demonstrated that lidocaine and bupivacaine inhibited the growth and metastasis of breast cancer cells. The anti-tumour properties of these LAs were partially attributed to the upregulation of *miR-187-5p*, which inhibited *MYB* signalling by directly binding to *MYB*. Screening for the possible targets of *miR-187-5p* using a dual-luciferase reporter assay revealed that the *DANCR* lncRNA directly targets *miR-187-5p*, suggesting that *DANCR* could act as a *miR-187-5p* sponge. In summary, we report that the *DANCR-miR-187-5p-MYB* axis may be activated by lidocaine and bupivacaine.

AUTHOR CONTRIBUTIONS

C-YL and L-CL: conception and design of experiments and manuscript preparation. C-YL and W-TT: performed experiments. C-YL and Y-YC: data analyses. L-CL, M-HT, and EC: contributed reagents, materials, and analytical tools. All the authors reviewed and approved the final version of the manuscript.

ACKNOWLEDGMENTS

The authors acknowledge the technical assistance provided by the Biomedical Resource Core at the 1st Core Facility Lab, NTU College of Medicine.

REFERENCES

1. Sessler DI, Pei L, Huang Y, Fleischmann E, Marhofer P, Kurz A, et al. Recurrence of breast cancer after regional or general anaesthesia: a randomised controlled trial. *Lancet.* (2019) 394:1807–15. doi: 10.1016/S0140-6736(19)32313-X
2. Wall T, Sherwin A, Ma D, Buggy DJ. Influence of perioperative anaesthetic and analgesic interventions on oncological outcomes: a narrative review. *Br J Anaesth.* (2019) 123:135–50. doi: 10.1016/j.bja.2019.04.062
3. Connolly C, Buggy DJ. Opioids and tumour metastasis: does the choice of the anesthetic-analgesic technique influence outcome after cancer surgery? *Curr Opin Anaesthesiol.* (2016) 29:468–74. doi: 10.1097/ACO.0000000000000360
4. Dockrell L, Buggy DJ. The role of regional anaesthesia in the emerging subspecialty of onco-anaesthesia: a state-of-the-art review. *Anaesthesia.* (2021) 76(Suppl. 1):148–59. doi: 10.1111/anae.15243
5. Li R, Xiao C, Liu H, Huang Y, Dilger JP, Lin J. Effects of local anesthetics on breast cancer cell viability and migration. *BMC Cancer.* (2018) 18:666. doi: 10.1186/s12885-018-4576-2
6. Xuan W, Zhao H, Hankin J, Chen L, Yao S, Ma D. Local anesthetic bupivacaine induced ovarian and prostate cancer apoptotic cell death and underlying mechanisms *in vitro. Sci Rep.* (2016) 6:26277. doi: 10.1038/srep26277
7. FitzGerald S, Odor PM, Barron A, Pawa A. Breast surgery and regional anaesthesia. *Best Pract Res Clin Anaesthesiol.* (2019) 33:95–110. doi: 10.1016/j.bpa.2019.03.003
8. D'Agostino G, Saporito A, Cecchinato V, Silvestri Y, Borgeat A, Anselmi L,, et al. Lidocaine inhibits cytoskeletal remodelling and human breast cancer cell migration. *Br J Anaesth.* (2018) 121:962–8. doi: 10.1016/j.bja.2018.07.015
9. Lucchinetti E, Awad AE, Rahman M, Feng J, Lou PH, Zhang L, et al. Antiproliferative effects of local anesthetics on mesenchymal stem cells: potential implications for tumor spreading and wound healing. *Anesthesiology.* (2012) 116:841–56. doi: 10.1097/ALN.0b013e31824babfe
10. Chamaraux-Tran TN, Piegeler T. The amide local anesthetic lidocaine in cancer surgery-potential antimetastatic effects and preservation of immune cell function? A narrative review. *Front Med.* (2017) 4:235. doi: 10.3389/fmed.2017.00235
11. Lirk P, Hollmann MW, Fleischer M, Weber NC, Fiegl H. Lidocaine and ropivacaine, but not bupivacaine, demethylate deoxyribonucleic acid in breast cancer cells *in vitro. Br J Anaesth.* (2014) 113(Suppl. 1):i32–8. doi: 10.1093/bja/aeu201
12. Sui H, Lou A, Li Z, Yang J. Lidocaine inhibits growth, migration and invasion of gastric carcinoma cells by up-regulation of miR-145. *BMC Cancer.* (2019) 19:233. doi: 10.1186/s12885-019-5431-9
13. Qu X, Yang L, Shi Q, Wang X, Wang D, Wu G. Lidocaine inhibits proliferation and induces apoptosis in colorectal cancer cells by upregulating mir-520a-3p and targeting EGFR. *Pathol Res Pract.* (2018) 214:1974–9. doi: 10.1016/j.prp.2018.09.012
14. Goodall GJ, Wickramasinghe VO. RNA in cancer. *Nat Rev Cancer.* (2021) 21:22–36. doi: 10.1038/s41568-020-00306-0
15. Barbieri I, Kouzarides T. Role of RNA modifications in cancer. *Nat Rev Cancer.* (2020) 20:303–22. doi: 10.1038/s41568-020-0253-2
16. Bracken CP, Scott HS, Goodall GJ. A network-biology perspective of microRNA function and dysfunction in cancer. *Nat Rev Genet.* (2016) 17:719–32. doi: 10.1038/nrg.2016.134
17. Han Li C, Chen Y. Small and long non-coding RNAs: Novel targets in perspective cancer therapy. *Curr Genomics.* (2015) 16:319–26. doi: 10.2174/138920291666615070715585l
18. Chan SH, Wang LH. Regulation of cancer metastasis by microRNAs. *J Biomed Sci.* (2015) 22:9. doi: 10.1186/s12929-015-0113-7
19. Salmena L, Poliseno L, Tay Y, Kats L, Pandolfi PP. A ceRNA hypothesis: the Rosetta Stone of a hidden RNA language? *Cell.* (2011) 146:353–8. doi: 10.1016/j.cell.2011.07.014
20. Li Y, Jin K, van Pelt GW, van Dam H, Yu X, Mesker WE, et al. c-Myb enhances breast cancer invasion and metastasis through the Wnt/beta-catenin/axin2 pathway. *Cancer Res.* (2016) 76:3364–75. doi: 10.1158/0008-5472.CAN-15-2302
21. Mitra P. Transcription regulation of MYB: a potential and novel therapeutic target in cancer. *Ann Transl Med.* (2018) 6:443. doi: 10.21037/atm.2018.09.62
22. Liu X, Xu Y, Han L, Yi Y. Reassessing the potential of Myb-targeted anti-cancer therapy. *J Cancer.* (2018) 9:1259–66. doi: 10.7150/jca.23992
23. Paraskevopoulou MD, Vlachos IS, Karagkouni D, Georgakilas G, Kanellos I, Vergoulis T, et al. DIANA-LncBase v2: indexing microRNA targets on non-coding transcripts. *Nucleic Acids Res.* (2016) 44:D231–8. doi: 10.1093/nar/gkv1270
24. Xia W, Wang L, Yu D, Mu X, Zhou X. Lidocaine inhibits the progression of retinoblastoma *in vitro* and *in vivo* by modulating the miR-520a-3p/EGFR axis. *Mol Med Rep.* (2019) 20:1333–42. doi: 10.3892/mmr.2019.10363
25. Ju C, Zhou J, Miao H, Chen X, Zhang Q. Bupivacaine suppresses the progression of gastric cancer through regulating circ_0000376/miR-145-5p axis. *BMC Anesthesiol.* (2020) 20:275. doi: 10.1186/s12871-020-01179-4
26. Mao M, Wu Z, Chen J. MicroRNA-187-5p suppresses cancer cell progression in non-small cell lung cancer (NSCLC) through down-regulation of CYP1B1. *Biochem Biophys Res Commun.* (2016) 478:649–55. doi: 10.1016/j.bbrc.2016.08.001
27. Gong J, Mou T, Wu H, Wu Z. Brg1 regulates murine liver regeneration by targeting miR-187-5p dependent on Hippo signalling pathway. *J Cell Mol Med.* (2020) 24:11592–602. doi: 10.1111/jcmm.15776
28. Li Z, Lin C, Zhao L, Zhou L, Pan X, Quan J, et al. Oncogene miR-187-5p is associated with cellular proliferation, migration, invasion, apoptosis and an increased risk of recurrence in bladder cancer. *Biomed Pharmacother.* (2018) 105:461–9. doi: 10.1016/j.biopha.2018.05.122
29. Lou Y, Liu L, Zhan L, Wang X, Fan H. miR-187-5p regulates cell growth and apoptosis in acute lymphoblastic leukemia via DKK2. *Oncol Res.* (2016) 24:89–97. doi: 10.3727/096504016X14597766487753
30. Uhr K, Prager-van der Smissen WJC, Heine AAJ, Ozturk B, van Jaarsveld MTM, Boersma AWM, et al. MicroRNAs as possible indicators of drug sensitivity in breast cancer cell lines. *PLoS ONE.* (2019) 14:e0216400. doi: 10.1371/journal.pone.0216400
31. Jia H, Wu D, Zhang Z, Li S. Regulatory effect of the MAFG-AS1/miR-150-5p/MYB axis on the proliferation and migration of breast cancer cells. *Int J Oncol.* (2021) 58:33–44. doi: 10.3892/ijo.2020.5150
32. Miao RY, Drabsch Y, Cross RS, Cheasley D, Carpinteri S, Pereira L, et al. MYB is essential for mammary tumorigenesis. *Cancer Res.* (2011) 71:7029–37. doi: 10.1158/0008-5472.CAN-11-1015
33. Ramsay RG, Gonda TJ. MYB function in normal and cancer cells. *Nat Rev Cancer.* (2008) 8:523–34. doi: 10.1038/nrc2439
34. Akhade VS, Pal D, Kanduri C. Long noncoding RNA: genome organization and mechanism of action. *Adv Exp Med Biol.* (2017) 1008:47–74. doi: 10.1007/978-981-10-5203-3_2
35. Volovat SR, Volovat C, Hordila I, Hordila DA, Mirestean CC, Miron OT, et al. MiRNA and lncRNA as potential biomarkers in triple-negative breast cancer: a review. *Front Oncol.* (2020) 10:526850. doi: 10.3389/fonc.2020.526850
36. Yan Y, Shi Q, Yuan X, Xue C, Shen S, He Y, et al. An emerging therapeutic target for cancer. *Am J Transl Res.* (2020) 12:4031–42.
37. Zhang KJ, Tan XL, Guo L. The long non-coding RNA DANCR regulates the inflammatory phenotype of breast cancer cells and promotes breast cancer progression via EZH2-dependent suppression of SOCS3 transcription. *Mol Oncol.* (2020) 14:309–28. doi: 10.1002/1878-0261.12622
38. Wang Y, Zeng X, Wang N, Zhao W, Zhang X, Teng S, et al. Long noncoding RNA DANCR, working as a competitive endogenous RNA, promotes ROCK1-mediated proliferation and metastasis via decoying of miR-335-5p and miR-1972 in osteosarcoma. *Mol Cancer.* (2018) 17:89. doi: 10.1186/s12943-018-0837-6
39. Liu H, Dilger JP, Lin J. Effects of local anesthetics on cancer cells. *Pharmacol Ther.* (2020) 212:107558. doi: 10.1016/j.pharmthera.2020.107558

11

Case Series: Video-Assisted Minimally Invasive Cardiac Surgery During Pregnancy

Anyi Lu[1,2†], *Yingxian Ye*[1†], *Jiaqi Hu*[1], *Ning Wei*[1], *Jinfeng Wei*[1], *Bimei Lin*[3] *and Sheng Wang*[1,4*]

[1] Department of Anesthesiology, Guangdong Cardiovascular Institute & Guangdong Provincial People's Hospital, Guangdong Academy of Medical Sciences, Guangzhou, China, [2] College of Medicine, Shantou University, Shantou, China, [3] Department of Operation Room, Guangdong Cardiovascular Institute & Guangdong Provincial People's Hospital, Guangdong Academy of Medical Sciences, Guangzhou, China, [4] Department of Anesthesiology, Linzhi People's Hospital, Linzhi, China

***Correspondence:**
Sheng Wang
shengwang_gz@163.com

† These authors have contributed equally to this work and share first authorship

Surgical intervention is expected to improve maternal outcomes in pregnant patients with heart disease once the conservative treatment fails. For pregnant patients with heart disease, the risk of cardiac surgery under cardiopulmonary bypass (CPB) must be balanced due to the high fetal loss. The video-assisted minimally invasive cardiac surgery (MICS) has been progressively applied and shows advantages in non-pregnant patients over the years. We present five cases of pregnant women who underwent a video-assisted minimally invasive surgical approach for cardiac surgery and the management strategies. In conclusion, the video-assisted MICS is feasible and safe to pregnant patients, with good maternal and fetal outcomes under the multidisciplinary assessment and management.

Keywords: minimally invasive cardiac surgery (MICS), video-assisted, pregnancy, cardiopulmonary bypass, perioperative management

INTRODUCTION

Heart diseases complicate 2–4% of pregnancies but account for up to 15% of maternal deaths (1). The cardiac potential to adapt hemodynamic change is impaired in women with structural heart disease, presented with reduced systolic and diastolic function (2). Once cardiac decompensation happens, cardiac surgery might be a solution for pregnant patients with structural heart diseases and compromised cardiac function. Maternal mortality after cardiac surgery during pregnancy is reported to be comparable to non-pregnant patients for about 11.2%, but the high fetal loss (33.1%) cannot be ignored (1). The management of these patients should be made with adequate multidisciplinary discussions, including cardiologists, anesthetists, and obstetricians, with aims to improve maternal and fetal outcomes.

The minimally invasive cardiac surgery (MICS) has been progressively applied in non-pregnant patients over the years and showed advantages, such as less transfusion rate and shorter postoperative ventilation support time as compared to that of mid-sternotomy approach thus, resulting to shorter ICU time and length of stay (3, 4). However, few MICS during pregnancy has been reported. This article presents a case series of five pregnant women who underwent a video-assisted MICS cardiac surgery during pregnancy in a tertiary medical center.

CASE SERIES

We retrospectively reviewed the records of all pregnancies with cardiac surgery in our hospital between 2019 and 2021. Only patients who underwent a video-assisted MICS ($n = 5$) were included. Informed consent has been obtained from all the patients. Baseline characteristics of all patients are shown in **Table 1**, and intraoperative and postoperative information of all patients are shown in **Tables 2, 3**.

PERIOPERATIVE MANAGEMENT STRATEGY

Perioperative management was discussed by the multidisciplinary team that included cardiologists, cardiac surgeons, anesthesiologists, perfusionists, and gynecologists. The operative procedure was conducted under general anesthesia with 35 F left double-lumen intubation to allow single lung ventilation. A central venous catheter was placed on the right internal jugular vein. A 16 Fr venous cannula was placed in the superior cava vein through the right jugular vein for cardiopulmonary bypass (CPB) venous return. Transesophageal echocardiography was routinely set up for intraoperative monitoring. The patient was placed in a supine position with elevated right chest. Propofol and rocuronium were used for anesthetic induction. Sevoflurane, propofol, dexmedetomidine, and rocuronium were used for anesthetic maintenance with certain level of Nacrotrend Bis values between 40 and 60. Sufentanil was intermittently given to ensure enough analgesia. Magnesium sulfate was used to inhibit uterine contraction. The fetal heart rate and uterine contraction were monitored by TEE and tocodynamometer. After heparinization, a 24 Fr venous cannula and 19 Fr arterial cannula were placed in the right femoral vein and artery. A right anterolateral 4th intercostal 3.5 cm incision was made and the thoracoscopy was inserted *via* the 5th intercostal space. The high-flow, high-pressure normothermic CPB was then started. Vacuum-assisted venous drainage was also utilized (maximum negative pressure 20–40 mmHg). Cold Del Nido cardioplegia solution (blood and crystalloid mixed formula) was used as anterograde. During CPB, the hematocrit was maintained between 25 and 29%, as well as normothermia. Post-bypass transesophageal echocardiography has ensured a satisfying surgical outcome and fetal survival. An intercostal nerve block with 0.5% ropivacaine combined with intravenous analgesia, was used for postoperative multimodal analgesia.

The patient was transferred to the intensive care unit temporarily for monitoring. Fetal status was ensured by Doppler echography and uterine contraction was monitored by the tocodynamometer after the surgery. Atosiban was used postoperatively to inhibit uterine contraction. Warfarin and/or low molecular weight heparin were administrated for anticoagulation for those patients who underwent mechanical valve replacement.

DISCUSSION

MICS During Pregnancy

Compared to standard sternotomy, the minimally invasive approach through thoracoscopy has been utilized in the past decades. However, there were few reports about occurrence of MICS with thoracoscopy during pregnancy. In one previous study, Nguyen et al. (5) reported a case of acute papillary muscle rupture during pregnancy. The minimally invasive mitral valve repair *via* the right thoracotomy was conducted, with main consideration on how morbidly obese this patient was. In our

TABLE 1 | Baseline characteristics of five patients undergoing minimally invasive cardiac surgery (MICS) during pregnancy.

Case no.	Age (years)	Gravida	Para	Weight (kg)	GA when cardiac surgery (weeks)	Diagnosis	NYHA grade	Preoperative transthoracic echocardiography	LVEF (%)	Pulmonary arterial systolic pressure (mmHg)	ECG
1	35	5	2	60	18	Rheumatic heart disease	II	Severe mitral stenosis with moderate regurgitation, and mild tricuspid and aortic regurgitation	62	45	Normal
2	27	2	1	40	22	Infective endocarditis	II	Moderate mitral stenosis and severe mitral regurgitation with abnormal vegetation echo	60	80	Sinus tachycardia
3	38	2	0	56	18	Rheumatic heart disease	II	Moderate-severe mitral valve stenosis with moderate-severe regurgitation, moderate tricuspid regurgitation	73	62	Normal
4	34	2	1	58	31	Rheumatic heart disease	III	Severe mitral stenosis and mild mitral regurgitation	76	60	Normal
5	32	5	2	54	18	Left atrial myxoma	II	A medium-echo 19 mm × 10 mm irregular mass with good mobility in the left atrium, with good mobility and the stalk adherent to the fossa ovalis, considered as a myxoma	66	<40	Normal

MICS, minimally invasive cardiac surgery; NYHA, New York Heart Association (NYHA) Classification; LVEF, left ventricular ejection fraction; ECG, electrocardiogram.

TABLE 2 | Intraoperative information of five patients undergoing MICS during pregnancy.

Case no.	Intervention	Intubation	Total operation time (minutes)	CPB time (minutes)	Aortic cross-clamp time (minutes)	Lowest core temperature (°C)	Pulsatile perfusion
1	Mitral valve replacement	Double lumen tube	145	75	47	36.0	Yes
2	Mitral valve replacement	Single lumen tube	165	92	64	36.0	Yes
3	Mitral valvuloplasty	Double lumen tube	170	88	68	36.0	Yes
4	Mitral valve replacement	Double lumen tube	133	67	43	36.0	No
5	Left atrial myxoma excision	Double lumen tube	135	46	21	35.7	No

TABLE 3 | Postoperative information of five patients undergoing MICS during pregnancy.

Case no.	Extubation time after surgery (hours)	Complication	Blood transfusion	Length of stay (days)	Maternal mortality	Gestational age when pregnancy termination (weeks)	Fetal outcomes
1	5	No	No	11	No	20	Abortion
2	5	No	No	13	No	35	Abortion due to fetal cerebral anomaly
3	5	No	No	18	No	37	Normal Term Infant
4	10	Atrial fibrillation*	No	22	No	37	Normal Term Infant
5	1	No	2U RBC	13	No	26	Abortion due to fetal chromosomal abnormality

**Four days after the surgery, the patient had an episode of acute atrial fibrillation with heart rate of 171 bpm. The sinus rhythm was returned with a heart rate of 92 bpm after the Valsava maneuver twice. One day after the first episode, the patients felt palpation with no reason and the ECG revealed a rapid onset of atrial fibrillation with a heart rate of 175 bpm. Antiarrhythmic drugs (12.5 mg beta-blocker and 0.2 mg deslanoside) were given and the episode was terminated. Beta-blocker was used to maintain the sinus rhythm.*

center, we conducted the MICS *via* video-assisted thoracoscopy, with the advantage of smaller operative incision, rather than the right thoracotomy. Also, favorable outcomes after the minimally invasive approach can be obtained more than that of standard sternotomy with less postoperative pain, faster recovery, less postoperative complication, and shorter length of stay in the hospital (6, 7). Qiu et al. (3) demonstrated that a full sternotomy was an independent risk factor for postoperative ventilation support. It was known that prolonged mechanical ventilation affects fetus morbidity and mortality in cardiac surgery during pregnancy (8). In our study, all fetuses remained alive after the cardiac surgery, supporting our supposition that the minimally invasive approach has its benefits to fetal survivals in pregnant women who underwent cardiac surgery under CPB. Also, sternal complications following a median sternotomy, including infection, sternal instability, and non-union, were reported by 1–8% worldwide (9). Sternal precautions were recommended for prevention of complication, which consisted of weight restrictions on the use of the upper limbs immediately after surgery for 6–12 weeks (10). This may interfere with normal maternal-infant bonding because motion restriction after median sternotomy may affect the mother in holding her child and in breastfeeding (5, 11). However, longer operation duration in the MICS should come into consideration for pregnant women as CPB time is reported as a risk factor for fetal mortality (12), but this may be solved by experienced surgeons. During MICS, single lung ventilation technique is required for a satisfactory field exposure. In our cases, we applied double lumen tube in four patients and single lumen tube in one patient. All surgical field remained satisfactory to the surgeons, including the one with single lumen intubation. Hypoxemia in the lung isolation after cardiopulmonary bypass (CPB) surgery might impair fetal oxygenation, and whether single lumen tube in MICS benefits to these patients still needs further investigation.

Cardiopulmonary Bypass During Pregnancy

Cardiopulmonary bypass can pose significant effects on both the fetus and the mother. Sustained uterine contraction during CPB is regarded as a risk factor to fetus survival. The cooling and rewarming process during CPB induces uterine contraction, especially after maternal hypothermia, which induces placental hypoperfusion and, consequently, fetal hypoxia. Hemodilution of progesterone during CPB also enhances uterine contraction (12, 13). In our study, we performed high perfusion pressure and normothermic CPB to ensure placental perfusion. It is thought that pulsatile perfusion can release endothelium-derived growth factors from the vascular endothelium and reduce uterine contractions, which may result to good fetal outcomes in pregnant women who undergo cardiac surgery (12, 14). In our study, non-pulsatile CPB was performed in two cases and both fetuses were alive after cardiac surgery, though 1 patient eventually has terminated pregnancy due to fetal chromosomal abnormality. Pulsatile perfusion was performed in three patients and one patient has terminated pregnancy due to fetal cerebral anomaly. In fact, there are few clinical data to support the advantage of pulsatile perfusion over non-pulsatile perfusion in pregnant women. In the cohort study of John et al. (15), there was a reported three fetal deaths among the 21 non-pulsatile CPB cases. Most of them (two fetal deaths) happened in women with other comorbidities. Further clinical research evidence is required to determine the beneficial application of pulsatile or non-pulsatile perfusion in cardiac surgery of pregnant women.

In the study of Jha et al. (1), the pooled rate of maternal complications was at 15%, maternal heart failure at 5.8%, and arrhythmia at 2.1%, respectively. In our study, only 1 patient experienced cardiovascular complication of acute onset of atrial fibrillation that requires treatment. Maternal mortality is comparable to that of CPB in non-pregnant women in the previous studies, with the estimated rate of 11% in the meta-analysis of Jha et al. (1). Maternal status with worse NYHA and emergency surgery contributed to unfavorable maternal outcomes in these patients. In our cases, all women survived and may benefit from good maternal NYHA status and semi-urgent surgery.

Management of Cardiac Surgery During Pregnancy

The decision to perform cardiac surgery during pregnancy should be thoroughly discussed within a multidisciplinary team of obstetricians, cardiologists, cardiac surgeons, anesthetists, and gynecologists. The Modified World Health Organization Classification of Cardiovascular Disease in Pregnancy is used as reference for risk stratification of maternal and neonatal complication (16). Compared to non-pregnant women, pregnant women are at higher risk of aspiration, difficult intubation, and thromboembolism, which made them require more attention in preoperative preparation (17). Once the patient is supine, the 15° position of left uterine displacement should be applied to avoid aortocaval compression after 18–20 weeks of gestation (18).

Pregnant patients are more sensitive to IV and inhalational medications. Propofol seems to be the preferred medication for induction in healthy pregnant patients. Mongardon et al. (19) demonstrated that the dose of propofol required in pregnant

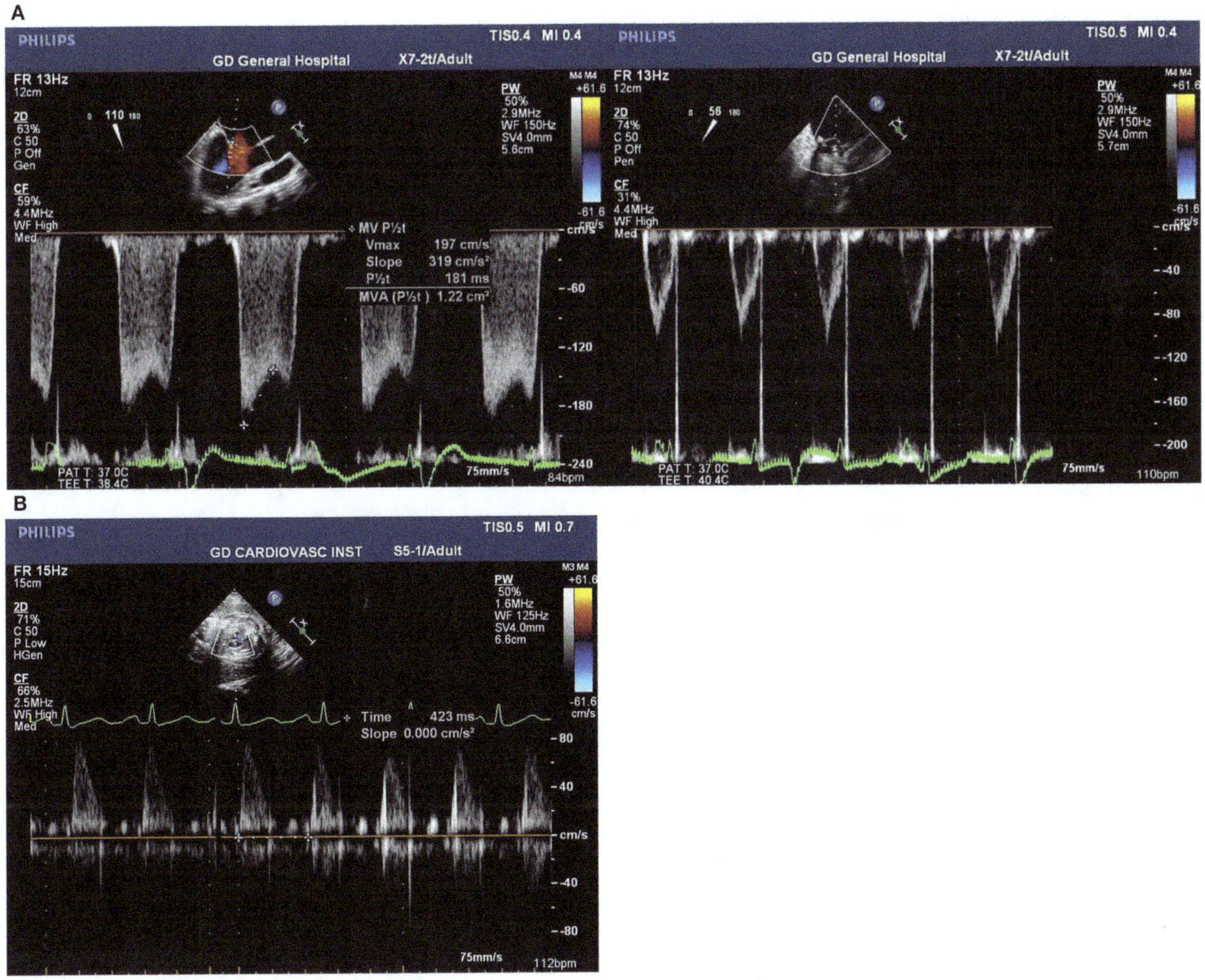

FIGURE 1 | (A) Pre and post-surgical mitral valve view of transesophageal echocardiogram images of mitral valve stenosis in Case 1. **(B)** Postoperative transesophageal echocardiogram images of Doppler of fetal blood flow in Case 3 presenting the fetal heart rate at 141 bpm.

women for loss of consciousness is 8% less than in non-pregnant patients. Inhalation medication, such as desflurane and sevoflurane, inhibits myometrial contractions during the operation, which may be beneficial to pregnant women undergoing cardiac surgery (20). It suggested a more rapid onset of neuromuscular block with vecuronium and rocuronium in pregnant women (18).

Sympathomimetic agents, such as phenylephrine and norepinephrine, are safe to maintain blood pressure. In comparison with phenylephrine, ephedrine may act on fetal metabolism and be associated with neonatal acidosis and, therefore, should be considered as secondary choice of vasopressor in pregnancy (16, 21).

Intraoperative monitoring for both the mother and the fetus is critically significant to favorable maternal and fetal outcomes. If uterine contractions are detected, increase maternal intravascular volume may be helpful and tocolytic treatment can be administrated (22). Fetal bradycardia is an important indicator of fetal distress during CPB, which usually occurs at the initiation of CPB caused by a decrease in systemic vascular resistance, thereby affected by hemodilution, and the release of vasoactive substances. It has been reported that fetal heart rate (FHR) monitoring with an external cardiotocography reduces fetal mortality to 7.5% in cardiac surgeries with CPB (23). In our cases, the tocodynamometer combined with TEE were used to monitor uterine contraction and fetal heart rate (**Figure 1**). FHR was measured intraoperatively by Doppler echocardiography across the fetal blood flow, which was available in all pregnant women in our cases whose gestational age ranged from 18 to 31 weeks.

Commonly tocolytic drugs include magnesium, beta-adrenergic drugs, nitroglycerin, and prostaglandin inhibitors (22). In our case, we chose magnesium sulfate, which is mainly used for pre-eclampsia control, to inhibit uterine contraction by decreasing acetylcholine transmission in motor nerve terminals (24). Also, it was reported that antenatal usage of magnesium sulfate may contribute to fetal neuroprotection and may reduce the risk of cerebral palsy or even death (25). However, magnesium may potentiate the activity of both depolarizing and non-depolarizing neuromuscular blocking agents (NMBA). Consequently, the dose of NMBA should be reduced (24). In a case of left atrial myxoma resection reported by Alexis et al. (26), a low dose of nicardipine, a calcium channel blocker, was used to inhibit uterine contractility and may show an advantage to restore FHR.

For these patients, postoperative monitoring is pivotal along with the assessment of fetus by using Doppler ultrasound, as well checking of uterine contraction with a tocodynamometer. If necessary, tocolytic drugs should be administrated in case of a preterm labor. The left lateral position should be maintained to prevent aortocaval compression (18). Furthermore, postoperative analgesia is important for pain control and can reduce the risk of premature labor. NSAIDs should be avoided in women as prenatal exposure to NSAIDs after 30 weeks gestational age is associated with an increased risk of premature closure of the fetal ductus arteriosus and oligohydramnios (27). In our center, multimodal analgesia was performed in every patient including intercostal nerve block with 0.5% ropivacaine and intravenous analgesia with opioids, resulting all patients to report a pain score <3 on a numeric rating scale (NRS).

CONCLUSION

The video-assisted MICS is feasible and safe with good maternal and fetal outcomes, which may be progressively applied in patients in the need for cardiac surgery during pregnancy. The multidisciplinary team for decision in the management of these patients is of vital importance to favorable outcome for both the mother and the fetus.

ETHICS STATEMENT

The studies involving human participants were reviewed and approved by Guangdong Provincial People's Hospital Ethics Committee. The patients/participants provided their written informed consent to participate in this study. Written informed consent was obtained from the individual(s) for the publication of any potentially identifiable images or data included in this article.

AUTHOR CONTRIBUTIONS

NW, YY, and JH collected and organized the information of patients. AL wrote the first draft of the manuscript. JW, YY, JH, BL, and NW wrote sections of the manuscript. All authors contributed to manuscript revision, read, and approved the submitted version.

REFERENCES

1. Jha N, Jha AK, Chand Chauhan R, Chauhan NS. Maternal and fetal outcome after cardiac operations during pregnancy: a meta-analysis. *Ann Thorac Surg.* (2018) 106:618–26. doi: 10.1016/j.athoracsur.2018.03.020
2. Cornette J, Ruys TP, Rossi A, Rizopoulos D, Takkenberg JJ, Karamermer Y, et al. Hemodynamic adaptation to pregnancy in women with structural heart disease. *Int J Cardiol.* (2013) 168:825–31. doi: 10.1016/j.ijcard.2012.10.005
3. Qiu Z, Chen X, Xu Y, Huang F, Xiao L, Yang T, et al. Does full sternotomy have more significant impact than the cardiopulmonary bypass

time in patients of mitral valve surgery? *J Cardiothorac Surg.* (2018) 13:29. doi: 10.1186/s13019-018-0719-4

4. Paparella D, Fattouch K, Moscarelli M, Santarpino G, Nasso G, Guida P, et al. Current trends in mitral valve surgery: a multicenter national comparison between full-sternotomy and minimally-invasive approach. *Int J Cardiol.* (2020) 306:147–51. doi: 10.1016/j.ijcard.2019.11.137
5. Nguyen S, Umana-Pizano JB, Donepudi R, Dhoble A, Nguyen TC. Minimally invasive mitral valve repair for acute papillary muscle rupture during pregnancy. *Ann Thorac Surg.* (2019) 107:e93–e5. doi: 10.1016/j.athoracsur.2018.06.048
6. Modi P, Hassan A, Chitwood WR Jr. Minimally invasive mitral valve surgery: a systematic review and meta-analysis. *Eur J Cardiothorac Surg.* (2008) 34:943–52. doi: 10.1016/j.ejcts.2008.07.057
7. Zhang QL, Chen Q, Lin ZQ, Yu LL, Lin ZW, Cao H. Thoracoscope-assisted mitral valve replacement with a small incision in the right chest: a Chinese single cardiac center experience. *Med Sci Monit.* (2018) 24:1054–63. doi: 10.12659/MSM.905855
8. Kapoor MC. Cardiopulmonary bypass in pregnancy. *Ann Card Anaesth.* (2014) 17:33–9. doi: 10.4103/0971-9784.124133
9. Cahalin LP, Lapier TK, Shaw DK. Sternal precautions: is it time for change? Precautions versus restrictions - a review of literature and recommendations for revision. *Cardiopulm Phys Ther J.* (2011) 22:5–15. doi: 10.1097/01823246-201122010-00002
10. Balachandran S, Lee A, Royse A, Denehy L, El-Ansary D. Upper limb exercise prescription following cardiac surgery *via* median sternotomy: a web survey. *J Cardiopulm Rehabil Prev.* (2014) 34:390–5. doi: 10.1097/HCR.0000000000000053
11. Taksaudom N, Traisrisilp K, Kanjanavanit R. Left atrial myxoma in pregnancy: management strategy using minimally invasive surgical approach. *Case Rep Cardiol.* (2017) 2017:8510160. doi: 10.1136/bcr-2017-219624
12. Patel A, Asopa S, Tang AT, Ohri SK. Cardiac surgery during pregnancy. *Tex Heart Inst J.* (2008) 35:307–12.
13. Yuan SM. Indications for cardiopulmonary bypass during pregnancy and impact on fetal outcomes. *Geburtshilfe Frauenheilkd.* (2014) 74:55–62. doi: 10.1055/s-0033-1350997
14. Jahangiri M, Clarke J, Prefumo F, Pumphrey C, Ward D. Cardiac surgery during pregnancy: pulsatile or nonpulsatile perfusion? *J Thorac Cardiovasc Surg.* (2003) 126:894–5. doi: 10.1016/S0022-5223(03)00607-X
15. John AS, Gurley F, Schaff HV, Warnes CA, Phillips SD, Arendt KW, et al. Cardiopulmonary bypass during pregnancy. *Ann Thorac Surg.* (2011) 91:1191–6. doi: 10.1016/j.athoracsur.2010.11.037
16. Carlier L, Devroe S, Budts W, Van Calsteren K, Rega F, Van de Velde M, et al. Cardiac interventions in pregnancy and peripartum - a narrative review of the literature. *J Cardiothorac Vasc Anesth.* (2020) 34:3409–19. doi: 10.1053/j.jvca.2019.12.021
17. Upadya M, Saneesh PJ. Anaesthesia for non-obstetric surgery during pregnancy. *Indian J Anaesth.* (2016) 60:234–41. doi: 10.4103/0019-5049.179445
18. Okeagu CN, Anandi P, Gennuso S, Hyatali F, Stark CW, Prabhakar A, et al. Clinical management of the pregnant patient undergoing non-obstetric surgery: review of guidelines. *Best Pract Res Clin Anaesthesiol.* (2020) 34:269–81. doi: 10.1016/j.bpa.2020.04.004
19. Mongardon N, Servin F, Perrin M, Bedairia E, Retout S, Yazbeck C, et al. Predicted propofol effect-site concentration for induction and emergence of anesthesia during early pregnancy. *Anesth Analg.* (2009) 109:90–5. doi: 10.1213/ane.0b013e3181a1a700
20. Yildiz K, Dogru K, Dalgic H, Serin IS, Sezer Z, Madenoglu H, et al. Inhibitory effects of desflurane and sevoflurane on oxytocin-induced contractions of isolated pregnant human myometrium. *Acta Anaesthesiol Scand.* (2005) 49:1355–9. doi: 10.1111/j.1399-6576.2005.00804.x
21. Veeser M, Hofmann T, Roth R, Klöhr S, Rossaint R, Heesen M. Vasopressors for the management of hypotension after spinal anesthesia for elective caesarean section. Systematic review and cumulative meta-analysis. *Acta Anaesthesiol Scand.* (2012) 56:810–6. doi: 10.1111/j.1399-6576.2011.02646.x
22. Chandrasekhar S, Cook CR, Collard CD. Cardiac surgery in the parturient. *Anesth Analg.* (2009) 108:777–85. doi: 10.1213/ane.0b013e31819367aa
23. Koh KS, Friesen RM, Livingstone RA, Peddle LJ. Fetal monitoring during maternal cardiac surgery with cardiopulmonary bypass. *Can Med Assoc J.* (1975) 112:1102–4.
24. Lu JF, Nightingale CH. Magnesium sulfate in eclampsia and pre-eclampsia: pharmacokinetic principles. *Clin Pharmacokinet.* (2000) 38:305–14. doi: 10.2165/00003088-200038040-00002
25. Magee LA, De Silva DA, Sawchuck D, Synnes A, von Dadelszen P. No. 376-Magnesium sulphate for fetal neuroprotection. *J Obstet Gynaecol Can.* (2019) 41:505–22. doi: 10.1016/j.jogc.2018.09.018
26. Alexis A, Origer P, Hacquebard JP, De Cannière D, Germay O, Vandenbossche JL, et al. Anesthetic management of a voluminous left atrial myxoma resection in a 19 weeks pregnant with atypical clinical presentation. *Case Rep Anesthesiol.* (2019) 2019:4181502. doi: 10.1155/2019/4181502
27. Antonucci R, Zaffanello M, Puxeddu E, Porcella A, Cuzzolin L, Pilloni MD, et al. Use of non-steroidal anti-inflammatory drugs in pregnancy: impact on the fetus and newborn. *Curr Drug Metab.* (2012) 13:474–90. doi: 10.2174/138920012800166607

12

A Thrombomodulin Promoter Gene Polymorphism, rs2239562, Influences Both Susceptibility to and Outcome of Sepsis

Eizo Watanabe [1,2], Osamu Takasu [3], Youichi Teratake [4], Teruo Sakamoto [3], Toshiaki Ikeda [5], Joji Kotani [6], Nobuya Kitamura [7], Masaaki Ohmori [1], Ayako Teratani [1], Goichi Honda [8], Masahiko Hatano [4], Benjamin Mayer [9], E. Marion Schneider [10] and Shigeto Oda [1]*

[1] Department of Emergency and Critical Care Medicine, Chiba University Graduate School of Medicine, Chiba, Japan, [2] General Medical Science, Chiba University Graduate School of Medicine, Chiba, Japan, [3] Department of Emergency and Critical Care Medicine, Kurume University School of Medicine, Kurume, Japan, [4] Biomedical Research Center, Chiba University, Chiba, Japan, [5] Division of Critical Care and Emergency Medicine, Tokyo Medical University Hachioji Medical Center, Hachioji, Japan, [6] Department of Emergency, Disaster and Critical Care Medicine, Hyogo College of Medicine, Nishinomiya, Japan, [7] Department of Emergency and Critical Care Medicine, Kimitsu Chuo Hospital, Kisarazu, Japan, [8] Medical Affairs Department, Asahi Kasei Pharma Corporation, Tokyo, Japan, [9] Institute for Epidemiology and Medical Biometry, Ulm Universtiy, Ulm, Germany, [10] Division of Experimental Anesthesiology, University Hospital Ulm, Ulm, Germany

***Correspondence:**
Eizo Watanabe
eizo-watanabe@umin.ac.jp*

Objective: Disseminated intravascular coagulation plays a key role in the pathophysiology of sepsis. Thrombomodulin is essential in the protein C system of coagulation cascade, and functional polymorphisms influence the human thrombomodulin gene (*THBD*). Therefore, we conducted a multicenter study to evaluate the influence of such polymorphisms on the pathophysiology of sepsis.

Methods: A collaborative case-control study in the intensive care unit (ICU) of each of five tertiary emergency centers. The study included 259 patients (of whom 125 displayed severe sepsis), who were admitted to the ICU of Chiba University Hospital, Chiba, Japan between October 2001 and September 2008 (discovery cohort) and 793 patients (of whom 271 patients displayed severe sepsis), who were admitted to the five ICUs between October 2008 and September 2012 (multicenter validation cohort). To assess the susceptibility to severe sepsis, we further selected 222 critically ill patients from the validation cohort matched for age, gender, morbidity, and severity with the patients with severe sepsis, but without any evidence of sepsis.

Results: We examined whether the eight *THBD* single nucleotide polymorphisms (SNPs) were associated with susceptibility to and/or mortality of sepsis. Higher mortality on severe sepsis in the discovery and combined cohorts was significantly associated with the CC genotype in a *THBD* promoter SNP (−1920*C/G; rs2239562) [odds ratio [*OR*] 2.709 (1.067–6.877), $P = 0.033$ and *OR* 1.768 (1.060–2.949), $P = 0.028$]. Furthermore, rs2239562 SNP was associated with susceptibility to severe sepsis [*OR* 1.593 (1.086–2.338), $P = 0.017$].

Conclusions: The data demonstrate that rs2239562, the *THBD* promoter SNP influences both the outcome and susceptibility to severe sepsis.

Keywords: genetic predisposition to disease, genetic testing, multicenter studies, disseminated intravascular coagulation, single nucleotide polymorphisms

INTRODUCTIONS

Sepsis is a global public death emergency, affecting millions of people worldwide, and representing one of the greatest global causes of mortality (1). Currently, numerous genetic polymorphisms are suggested to be associated with susceptibility to and/or outcome of sepsis, and we discovered several polymorphisms related to sepsis pathophysiology (2). One of the purposes of investigating the effects of genetic polymorphisms on the clinical course of diseases is to examine the association of particular molecular pathways, that is, cytokine networks (3, 4), cell death (5, 6), and coagulation/fibrinolysis systems among others (7–9).

Recently, precision medicine has gained attention, particularly for multifactorial diseases in the critical care field, and disseminated intravascular coagulation (DIC) in the pathophysiology of sepsis has of late been increasingly recognized to play a key role as well as to be a therapeutic target (10). Thrombomodulin is an integral membrane protein expressed on the surface of endothelial cells and serves as a cofactor for thrombin, having a pivotal role in the protein C system through the extracellular domain, which binds to thrombin. Thereby, thrombomodulin activates protein C and prevents excessive coagulation (11). Therefore, the recombinant agent is thought to be a promising drug for sepsis-induced coagulopathy (12–14). A recent clinical trial using recombinant human thrombomodulin (ART-123) still showed a tendency of survival benefit in phase three multicenter study (14). Activated protein C (APC) decomposes the coagulation factors Va and VIIIa, thus exerting the anti-coagulative properties (15). The pathophysiology of sepsis-induced DIC is recognized as a perfusion abnormality by fibrin clotting, against which APC has therapeutic potential. Additionally, APC acts both by activating the endothelial receptors, such as protease-activated receptor-1and endothelial protein C receptor, as well as by degrading histones (16). Although the polymorphisms of protein C genes, for example, PROC(−1641), are already demonstrated to be associated with the mortality and organ failures of sepsis (9), there is only limited investigation of the thrombomodulin gene *THBD*.

Accordingly, we postulated that some of the *THBD* single nucleotide polymorphisms (SNPs) are associated with susceptibility to and/or mortality of sepsis. In addition, the present study aimed to evaluate the role of thrombomodulin in the pathophysiology of sepsis through a genetic association study with Japanese multicenter cohorts, focusing on the *THBD* gene polymorphisms.

MATERIALS AND METHODS

Patient Selection

The subjects were recruited as part of a prospective, observational study of adults admitted during 2001–2012 into a network of Japanese intensive care units (ICUs). The study using these subjects has been reported elsewhere (6). The protocol was approved by the institutional Ethics Committees at all the five participating institutes [the Ethics Committee of Chiba University School of Medicine (permission number 205), the Ethical Committee of Kurume University (bioethics permission number 49), the Medical Research Ethics Committee of Tokyo Medical University, the Ethics Review Board of Hyogo College of Medicine (permission number 208), and the Ethics Committee of Kimitsu Chuo Hospital (permission number 120)]. Following approval by the institutional ethics committees, a written informed consent was obtained from the patients or their next of kin. **Figure 1** summarizes the patient inclusion process.

Discovery Cohort

In total, 259 critically ill patients admitted to the ICU of Chiba university hospital in Chiba, Japan, between October 2001 and September 2008 were included (**Table 1**). The inclusion criteria were as follows: admission to the ICU, aged 20 years or older, and the patients able to provide informed written consent or obtainable from a family member or the legal representative. The exclusion criteria are as follows: pregnancy, treatment for hematologic malignancies, the patients receiving radiation treatment and chemotherapy, a history of genetic therapy, and being outside the scope of active treatment. The blood samples were obtained immediately after admission to the ICU. The genomic DNA was extracted from the whole blood cells.

Multicenter Validation Cohort

In the multicenter validation cohort, 793 critically ill patients admitted to the general ICU of each of the five tertiary emergency centers of Kurume University Hospital, Tokyo Medical University Hachioji Medical Center, Hyogo College of Medicine, Kimitsu Chuo Hospital, and Chiba University Hospital (updated permission number 457) from October 2008 to September 2012 were included (**Table 1**). The inclusion and exclusion criteria were the same as for the discovery cohort. The blood cells were refrigerated and transferred to the Chiba University Hospital, where the genomic DNA was subsequently extracted.

Propensity Score Matching in Multicenter Cohort

We conducted a case-cohort study to compare the *THBD* genotypic distributions in whole blood genomic DNA from the critically ill patients with severe sepsis vs. non-sepsis with similar age, gender, severity of illness, and mortality to assess the genetic association for susceptibility to sepsis between the similar severity of critically ill patients. The patients with sepsis tend to die than the patients with non-sepsis do. Therefore, propensity score matching was implemented to compare *THBD* genotypic distributions between the severe sepsis and non-sepsis having similar severity, such as mortality. Controls were matched as follows: the participating centers submitted similar blood samples from critically ill patients who were not known to have sepsis. All the patients who did not meet severe sepsis criteria were placed into the matching pool, and those who had any evidence of sepsis were then excluded. Each patient with sepsis was tentatively matched

TABLE 1 | Baseline characteristics of the study population.

	Discovery cohort				Multicenter validation cohort			
	All $n = 259$	**Non-sepsis patients** $n = 104$	**SS patients** $n = 125$	***P***	**All** $n = 793$	**Non-sepsis patients** $n = 454$	**SS patients** $n = 271$	***P***
Age (years), mean ± SD	56.8 ± 17.4	56.5 ± 17.5	57.6 ± 17.3	0.492*	63.9 ± 17	62.5 ± 17.9	66.6 ± 15.0	0.0008*
Male/female gender, *n*	146/113	60/44	69/56	0.659**	517/276	296/158	176/95	0.915**
Length of ICU stay (days), median (IQR)	6 (3–15)	3 (1–7)	13 (7–15)	<0.0001*	9 (4–19)	7 (4–14)	15 (7–29.3)	<0.0001*
SOFA score, median (IQR)	6 (3–11)	3 (1–6)	10 (7–13)	<0.0001*	6 (3–9)	4 (2–6)	9 (6–12)	<0.0001*
APACHE II score, median (IQR)	15 (9.3–22)	10 (6–14)	21 (17–27)	<0.0001*	16 (10–23)	13 (8–19.8)	21 (16–26)	<0.0001*
Severe sepsis morbidity (%)	48.3				33.8			
Mortality (%)	17	5.71	29.6	<0.0001**	12.2	5.4	25.3	<0.0001**
Post-surgical operation								
Post-cardiovascular surgery, *n* (%)	28 (10.8)	24 (23.0)	4 (3.2)	<0.0001**	21 (2.6)	5 (1.1)	12 (4.4)	0.009**
Post-gastrointestinal surgery, *n* (%)	33 (12.7)	11 (10.6)	15 (12.0)	0.835**	79 (10.0)	25 (5.5)	43 (15.9)	<0.0001**
Others, *n* (%)	20 (7.7)	12 (11.5)	6 (4.8)	0.083**	6 (0.8)	3 (0.7)	3 (1.1)	0.677**
Intracranial disease (ICH/CI), *n* (%)	5 (2.0)	0 (0)	4 (3.2)	0.128**	68 (8.6)	62 (13.7)	3 (1.1)	<0.0001**
Respiratory failure, *n* (%)	28 (10.8)	4 (3.8)	22 (17.6)	0.001**	77 (9.7)	15 (3.3)	51 (18.8)	<0.0001**
Heart failure, *n* (%)	10 (3.9)	4 (3.8)	3 (2.4)	0.705**	72 (9.1)	61 (13.4)	8 (3.0)	<0.0001**
Endogenous abdominal disease								
Acute pancreatitis, *n* (%)	22 (8.5)	16 (15.4)	6 (4.8)	0.012**	39 (4.9)	22 (4.8)	14 (5.2)	0.861**
Gastrointestinal bleeding, *n* (%)	5 (2.0)	2 (1.9)	3 (2.4)	>0.9999**	36 (4.5)	33 (7.3)	2 (0.7)	<0.0001**
Hepatic failure, *n* (%)	7 (2.7)	3 (2.9)	4 (3.2)	>0.9999**	19 (2.4)	7 (1.5)	9 (3.3)	0.124**
Others, *n* (%)	13 (5.0)	1 (1.0)	9 (7.2)	0.024**	34 (4.3)	10 (2.2)	21 (7.7)	0.001**
CPAOA, *n* (%)	4 (1.5)	2 (1.9)	2 (1.6)	>0.9999**	39 (4.9)	32 (7.0)	4 (1.5)	0.001**
Trauma, *n* (%)	11 (4.3)	9 (8.7)	0 (0)	0.001**	119 (15.0)	105 (23.1)	8 (3.0)	<0.0001**
Intoxication, *n* (%)	8 (3.1)	4 (3.8)	4 (3.2)	>0.9999**	23 (2.9)	17 (3.7)	6 (2.2)	0.283**
Burn, *n* (%)	2 (0.8)	1 (1.0)	0 (0)	0.454**	12 (1.5)	7 (1.5)	4 (1.5)	>0.9999**
Others, *n* (%)	63 (24.3)	11 (10.6)	43 (34.4)	<0.0001**	149 (18.8)	50 (11.0)	83 (30.6)	<0.0001**

P values (non-sepsis patients vs. severe sepsis/septic shock patients) were calculated with Student's t-test or Mann-Whitney U-test and Fisher's exact test**.*
ICH, intracranial hemorrhage; CI, cerebral infarction; CPAOA, cardiopulmonary arrest on arrival; SS, severe sepsis/septic shock; SOFA, sequential organ failure assessment; APACHE II, the acute physiology and chronic health evaluation; SD, standard deviation, IQR, interquartile range. Discovery and validation cohorts include 30 and 68 mild sepsis patients (non-severe), respectively.

with all the patients in the pool of the same gender and hospital discharge status (alive vs. dead). Then, each patient with severe sepsis was matched with one patient from its set of potential non-sepsis matches. The patient selection above was performed employing the propensity score matching method with a Greedy 5-to-1 digit-matching algorithm for the clinical factors, that is, age, gender, severity scores, and hospital discharge status. Once all the propensity-score matching was performed, we compared the baseline covariates between the two groups. Ultimately, 444 patients (222 with severe sepsis/septic shock (SS) while 222 displayed non-sepsis) were selected (**Table 2**).

TABLE 2 | Propensity score-matched patients with severe sepsis and without any evidence of sepsis in the validation cohort (post-matching results).

	Non-sepsis patients $n = 222$	**SS patients** $n = 222$
Age (years), mean ± SD	66.7 ± 16.4	66.2 ± 14.9
Male/female gender, *n*	194/222	191/222
SOFA score, mean ± SD	6.6 ± 3.7	9.1 ± 4.1
APACHE II score, mean ± SD	21.0 ± 7.7	20.8 ± 7.6
Mortality (%)	35.4	35.9

SS, severe sepsis/septic shock; SOFA, sequential organ failure assessment; APACHE II, the acute physiology and chronic health evaluation; SD, standard deviation.

Data Collection

The baseline characteristics (age and gender) and clinical data, such as length of ICU stay, Sequential Organ Failure Assessment (SOFA) scores (17), Acute Physiology and Chronic Health Evaluation (APACHE) II scores (18), morbidity of severe sepsis and septic shock, and ICU mortality, were obtained after the patients were documented at study entry. The APACHE II scores and SOFA scores were calculated during the first 24 h after admission. The diagnosis of sepsis, severe sepsis, and septic shock was based on the criteria presented at the American College of Chest Physicians/Society of Critical Care Medicine Consensus Conference in 1992 (19). In the present study, both the severe sepsis and septic shock are expressed together as the SS group.

SNP Selection and Genotyping

Genomic DNA was isolated from the banked whole blood specimens collected on ICU admission. We genotyped eight markers from the region surrounding *THBD* (**Supplementary Table 1**). Genotyping of SNPs was performed using the APEX testing methods, an outsourced service provided by Asper Biogene (Tartu, Estonia, https://www.asperbio.com/, accessed on 2021/5/25). Eight SNPs distributed in *THBD* and its promoter region (rs2239562, rs3216183, rs121918667, rs1800577, rs1042579, rs41348347, rs1042580, and rs3176123) were investigated. We were able to assign the genotype in >95% of typed samples. To verify the genotypes of the SNPs, some were tested in a set of earlier Japanese samples (6). The allelic statuses were determined employing the PCR with sequence-specific primers, using the TaqMan® probe (Applied Biosystems, Foster City, CA, USA). The genotyped SNPs can be found at dbSNP (http://www.ncbi.nlm.nih.gov/SNP/). The SNP genotyping matching rate was 100%, according to the earlier results (6).

Statistical Analysis

The primary endpoint was a mortality of severe sepsis, and the secondary endpoint was susceptibility to severe sepsis concerning the *THBD* SNP. Hardy–Weinberg equilibrium (HWE) for the population distribution of the variant alleles was determined according to the approach described by Guo and Thompson (20). The allelic *chi*-square tests were applied for each SNP. The statistical analyses for the genetic association tests were performed using the SNP & Variation Suite 8.8.3 software (Golden Helix, Bozeman, MT, USA). Significant differences in the mean ± SD or median (interquartile range; IQR) values between the two groups were evaluated by using the Student's *t*-test or Mann–Whitney *U*-test, depending on the variables. The statistical analyses were performed using the GraphPad PRISM 8, version 8.3.0 (GraphPad Software, San Diego, CA, USA) for Windows. We considered differences to be significant at $P < .05$.

RESULTS

The Baseline Characteristics of the Discovery and Multicenter Validation Cohorts

Table 1 summarizes the baseline characteristics of the discovery cohort ($n = 259$) and the multicenter validation cohort ($n = 793$). Mortality and the SOFA and APACHE II scores were significantly higher in the SS group than those in the non-sepsis group in both the cohorts ($P < 0.0001$, **Table 1**). In the validation cohort, the SS patients were significantly older than the non-septic controls ($P = 0.0008$, **Table 1**). By contrast, no significant difference in the SOFA or APACHE II scores was detectable between the SS groups of the two cohorts ($P = 0.1126$, 0.8714, respectively), which indicated that there was no marked difference in severity in the SS patients between the two cohorts. In the validation cohort, trauma, heart failure, and intracranial diseases were overrepresented in the non-sepsis group.

Genotype Distributions of Eight *THBD* SNPs Related to the Outcome of Severe Sepsis

To determine the frequencies of eight SNPs of *THBD*, which are associated with the mortality of severe sepsis, genotyping of these polymorphisms was performed in the discovery cohort. The observed allele frequencies and genotypic distributions for the investigated polymorphisms are summarized in **Supplementary Table 2** (discovery cohort), **3** (validation cohort), and **4** (combined cohort). The distributions of genotypes for all the investigated polymorphisms conformed to the HWE test ($P > 0.01$).

The genotype call rate of the eight SNPs was 96.3–100%, although the genotypic distributions in rs1042579 diverged from the HWE in the studied subjects ($P = 0.005$, **Supplementary Table 4**). Among the eight SNPs, a *THBD* promoter SNP (−1920*C/G; rs2239562) was found to be most significantly associated with mortality of SS group in the discovery cohort [odds ratio (*OR*) 2.709 (range of lower and upper confidence bound; 1.067–6.877), $P = 0.033$ in a dominant model with the trend test, **Figure 2A**] and the trend was maintained in the validation cohort [*OR* 1.446 (0.782–2.675), $P = 0.249$, **Figure 2A**]. As a result, the association was statistically strengthened in the combined cohort [*OR* 1.768 (1.060–2.949), $P = 0.028$ in a dominant model with the trend test, **Figure 2A**]. Consequently, the carriage of the CC genotype was significantly associated with a worse outcome of SS group. All the genotypic distributions in relation to a mortality of SS of both the cohorts are presented in **Supplementary Tables 2–4**.

Genotypic Distributions of Eight *THBD* SNPs Related to Susceptibility to Severe Sepsis

Because of the retrospective nature of the study, the baseline imbalances between the SS and non-sepsis existed; therefore, we identified 222 subjects from each of the SS and non-sepsis groups from the validation cohort by propensity score matching (17) to equalize morbidity of severe sepsis and severity of illness of both the cohorts (**Table 2**). **Figure 1** summarizes the patient inclusion process. By matching with the Propensity Score in the multicenter validation cohort, 222 patients with severe sepsis and the same number of controls with a similar number of ICU deaths, the severity of illness (APACHEII), and age and gender-matched without evidence of any infection also admitted to the ICUs were included (**Table 2**). The genotypic distributions of the *THBD* promoter SNP (rs2239562) and the *THBD* exon 1 SNP (rs41348347) were significantly different between the SS and non-sepsis groups with similar severity of illness [*OR* 1.593 (1.086–2.338), $P = 0.017$ and *OR* 0.107 (0.013–0.853), $P = 0.011$, respectively in a dominant model with the trend test, **Figure 2B**]. By contrast, the minor allele

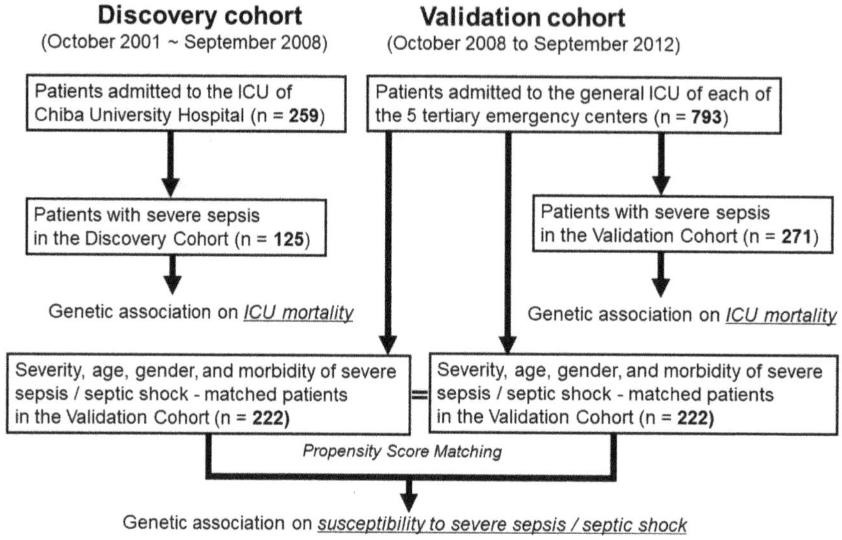

FIGURE 1 | Flow diagram of patient inclusion.

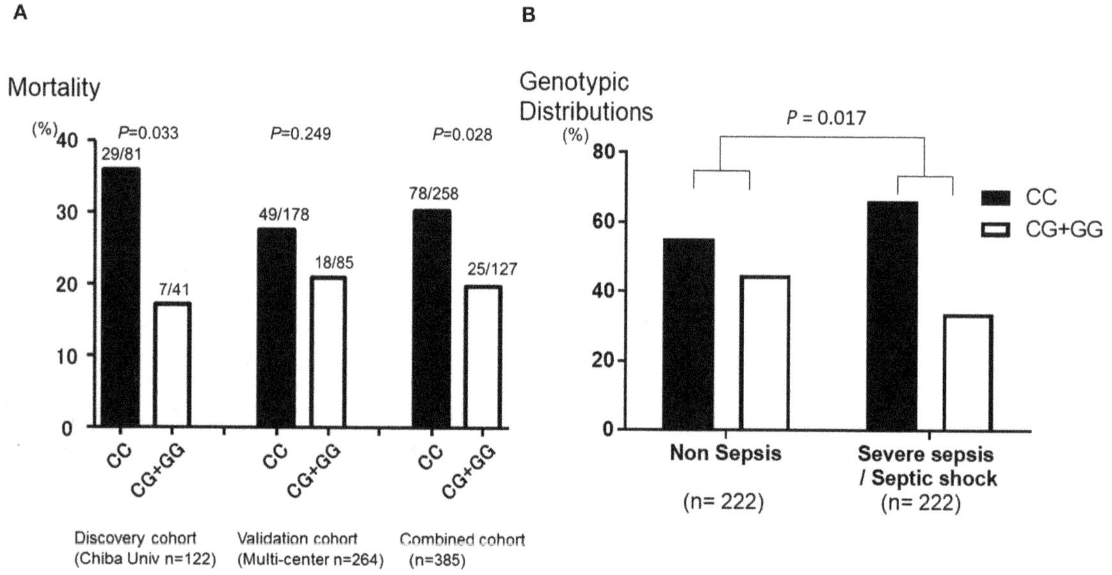

FIGURE 2 | Mortality and morbidity of severe sepsis in genotype categories of *thrombomodulin gene (THBD)* single nucleotide polymorphisms (SNPs) rs2239562. **(A)** The *Y*-axis of the graph shows the mortality of severe sepsis in the SNPs that is in the promoter region of *THBD* (−1920*C/G; rs2239562). The patients with the CC genotype of rs2239562 were significantly associated with worse outcome of severe sepsis than the CG + GG genotype of the SNP in the discovery cohort ($P = 0.033$). The trend was maintained in the validation cohort ($P = 0.249$), and the association was strengthened in the combined cohort ($P = 0.028$). **(B)** The *Y*-axis of the graph shows the genotypic distributions of the SNP that is in the promoter region of *THBD* (−1920*C/G; rs2239562) in the patients with severe sepsis and without any evidence of sepsis (non-sepsis). The percentage of patients with the CC genotype of rs2239562 was significantly higher in the SS group than those in the non-sepsis group ($P = 0.017$). *The P* values for the SNP were evaluated with the chi-square test on the dominant model analysis with the correlation/trend test.

frequency of the exon SNP rs41348347 was too low to reveal the clinical implications (1.14%), and this SNP was found not to be related to the outcome of SS patients in the previous analysis (**Supplementary Tables 2–4**). Therefore, the association between rs2239562 and susceptibility to SS was confirmed, even though both the groups were similar for severity and the other background characteristics. The genotype call rate of the eight SNPs was 93.9–100%, and the genotypic distributions in all the eight SNPs did not diverge from the HWE in the studied subjects (**Supplementary Table 5**).

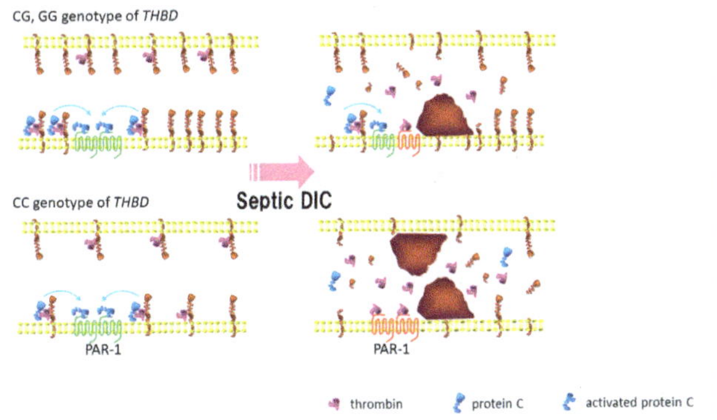

FIGURE 3 | *Thrombomodulin gene* promotor may influence thrombomodulin guided activated protein C (APC) function and limit endothelial cell damage in sepsis. In the blood stream, the thrombomodulin levels influence APC and antiinflammatory PAR-1 signaling. Bottom right: restricted thrombomodulin (due to carriage of CC genotype of rs2239562) promote thrombin induced inflammation and endothelial cell damage. APC, activated protein C; PAR-1, protease-activated receptor-1; DIC, disseminated intravascular coagulation.

DISCUSSIONS

The coagulation disorders are common in sepsis, and the patients frequently progress to develop DIC. The present study indicated that a coagulopathy-associated *THBD* promoter SNP, rs2239562, had a significant influence on the outcome as well as the progress of severe sepsis/septic shock. First, we determined the worse outcome of severe sepsis to be associated with the CC (major) allele homozygotes of rs2239562. Intriguingly, the frequency of the CC carriers was also augmented in the SS in a propensity-matched patient cohort. In the pathophysiology of sepsis, *THBD* promotor may influence the thrombomodulin-guided APC function and limit endothelial cell damage (**Figure 3**). In the bloodstream, the thrombomodulin levels influence APC and antiinflammatory protease-activated receptor-1 (PAR-1) signaling. The restricted thrombomodulin (due to carriage of CC genotype of rs2239562) promotes thrombin-induced inflammation and endothelial cell damage.

Some drugs in development aim to regulate sepsis-induced coagulopathy or when inflammation has been initiated. One of the promising drugs is ART-123, a recombinant form of the anticoagulant protein thrombomodulin from Asahi Kasei Pharma that is currently in a global clinical trial (14, 21). Emerging evidence is accumulating, which demonstrates the therapeutic efficacy of ART-123 (22, 23), and the mechanisms of thrombomodulin of not only anticoagulation but also anti-inflammation through the adsorption of high-mobility group-B1 (HMG-B1) have been advocated (24). In the recently published Japanese Guidelines, ART-123 has been weakly recommended for the patients with sepsis with DIC (25). From a practical point, the proper use of ART-123, such as target-illness severity and dosage for the patients with sepsis-induced DIC, remains unclear, particularly for those with renal impairment (26) as well as for those on continuous hemodiafiltration (27). Because of the anticoagulant properties of ART-123, the most critical concern in treating the patients with DIC, who are susceptible to bleeding, is a severe hemorrhage due to abrupt increases in plasma concentration of this drug. The present study results should shed light on the precision medicine for sepsis-induced DIC utilizing the pharmacogenetics associated with the coagulation system.

An earlier study reported soluble thrombomodulin concentrations and deep venous thrombosis associated with 2729A>C and A455V missense mutations in the Japanese (28). The *THBD* 1418T allele in rs1042579 SNP was associated with the lower soluble thrombomodulin levels, both in plasma and in HUVEC-conditioned medium, and with an increase in functional membrane-bound thrombomodulin in HUVEC, explaining the increased APC levels and the reduced venous thromboembolism risk (29). Interestingly, *THBD* is also recognized as a pathogenic gene of the atypical hemolytic uremic syndrome (aHUS) (30), caused by complement dysregulation and may occasionally be triggered by a septic insult. Therefore, the present data indicating that a *THBD* polymorphism influenced the susceptibility, as well as the outcome of sepsis, might be key in the pathogenesis of aHUS. To counteract sepsis-triggered aHUS, the continued accumulation of knowledge regarding the patterns of disease onset and response to the treatments under different genetic backgrounds, such as *THBD*, will be essential for developing future treatment strategies (31). Further, a recent study demonstrated that one of the *THBD* SNPs, rs1962, was related to the risk of death in the patients with sepsis (32). The above reports support the deep association between the *THBD* SNPs and the pathophysiology of sepsis-induced organ dysfunctions.

Our work has several limitations. First, we used the criteria of the 2013 surviving sepsis campaign guidelines to include patients because this work was initiated before introducing the SEPSIS-3 diagnostic criteria (33). Second, the statistical significance of the results of the *THBD* genetic association was relatively weak because the patient characteristics were very heterogeneous, such that it was challenging to show the influence on an outcome with the present sample volume. Interestingly, a recent study demonstrates that phenotype γ and δ reveals the characteristics of hematologic dysfunctions, such as coagulopathy (34). A survey in Japan conducted by the Japanese Association for Acute Medicine reported that the incidence of DIC is high and exceeded 50% in sepsis (35). At least in part, these may explain the lack of significance concerning the association between the *THBD* SNP and the incidence of SS in "the less severe" validation cohort. More studies along these lines will clarify these questions. Third, neither the gene expression nor biomarker values can be recruited since we performed piggyback evaluation using the DNA samples from an earlier genetic association study of sepsis (6). Ideally, we might have examined the concentrations of soluble thrombomodulin as a phenotype parameter of the rs2239652 SNP promotor influence. However, it is also true that the concentrations do not always correlate with sepsis severity (36). Finally, any data on site of infection, administered antimicrobials, microbiology, and coagulopathy markers were not provided. Although we used a prospective registry of the genetic association study for the critically ill patients, the data were not mandatory in the long-continued cohorts. Even in such miscellaneous populations, the rs2239562 *THBD* SNP was associated with susceptibility to and outcome of SS. This suggests the crucial role of the coagulation system in the pathophysiology of sepsis.

CONCLUSIONS

Our mid-scale population association study supports the hypothesis that the genetic predispositions to severe sepsis as well as to the worse outcome of sepsis exist. Consequently, a variation in the promoter region of the *THBD* appears to explain, in part, the susceptibility to severe sepsis/septic shock in the Japanese multicenter ICU. Whole-genome sequencing targeting *THBD* with a more extensive study population is warranted to be able to transfer the present data to the clinical settings.

ETHICS STATEMENT

The studies involving human participants were reviewed and approved by the Ethics Committee of Chiba University School of Medicine (permission number 205), the Ethical Committee of Kurume University (bioethics permission number 49), the Medical Research Ethics Committee of Tokyo Medical University, the Ethics Review Board of Hyogo College of Medicine (permission number 208), and the Ethics Committee of Kimitsu Chuo Hospital (permission number 120). The patients/participants provided their written informed consent to participate in this study.

AUTHOR CONTRIBUTIONS

EW, MH, and SO: conceived and designed the experiments. YT, MO, and AT: performed the experiments. EW, YT, MO, BM, and MH: analyzed the data. OT, TS, TI, JK, NK, and EMS: contributed reagents, materials, and analysis tools. EW and GH: wrote the paper. All authors contributed to the article and approved the submitted version.

ACKNOWLEDGMENTS

We thank the Asahi Kasei Pharma Corporation for providing funding for genetic testing. We also thank Ms. Yoshiko Ohashi for her excellent secretarial assistance. We are pleased to acknowledge the dedication and participation of the following individuals and institutions: Tomonori Kimura, Yoshihisa Tateishi, the Chiba University Graduate School of Medicine, Chiba University, Chiba; Mariko Yamada, the Hyogo College of Medicine; Evelyn Pihla, Piret Põiklik, Asper Biogene, and Julian Schneider.

REFERENCES

1. Fleischmann C, Scherag A, Adhikari NK, Hartog CS, Tsaganos T, Schlattmann P, et al. International forum of acute care T: assessment of global incidence and mortality of hospital-treated sepsis. Current estimates and limitations. *Am J Respir Crit Care Med.* (2016) 193:259–72. doi: 10.1164/rccm.201504-0781OC
2. Cohen J, Vincent JL, Adhikari NK, Machado FR, Angus DC, Calandra T, et al. Sepsis: a roadmap for future research. *Lancet Infect Dis.* (2015) 15:581–614. doi: 10.1016/S1473-3099(15)70112-X
3. Watanabe E, Hirasawa H, Oda S, Matsuda K, Hatano M, Tokuhisa T. Extremely high interleukin-6 blood levels and outcome in the critically ill are associated with tumor necrosis factor- and interleukin-1-related gene polymorphisms. *Crit Care Med.* (2005) 33:89–97; discussion 242–243. doi: 10.1097/01.CCM.0000150025.79100.7D
4. Watanabe E, Buchman TG, Hirasawa H, Zehnbauer BA. Association between lymphotoxin-alpha (tumor necrosis factor-beta) intron polymorphism and predisposition to severe sepsis is modified by gender and age. *Crit Care Med.* (2010) 38:181–93. doi: 10.1097/CCM.0b013e3181bc805d
5. Frank AJ, Sheu CC, Zhao Y, Chen F, Su L, Gong MN, et al. BCL2 genetic variants are associated with acute kidney injury in septic shock*. *Crit Care Med.* (2012) 40:2116–23. doi: 10.1097/CCM.0b013e3182514bca
6. Kimura T, Watanabe E, Sakamoto T, Takasu O, Ikeda T, Ikeda K, et al. Autophagy-related IRGM polymorphism is associated with mortality of patients with severe sepsis. *PLoS ONE.* (2014) 9:e91522. doi: 10.1371/journal.pone.0091522
7. Haralambous E, Hibberd ML, Hermans PW, Ninis N, Nadel S, Levin M. Role of functional plasminogen-activator-inhibitor-1 4G/5G promoter polymorphism in susceptibility, severity, and outcome of meningococcal disease in Caucasian children. *Crit Care Med.* (2003) 31:2788–93. doi: 10.1097/01.CCM.0000100122.57249.5D
8. Madach K, Aladzsity I, Szilagyi A, Fust G, Gal J, Penzes I, et al. 4G/5G polymorphism of PAI-1 gene is associated with multiple organ dysfunction and septic shock in pneumonia induced severe sepsis: prospective, observational, genetic study. *Crit Care.* (2010) 14:R79. doi: 10.1186/cc8992
9. Walley KR, Russell JA. Protein C−1641 AA is associated with decreased survival and more organ dysfunction in severe sepsis. *Crit Care Med.* (2007) 35:12–7. doi: 10.1097/01.CCM.0000249823.44726.4E
10. Vincent JL, Castro P, Hunt BJ, Jorres A, Praga M, Rojas-Suarez J, et al. Thrombocytopenia in the ICU: disseminated intravascular coagulation and thrombotic microangiopathies-what intensivists need to know. *Crit Care.* (2018) 22:158. doi: 10.1186/s13054-018-2073-2
11. Mohri M, Sugimoto E, Sata M, Asano T. The inhibitory effect of recombinant human soluble thrombomodulin on initiation and extension of coagulation–a comparison with other anticoagulants. *Thromb Haemost.* (1999) 82:1687–93. doi: 10.1055/s-0037-1614900
12. Vincent JL, Ramesh MK, Ernest D, LaRosa SP, Pachl J, Aikawa N, et al. A randomized, double-blind, placebo-controlled, Phase 2b study to evaluate the safety and efficacy of recombinant human soluble thrombomodulin, ART-123, in patients with sepsis and suspected disseminated intravascular coagulation. *Crit Care Med.* (2013) 41:2069–79. doi: 10.1097/CCM.0b013e31828e9b03
13. Yoshihiro S, Sakuraya M, Hayakawa M, Ono K, Hirata A, Takaba A, et al. Recombinant human soluble thrombomodulin contributes to reduced mortality in sepsis patients with severe respiratory failure: a retrospective observational study using a multicenter dataset. *Shock.* (2018) 51:174–9. doi: 10.1097/SHK.0000000000001148
14. Vincent JL, Francois B, Zabolotskikh I, Daga MK, Lascarrou JB, Kirov MY, et al. Effect of a recombinant human soluble thrombomodulin on mortality in patients with sepsis-associated coagulopathy: the SCARLET randomized clinical trial. *JAMA.* (2019) 321:1993–2002. doi: 10.1001/jama.2019.5358

15. Schouten M, Wiersinga WJ, Levi M, van der Poll T. Inflammation, endothelium, and coagulation in sepsis. *J Leukoc Biol.* (2008) 83:536–45. doi: 10.1189/jlb.0607373
16. Chaput C, Zychlinsky A. Sepsis: the dark side of histones. *Nat Med.* (2009) 15:1245–6. doi: 10.1038/nm1109-1245
17. Vincent JL, de Mendonca A, Cantraine F, Moreno R, Takala J, Suter PM, et al. Use of the SOFA score to assess the incidence of organ dysfunction/failure in intensive care units: results of a multicenter, prospective study. Working group on "sepsis-related problems" of the European Society of Intensive Care Medicine. *Crit Care Med.* (1998) 26:1793–800. doi: 10.1097/00003246-199811000-00016
18. Knaus WA, Draper EA, Wagner DP, Zimmerman JE. APACHE II: a severity of disease classification system. *Crit Care Med.* (1985) 13:818–29. doi: 10.1097/00003246-198510000-00009
19. American College of Chest Physicians/Society of Critical Care Medicine Consensus Conference: definitions for sepsis and organ failure and guidelines for the use of innovative therapies in sepsis. *Crit Care Med.* (1992) 20:864–74. doi: 10.1097/00003246-199206000-00025
20. Guo SW, Thompson EA. Performing the exact test of Hardy-Weinberg proportion for multiple alleles. *Biometrics.* (1992) 48:361–72. doi: 10.2307/2532296
21. Williams SC. After Xigris, researchers look to new targets to combat sepsis. *Nat Med.* (2012) 18:1001. doi: 10.1038/nm0712-1001
22. Yoshimura J, Yamakawa K, Ogura H, Umemura Y, Takahashi H, Morikawa M, et al. Benefit profile of recombinant human soluble thrombomodulin in sepsis-induced disseminated intravascular coagulation: a multicenter propensity score analysis. *Crit Care.* (2015) 19:78. doi: 10.1186/s13054-015-0810-3
23. Yamakawa K, Levy JH, Iba T. Recombinant human soluble thrombomodulin in patients with sepsis-associated coagulopathy (SCARLET): an updated meta-analysis. *Crit Care.* (2019) 23:302. doi: 10.1186/s13054-019-2587-2
24. Abeyama K, Stern DM, Ito Y, Kawahara K, Yoshimoto Y, Tanaka M, et al. The N-terminal domain of thrombomodulin sequesters high-mobility group-B1 protein, a novel antiinflammatory mechanism. *J Clin Invest.* (2005) 115:1267–74. doi: 10.1172/JCI22782
25. Egi M, Ogura H, Yatabe T, Atagi K, Inoue S, Iba T, et al. The Japanese clinical practice guidelines for management of sepsis and septic shock 2020 (J-SSCG 2020). *Acute Med Surg.* (2021) 8:e659. doi: 10.1186/s40560-021-00555-7
26. Hayakawa M, Kushimoto S, Watanabe E, Goto K, Suzuki Y, Kotani T, et al. Pharmacokinetics of recombinant human soluble thrombomodulin in disseminated intravascular coagulation patients with acute renal dysfunction. *Thromb Haemost.* (2017) 117:851–9. doi: 10.1160/TH16-07-0547
27. Watanabe E, Yamazaki S, Setoguchi D, Sadahiro T, Tateishi Y, Suzuki T, et al. Pharmacokinetics of standard- and reduced-dose recombinant human soluble thrombomodulin in patients with septic disseminated intravascular coagulation during continuous hemodiafiltration. *Front Med.* (2017) 4:15. doi: 10.3389/fmed.2017.00015
28. Sugiyama S, Hirota H, Kimura R, Kokubo Y, Kawasaki T, Suehisa E, et al. Haplotype of thrombomodulin gene associated with plasma thrombomodulin level and deep vein thrombosis in the Japanese population. *Thromb Res.* (2007) 119:35–43. doi: 10.1016/j.thromres.2005.12.012
29. Navarro S, Medina P, Bonet E, Corral J, Martinez-Sales V, Martos L, et al. Association of the thrombomodulin gene c.1418C>T polymorphism with thrombomodulin levels and with venous thrombosis risk. *Arterioscler Thromb Vasc Biol.* (2013) 33:1435–40. doi: 10.1161/ATVBAHA.113.301360
30. Delvaeye M, Noris M, De Vriese A, Esmon CT, Esmon NL, Ferrell G, et al. Thrombomodulin mutations in atypical hemolytic-uremic syndrome. *N Engl J Med.* (2009) 361:345–57. doi: 10.1056/NEJMoa0810739
31. Riedl M, Fakhouri F, Le Quintrec M, Noone DG, Jungraithmayr TC, Fremeaux-Bacchi V, et al. Spectrum of complement-mediated thrombotic microangiopathies: pathogenetic insights identifying novel treatment approaches. *Semin Thromb Hemost.* (2014) 40:444–64. doi: 10.1055/s-0034-1376153
32. Li Q, Yang W, Zhao K, Sun X, Bao L. Thrombomodulin gene polymorphism and the occurrence and prognostic value of sepsis acute kidney injury. *Medicine.* (2021) 100:e26293. doi: 10.1097/MD.0000000000026293
33. Singer M, Deutschman CS, Seymour CW, Shankar-Hari M, Annane D, Bauer M, et al. The third international consensus definitions for sepsis and septic shock (Sepsis-3). *JAMA.* (2016) 315:801–10. doi: 10.1001/jama.2016.0287
34. Seymour CW, Kennedy JN, Wang S, Chang CH, Elliott CF, Xu Z, et al. Derivation, validation, and potential treatment implications of novel clinical phenotypes for sepsis. *JAMA.* (2019) 321:2003–17. doi: 10.1001/jama.2019.5791
35. Gando S, Shiraishi A, Yamakawa K, Ogura H, Saitoh D, Fujishima S, et al. Role of disseminated intravascular coagulation in severe sepsis. *Thromb Res.* (2019) 178:182–8. doi: 10.1016/j.chest.2019.08.1025
36. Reinhart K, Bayer O, Brunkhorst F, Meisner M. Markers of endothelial damage in organ dysfunction and sepsis. *Crit Care Med.* (2002) 30(5 Suppl):S302–12. doi: 10.1097/00003246-200205001-00021

13

The Amplitude of Diaphragm Compound Muscle Action Potential Correlates with Diaphragmatic Excursion on Ultrasound and Pulmonary Function After Supraclavicular Brachial Plexus Block

Xiuxia Bao [1], Tao Liu [2], Haorong Feng [3], Yeke Zhu [1], Yingying Wu [4], Xianghe Wang [5] and Xianhui Kang [1]**

[1] Department of Anesthesiology, The First Affiliated Hospital, Zhejiang University School of Medicine, Hangzhou, China, [2] Department of Anesthesiology, The First People' Hospital of Huzhou, Huzhou, China, [3] Department of Anesthesiology, South Taihu Hospital of Huzhou, Huzhou, China, [4] Department of Anesthesiology, Huzhou Fourth Hospital, Huzhou, China, [5] Department of Anesthesiology, The 98th Clinical College of People's Liberation Army (PLM), Anhui Medical University, Huzhou, China

***Correspondence:**
Xianhui Kang
kxhui66@zju.edu.cn
Xianghe Wang
863097@sina.com

Objective: This prospective, double-blind, randomized study assessed (1) the associations between diaphragm compound muscle action potential (CMAP), hemidiaphragmatic excursion, and pulmonary function after supraclavicular brachial plexus block (SCBPB) and (2) diagnostic efficacy of pulmonary function for hemidiaphragmatic paralysis evidenced by diaphragm CMAP as an assessment of diaphragm strength was evaluated.

Methods: Eighty-six patients were scheduled for the removal of hardware after healing of a right upper limb fracture distal to the shoulder who were randomly assigned in a 1:1 ratio to two groups: Group A (diaphragmatic excursion), or Group B (pulmonary function). Phrenic nerve conduction studies (PNCSs), M-mode ultrasonography of the diaphragm, and pulmonary function tests (PFTs) were performed before and 30 min after SCBPB. PNCSs were used to determine the latency and amplitude of diaphragm CMAP. Ultrasonography of the diaphragm was performed with patients in a supine position using a low-frequency probe over the subcostal space at the midclavicular line. The diaphragmatic excursion was measured during quiet breathing and deep breathing. Pulmonary function, i.e., forced vital capacity (FVC), predicted value of FVC, and forced expiratory flow in the first second (FEV1), was measured with spirometry. Receiver Operating Characteristic (ROC) curve analysis was used to assess the diagnostic efficacy of pulmonary function for hemidiaphragmatic paralysis evidenced by diaphragm CMAP as an assessment of diaphragm strength.

Results: There were significant associations between the reduction in amplitude of diaphragm CMAP and reductions in diaphragmatic excursion during quiet breathing ($r = 0.70$, $p < 0.01$) and deep breathing ($r = 0.63$, $p < 0.01$) when expressed as a percentage of baseline values. There were significant associations between the reduction in amplitude of diaphragm CMAP and reductions in FVC ($r = 0.67$, $p < 0.01$), FVC% ($r = 0.67$, $p < 0.01$), and FEV1 ($r = 0.62$, $p < 0.01$), when expressed as percentage of baseline values. The area under the ROC curve for FVC was 0.86. A decrease of >8.4% in FVC compared to pre-block predicted hemidiaphragmatic paralysis (determined by diaphragm CMAP) with sensitivity and specificity of 79.2 and 100%, respectively.

Conclusions: The relative reduction in diaphragm CMAP amplitude after SCBPB was correlated with relative reductions in diaphragmatic excursion and pulmonary function. FVC has potential as a useful diagnostic indicator of hemidiaphragmatic paralysis, evidenced by diaphragm CMAP, after SCBPB. These data establish diaphragm CMAP as a direct and objective index of diaphragmatic paralysis after SCBPB.

Keywords: diaphragm compound muscle action potential (CMAP), supraclavicular brachial plexus block, phrenic nerve conduction studies, hemidiaphragmatic excursion, pulmonary function

INTRODUCTION

Brachial plexus block is an effective method for providing anesthesia and post-operative analgesia in patients who underwent surgery of the upper limb. Compared to general anesthesia, brachial plexus block is associated with reduced opioid consumption and opioid-related side effects, decreased length of stay in the post-anesthesia care unit (PACU), and improved patient satisfaction (1). However, brachial plexus block may result in ipsilateral phrenic nerve block and hemidiaphragmatic paresis (2). The incidence of ipsilateral hemidiaphragmatic palsy in the interscalene brachial plexus block is almost 100% (3). However, the distance between the phrenic nerve and the brachial plexus increases caudally to the cricoid cartilage; therefore, the incidence of ipsilateral hemidiaphragmatic palsy in supraclavicular brachial plexus block (SCBPB) is 36–67% (2).

The diaphragm is a main inspiratory muscle, accounting for 75% of the total tidal volume in quiet breathing (4). Healthy individuals at rest are able to tolerate hemidiaphragmatic paresis, but they may experience exercise-associated dyspnea and reduced exercise tolerance (5–8). Patients with unilateral paralysis of the diaphragm usually have no symptoms, as the contralateral diaphragm can compensate. In some patients, clinical signs of respiratory failure after diaphragmatic paralysis cannot be resolved through compensation by the contralateral diaphragm. In one report, a patient with no obesity or history of respiratory disease experienced dyspnea in the post-operative recovery unit after total shoulder replacement (9). In patients with obesity and respiratory diseases, dyspnea and decreased blood oxygen saturation may be more serious.

Diagnosis of diaphragmatic paralysis is essential to avoid respiratory morbidity and can be achieved with a variety of tests. Spirometry techniques are commonly used to measure pulmonary function by assessing forced vital capacity (FVC), predicted value of FVC, and forced expiratory flow in the first second (FEV1). The quality of the spirometry test is influenced by the effort and cooperation of a patient. With the evolution of ultrasound technology, M-mode imaging has been used to identify abnormal diaphragm movement/position during quiet or deep breathing (4); however, ultrasound does not account for the influence of the contralateral diaphragm and accessory respiratory muscles. Phrenic nerve conduction can overcome these challenges. Phrenic nerve conduction is an emerging technique that can be used to evaluate diaphragmatic dysfunction (10, 11) by measuring the change of diaphragm compound muscle action potentials (CMAPs).

Physicians should be aware of diaphragmatic paralysis caused by brachial plexus block, diagnosis of diaphragmatic paralysis, and that early detection of diaphragmatic paralysis can prevent the onset of dyspnea (9). The objective of this prospective, double-blind, randomized study was to assess the associations between diaphragm CMAP, hemidiaphragmatic excursion, and pulmonary function after SCBPB. The diagnostic efficacy of pulmonary function for hemidiaphragmatic paralysis evidenced by diaphragm CMAP as an assessment of diaphragm strength was evaluated.

METHODS

Patients

Patients scheduled for the removal of hardware after healing of right upper limb fracture distal to the shoulder between September 1, 2019 and January 30, 2020 at the 98th Hospital of the People's Liberation Army (PLA) were eligible for this study. Inclusion criteria were as follows: (1) aged 18–60 years; (2) American Society of Anesthesiologists physical status class I or II; (3) body weight 45–85 kg; and (4) consented to SCBPB. Exclusion criteria were as follows: (1) history of the cardiopulmonary disease; (2) body mass index (BMI) >30 kg/m^2; (3) sensory or motor impairment; (4) coagulopathy or severe renal or hepatic failure; (4) known allergy to local anesthetics; (5) extremely atypical diaphragm CMAP; or (6) mild block.

Included patients were randomly assigned in a 1:1 ratio (using a computer-generated random number table and the sealed envelope system for allocation concealment) to two groups: Group A, in which diaphragm CMAP and diaphragmatic excursion were measured, or Group B, in which diaphragm

CMAP and pulmonary function were measured. Two groups of patients were required as it takes 2 min to measure diaphragmatic excursions and 3 min to measure pulmonary function. We could not adjust for the differences in the time it takes to obtain these measurements; therefore, both measurements could not be obtained from a single group of patients.

This prospective, double-blind, randomized study was approved by the Medical Ethics Committee of the 98th Hospital of the PLA. Written informed consent was obtained from all patients before enrollment. This study was an extension of a clinical trial registered on the Chinese Clinical Registry (http://www.chictr.org.cn/showproj.aspx?proj=16992; ChiCTR-IND-17012166, 2017/7/27).

Supraclavicular Brachial Plexus Block

Patients were routinely prepared for surgery. Intravenous access was established prior to the brachial plexus block. ECG, oximetry (SPO_2), and blood pressure (non-invasive) monitoring were performed while patients breathed room air. The patients, the anesthesiologist who managed the patients in the surgery preparation room, and the researchers who collected and analyzed data were blinded to the group allocation.

All the patients were placed in the supine position with the head rotated in the contralateral direction. After sterile skin preparation with 2% chiorhexidine, an ultrasound probe was placed in the supraclavicular fossa to view the brachial plexus and subclavian artery. The skin and subcutaneous tissues were infiltrated with 1 ml of 2% lidocaine. Using the in-plane approach, 0.375% ropivacaine was injected in a lateral-to-medial direction with a sterile 22-gauge, 50-mm insulated nerve stimulating needle. Initially, 15 ml of 0.375% ropivacaine was injected into the "corner pocket" at the junction of the subclavian artery and first rib or pleura (12). The remaining 15 ml of 0.375% ropivacaine was injected into the most superficial portion of the lateral aspect of the cluster formed by the brachial plexus trunks and divisions (13). Adverse events associated with performing the block, such as vascular puncture and dyspnea, were recorded.

The success of the block was assessed after 30 min by an anesthetist who was blinded to the group allocation. The anesthetic effect was categorized as excellent, moderate, or mild. Excellent was defined as no need for supplemental local anesthetics and/or opioids or conversion to general anesthesia. Moderate was defined as the patient can undergo surgery with the need for 1–2 μg/kg fentanyl (14). Mild was defined as the patient was unable to tolerate the pain caused by the skin incision at the initiation of surgery or fentanyl administration did not increase the pain. Patients were followed up for 24 h after completion of infiltration of local anesthetic. Adverse events, such as local anesthetic toxicity, lack of return of normal motor and sensory function, SpO_2 decline (accounting for a 5% decrease as the patient was breathing room air), difficulty in breathing, and hoarseness, were recorded.

Diaphragm CMAP With Phrenic Nerve Conduction

Phrenic nerve conduction studies (PNCSs) were performed by a single technician using Cascade software (Cadwell Laboratories, Kennewick, WA, USA) according to previously published protocols (15–17). The patient was placed in the supine position with the head slightly elevated and rotated 30° in the contralateral direction. A bipolar surface stimulating electrode was placed at the posterior border of the right sternomastoid muscle at the level of the cricoid cartilage. One needle was inserted into the diaphragm at the xiphoid process, 16 cm from a second needle that was placed at the ipsilateral costal margin. A ground disc electrode was placed between the stimulator and the recording electrode. The right phrenic nerve was stimulated at end-expiration using rectangular pulses of 0.2 ms duration. The intensity of the stimulus was increased until reproducible response and maximal diaphragm CMAP amplitude were obtained (maximal stimulation). The phrenic nerve was supramaximally stimulated to 10–20% above maximal stimulation. The latency of the diaphragm CMAP, expressed as phrenic nerve conduction time (PNCT), was measured from stimulus to CMAP onset in milliseconds (ms). The amplitude of the diaphragm CMAP was measured from the negative peak to the positive peak of the waveform in microvolts (μV). Mean latency and amplitude of the diaphragm CMAP measured on three tests before and 30 min after SCBPB were used in the analyses. Paralysis of the diaphragm was defined as >50% reduction in the amplitude of the diaphragm CMAP.

Diaphragm CMAP with phrenic nerve conduction was performed after an ultrasound of the diaphragm and spirometry.

Ultrasound of the Diaphragm

Measurements were performed with the patient in the supine position with the head of the bed at a 30° angle (18) using a SonoSite M-Turbo system with a 2–5 MHz convex transducer. The right hemidiaphragm was visualized by placing the probe over the right anterior subcostal region between the midclavicular and anterior axillary lines. The probe was directed cranially at 30° to the coronal plane. Initially, the right hemidiaphragm was visualized in 2-dimensional (2D) mode with the liver serving as an acoustic window to the right. Subsequently, the probe was raised to the apex of the diaphragmatic dome, and M-mode was used to measure the amplitude of the diaphragmatic excursion during quiet and deep breathing. The means of 3 consecutive measurements before and 30 min after SCBPB were used in the analyses. "Complete paralysis" was defined as >75% reduction in diaphragmatic movement. "Partial paralysis" was defined as a 25–75% reduction in diaphragmatic movement, and "no paralysis" was defined as a <25% reduction in diaphragmatic movement. The number of patients with "paralysis" (partial or complete paralysis) or "no paralysis" was recorded.

Spirometry

Spirometry (Multi-Functional Spirometer H1-701, Japan) was performed in the surgery preparation room according to the recommendations of the American Thoracic Society (19, 20). Patients were placed in the seated position with the head of the bed at a 90° angle and instructed how to perform the test. The FVC, predicted value for FVC, and FEV1 were measured three times at 2-min intervals before and 30 min after SCBPB. The means of 3 acceptable measurements before and 30 min after SCBPB were used in the analyses.

Statistical Analysis

Statistical analyses were performed using IBM SPSS Statistics, version 22. Variables are reported as mean ± SD or medians and interquartile range (IQR). Between-group comparisons of baseline demographic and clinical characteristics were conducted using the Student's *t*-test. Associations between diaphragm CMAP amplitude, diaphragmatic excursion, and pulmonary function were evaluated using Pearson correlation analysis. The diagnostic efficacy of pulmonary function for hemidiaphragmatic paralysis determined by diaphragm CMAP was evaluated with Receiver Operating Curve (ROC) analysis. $p < 0.05$ was considered statistically significant.

The sample size required to obtain minimum correlation coefficients between reduction in amplitude of diaphragm CMAP and diaphragmatic excursion during quiet breathing and deep breathing of 0.75 and 0.53, respectively, in Group A and minimum correlation coefficients between reduction in amplitude of diaphragm CMAP and FVC, FVC%, and FEV1 of 0.6, 0.6, and 0.7, respectively, in Group B was calculated using the following formula ($n = 4 \times \left[(u_\alpha + u_\beta)/\ln(\frac{1+r}{1-r})\right]^2 + 3$,

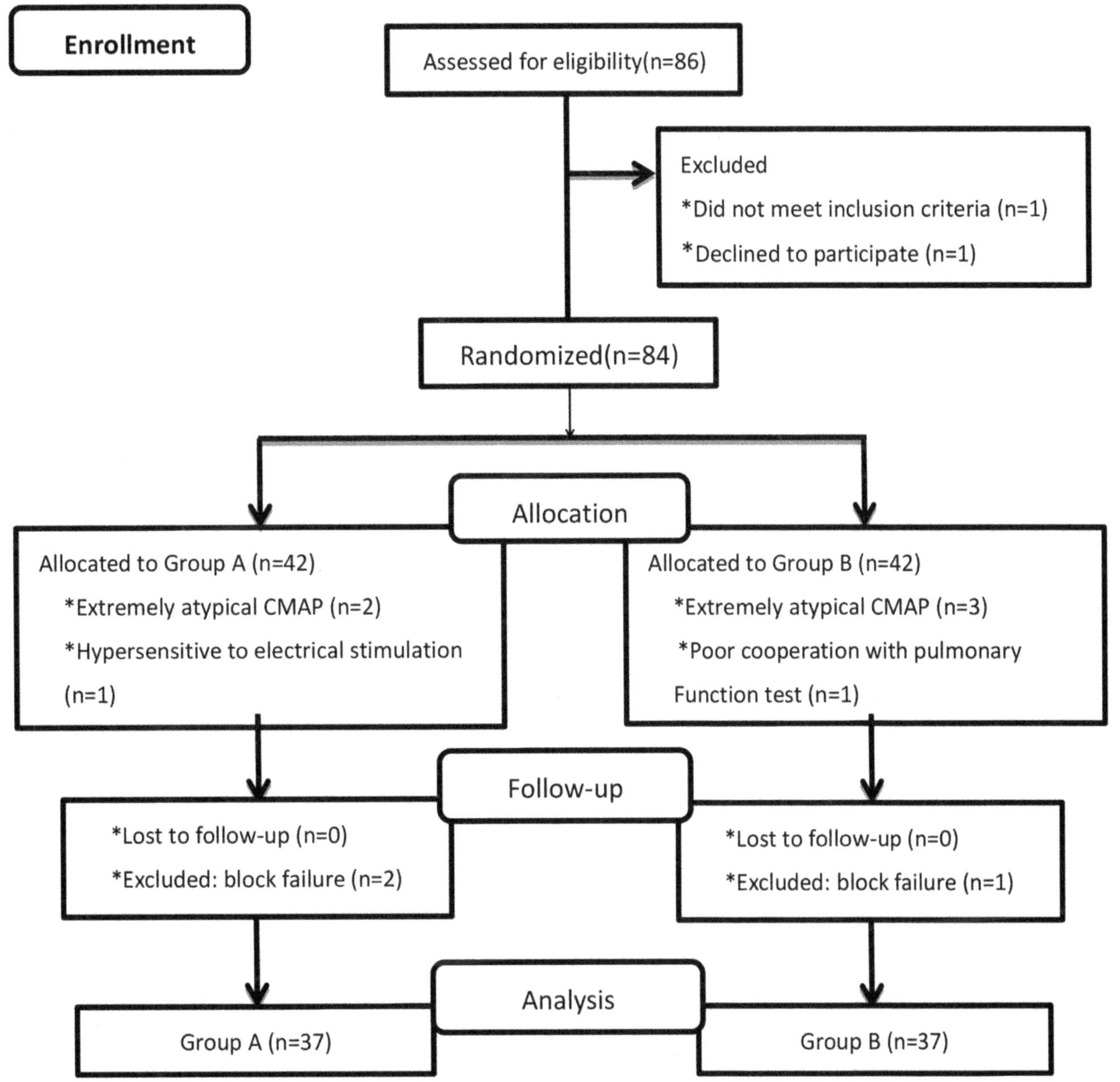

FIGURE 1 | Flowchart of patient selection. CMAP, compound muscle action potential.

$u_\alpha = 1.96, u_\beta = 1.282$). In total, 34 patients were required in each group. Assuming that 20% of study participants were lost to follow-up or dropped out, 86 patients were enrolled in the study.

The sample size for ROC curve analysis was determined using Power Analysis Software (PASS 11). Based on a preliminary study with 10 patients in each group, to obtain an area under the ROC curve of 0.75 with a statistical power of 80%, an alpha error of 0.05, and assuming that 20% of study participants were lost to follow-up or dropped out, 32 patients were required in Group B.

RESULTS

Patient Population

A total of 86 patients were randomized, and data for 74 patients were included in the analyses ($n = 37$ in each group; **Figure 1**). The demographic and clinical characteristics of the patients in Groups A and B were similar (**Table 1**).

Overall, 49 of the 74 (66.2%) patients experienced hemidiaphragmatic paralysis evidenced by diaphragm CMAP as the reference standard. Two patients in Group A and one patient in Group B were converted to general anesthesia because the anesthetic effect of the block was mild. The latency and amplitude of the diaphragm CMAP were extremely atypical in two patients in Group A and three patients in Group B, possibly due to stimulation of the brachial plexus. Among these, one patient in Group A was hypersensitive to the electrical stimulation as the amplitude of the diaphragm CMAP was >3,000 μV. This may be because the long thoracic, lateral pectorals, and/or medial pectoral nerves, which are derived from the brachial plexus, were stimulated.

Associations Between Diaphragm CMAP, Hemidiaphragmatic Excursion, and Pulmonary Function After SCBPB

Respiratory function, diaphragmatic excursion, and diaphragm CMAP are presented in **Table 1**. There were no differences in the effectiveness of SCBPB between Groups A and B. In

TABLE 1 | Baseline demographic and clinical characteristics of the study population.

	All patients ($N = 74$)	Group A ($n = 37$)	Group B ($n = 37$)	*P*-value (A vs. B)
Age (years)	41.95 ± 11.32	42.73 ± 11.86	41.16 ± 10.85	$P = 0.81$
Weight (kg)	62.81 ± 11.68	61.19 ± 11.41	64.43 ± 11.87	$P = 0.78$
Height (cm)	166.55 ± 7.66	165.57 ± 7.86	167.54 ± 7.43	$P = 0.31$
BMI(kg/m^2)	22.52 ± 3.13	22.22 ± 3.15	22.82 ± 3.12	$P = 0.68$
Sex (F/M)	17/57	10/27	7/30	$P = 0.41$
ASA physical status (I/II)	25/49	11/26	14/23	$P = 0.46$
Amplitude (μV)	1034.91 ± 497.96	1039.19 ± 511.06	1030.64 ± 491.52	$P = 0.61$
Amplitude (μV) of diaphragm CMAP after block	382.25 ± 303.77	385.10 ± 334.45	379.40 ± 274.31	$P = 0.48$
Latency (ms)	5.78 ± 1.65	5.69 ± 1.42	5.87 ± 1.86	$P = 0.15$
Quiet excursion (cm)		1.53 ± 0.29 ($P = 0.16$)		
Deep excursion (cm)		7.05 ± 1.03 ($P = 0.11$)		
FVC			3.44 ± 0.75 ($P = 0.2$)	
FVC%			84.48 ± 9.37 ($P = 0.2$)	
FEV1			2.98 ± 0.65 ($P = 0.17$)	

Values are mean ± SD or number. Group A, diaphragm excursion; Group B, pulmonary function; ASA, American Society of Anesthesiologists; FVC, forced vital capacity; FVC%, predicted value of FVC; FEV1, forced expiratory flow in the first second.

TABLE 2 | Diaphragm compound muscle action potential, diaphragm excursion during SCBPB, and respiratory function post-SCBPB.

	All patients ($N = 74$)	Group A	Group B	*P*-value
ΔCMAP pre-block to post-block	−73.6% (−86.1∼−30.4%)	−73.1% (−87.1∼−38.3%)	−74.6% (−84.5∼−27.2%)	0.95
ΔPNCT pre-block to post-block	25.1% (4.1∼67.6%)	24.2% (4.0∼60.6%)	27.7% (4.6∼70.3%)	0.67
Δquiet excursion pre-block to post-block		−40.0% (−100∼−6.5%)		
Δdeep excursion pre-block to post-block		−43.4% (−57.7∼−6.8%)		
ΔFVC pre-block to post-block			−11.9% (−31.2∼−4.2%)	
ΔFVC% pre-block to post-block			−11.9% (−31.2∼−4.3%)	
ΔFEV$_1$ pre-block to post-block			−13.2% (−30.7∼−5.1%)	

SCBPB, supraclavicular brachial plexus block; ΔCMAP, percent reduction in diaphragm compound muscle action potential pre-block to post-block; ΔPNCT, percent reduction in phrenic nerve conduction time pre-block to post-block; Δquiet excursion, percent reduction in quiet breath excursion pre-block to post-block; Δdeep excursion, percent reduction in deep breath excursion pre-block to post-block; ΔFVC, percent reduction in forced vital capacity pre-block to post-block; ΔFVC%, percent reduction in predicted FVC pre-block to post-block; ΔFEV1, the percent reduction in forced expiratory flow in the first second.

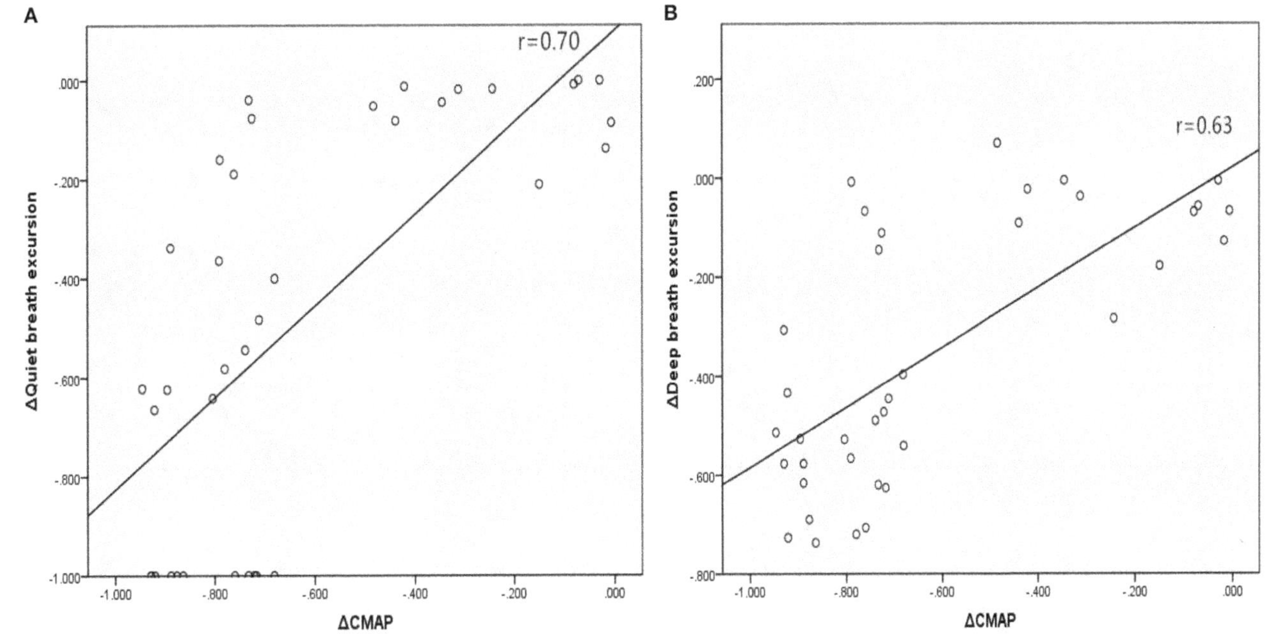

FIGURE 2 | Associations between relative changes (Δ) in diaphragm CMAP amplitude and diaphragmatic excursions during quiet breathing **(A)** and deep breathing **(B)** before and 30 min after SCBPB in Group A. CMAP, compound muscle action potential.

Group A (−73.1%) and Group B (−74.6%), the amplitude of diaphragm CMAP was decreased 30 min after SCBPB compared to baseline. In Group A, hemidiaphragmatic excursions during quiet breathing (−40.0%) and deep breathing (−43.4%) were decreased 30 min after SCBPB compared to baseline. In Group B, FVC (−11.9%), FVC% (−11.9%), and FEV1 (−13.2%) were decreased 30 min after SCBPB compared to baseline (**Table 2**).

Five patients (13.5%) in Group A vs. three patients (8.1%) in Group B reported transient dyspnea and oxygen desaturation 10 min after SCBPB. Symptoms were significantly improved after oxygen inhalation through a nasal catheter.

In Group A, there were significant associations between the reduction in amplitude of diaphragm CMAP and reductions in diaphragmatic excursion during quiet breathing (**Figure 2A**; $r = 0.70$, $p < 0.001$) and deep breathing (**Figure 2B**; $r = 0.63$, $p < 0.001$), when expressed as a percentage of baseline values. In Group B, there were significant associations between the reduction in amplitude of diaphragm CMAP and reductions in FVC (**Figure 3A**; $r = 0.67$, $p < 0.001$), FVC% (**Figure 3B**; $r = 0.67$, $p < 0.001$), and FEV1 (**Figure 3C**; $r = 0.62$, $p < 0.001$), when expressed as a percentage of baseline values.

Diagnostic Efficacy of Pulmonary Function for Hemidiaphragmatic Paralysis

In Group B, 24 of the 37 (64.9%) patients experienced hemidiaphragmatic paralysis. ROC curve analysis was used to assess the diagnostic efficacy of pulmonary function for hemidiaphragmatic paralysis evidenced by diaphragm CMAP as an assessment of diaphragm strength (**Figure 4**). The area under the ROC curve for FVC was 0.86. At a cut-off of 0.084, FVC predicted hemidiaphragmatic paralysis (determined by diaphragm CMAP) with sensitivity and specificity of 79.2 and 100%, respectively.

DISCUSSION

This study assessed the associations between diaphragm CMAP, hemidiaphragmatic excursion, and pulmonary function after SCBPB. The efficacy of pulmonary function for diagnosing hemidiaphragmatic paralysis evidenced by diaphragm CMAP as an assessment of diaphragm strength was evaluated. To date, the pulmonary function has not been used to indicate diaphragmatic paralysis. A decrease of >8.4% in FVC compared to pre-block has predicted hemidiaphragmatic paralysis (determined by diaphragm CMAP) with sensitivity and specificity of 79.2 and 100%, respectively.

The brachial plexus nerve is anatomically adjacent to the phrenic nerve and originates from the anterior rami of C5 ≈ 8 and T1. The phrenic nerve originates from the anterior rami of C3 to C5 and passes over the anterior surface of the anterior scalene. The accessory phrenic nerve originates from the anterior rami of C5 ≈ 6. The accessory phrenic nerve is a common anatomic variant that is present in up to 75% of individuals. Local anesthetic blockade of the accessory phrenic nerve may lead to diaphragmatic paralysis during brachial plexus block. Diaphragmatic paralysis may be a temporary or persistent phenomenon. The incidence of diaphragmatic paralysis after SCBPB in our patient population was high. Eight patients reported transient dyspnea and oxygen desaturation 10 min after SCBPB. These data highlight the unmet clinical need to raise

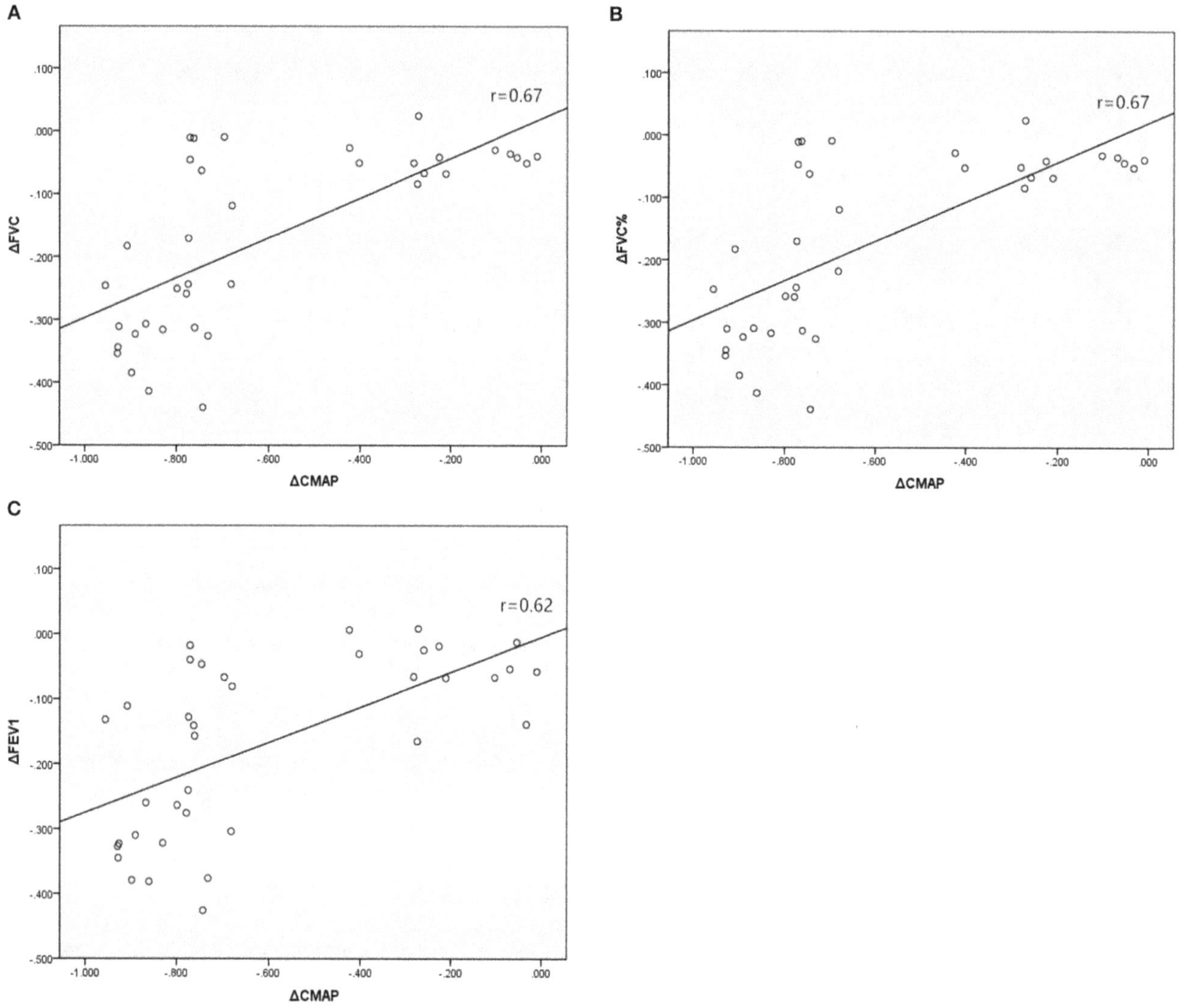

FIGURE 3 | Associations between relative changes (Δ) in diaphragm CMAP amplitude and FVC **(A)**, FVC% **(B)**, and FEV1 **(C)** before and 30 min after SCBPB in Group B. CMAP, compound muscle action potential; FVC, forced vital capacity; FVC%, predicted value of FVC; FEV1, forced expiratory flow in the first second.

awareness about diaphragmatic paralysis as a complication of brachial plexus block and identify novel methods to measure diaphragmatic paralysis. Previously, we explored the effect of 20 and 30 ml of 0.375% ropivacaine on electromyography of the diaphragm and pulmonary function before and after ultrasound-guided SCBPB (21).

In the present study, we showed a significant association between the reduction in amplitude of diaphragm CMAP after SCBPB, measured by PNCS, and the reductions in a diaphragmatic excursion on quiet and deep breathing, visualized on the ultrasound, when expressed as a percentage of baseline values. The association was better during quiet breathing compared to deep breathing. The diaphragm is responsible for 75% of tidal volume during quiet inspiration (22). This percentage is reduced during deep breathing due to the assistance of extrinsic musculature, which increases the volume of the thorax and expands the lungs (23).

In addition, there was a significant association between the reduction in amplitude of diaphragm CMAP after SCBPB and the reduction in pulmonary function (FVC, FVC%, and FEV1), when expressed as a percentage of baseline values. It is well-established that diaphragmatic paralysis is related to a restricted breathing pattern and reduced ability of the lung to expand, which is characterized by reduced FVC and FVC% (24). There was a moderate association between the pre-block and post-block changes in diaphragm CMAP and FVC, FVC%, and FEV1. During unilateral diaphragmatic paralysis, the contralateral diaphragm may compensate for the dysfunction of the paralyzed hemidiaphragm, and patients can maintain normal ventilation at rest and during mild exercise. Patients may not have signs or symptoms until FVC falls to 38% of predicted due to physiological compensation (25, 26).

Results of our ROC curve analysis imply that hemidiaphragmatic paralysis after SCBPB, evidenced by diaphragm CMAP as an assessment of diaphragm strength,

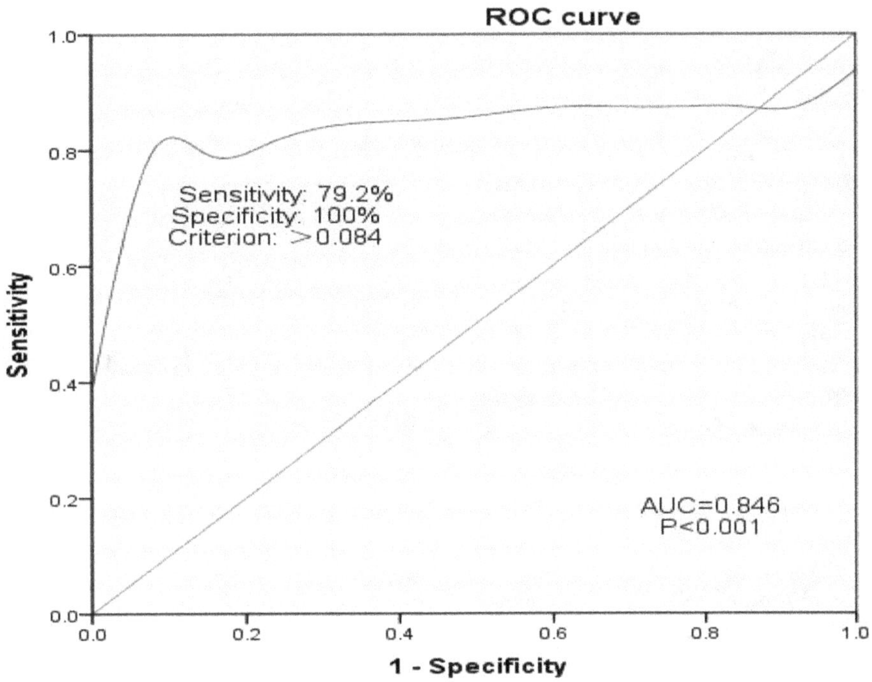

FIGURE 4 | ROC curve analysis assessing the efficacy of pulmonary function for diagnosing hemidiaphragmatic paralysis evidenced by diaphragm CMAP as an assessment of diaphragm function. CMAP, compound muscle action potential. Sensitivity = True Positives/(True Positives + False Negatives). False Positive Rate = 1 - Specificity, where specificity = True Negatives/(True Negatives + False Positives).

may be diagnosed when FVC falls below 0.084. The area under the ROC curve was 0.85, and sensitivity and specificity were 79.2 and 100%, respectively. Consistent with this, Ming-Lung et al. reported that phrenic nerve transfer for the repair of avulsed brachial plexus injury resulted in permanent ipsilateral diaphragmatic paralysis accompanied by an estimated 8% decrease in inspiratory capacity, FVC, and total lung capacity (27).

Several methods have been used to diagnose hemidiaphragmatic paresis after the brachial blockade, such as fluoroscopy, maximum transdiaphragmatic pressure, PNCS CMAP amplitude, and ultrasound of the diaphragm. Each method has its advantages and disadvantages. Ultrasound of the diaphragm has advantages over diaphragm CMAP as it is easy to apply. However, ultrasound does not account for the influence of the contralateral diaphragm and accessory respiratory muscles. PNCS can overcome these deficiencies. In this study, we used needles instead of surface electrodes to collect diaphragm CMAP. As surface electrodes are distant from the deep target muscle, the signal can be influenced by factors, such as lung inflation, skin thickness, the amount of subcutaneous tissue, and the depth of lung tissue separating the recording electrode from the diaphragm. Needles are not prone to interference from activity in neighboring muscles and are considered safe (17); however, this approach can be technically challenging. Inaccurate placement of needles can make it difficult to collect diaphragmatic needle electromyographic recordings, providing inaccurate measurements of the latency and amplitude of the diaphragm CMAP.

Pulmonary function is widely used to evaluate the effect of brachial plexus block on respiratory function. It is simple and easy to perform, but the quality of the spirometry test is influenced by patient efforts and cooperation, and there are no diagnostic criteria for diaphragmatic paralysis. Diaphragm CMAP has been applied in the diagnosis of respiratory insufficiency due to amyotrophic lateralizing sclerosis and other neuromuscular disorders (28), but data describing the use of diaphragm CMAP to diagnose diaphragmatic paralysis after SCBPB are limited. The majority of previous reports have used ultrasound to diagnose hemidiaphragmatic paralysis after SCBPB. With the rapid development and decreasing cost of ultrasound technology, real-time 2-dimensional visualization of the diaphragm can be easily performed at the bedside (29). However, ultrasound may misdiagnose complete paralysis of the phrenic nerve as diaphragmatic movement on the ipsilateral side can be affected by movement from the contralateral diaphragm and accessory respiratory muscles (30). PNCS of the affected hemidiaphragm is needed to confirm complete paralysis of the phrenic nerve. The phrenic nerve is the only source of motor innervation to the diaphragm (24). Therefore, the electrophysiological function of the diaphragm can be analyzed without being affected by other respiratory muscles.

This study was associated with several limitations. First, the latency and amplitude of the diaphragm CMAP were extremely atypical in several patients. This may have been due to interference caused by stimulation of the brachial plexus. Second, patients with a high BMI or cardiopulmonary disease were excluded from this study. This may limit the generalizability of our findings, as these patients are most likely to be affected by diaphragmatic paralysis. Third, the left hemidiaphragm is lower than the right hemidiaphragm, but the motion of the left hemidiaphragm is greater than the right hemidiaphragm (24); therefore, measurements from the right hemidiaphragm cannot be extrapolated to the left. Fourth, it takes 2 min to measure diaphragmatic excursions and 3 min to measure pulmonary function. As we could not adjust for the differences in the time it takes to obtain these measurements, we did not explore the relationship between diaphragmatic excursion and pulmonary functions. Although diaphragm dysfunction (CMAP) was identified by two different approaches [ultrasound and pulmonary function tests (PFTs)] in two groups of patients, the characteristics of the patients in Groups A and B were similar, allowing for a relevant extrapolation of data.

CONCLUSIONS

Diaphragm CMAP, determined by PNCS, diaphragmatic excursion during quiet and deep breathing, and pulmonary function (FVC, FVC%, and FEV1) were decreased after SCBPB, implying these three methods can be used to diagnose diaphragmatic paralysis. The pulmonary function can directly reflect the influence of diaphragmatic paralysis on respiratory function after SCBPB. A decrease of >8.4% in FVC compared to pre-block has predicted hemidiaphragmatic paralysis (determined by diaphragm CMAP). The relative reduction in diaphragm CMAP amplitude was correlated well with the relative reductions in diaphragmatic excursion and pulmonary functions. These data establish diaphragm CMAP as an accurate and objective index of diaphragmatic paralysis.

ETHICS STATEMENT

The studies involving human participants were reviewed and approved by Ethical Committee of 98th Hospital of PLA. The patients/participants provided their written informed consent to participate in this study.

AUTHOR CONTRIBUTIONS

XB is responsible for conducting this study and the manuscript writing. Data collection and analysis were completed by TL and YZ. YW is responsible for implementation of clinical trials. This study was designed by XK. After completing this clinical study and article writing, XW was responsible for the revision of the manuscript. All authors contributed to the article and approved the submitted version.

ACKNOWLEDGMENTS

The authors would like to express gratitude to XW and XK, supervisors, for their constant encouragement and guidance, to statistics teacher Jiantong Shen, and to beloved family for their loving considerations and great confidence all through this year.

REFERENCES

1. Hadzic A, Williams BA, Karaca PE, Hobeika P, Unis G, Dermksian J, et al. For outpatient rotator cuff surgery, nerve block anesthesia provides superior same-day recovery over general anesthesia. *Anesthesiology.* (2005) 102:1001–7. doi: 10.1097/00000542-200505000-00020
2. Marhofer P, Harrop-Griffiths W, Willschke H, Kirchmair L. Fifteen years of ultrasound guidance in regional anaesthesia: part 2-recent developments in block techniques. *Br J Anaesth.* (2010) 104:673–83. doi: 10.1093/bja/aeq086
3. Urmey WF, Talt KH, Sharrock NE. One hundred percent incidence of hemidiaphragmatic paresis associated with interscalene brachial plexus anesthesia as diagnosed by ultrasonography. *Anesth Analg.* (1991) 72:498–503. doi: 10.1213/00000539-199104000-00014
4. Gerscovich EO, Cronan M, McGahan JP, Jain K, Jones CD, McDonald C. Ultrasonographic evaluation of diaphragmatic motion. *J Ultrasound Med.* (2001) 20:597–604. doi: 10.7863/jum.2001.20.6.597
5. Kumar N, Folger WN, Bolton CF. Dyspnea as the predominant manifestation of bilateral phrenic neuropathy. *Mayo Clin Proc.* (2004) 79:1563–5. doi: 10.4065/79.12.1563
6. Laroche CM, Mier AK, Moxham J, Green M. Diaphragm strength in patients with recent hemidiaphragm paralysis. *Thorax.* (1988) 43:170–4. doi: 10.1136/thx.43.3.170
7. Hart N, Nickol AH, Cramer D, Ward SP, Lofaso F, Pride NB, et al. Effect of severe isolated unilateral and bilateral diaphragm weakness on exercise performance. *Am J Respir Crit Care Med.* (2002) 165:1265–70. doi: 10.1164/rccm.2110016
8. Lisboa C, Paré PD, Pertuzé J, Contreras G, Moreno R, Guillemi S, et al. Inspiratory muscle function in unilateral diaphragmatic paralysis. *Am Rev Respir Dis.* (1986) 134:488–92.
9. Baixauli PK, Gimillo PR, Gosalvez JB, Ibáñez JA. Usefulness of diaphragmatic ultrasound in the early diagnosis of phrenic nerve palsy after shoulder surgery in the prevention of post-operative respiratory complications. *Rev Esp Anestesiol Reanim.* (2018) 65:593–6. doi: 10.1016/j.redare.2018.11.001
10. Zoumot Z, Jordan S, Hopkinson NS, Polkey MI. Twitch transdiaphragmatic pressure morphology can distinguish diaphragm paralysis from a diaphragm defect. *Am J Respir Crit Care Med.* (2013) 188:e3. doi: 10.1164/rccm.201207-1185IM
11. Reynaud V, Prigent H, Mulliez A, Durand M-C, Lofaso F. Phrenic nerve conduction study to diagnose unilateral diaphragmatic paralysis. *Muscle Nerve.* (2021) 63:327–35. doi: 10.1002/mus.27144
12. Soares LG, Brull R, Lai J, Chan VW. Eight ball, corner pocket: the optimal needle position for ultrasound-guided supraclavicular block. *Reg Anesth Pain Med.* (2007) 32:94–5. doi: 10.1097/00115550-200701000-00019
13. Roy M, Nadeau MJ, Côté D, Levesque S, Dion N, Nicole PC, et al. Comparison of a single- or double-injection technique for ultrasound-

guided supraclavicular block: a prospective, randomized, blinded controlled study. *Reg Anesth Pain Med.* (2012) 37:55–9. doi: 10.1097/AAP.0b013e3182367b97

14. Perlas A, Lobo G, Lo N, Brull R, Chan RWS, Karkhanis R. Ultrasound-guided supraclavicular block: outcome of 510 consecutive cases. *Reg Anesth Pain Med.* (2009) 34:171–6. doi: 10.1097/AAP.0b013e31819a3f81
15. El-tantawi GAY, Imam MH, Morsi TS. Phrenic nerve conduction abnormalities correlate with diaphragmatic descent in chronic obstructive pulmonary disease. *COPD.* (2015) 12:516–24. doi: 10.3109/15412555.2014.993465
16. Podnar S, Harlander M. Phrenic nerve conduction studies in patients with chronic obstructive pulmonary disease. *Muscle Nerve.* (2013) 47:504–9. doi: 10.1002/mus.23617
17. de Carvalho M, Pinto P, Swash M. Diaphragm motor responses to phrenic nerve stimulation in ALS: surface and needle recordings. *Clin Neurophysiol.* (2018) 129:349–53. doi: 10.1016/j.clinph.2017.11.019
18. Mariani LF, Bedel J, Gros A, Lerolle N, Milojevic K, Laurent V, et al. Ultrasonography for screening and follow-up of diaphragmatic dysfunction in the ICU: a pilot study. *J Intensive Care Med.* (2016) 31:338–43. doi: 10.1177/0885066615583639
19. Miller MR, Crapo R, Hankinson J, Brusasco V, Burgos F, Casaburi R, et al. General considerations for lung function testing. *Eur Respir J.* (2005) 26:153–61. doi: 10.1183/09031936.05.00034505
20. Miller MR, Hankinson J, Brusasco V, Burgos F, Casaburi R, Coates A, et al. Standardisation of spirometry. *Eur Respir J.* (2005) 26:319–38. doi: 10.1183/09031936.05.00034805
21. Bao X, Huang J, Feng H, Qian Y, Wang Y, Zhang Q, et al. Effect of local anesthetic volume (20 mL vs 30 mL ropivacaine) on electromyography of the diaphragm and pulmonary function after ultrasound-guided supraclavicular brachial plexus block: a randomized controlled trial. *Reg Anesth Pain Med.* (2019) 44:69–75. doi: 10.1136/rapm-2018-000014
22. Nason LK, Walker CM, McNeeley MF, Burivong W, Fligner CL, Godwin JD. Imaging of the diaphragm: anatomy and function. *Radiographics.* (2012) 32:E51–70. doi: 10.1148/rg.322115127
23. de la Quintana Gordon FB, Nacarino Alcorta B, Fajardo Pérez M. Ultrasound evaluation of diaphragm function and its application in critical patients, mechanical ventilation and brachial plexus block. *Rev Esp Anestesiol Reanim.* (2017) 64: 513–521. doi: 10.1016/j.redare.2017.07.002
24. Gordon D C, Richmond F J. Topography in the phrenic motoneuron nucleus demonstrated by retrograde multiple-labelling techniques. *J Comp Neurol.* (1990) 292:424–34. doi: 10.1002/cne.902920308
25. Similowski T, Attali V, Bensimon G, Salachas F, Mehiri S, Arnulf I, et al. Diaphragmatic dysfunction and dyspnoea in amyotrophic lateral sclerosis. *Eur Respir J.* (2000) 15:332–7. doi: 10.1034/j.1399-3003.2000.15b19.x
26. Caleffi-Pereira M, Pletsch-Assunção R, Cardenas LZ, Santana PV, Ferreira JG, Iamonti VC, et al. Unilateral diaphragm paralysis: a dysfunction restricted not just to one hemidiaphragm. *BMC Pulm Med.* (2018) 18:126. doi: 10.1186/s12890-018-0698-1
27. Chuang ML, Chuang DC, Lin IF, Vintch JR, Ker JJ, Tsao TC. Ventilation and exercise performance after phrenic nerve and multiple intercostal nerve transfers for avulsed brachial plexus injury. *Chest.* (2005) 128:3434–9. doi: 10.1378/chest.128.5.3434
28. Swenson MR, Rubenstein RS. Phrenic nerve conduction studies. *Muscle Nerve.* (1992) 15:597–603. doi: 10.1002/mus.880150511
29. Sarwal A, Walker FO, Cartwright MS. Neuromuscular ultrasound for evaluation of the diaphragm. *Muscle Nerve.* (2013) 47:319–29. doi: 10.1002/mus.23671
30. Mak PH, Irwin MG, Ooi CG, Chow BF. Incidence of diaphragmatic paralysis following supraclavicular brachial plexus block and its effect on pulmonary function. *Anaesthesia.* (2001) 56:352–6. doi: 10.1046/j.1365-2044.2001.01708-2.x

14

Association Between Platelet Levels on Admission and 90-day Mortality in Patients with Exertional Heatstroke, a 10 Years Cohort Study

Li Zhong[1†], *Ming Wu*[2†], *Jingjing Ji*[3], *Conglin Wang*[3,4] *and Zhifeng Liu*[3,4*]

[1] Department of Critical Care Medicine, The First Affiliated Hospital, Guizhou University of Chinese Medicine, Guiyang, China, [2] Department of Critical Care Medicine and Infection Prevention and Control, The Second People's Hospital of Shenzhen & First Affiliated Hospital of Shenzhen University, Health Science Center, Shenzhen, China, [3] Department of Critical Care Medicine, General Hospital of Southern Theater Command of PLA, Guangzhou, China, [4] The First School of Clinical Medicine, Southern Medical University, Guangzhou, China

***Correspondence:**
Zhifeng Liu
Zhifengliu7797@163.com

These authors have contributed equally to this work

†

Background: Heatstroke is a common clinical symptom in summer with high mortality requiring identification of appropriate and rapid methods of assessment.

Method: This is a retrospective study that included the recent 10 years clinical data of heatstroke patients. A total of $n = 186$ patients were included in this study and grouped based on platelet (PLT) abnormality observed on admission.

Results: In the study group, $n = 120$ patients (64.5%) patients had normal PLT and $n = 66$ patients (35.5%) had abnormal PLT. Compared with PLT-normal group, PLT-abnormal group had higher Acute Physiology and Chronic Health Evaluation II (APACHE II) scores [median 15.0 (IQR 11.5–21.5) vs. 9.0 (IQR 7.0–12.5)] and SOFA scores [median 6.0 (IQR 4.0–10.0) vs. 2.0 (IQR 2.0–4.0)], lower Sequential Organ Failure Assessment (GCS)[median 8.0 (IQR 5.0–12.0) vs. 13.0 (IQR 9.0–14.0)]. The PLT-abnormal group had severe organ damage, including damage to the coagulation system, liver, and kidney (all $p < 0.05$). Significant differences were noted in 90-day survival between the two groups even after correction for Age, GCS, White blood cell count (WBC), Neutrophil, International normalized ratio (INR), Activated partial thromboplastin time (APTT), Procalcitonin (PCT), Alanine aminotransferase (ALT), Creatine (CR), D-Dime (D-D) (Before correction $P < 0.001$; After correction $P = 0.009$).The area under the ROC curve for the prediction of mortality based on PLT was 80.7% (95% CI 0.726–0.888, $P < 0.001$), the optimal cutoff value was 94, the sensitivity was 77.3%, and the specificity was 82.6%.

Conclusion: Patients with heatstroke with platelet abnormalities during admission have more severe organ impairment and a lower 90-day survival rate even when adjusted for other factors.

Keywords: heatstroke, platelets, APACHE II scores, SOFA scores, mortality

INTRODUCTION

Heatstroke is a common clinical symptom in any season especially in summer, manifesting as multi-system inflammation caused by central hyperthermia and eventually multi-organ dysfunction, mortality up to 40% (1, 2). Heatstroke can be clarified in exertional heatstroke or classic heatstroke. Classic heatstroke occurs mostly in older patients, especially those with chronic diseases, they have weak ability to regulate thermal stimulation and are easily affected by high temperature stimulation. Exertional heatstroke usually occurs in athletes, soldiers or worker engaged in outdoor physical labor and it usually occurs under the condition of continuous high temperature and high intensity exercise. The best way to diagnose heatstroke is with rapid body temperature assessment and evaluation of central nervous system status. Since much of the research on exertional heatstroke indicates cellular damage occurs when body temperature exceeds 40.5 C for 30 min. It is very important to find an effective indicator to quickly evaluate the severity and prognosis of the disease. Platelets stop bleeding and participate in thrombosis (3). Platelet abnormality is a risk factor for evaluating the prognosis of a variety of diseases (4–6). Hence this study, retrospectively analyzed the clinical data of patients admitted to hospital for severe heatstroke in the past 10 years, and evaluated early platelet changes on the prognosis of patients with heatstroke for timely and effective clinical treatment.

METHODS

Study Design and Participants

This single-center retrospective case-control study collected all patients with heatstroke admitted to the ICU of the General Hospital of Southern Theater Command in China from October 2008 to May 2019.

The inclusion criteria were as follows: (1) age > = 18 years old; (2) met the diagnostic criteria of severe heatstroke described below; (3) The diagnostic criteria for heatstroke were as follows: classic or exertional heatstroke with a history of exposure to hot and humid weather or strenuous activity, concurrent hyperthermia (central temperature above 40°C), and neurological dysfunction, including delirium, cognitive disorders, and disturbed consciousness. The exclusion criteria were as follows: (1) existing irreversible underlying diseases affecting mortality and (2) pregnancy or breastfeeding.

Research Procedures

The base data of patients were collected, including inflammatory and organ function parameters on admission. Patients were divided into the PLT-normal and PLT-abnormal group according to whether their PLT is normal or not. The main result was 90-day mortality. Survival curve analysis was also performed and ROC curve analysis of PLT to assess the 90-day mortality of heatstroke patients. The PLT-abnormal group was further divided into the Survivors subgroup and Non-survivors subgroup, and the characteristics of the subgroups were compared.

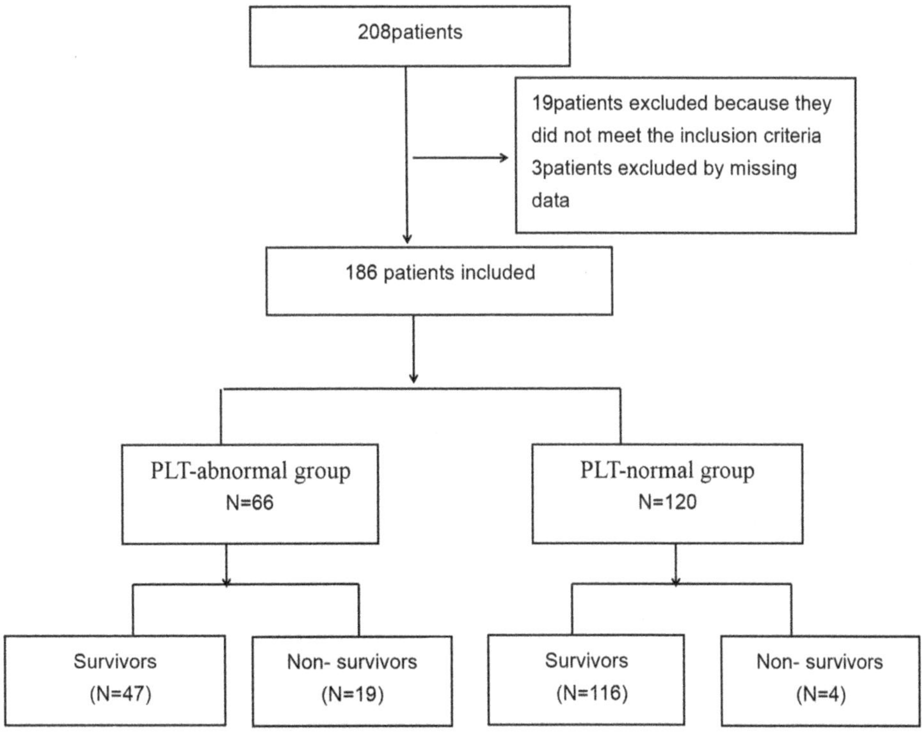

FIGURE 1 | Flowchart of all excluded and included patients.

Definitions

Diagnostic criteria for platelet abnormalities: platelet count (PLT) $<100(1 \times 10^9/L)$ or platelet count $>300(1 \times 10^9/L)$.

Statistical Analysis

The categorical data are expressed as numbers and percentages, and intergroup comparisons were performed with the Mann-Whitney U test, χ^2 test, or Fisher's exact test. Continuous variables are expressed as the medians and interquartile ranges. Continuous data with a Gaussian distribution were compared with Student's *t*-test or one-way ANOVA, and those with a non-Gaussian distribution were compared with the Wilcoxon rank-sum test. The patient endpoint event was death within 90 days after onset. The survival curve was drawn using the Kaplan-Meier method. Significant indicators were identified using single-factor analysis, ROC curves were used to predict the prognosis of patients according to PLT. Statistical analyses were performed using the SPSS Windows version 11.0 statistical package (SPSS Inc, Chicago, IL), and *P* values (two-tailed) <0.05 were considered statistically significant.

RESULTS

Demographics and Baseline Characteristics

A total of 208 patients were included. After screening, 28 patients were excluded because they did not meet the inclusion criteria,

TABLE 1 | Baseline characteristics of clinical and laboratory findings in PLT-normal group and PLT-abnormal group.

	Total (*N* = 186)	PLT-normal (*N* = 120)	PLT-abnormal (*N* = 66)	*P* value
APACHII score, median (IQR)	11.0 (8.0–16.0)	9.0 (7.0–12.5)	15.0 (11.5–21.5)	< 0.001
SOFA score, median (IQR)	3.0 (2.0–6.0)	2.0 (2.0–4.0)	6.0 (4.0–10.0)	< 0.001
GCS score, median (IQR)	12.0 (7.0–14.0)	13.0 (9.0–14.0)	8.0 (5.0–12.0)	< 0.001
Age (years), median (IQR)	21.0 (19.0–27.0)	20.0 (19.0–25.0)	23.0 (19.8–37.3)	0.003
WBC (1 × 10^9/L), median (IQR)	11.4 (8.6–14.7)	11.7 (9.0–15.6)	10.1 (7.9–13.3)	0.020
Neutrophil (1 × 10^9/L), median (IQR)	8.9 (6.5–12.5)	9.3 (6.6–13.2)	8.6 (6.5–10.9)	0.237
Lymphocyte (1 × 10^9/L), median (IQR)	1.1 (0.6–1.9)	1.4 (0.8–2.2)	0.6(0.4–1.4)	< 0.001
Monocytes (1 × 10^9/L), median (IQR)	0.7 (0.4–1.0)	0.8 (0.4–1.1)	0.6 (0.3–0.7)	0.001
Platelets (1 × 10^9/L), median (IQR)	165.0 (81.5–219.0)	187.0 (158.0–226.8)	62.0 (34.5–86.8)	< 0.001
Mean platelet volume (%)	10.7 (10.1–11.5)	10.6 (10.1–11.1)	10.9 (10.2–11.7)	< 0.001
Platelet distribution width (%)	12.5 (11.5–13.8)	12.0 (11.2–13.3)	13.5 (11.8–15.2)	< 0.001
TBIL (μmol/L), median (IQR)	15.9 (10.1–29.5)	11.8 (8.7–18.8)	31.2 (16.1–65.3)	< 0.001
ALT (U/L), median (IQR)	34.5 (20.0–228.8)	26.0 (17.0–47.0)	221.0 (53.8–1,606.3)	< 0.001
AST (U/L), median (IQR)	66.5 (34.3–228.0)	44.0 (28.0–84.5)	290.0 (110.0–1,587.0)	< 0.001
BUN (mmol/L), median (IQR)	5.8 (4.5–7.6)	5.6 (4.2–6.8)	6.4 (5.0–8.7)	0.009
CR (μmol/L), median (IQR)	127.5 (92.0–163.0)	125.0 (94.0–146.0)	147.5(87.8–223.5)	0.009
Cystatin C (mg/L)	1.0 (0.9–1.2)	1.0 (0.8–1.2)	1.1 (0.9–1.5)	0.003
CK (U/L), median (IQR)	912.0 (341.0–2,554.0)	585.5 (252.0–1,601.8)	1,688.5 (814.5–5,465.8)	< 0.001
CKMB (ng/ml), median (IQR)	8.9(4.5–20.4)	5.7(3.8–14.8)	18.0(8.4–37.7)	< 0.001
Mb (ng/ml), median (IQR)	468.9 (122.0–1,000.0)	265.4 (69.2–840.9)	789.0 (219.0–1,000.0)	0.001
CTNI (ng/ml), median (IQR)	0.11 (0.02–0.43)	0.06 (0.01–0.2)	0.28 (0.11–1.11)	< 0.001
PT (s), median (IQR)	15.9 (14.1–20.6)	15.0 (13.9–16.3)	23.5 (16.6–37.4)	< 0.001
INR median (IQR)	1.3 (1.1–1.8)	1.2 (1.1–1.3)	2.0 (1.3–3.7)	< 0.001
APTT (s), median (IQR)	39.0 (33.5–49.5)	35.6 (32.2–40.9)	58.1 (41.4–99.9)	< 0.001
TT(s), median (IQR)	17.6 (16.6–21.3)	17.2 (16.3–18.0)	22.6 (17.6–54.0)	< 0.001
FIB (g/L), median (IQR)	2.5 (2.0–2.9)	2.5 (2.2–3.1)	2.2 (1.5–2.8)	0.003
D-D (mg/L), median (IQR)	1.7 (0.5–7.0)	0.8 (0.4–2.7)	6.6 (2.0–13.3)	< 0.001
CRP (mg/dl), median (IQR)	3.3 (1.4–6.6)	3.2 (0.7–5.6)	3.4 (3.2–9.8)	0.016
PCT (ng/ml), median (IQR)	1.9 (0.8–4.3)	1.3 (0.6–3.3)	3.2 (1.4–5.9)	< 0.001
RM	83/174(47.7%)	40 (48.2%)	43 (51.8%)	< 0.001
AKI	80/185 (43.2%)	41 (51.2%)	39 (48.8%)	0.001
RM&AKI	40/181 (22.1%)	13 (32.5%)	27 (67.5%)	< 0.001

IQR, Inter-Quartile Range; APACHE II, Acute Physiology and Chronic Health Evaluation II score; SOFA, Sequential Organ Failure Assessment; GCS, Glasgow Coma Score; WBC, White blood cell count; TBIL, Total bilirubin; ALT, Alanine aminotransferase; AST, Aspartate aminotransferase; BUN, Blood urea nitrogen; CR, Creatine; CK, Creatine Kinase; CK-MB, Creatine kinase isoenzymes; CTNI, Cardiac troponin I; PT, Prothrombin time; INR, International normalized ratio; APTT, Activated partial thromboplastin time; TT, Thrombin time; FIB, Fibrinogen; D-D:D-Dimer; CPR, C-reactive protein; PCT, Procalcitonin.

3 patients were excluded by missing data, 19 patients excluded because they did not meet the inclusion criteria, and 186 patients were finally included (**Figure 1**). All 186 patients were male, with a mean age of 21.0 years (IQR 19.0–27.0), Acute Physiology and Chronic Health Evaluation II (APACHE II) scores of 11.0 (IQR 8.0–16.0), Sequential Organ Failure Assessment (SOFA) scores of 3.0 (IQR 2.0–6.0), and GCS score of 12.0 (IQR 7.0–14.0). There were 120 patients (64.5%) patients with normal PLT and 66 patients (35.5%) with abnormal PLT.

Comparison of Groups

Compared with PLT-normal group, PLT-abnormal group had higher APACHE II scores [median 15.0 (IQR 11.5–21.5) vs. 9.0 (IQR 7.0–12.5)] and SOFA scores [median 6.0 (IQR 4.0–10.0) vs. 2.0 (IQR 2.0–4.0)], lower GCS [median 8.0 (IQR 5.0–12.0) vs. 13.0 (IQR 9.0–14.0)]. PLT-abnormal group had severe organ damage, including damage to the coagulation system, liver and kidney (all $p < 0.05$) (**Table 1**).

Main Outcomes

The 90-day mortality rate of the PLT-abnormal group was 29% (19/66), while that of the PLT-normal group was 3.3% (4/120). There were statistically significant differences in 90-day survival between the two groups even after correction for Age, GCS, White blood cell count (WBC), Neutrophil, International normalized ratio (INR), Activated partial thromboplastin time (APTT), Procalcitonin (PCT), Alanine aminotransferase (ALT), Creatine (CR), D-Dime (D-D) (Before correction $P < 0.001$; After correction $P = 0.009$) (**Table 2**). Survival analysis showed that the 90-day survival time of patients with PLT-abnormal group was shorter than that of the PLT-normal group ($P < 0.001$) (**Figure 2**).

Subgroup Analysis

In the subgroup analysis of the PLT-abnormal group, there were 47 survivors (71.2%) and 19 Non-survivors (28.8%).Compared with survivors, non-survivors had higher APACHE II scores [median 22.0 (IQR 17.8–23.5) vs. 14.0 (IQR 10.0–18.0)], higher SOFA scores [median 13.5 (IQR 8.8–15.0) vs. 6.0 (IQR 3.0–7.0)], lower GCS [median 4.0 (IQR 3.0–7.3) vs. 10.0 (IQR 6.0–14.0)]. In addition, kidney and blood coagulation system was more serious in the non-survivors ($P < 0.05$), (**Table 3**).

Risk Factor Analysis

The area under the ROC curve for the prediction of mortality based on PLT was 80.7% (95% CI 0.726–0.888, $P < 0.001$), the optimal cutoff value was 94 (1×10^9/L), the sensitivity was 77.3%, and the specificity was 82.6% (**Figure 3**).

TABLE 2 | Outcomes of PLT-normal group and PLT-abnormal group.

All cohort	PLT-normal ($n = 120$)	PLT-abnormal ($n = 66$)	*P*-value	*P*-value*
90-day fatality			< 0.001	0.009
Survivor	116(96.7%)	47(71%)		
Non-survivor	4(3.3%)	19(29%)		

**Adjusted: Age, GCS, WBC, Neutrophil, INR, APTT, PCT, ALT, SCR, D-D.*

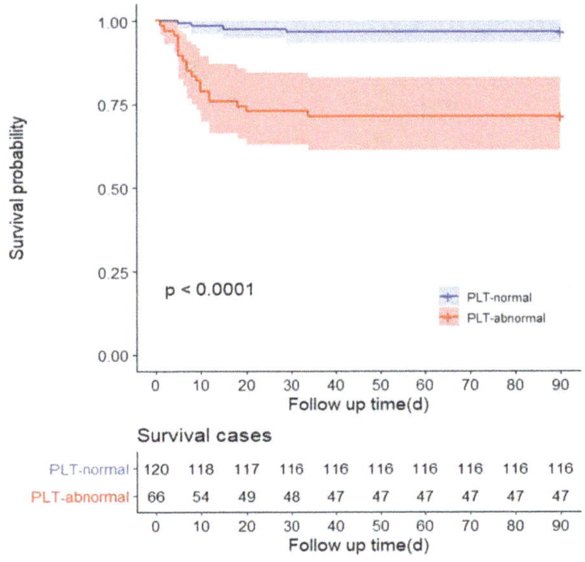

FIGURE 2 | Survival curves of 90-day mortality rate in PLT-abnormal group and PLT-normal group.

DISCUSSION

In this retrospective cohort study, patients with heat stroke and abnormal platelets at the time of admission had more serious organ function damage, mainly blood coagulation, liver, and kidney damage. Compared with patients without platelet abnormalities, patients with platelet abnormalities had a reduced 90-day survival rate. The cut-off value of PLT predicted by the ROC curve was 94(1×10^9/L), the sensitivity was 77.3%, and the specificity was 82.6%.

In our study, it was found that 35.5% of heatstroke patients had abnormal platelets, of which thrombocytopenia was the majority. Those with platelet abnormalities will suffer more severe organ function damage, mainly blood clotting, liver, and kidney damage, which is consistent with previous studies (7). Platelet count and function play an important role in the coagulation lesions of heatstroke, and platelet activation is triggered by heat and/or endothelial injury (7). Heatstroke can lead to inflammation, coagulation, and direct cytotoxic effects, damage to endothelial cells, leading to microthrombosis, and eventually platelet depletion, which can lead to coagulation disorders and even DIC (8). Thrombocytopenia is an important finding in the development of HS-induced Acute kidney injury (AKI) (9, 10). AKI patients are combined with renal blood flow reduction, renal tissue ischemia, and hypoxia, fibrinolytic system disorders, causing abnormal coagulation, that are mainly manifested as platelet function loss (11). Heatstroke can lead to dysfunction of multiple organs, including liver damage. Serotonin from platelets are released and involved

TABLE 3 | Baseline characteristics of survivors and non-survivors in patients with PLT-abnormal.

	Total (*N* = 66)	Survivors (*N* = 47)	Non-survivors (*N* = 19)	*P* value
APACHII score, median (IQR)	15.0 (11.5–21.5)	14.0 (10.0–18.0)	22.0 (17.8–23.5)	0.001
SOFA score, median (IQR)	6.0 (4.0–10.0)	6.0 (3.0–7.0)	13.5 (8.8–15.0)	< 0.001
GCS score, median (IQR)	8.0 (5.0–12.0)	10.0 (6.0–14.0)	4.0 (3.0–7.3)	0.002
Age (years), median (IQR)	23.0 (19.8–37.3)	26.0 (20.0–39.0)	22.0 (18.0–24.0)	0.077
WBC (1×10^9/L), median (IQR)	10.1 (7.9–13.3)	10.1 (8.3–12.5)	9.8 (7.6–14.2)	0.927
Neutrophil (1×10^9/L), median (IQR)	8.6 (6.5–10.9)	8.6 (6.8–10.9)	7.4 (5.9–11.8)	0.620
Lymphocyte (1×10^9/L), median (IQR)	0.6 (0.4–1.4)	0.6 (0.4–1.1)	0.5 (0.3–3.1)	0.788
Monocytes (1×10^9/L), median (IQR)	0.6 (0.3–0.7)	0.5 (0.3–0.7)	0.7 (0.2–0.8)	0.854
Platelets (1×10^9/L), median (IQR)	62.0 (34.5–86.8)	59.0 (37.0–91.0)	71.0 (29.0–84.0)	0.600
Mean platelet volume (%)	11.2 (10.5–11.8)	11.2 (10.4–11.9)	11.1 (10.5–11.9)	0.837
Platelet distribution width (%)	13.3 (11.8–15.2)	13.3 (11.5–11.4)	13.2 (12.0–16.6)	0.430
TBIL (μmol/L), median (IQR)	31.2 (16.1–65.3)	27.6 (15.1–61.6)	37.4 (21.2–127.8)	0.183
ALT (U/L), median (IQR)	221.0 (53.8–1,606.3)	162.0 (44.0–1,314.0)	246.0 (87.0–1,897.0)	0.350
AST (U/L), median (IQR)	290.0 (110.0–1,587.0)	190.0 (81.0–160.0)	406.5 (112.5–2,270.0)	0.315
BUN (mmol/L), median (IQR)	6.4 (5.0–8.7)	5.8 (4.9–7.7)	8.1 (6.2–10.0)	0.058
CR (μmol/L), median (IQR)	147.5 (87.8–223.5)	109.0 (81.0–160.0)	228.0 (187.0–286.0)	< 0.001
Cystatin C (mg/L)	1.1 (0.9–1.5)	1.0 (0.8–1.3)	1.5 (1.1–3.4)	0.001
CK (U/L), median (IQR)	1,688.5 (814.5–5,465.8)	1,796.5.0 (799.3–4,572.3)	1,672.0 (863.3–8,240.5)	0.500
CKMB (ng/ml), median (IQR)	18.0 (8.4–37.7)	16.4 (7.8–31.9)	19.9 (9.7–50.4)	0.299
Mb (ng/ml), median (IQR)	789.0 (219.0–1,000.0)	456.2 (124.3–1,000.0)	1,000.0 (935.1–1,000.0)	0.003
CTNI (ng/ml), median (IQR)	0.28 (0.11–1.11)	0.16 (0.02–0.46)	1.9 (0.90–3.86)	< 0.001
PT (s), median (IQR)	23.5 (16.6–37.4)	20.3 (17.0–35.4)	37.5 (25.6–45.6)	0.003
INR median (IQR)	2.0 (1.3–3.7)	1.7 (1.3–2.5)	3.8 (2.4–5.0)	0.001
APTT (s), median (IQR)	58.1 (41.4–99.9)	46.3 (39.2–77.9)	91.2 (76.1–124.8)	0.003
TT (s), median (IQR)	22.6 (17.6–54.0)	20.3 (17.0–35.4)	38.7 (27.2–82.5)	0.004
FIB (g/L), median (IQR)	2.2 (1.5–2.8)	2.5 (1.9–2.8)	1.3 (0.9–2.1)	0.003
D-D (mg/L), median (IQR)	6.6 (2.0–13.3)	3.9 (0.9–11.4)	10.1 (9.8–20.0)	0.001
CRP (mg/dl), median (IQR)	3.4 (3.2–9.8)	3.4 (2.5–11.0)	3.4 (3.3–6.7)	0.886
PCT (ng/ml), median (IQR)	3.2 (1.4–5.9)	2.9 (1.2–5.4)	3.8 (1.7–8.8)	0.182

IQR, Inter-Quartile Range; APACHE II, Acute Physiology and Chronic Health Evaluation II score; SOFA, Sequential Organ Failure Assessment; GCS, Glasgow Coma Score; WBC, White blood cell count; TBIL, Total bilirubin; ALT, Alanine aminotransferase; AST, Aspartate aminotransferase; BUN, Blood urea nitrogen; CR, Creatine; CK, Creatine Kinase; CK-MB, Creatine kinase isoenzymes; CTNI, Cardiac troponin I; PT, Prothrombin time; INR, International normalized ratio; APTT, Activated partial thromboplastin time; TT, Thrombin time; FIB, Fibrinogen; D-D, D-Dimer; CPR, C-reactive protein; PCT, Procalcitonin.

in pathophysiological processes such as liver injury response, regulation of liver function, and regeneration (12).

PLT has been evaluated in sepsis, diabetes, cardiovascular disease, and other diseases, and is correlated with disease severity and prognosis (13–16). PLT count is also part of the scoring for heatstroke patients (17). What makes our study different from other studies is that we investigated the effect of early platelet changes on 90-day prognosis in a population with exertional heat stroke, not limited to patients with AKI. In addition, we had a relatively long follow-up period, and prognostic parameters were adjusted for statistical analysis. The clinical characteristics of patients with platelet abnormality were analyzed in detail, which was not mentioned in other literatures. ROC curve analysis of platelets, and prediction of cut-off values, which further clarified the prognostic value of platelets for heatstroke patients. In our study, it was also found that compared with patients without platelet abnormality, the 90-day survival rate of patients with platelet abnormality was lower, and the sensitivity and specificity were 77.3% and 82.6% when the PLT of 94 (1×10^9/L) was taken as the critical point for predicting the 90-day death of patients with severe heatstroke. In the pathophysiological process of heatstroke, the relationship between heatstroke and platelets is very complex. Heatstroke damages platelets through heat stress and inflammation, and platelets aggravate the condition by activating coagulation response and further amplifying inflammation response (18). Therefore, platelets can assess the severity of heatstroke patients to a certain extent, contribute to the evaluation of the prognosis of heatstroke patients, and provide a reference for the selection of clinical treatment options.

This study has some limitations. First, it is a single-center cohort study with a relatively small number of cases. A multi-center study will be conducted in the later stage to increase the sample size and increase the statistical reliability. Second, exertional heatstroke is a special disease that occurs mainly in

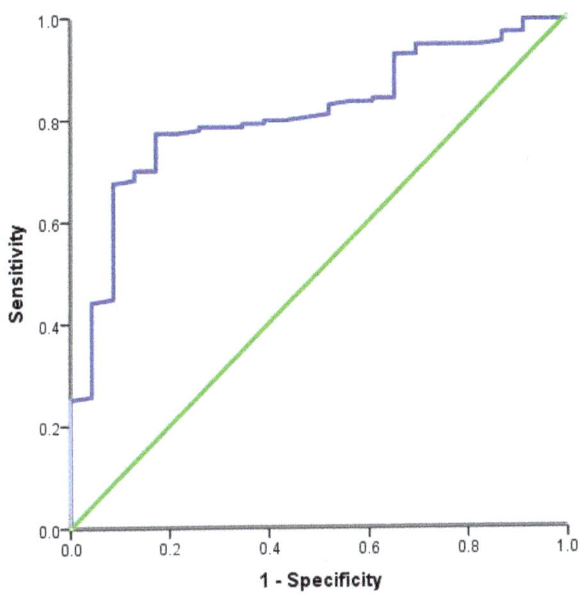

FIGURE 3 | ROC curve analysis of PLT to assess the 90-day mortality of heat stroke patients.

people who are engaged in heavy physical labor and exercise, often in a predominantly male group. In addition, due to estrogen protection and other factors, women under equal conditions rarely develop heatstroke. Therefore, our study subjects are also mainly male and may not fully reflect the changes of platelets in the overall population. Third, it is true that early recognition and treatment is crucial for heatstroke survivability, and the patients in our study usually received basic treatment before admission, including simple cooling and symptomatic support therapy. However, these information were pre hospital data. This study is a retrospective study, so we can not accurately obtain all these information, which is also one of the limitations of this study.

CONCLUSION

Patients with heatstroke who are admitted to hospital with platelet abnormalities have more severe organ impairment and a lower 90-day survival rate even when adjusted for other factors.

ETHICS STATEMENT

The studies involving human participants were reviewed and approved by Medical Ethics Committee of the Southern Theater General Hospital. Written informed consent for participation was not required for this study in accordance with the national legislation and the institutional requirements.

AUTHOR CONTRIBUTIONS

LZ and MW: data collection and analysis and manuscript preparation. JJ and CW: data collection and analysis. ZL: study designed, data collection and analysis, manuscript preparation, and review. All authors read and approved the final manuscript.

REFERENCES

1. Morris A, Patel G. "Heat Stroke," In: *StatPearls*. Treasure Island (FL): StatPearls Publishing Copyright © (2020) StatPearls Publishing LLC., 2020.
2. Gauer R, Meyers BK. Heat-related illnesses. *Am Fam Physician.* (2019) 99:482–9. doi: 10.13201/j.issn.1009-5918.2017.05.005
3. Krishnegowda M, Rajashekaraiah V. Platelet disorders: an overview. *Blood Coagul Fibrinolysis.* (2015) 26:479–91. doi: 10.1097/01.mbc.0000469521.23628.2d
4. Wang JJ, Wang YL, Ge XX, et al. Prognostic values of platelet-associated indicators in resectable lung cancers. *Technol Cancer Res Treat.* (2019) 18:1533033819837261. doi: 10.1177/1533033819837261
5. Yang W, Chen YY Bi C, et al. Predictive and prognostic values of preoperative platelet parameters in patients with gynecological tumors. *J Clin Lab Anal.* (2020) 34:e23295. doi: 10.1002/jcla.23295
6. Budak YU, Polat M, Huysal K. The use of platelet indices, plateletcrit, mean platelet volume and platelet distribution width in emergency non-traumatic abdominal surgery: a systematic review. *Biochem Med.* (2016) 26:178–93. doi: 10.11613/BM.2016.020
7. Gader AM. Heat stroke and platelets. *Platelets.* (1992) 3:125–8. doi: 10.3109/09537109209013172
8. Al-Mashhadani SA, Gader AM, Al Harthi S. The role of platelets in the coagulopathy of heatstroke—a study of platelet aggregation in heatstroke patients during the Makkah pilgrimage (Haj) to Makkah. *Platelets.* (1997) 8:37–42. doi: 10.1080/09537109777528
9. Fan H, Zhao Y, Zhu JH, et al. Thrombocytopenia as a predictor of severe acute kidney injury in patients with heat stroke. *Ren Fail.* (2015) 37:877–81. doi: 10.3109/0886022X.2015.1022851
10. Xing L, Liu SY, Mao HD, Zhou KG, Song Q, Cao QM. The prognostic value of routine coagulation tests for patients with heat stroke. *Am J Emerg Med.* (2021) 44:366–72. doi: 10.1016/j.ajem.2020.04.062
11. Celep RB, Unlu BS. Retrospective platelet values measurement. Is it acceptable to discuss? *Eur Rev Med Pharmacol Sci.* (2014) 18:1108.
12. Nocito A, Georgiev P, Dahm F, et al. Platelets and platelet-derived serotonin promote tissue repair after normothermic hepatic ischemia in mice. *Hepatology.* (2007) 45:369–76. doi: 10.1002/hep.21516

13. Guclu E, Durmaz Y, Karabay O. Effect of severe sepsis on platelet count and their indices. *Afr Health Sci.* (2013) 13:333–8. doi: 10.4314/ahs.v13i2.19
14. Laursen MA, Larsen JB, Larsen KM, et al. Platelet function in patients with septic shock. *Thromb Res.* (2020) 185:33–42. doi: 10.1016/j.thromres.2019.11.011
15. Strauss R, Wehler M, Mehler K, et al. Thrombocytopenia in patients in the medical intensive care unit: bleeding prevalence, transfusion requirements, and outcome. *Crit Care Med.* (2002) 30:1765–71. doi: 10.1097/00003246-200208000-00015
16. Zeng Z, Xia L, Fan X, et al. Platelet-derived miR-223 promotes a phenotypic switch in arterial injury repair. *J Clin Invest.* (2019) 129:1372–86. doi: 10.1172/JCI124508
17. Yang MM, Wang L, Zhang Y, Yuan R, Zhao Y, Hu J, et al. Establishment and effectiveness evaluation of a scoring system for exertional heat stroke by retrospective analysis. *Mil Med Res.* (2020) 7:40. doi: 10.1186/s40779-020-00269-1
18. Huimei Y, Huasheng T. Research progress on the pathogenesis of platelet injury and heat stroke. *J Clinic Emerg Med.* (2017) 18:342–4.

15

Effectiveness of Combined Strategies for the Prevention of Hypothermia Measured by Noninvasive Zero-Heat Flux Thermometer During Cesarean Section

Antonella Cotoia [1], Paola Sara Mariotti [1], Claudia Ferialdi [1], Pasquale Del Vecchio [1], Renata Beck [1], Simona Zaami [2] and Gilda Cinnella [1]*

[1] Department of Medical and Surgical Sciences, Anesthesia and Intensive Care Unit, University of Foggia, Foggia, Italy,
[2] Department of Anatomical, Histological, Forensic, and Orthopedic Science, Sapienza University of Rome, Rome, Italy

***Correspondence:**
Antonella Cotoia
antonella.cotoia@unifg.it*

Background: Perioperative hypothermia (body temperature <36°C) is a common complication of anesthesia increasing the risk for maternal cardiovascular events and coagulative disorders, and can also influence neonatal health. The aim of our work was to evaluate the impact of combined warming strategies on maternal core temperature, measured with the SpotOn. We hypothesized that combined modalities of active warming prevent hypothermia in pregnant women undergoing cesarean delivery with spinal anesthesia.

Methods: Seventy-eight pregnant women were randomly allocated into three study groups receiving warmed IV fluids and forced-air warming (AW), warmed IV fluids (WF), or no warming (NW). Noninvasive core temperature device (SpotOn) measured maternal core temperature intraoperatively and for 30 min after surgery. Maternal mean arterial pressure, incidence of shivering, thermal comfort and newborn's APGAR, axillary temperature, weight, and blood gas analysis were also recorded.

Results: Incidence of hypothermia was of 0% in AW, 4% in WF, and 47% in NW. Core temperature in AW was constantly higher than WF and NW groups. Incidence of shivering in perioperative time was significantly lower in AW and WF groups compared with the NW group ($p < 0.04$). Thermal comfort was higher in both AW and WF groups compared with NW group ($p = 0.02$ and $p = 0.008$, respectively). There were no significant differences among groups for the other evaluated parameters.

Conclusion: Combined modalities of active warming are effective in preventing perioperative hypothermia. The routine uses of combined AW are suggested in the setting of cesarean delivery.

Keywords: spinal anesthesia, core temperature, perioperative hypothermia, SpotOn, cesarean delivery (CD)

INTRODUCTION

The inadvertent perioperative hypothermia (PH) is the unintentional cooling of a patient's core temperature (CT°) >36°C (1).

Perioperative hypothermia is estimated to occur in >60% of patients receiving spinal anesthesia for cesarean delivery (2–4), in whom it significantly impairs thermal autoregulation by inhibiting the vasomotor and shivering responses even above the level of the sensory block and causes a thermal redistribution of heat from core to peripheral tissues (5–9).

In absence of strategies for preserving normothermia, patients become hypothermic in the early 30–40 min of surgery, and they remain hypothermic during postoperative time (10).

Hypothermia increases the risk of cardiovascular events, such as myocardial ischemia, arrhythmias, and coagulative disorders, greater blood loss with a need of transfusions, wounds infection with delayed healing due to decreased antibody- and cell-mediated immune responses, and also oxygen availability in the peripheral wound tissues. PH changes the kinetics and action of various anesthetic and paralyzing agents, increases thermal discomfort, and is associated with delayed postanesthetic recovery (2, 11–14).

Moreover, PH can increase oxygen consumption and catecholamines release, which are responsible of intraoperative complications, such as hypoxia and increased pulmonary vascular resistances, and postoperative shivering can increase the metabolic rate leading to an increased incidence of early postoperative myocardial ischemia, especially in high risk-patients (15, 16).

Maternal hypothermia during cesarean delivery can also influence the APGAR score of newborns, neonatal temperature, umbilical vein blood gas analysis (BGA), and blood coagulation (13). Those consequences are particularly relevant in light of the fact that failure to identify and treat perioperative hypothermia is starting to be acknowledged as a potential cause of malpractice lawsuits, in case adverse outcomes arise. It is worth bearing in mind that if a claim should be filed based on alleged medical malpractice stemming from negligence, courts (particularly under tort law statutes) are likely to hold doctors and facilities liable, if the patient medical records and informed consent documentation process turn out to be inaccurate or lacking in any measure. Such inconsistencies may be viewed by the court as resulting from negligent practices rather than unavoidable clinical complications. Overall, any failure to comply with surgical safety protocols or to produce documentation proving adherence to guidelines issued by recognized scientific societies and bodies, and therefore deemed reliable, will likely result in unfavorable rulings for doctors and hospitals (17–19).

Core temperature is the best single indicator of thermal status in humans. There are several methods to detect the body CT°, including: noninvasive, such as tympanic thermometer and rectal probe; and invasive, such as pulmonary artery catheter (PAC), esophageal and nasopharyngeal probes. All the studies on perioperative hypothermia used noninvasive CT° monitoring devices, especially tympanic thermometers.

A new skin temperature monitoring system, the SpotOn, measures the heat flux in a temporal artery and is a very reliable device in comparison with PAC, which is the gold standard.

The warming systems currently used to prevent and treat hypothermia, are classified into passive and active. Among the active warming methods, the most used are heated infusion fluids and forced air-warming systems; the latter can be applied on superior and/or lower extremities.

The multimodal approach of combined warming modalities (intravenous fluid infusion and forced air warming), temperature measurements, type of neuraxial anesthesia, duration, and time of warming (preoperative, preanesthetic, intraoperative) (2, 20, 21) have provided a series of interesting studies, but with no total consensus on the best management of perioperative hypothermia (2, 11, 12, 22).

Multiple studies used a single-modality warming intervention (warmed IV fluids (WF) or forced-air warming alone) and have shown little efficacy in preventing perioperative hypothermia during cesarean delivery (4, 20, 21, 23–27).

The aim of our prospective randomized controlled study is to evaluate the impact of combined strategies of warming in pregnant women undergoing cesarean delivery in terms of maternal CT° using the SpotOn.

METHODS

Study Design and Patient Population

After ethical approval, our prospective randomized, controlled study was performed at the Obstetrics and Gynecology Department of the University Hospital of Foggia, Italy (ClinicalTrials.gov registration number: NCT03473470).

Consecutive patients with the following inclusion criteria were considered for enrollment: healthy pregnant women (ASA 1-2), age from 18 to 40 years, at term gestation (≥ 37 weeks), and elective cesarean delivery with spinal anesthesia. Exclusion criteria included conditions, such as fever, diabetes mellitus, BMI > 40 kg/m, coagulative disorders, preeclampsia, and all those factors that can cause intraoperative bleeding (placental abruption or history of placenta previa). Before data collection, the purpose of the work was carefully explained and a written informed consent was obtained from each participant, according to the Helsinki declaration. From the original sample of 93 pregnant women, only 78 were enrolled in the work.

Women were randomly assigned, by a computer-generated randomization, to three study groups (26 patients each) to receive WF alone, warmed IV fluids and forced-air warming (AW), or IV fluids at room temperature with further no warming (NW).

Abbreviations: ASA, American society of anesthesiologists; AW, warmed IV fluids and forced-air warming; BGA, blood gas analysis; BMI, body mass index; BSAS, bedside shivering assessment scale; CD, cesarean delivery; CT°, core temperature (°C); MAP, mean arterial pressure; NW, no warming; OR, operating room; P, p-value; PAC, pulmonary artery catheter; PH, perioperative hypothermia; SD, standard deviation; T° OR, temperature in the operating room; T5-15-20-25-35-40-45-55, time at 5-15-20-25-35-40-45-55 min from baseline; TCS, thermal comfort score; WF, warmed IV fluids.

Study Protocol

Demographic data, vital signs (heart rate, mean arterial pressure, and pulse oximetry), and CT° were obtained in the preoperative holding area. CT° was obtained using the 3M™SpotOn™ monitoring System (Model 370, 3M Science, St.Paul, MN, USA), where the single-use sensor was placed on the patient's forehead before surgery which provided a continuous noninvasive CT° monitoring. In this study, we refer to maternal hypothermia as core body temperature <36°C, according to the 2017 SIAARTI Best Clinical Practice on Perioperative Normothermia (28). Spinal anesthesia was performed with intrathecal isobaric 8 mg levobupivacaine and 20 µg fentanyl, administered *via* a 27-gauge Whitacre needle, inserted at the L2–L3 or L3–L4 intervertebral space. After the spinal anesthesia, patients were immediately positioned supine, and the uterus was manually displaced to the left. Intravenous crystalloid preloading (Ringer's lactate solution, 10 ml/kg) was infused 10 min before the lumbar puncture. Thereafter, a coload of 10 ml/kg/h Ringer's lactate solution was administered.

The WF group received the IV fluids coload warmed to 41°C through a 3M Ranger™ Fluid Warmer (Model 245, Arizant Healthcare, Maplewood, MN, USA). The AW group received WF, and a thermal blanket (forced-air warming system) was placed after spinal anesthesia all over the upper extremities and attached to the convective temperature management system 3M Bair Hugger™ (Model 505); the device was set to "high" (43°C) in the AW group and "ambient" in the WF and NW groups. NW group received IV fluid at room temperature (fluid warmer set to "off"), no active warming was administered, but routine care with blankets was provided.

Room Temperature Was Measured in the Operative Room (OR) on the Arrival of Patients

Core temperature ° and mean arterial pressure (MAP) were recorded on the arrival of patient in the operating room (baseline), 5 min postspinal anesthesia (T5), every 10 min during surgery until the end of the cesarean delivery, and 30 min after the surgery (discharge).

Patients were also asked to report the severity of shivering using the Bedside Shivering Assessment Scale (BSAS) from 0 to 3 (0 = no shivering, 1 = shivering localized to the core and neck, 2 = shivering including the upper extremities, 3 = total body shivering) and the thermal comfort scores (TCS) obtained by using a visual analog scale from 0 to 100 (0 mm= worst imaginable cold, 50 mm = thermos-neutrality, and 100 mm = insufferably hot); these data were taken at 20 and 40 min (T20, T40) from baseline and at discharge from the OR.

Total volume of estimated blood losses during surgery was recorded at the end of surgery.

Apgar scores and axillary neonatal temperature were recorded at 1 and 5 min after birth, and umbilical vein BGA was obtained for analysis from a double-clamped umbilical cord.

Statistical Analysis

The power analysis suggested that a sample size of 21 parturients/group was required to detect a 0.5°C difference among groups in maternal CT (assuming $\alpha = 0.01$ and power = 0.95) (29). The number was then increased to 26 per group to allow for a 20% patients drop-out rate.

The normality of distribution was assessed by Shapiro–Wilkinson test. Since we found almost all of the data normally distributed, the data were expressed as mean ± SD values or number as appropriate. Data were analyzed using repeated measurements analysis of variance (RANOVA). Differences between the groups at each time point were examined *post hoc* using an independent sample *t*-test. A paired sample *t*-test was used to detect changes within the groups. Categorical data were analyzed by Chi-squared test (χ^2). Level of statistical significance was chosen to be at $p < 0.05$. Statistical analysis was performed by Statistical Package for the Social Sciences (SPSS Inc., Chicago, IL, USA) version 15.0 for Windows.

RESULTS

We recruited 93 pregnant women of whom 78 were enrolled in the study and divided them into three groups of 26 patients each (**Figure 1**). There were no significant differences among the three groups as regards age, height, weight, BMI, gestational age, baseline temperature, and surgery duration (from surgical incision to skin closure) (**Table 1**).

At the arrival of the patients, the operative room temperature (T°OR) was 23.4°C ± 1.4°C in the NW, 24.25°C ± 1.8°C in the WF group, and 22.5°C ± 0.4°C in the AW group, with no significant difference between the study groups.

Intergroup analysis showed that at baseline, the patient CT° was 36.9°C ± 0.4°C in the NW group; 37°C ± 0.5°C in the WF group, and 37°C ± 0.5°C in the AW group ($p = 0.80$).

At T25, the CT° of NW, WF, and AW groups were respectively 36.4°C ± 0.4°C, 36.6°C ± 0.3°C, and 36.8°C ± 0.3°C; CT° in AW group was significantly higher than WF group and NW group (AW vs. WF: $p = 0.023$; AW vs. NW: $p = 0.001$).

At T35, the CT° of NW, WF, and AW groups were respectively 36.3°C ± 0.5°C, 36.5°C ± 0.3°C, and 36.7°C ± 0.3°C; CT° in AW group was significantly higher than WF group and NW group (AW vs. WF: $p = 0.025$; AW vs. NW: $p < 0.001$). The CT° in WF group was also statistically higher than the NW group ($p = 0.047$).

At T45, the CT° of NW, WF, and AW groups were respectively 36.2°C ± 0.3°C, 36.5°C ±0.3°C, and 36.7°C ± 0.3; CT° in AW and WF groups was significantly higher than the NW group (AW vs. NW: $p < 0.001$; WF vs. NW: $p = 0.004$).

At discharge, the CT° of NW, WF, and AW groups were respectively 36.2°C ± 0.3°C, 36.4°C ± 0.3°C, and 36.7°C ± 0.3°C; CT° in the AW group was significantly higher than WF group and NW group (AW vs. WF: $P = 0.001$; AW vs. NW: $p < 0.00$).

Intragroup analysis showed that the CT° gradually decreased in perioperative time in all the three groups and with significant difference from baseline to discharge (NW and WF: $p < 0.001$;

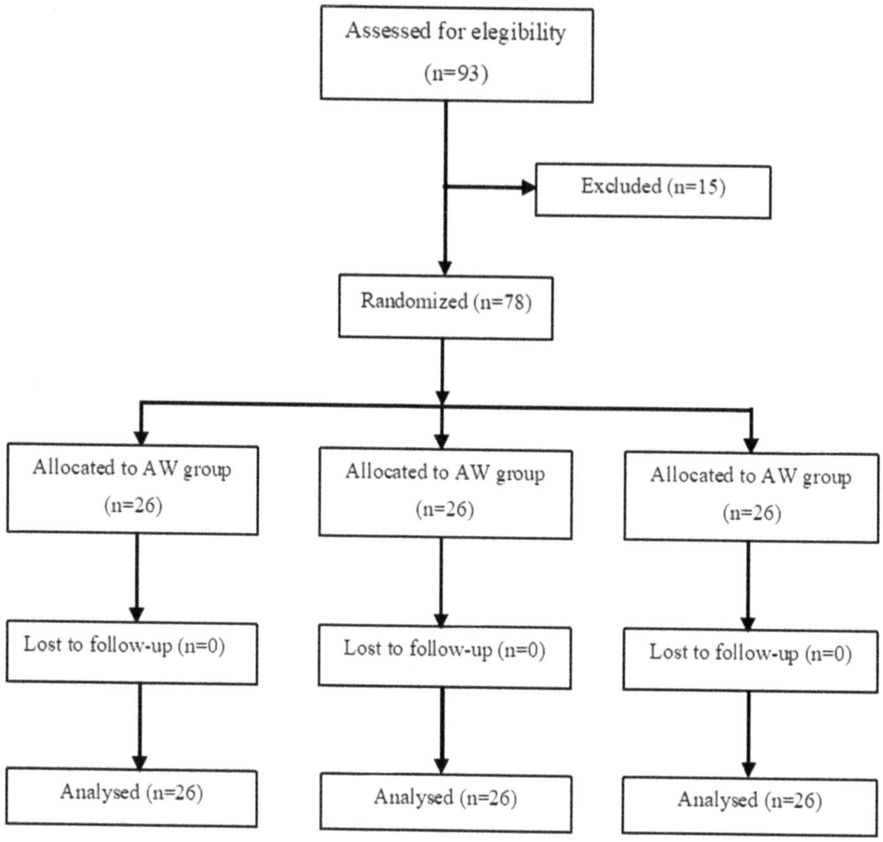

FIGURE 1 | Flowchart of patient's enrolment.

AW: $p = 0.045$). CT° in our study was never < 36°C in the AW group (**Table 2**, **Figure 2**).

As regards the MAP, no differences were observed among the three groups during the study period.

Blood loss in perioperative time was 258 ± 80 ml in the NW, 218 ± 90 ml in the WF group, and 227 ± 55 ml in the AW group, with no significant difference between these groups.

The other two statistically relevant outcomes were the BSAS (**Table 3**) and the maternal TCS (**Figure 3**).

At T20 and T40, the incidence of shivering was significantly higher in the NW than in the AW and WF groups (respectively, at T20: $p = 0.04$; at T40: $p < 0.001$).

At discharge, no shivering was observed. No patient had severe shivering (BSAS 3) in either group.

As far as thermal comfort is concerned, at T20, the TCS in the NW, WF, and AW groups were respectively 49 ± 6 mm, 51.5 ± 4 mm, and 51 ± 3 mm; TCS in NW group was lower only with respect to the WF group (NW vs. WF: $p = 0.04$).

At T40, the TCS in the NW, WF, and AW groups were respectively 46 ± 7 mm, 52 ± 5 mm, and 50 ± 2 mm; TCS in NW group was lower than WF and AW groups (NW vs WF: $p < 0.001$; NW vs. AW: $p = 0.007$).

At discharge, the TCS in the NW, WF, and AW groups were respectively 47 ± 7 mm, 50 ± 2 mm, and 50 ± 0 mm; TCS in NW group was lower than WF and AW groups (NW vs. WF: $p = 0.008$; NW vs. AW: $p = 0.02$). No patient reported insufferable hot during warming.

There were no significant differences among the three groups in terms of APGAR score and neonatal body temperature at 1 and 5 min from birth, birth weight, and umbilical cord vein BGA (**Table 4**).

No infant had complications or died.

DISCUSSION

The main results of our study demonstrated that the combination of AW is effective in reducing the loss of maternal CT° and the incidence of shivering during cesarean delivery (CD) in patients undergoing spinal anesthesia.

Warmed IV fluids, when used alone, are useful in maintaining a higher temperature during surgery and in postoperative time compared with no use of warming systems (NW), but they provided the worst results, in terms of incidence of shivering, compared with AW.

Perioperative hypothermia (PH), defined as a CT below 36°C, is one of the most common phenomena in surgical patients (30). Hypothermia during surgery can be generated by various factors,

TABLE 1 | Demographic and obstetric data of the study population.

	NW group (*n* = 26)	WF group (*n* = 26)	AW group (*n* = 26)	*P*
Age (years)	34 ± 5	33 ± 7	36 ± 63	0.756
Height (cm)	163 ± 6	162 ± 6	163 ± 5	0.926
Weight (kg)	73 ± 11	75 ± 16	79± 14	0.227
BMI (kg/m²)	27 ± 3	28 ± 6	29 ± 5	0.194
Gestational age (weeks)	38 ± 7	38 ± 1	38 ± 1	0.205
Baseline CT° (°C)	36.9 ± 0.4	37 ± 0.4	37 ± 0.4	0.807
Duration of surgery (min)	52 ± 10	52 ± 10	48 ± 6	0.207
T°OR (°C)	23 ± 1	24 ± 2	23 ± 0.4	0.103

Data are expressed in terms of mean ± standard deviation.
NW, IV fluids at room temperature and no forced-air warming; WF, warmed IV fluids; AW, warmed IV fluids and forced-air warming; P, p-value; CT, core temperature (°C); T°OR, temperature in the operating room (°C).

TABLE 2 | Maternal PH incidence.

Outcome	NW group (*N* = 26) *n* (%)	WF group (*N* = 26) *n* (%)	AW group (*N* = 26) *n* (%)	*P*
Peri-operative hypothermia (PH)	(47%)* °	1 (4%)* #	0 (0%)# °	0.04*
				0.31#
				0.009°

Data are expressed in terms of % of women with PH for each study group.
PH, peri-operative hypothermia; NW, IV fluids at room temperature and no forced-air warming; WF, warmed IV fluids; AW, warmed IV fluids and forced-air warming; P, p-value.
**, NW vs WF (P = 0.04); #, WF vs AW (P = 0.31); °, NW vs AW (P = 0.009).*

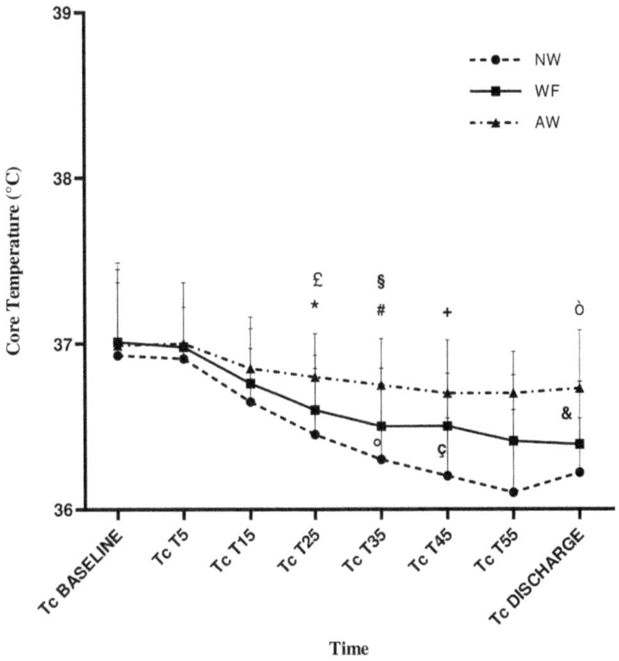

FIGURE 2 | Core temperature (CT°) variation during the perioperative time. Data are expressed in terms of mean ± standard deviation. NW, IV fluids at room temperature and no forced-air warming; WF, warmed IV fluids; AW, warmed IV fluids and forced-air warming; P, p-value; CT°, core temperature, expressed in °C; T°OR, temperature in the operating room, expressed in °C; CT°, core temperature; T5, T15, T25, T35, T45, and T55: 5, 15, 25, 35, 45, and −55 min from baseline, respectively. £, AW vs. WF (p = 0.023); *, AW vs. NW (p = 0.001); #, AW vs WF (p = 0.025); §, AW vs NW (p < 0.001); °, WF vs NW (p = 0.047); +, AW vs NW (p < 0.001); ç, WF vs NW (p = 0.004); ò, AW vs. NW (p < 0.001); &, AW vs. WF (p = 0.001).

such as exposure to the surgical environment, thermoregulatory dysfunction, and medications.

The primary mechanism of perioperative hypothermia during CD, after neuraxial anesthesia, is the redistribution of intravascular volume from the core to the peripheral compartment. Moreover, after a drop of CT, hypothermia triggers vasoconstriction and shivering in unblocked regions.

Perioperative hypothermia leads to intraoperative blood loss, cardiac events, coagulopathy, an increase in hospital stay and associated costs (31). Excluding therapeutic uses of hypothermia, such as in cardiac arrest patients and neonatal hypoxic-ischemic encephalopathy, perioperative PH should be avoided (32, 33).

Currently, a plethora of patient warming devices is utilized to reduce the incidence of intraoperative hypothermia; the most used are forced-air warming systems, which warm the patient from the outside, and WF, which may prevent a decrease in body temperature in the setting of redistribution hypothermia (3). Several studies have shown that WF, as a single modality of warming, are effective in minimizing maternal PH, but did not reduce the incidence of shivering (23, 31, 34, 35).

In other studies, forced-air warming was used as the only warming method. Butwick et al. applied the forced-air warming on the lower extremities to warm the peripheral compartment below the level of sympathetic inhibition, but they found no improvements in preventing PH and shivering (4). Fallis and Horn et al. used forced-air warming on the upper extremities, but they obtained contrasting results in terms of maternal CT° and shivering (20, 21). Therefore, the optimal area of application (upper or lower) for forced-air warming still needs be determined.

In the last few years, many groups focused their study on the effects of combining AW on maternal CT° and shivering incidence.

Cobb et al. used combined intraoperative WF and lower body forced-air warming, and they found good results compared with no warmed control group in reducing the trend of maternal CT° decline and greater maternal thermal comfort, but they still observed high incidence of PH and no decrease in shivering incidence (2).

In contrast with our study, patients were hypothermic in AW group. A potential explanation could be that our surgeons were faster in performing CD.

In regards to the timing of application of warming systems, some studies demonstrated that prewarming is effective in preventing redistribution hypothermia after both neuraxial and general anesthesia (20, 36).

TABLE 3 | Bedside shivering assessment scale evaluation (BSAS) during the perioperative time.

BSAS time	score	NW group (N = 26) n (%)	WF group (N = 26) n (%)	AW group (N = 26) n (%)	P
BSAS T20	0	22 (85%)*+	26 (100%)*	26 (100% +	0.04*+
	1	1 (4%)	0 (0%)	0 (0%)	
	2	3 (11%)	0 (0%)	0 (0%)	
BSAS T40	0	12 (46%)#ç	24 (92%)#	26 (100%) ç	<0.001#ç
	1	10 (38%)	2 (8%)	0 (0%)	
	2	4 (16%)	0 (0%)	0 (0%)	
BSAS discharge	0	23 (88%)	25 (96%)	26 (100%)	0.383
	1	3 (12%)	1 (4%)	0 (0%)	
	2	0 (0%)	0 (0%)	0 (0%)	

Bedside shivering assessment scale evaluation. Data are expressed in terms of mean ± standard deviation.
BSAS, bed shivering assessment scale; NW, IV fluids at room temperature and no forced-air warming; WF, warmed IV fluids; AW, warmed IV fluids and forced-air warming; T20, at 20 min from baseline; T40, at 40 min from baseline.
**, NW vs. WF (p = 0.04); +, NW vs. AW (p = 0.04); #, NW vs. WF (p < 0.001); ç, NW vs. AW (p < 0.001).*

With the aim of reducing redistribution hypothermia and core-to-periphery temperature gradient, Jun et al. treated patients with forced-air warming placed over the entire body 15 min before starting anesthesia and WF coload during surgery (11). This strategy yielded only little efficacy in preventing perioperative CT° decline and shivering in the warmed group with respect to no warmed control. Our work demonstrated that the combination of AW was effective when active warming interventions are applied during the intraoperative time, when forced-air warming started soon after the spinal anesthesia and continued for the whole time of surgery.

Horn et al. applied forced-air warming on the upper extremities 15 min before anesthesia, showing an additional efficacy when it was combined with WF in the setting of epidural anesthesia and CD (20). Differently, we applied forced-air warming after spinal anesthesia.

Furthermore, Meghana et al. compared the use of combined lower extremities AW to only forced-air warming modality. They observed that combined warming methods preserved maternal CT° and reduced shivering in patients undergoing CD and spinal anesthesia, recommending the use of active warming methods in the operation theater (22).

In our work, the combined AW interventions dampened the decline in CT° in perioperative time and decreased the incidence of shivering more than WF group, although the difference was not significant, and we cannot make a strong suggestion for AW strategy as routine care during CD.

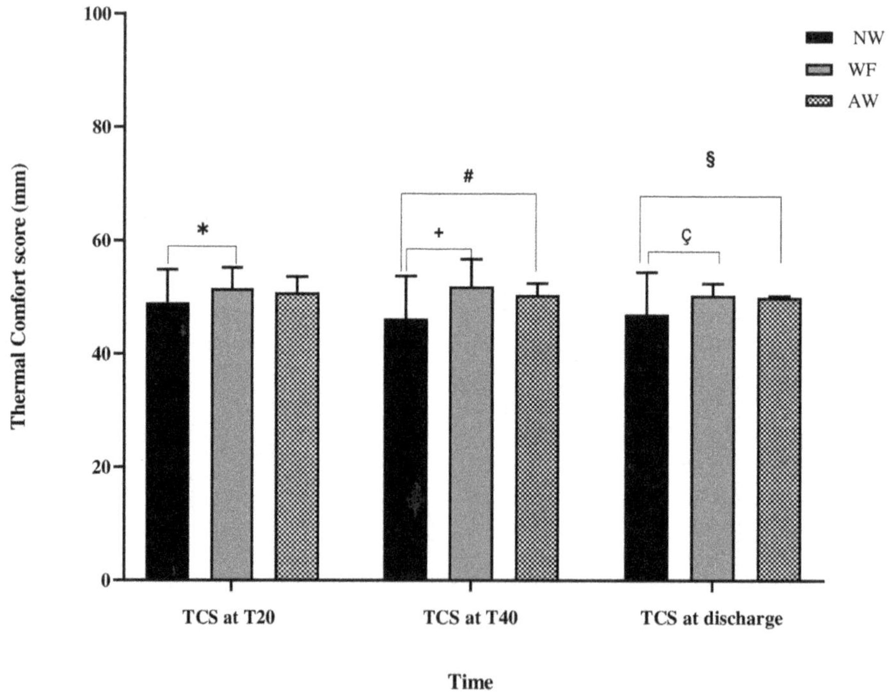

FIGURE 3 | Thermal comfort score evaluation (TCS) during the perioperative time. Thermal comfort score evaluation. Data are expressed in terms of mean ± standard deviation. TCS, thermal comfort score (mm); NW, IV fluids at room temperature and no forced-air warming; WF, warmed IV fluids; AW, warmed IV fluids and forced-air warming; T20, at 20 min from baseline; T40, at 40 min from baseline. *, NW vs. WF (p = 0.04); #, NW vs. AW (p = 0.007); +, NW vs. WF (p < 0.001); §, NW vs. AW (p = 0.02); ç, NW vs. WF (p = 0.008).

TABLE 4 | Neonatal demographics, APGAR scores, umbilical cord vein BGA, and temperature data.

	NW group (*N* = 26)	WF group (*N* = 26)	AW group (*N* = 26)	*P*
APGAR score 1 m	8 ± 8	8 ± 5	8 ± 3	0.948
APGAR score 5 m	8.9 ± 2	8.9 ± 3	9 ± 1	0.099
Temperature (°C) 1 m	35.9 ± 4	35 ± 7	36.6 ± 2	0.430
Temperature (°C) 5 m	35.9 ± 3	34.9 ± 7	36.6 ± 2	0.364
Birth weight (g)	2,966 ± 433	3,245 ± 597	3,087 ± 314	0.104
Umbilical cord vein BGA	7.32 ± 0.05	7.34 ± 0.05	7.33 ± 0.06	0.454

Data are expressed in terms of mean ± standard deviation.
NW, IV fluids at room temperature and no forced-air warming; WF, warmed IV fluids; AW, warmed IV fluids and forced-air warming; p, p-value; BGA, blood gas analysis.

As far as concern blood losses during surgery, a recent metaanalysis indicates that even mild hypothermia (CT° 34–36°C) increases blood loss and the relative risk of transfusion by small but significant amounts compared with normothermic surgical patients (37, 38). In our work, we did not observe a significant difference in blood loss among the three study groups.

Previous studies used infrared tympanic thermometer or oral probes whose reliability has been questioned (39). In our work, we used the SpotOn which is a new noninvasive, skin temperature monitoring system that measures the heat-flux in temporal artery by using a single-use sensor placed on the patient's forehead. Indeed, the SpotOn is much more sensitive to temperature changes when compared with other noninvasive devices.

In this work, our primary goals were the evaluation of maternal CT°, the incidence of shivering, and the maternal thermal comfort in perioperative period for women undergoing CD.

Secondary goals included blood loss evaluation and neonatal outcomes (Apgar score, axillary temperature, birth weight, and umbilical cord vein BGA), neither of them showing significant variation; these latter results are not surprising given our limited measures of neonatal well-being.

One potential limitation of our study consisted of the use of a nonvalidated visual analog scale for thermal comfort quantification. We used the same scale devised by Horn et al. (20) (0 mm = worst imaginable cold, 50 mm = thermoneutrality, and 100 mm = insufferable hot), which was not validated and was a little confusing to patients. Nevertheless, this scale can well differentiate between the hot and cold spectrum of discomfort compared with the one used by other studies that indicate with a verbal numerical scale the thermal comfort in terms of maternal satisfaction (0 = completely unsatisfied and 100 = completely satisfied) (2, 11).

Another limitation consisted of newborn CT° measured with axillary thermometer rather than the SpotOn system, which has a low level of accuracy as a method of monitoring body CT° in pediatric patients (<10 kg) (40).

CONCLUSIONS

In summary, our study showed that the combination of AW systems for elective CD under spinal anesthesia increases maternal CT°, prevents PH, and reduces the overall perioperative CT° decline and the incidence of shivering compared with the use of only WF or no interventions.

Based on the study findings, identification of women at risk of developing perioperative hypothermia may allow for more targeted AW strategies.

ETHICS STATEMENT

The studies involving human participants were reviewed and approved by Comitato Etico Area 1-Azienda Ospedaliera Riuniti di Foggia (DDG n. 363 del 25.10.2016 e s.m.i. DDG n. 318 del 14.6.2019). The patients/participants provided their written informed consent to participate in this study.

AUTHOR CONTRIBUTIONS

AC was responsible for the conception and design of the study, analyzed the data of the study, and wrote the manuscript. PM analyzed the data and wrote the manuscript. CF organized the database. PD performed the study. RB and SZ wrote a section of the manuscript. GC revised the final manuscript. AC, PM, CF, PD, RB, SZ, and GC approved the final manuscript. All authors contributed to the article and approved the submitted version.

REFERENCES

1. Allen TK, Habib AS. Inadvertent perioperative hypothermia induced by spinal anesthesia for cesarean delivery might be more significant than we think: are we doing enough to warm our parturients? *Anesth Analg.* (2018) 126:7–9. doi: 10.1213/ANE.0000000000002604
2. Cobb B, Cho Y, Hilton G, Ting V, Carvalho B. Active warming utilizing combined IV fluid and forced-air warming decreases hypothermia and improves maternal comfort during cesarean delivery: a randomized control trial. *Anesth Analg.* (2016) 122:1490–7. doi: 10.1213/ANE.0000000000001181
3. Sultan P, Habib AS, Cho Y, Carvalho B. The Effect of patient warming during Caesarean delivery on maternal and neonatal outcomes: A meta-analysis. *Br J Anaesth.* (2015). doi: 10.1093/bja/aev325
4. Butwick AJ, Lipman SS, Carvalho B. Intraoperative forced air-warming during cesarean delivery under spinal anesthesia does not prevent maternal hypothermia. *Anesth Analg.* (2007) 105:1413–9. doi: 10.1213/01.ane.0000286167.96410.27
5. Matsukawa T, Sessler DI, Sessler AM, Schroeder M, Ozaki M, Kurz A, et al. Heat flow and distribution during induction of general anesthesia. *Anesthesiology.* (1995) 82:662–73. doi: 10.1097/00000542-199503000-00008
6. Kim JS, Ikeda T, Sessler DI, Turakhia M, Jeffrey R. Epidural anesthesia reduces the gain and maximum intensity of shivering. *Anesthesiology.* (1998) 88:851–7. doi: 10.1097/00000542-199804000-00002
7. Sessler DI. Perioperative heat balance. *Anesthesiology.* (2000) 92:578–96. doi: 10.1097/00000542-200002000-00042

8. Sessler DI. Complications and treatment of mild hypothermia. *Anesthesiology.* (2001) 95:531–43. doi: 10.1097/00000542-200108000-00040
9. Kurz A, Sessler DI, Lenhardt R. Perioperative normothermia to reduce the incidence of surgical-wound infection and shorten hospitalization. Study of Wound Infection and Temperature Group. *N Engl J Med.* (1996) 334:1209–15. doi: 10.1056/NEJM199605093341901
10. NICE. Inadvertent perioperative hypothermia: the management of inadvertent perioperative hypothermia in adults NICE guideline. London: National Collaborating Centre for Nursing and SupportiveCare. (2007).
11. Jun J-H, Chung MH, Jun I-J, Kim Y, Kim H, Kim JH, et al. Efficacy of forced-air warming and warmed intravenous fluid for prevention of hypothermia and shivering during caesarean delivery under spinal anaesthesia: A randomised controlled trial. *Eur J Anaesthesiol.* (2019) 36:442–8. doi: 10.1097/EJA.0000000000000990
12. Munday J, Hines S, Wallace K, Chang AM, Gibbons K, Yates P, et al. systematic review of the effectiveness of warming interventions for women undergoing cesarean section. *Worldviews Evid Based Nurs.* (2014) 11:383–93. doi: 10.1111/wvn.12067
13. Mirabella L, Mollica G, Mariano K, Dambrosio M. Reference values for coagulation assessment in full-term newborns. *Minerva Anestesiol.* (2017) 83:6. doi: 10.23736/S0375-9393.16.11375-6
14. Rauch S, Miller C, Bräuer A, Wallner B, Bock M, Paal P. Perioperative hypothermia—a narrative review. *Int J Environ Res Public Health.* (2021) 18:8749. doi: 10.3390/ijerph18168749
15. D'Ambrosio A, Cotoia A, Beck R, Salatto P, Zibar L, Cinnella G. Impedance cardiography as tool for continuous hemodynamic monitoring during cesarean section: Randomized, prospective double blind study. *BMC Anesthesiol.* (2018) 18:32. doi: 10.1186/s12871-018-0498-4
16. Frank SM, Beattie C, Christopherson R, Norris EJ, Perler BA, Williams GM, et al. Unintentional hypothermia is associated with postoperative myocardial ischemia. The Perioperative Ischemia Randomized Anesthesia Trial Study Group. *Anesthesiology.* (1993) 78:468–76. doi: 10.1097/00000542-199303000-00010
17. Iden T, Höcker J. Vermeidung unbeabsichtigter perioperativer Hypothermie: ein Leitfaden. *AINS - Anästhesiol Intensivmed Notfallmedizin Schmerzther.* (2017) 52:554–62. doi: 10.1055/s-0041-103653
18. Torossian A, Bräuer A, Höcker J, Bein B, Wulf H, Horn E-P. Preventing Inadvertent Perioperative Hypothermia. *Dtsch Ärztebl Int.* (2015) 112:166–72. doi: 10.3238/arztebl.2015.0166
19. Adoption of the ASPAN Clinical Guideline for the Prevention of Unplanned Perioperative Hypothermia: A Data Collection Tool - Journal of PeriAnesthesia Nursing. Available online at:: https://www.jopan.org/article/S1089-9472(06)00128-6/fulltext (accessed June 24, 2021).
20. Horn EP, Schroeder F, Gottschalk A, Sessler DI, Hiltmeyer N, Standl T, et al. Active warming during cesarean delivery. *Anesth Analg.* (2002) 94:409–14 doi: 10.1213/00000539-200202000-00034
21. Fallis WM, Hamelin K, Symonds J, Wang X. Maternal and newborn outcomes related to maternal warming during cesarean delivery. *JOGNN - J Obstet Gynecol Neonatal Nurs.* (2006) 35:324-31. doi: 10.1111/j.1552-6909.2006.00052.x
22. Meghana V, Vasudevarao S, Kamath S. The effect of combination of warm intravenous fluid infusion and forced air warming versus forced air warming alone on maternal temperature and shivering during cesarian delivery under spinal anesthesia. *Ann Afr Med.* (2020) 19:137–43. doi: 10.4103/aam.aam_58_19
23. Yokoyama K, Suzuki M, Shimada Y, Matsushima T, Bito H, Sakamoto A. Effect of administration of pre-warmed intravenous fluids on the frequency of hypothermia following spinal anesthesia for Cesarean delivery. *J Clin Anesth.* (2009) 21:242–8. doi: 10.1016/j.jclinane.2008.12.010
24. Kundra S, Grewal A, Singh Mr, Goyal P, Sharma S, Kaul T. Efficacy of intravenous fluid warming for maintenance of core temperature during lower segment cesarean section under spinal anesthesia. *J Obstet Anaesth Crit Care.* (2011) 1:73–7. doi: 10.4103/2249-4472.93990
25. Chung SH, Lee BS, Yang HJ, Kweon KS, Kim HH, Song J, et al. Effect of preoperative warming during cesarean section under spinal anesthesia. *Korean J Anesthesiol.* (2012) 62:454–60. doi: 10.4097/kjae.2012.62.5.454
26. Woolnough M, Allam J, Hemingway C, Cox M, Yentis SM. Intraoperative fluid warming in elective cesarean section: a blinded randomized controlled trial. *Obstet Anesth Dig.* 18:346–51. (2010) doi: 10.1097/01.aoa.0000386826.89761.80
27. Jørgensen HS, Bach LF, Helbo-Hansen HS, Nielsen PA. Warm or cold saline for volume preload before spinal anaesthesia for caesarean section? *Int J Obstet Anesth.* (2000) 9:20–5. doi: 10.1054/ijoa.1999.0331
28. Buone-Pratiche-Cliniche-SIAARTI-Normotermia-perioperatoria1.pdf. Available online at: http://www.ipotermia.org/wp-content/uploads/2017/10/Buone-Pratiche-Cliniche-SIAARTI-Normotermia-perioperatoria1.pdf (accessed June 24, 2021).
29. Wittes J. Sample Size Calculations for Randomized Controlled Trials. *Epidemiol Rev.* (2002) 24:39–53. doi: 10.1093/epirev/24.1.39
30. Ackermann W, Fan Q, Parekh AJ, Stoicea N, Ryan J, Bergese SD. Forced-air warming and resistive heating devices. Updated perspectives on safety and surgical site infections. *Front Surg.* (2018) 5:64. doi: 10.3389/fsurg.2018.00064
31. John M, Crook D, Dasari K, Eljelani F, El-Haboby A, Harper CM. Comparison of resistive heating and forced-air warming to prevent inadvertent perioperative hypothermia. *Br J Anaesth.* (2016) 116:249–54. doi: 10.1097/01.sa.0000504596.04838.dd
32. Crippa IA, Vincent J-L, Zama Cavicchi F, Pozzebon S, Annoni F, Cotoia A, et al. Cerebral autoregulation in anoxic brain injury patients treated with targeted temperature management. *J Intensive Care.* (2021) 9:67. doi: 10.1186/s40560-021-00579-z
33. Sakr M, Balasundaram P. Neonatal Therapeutic Hypothermia. In: StatPearls. Treasure Island (FL): StatPearls Publishing. (2021). Available online at: http://www.ncbi.nlm.nih.gov/books/NBK567714/ (accessed June 24, 2021).
34. Badjatia N, Strongilis E, Gordon E, Prescutti M, Fernandez L, Fernandez A, et al. Metabolic impact of shivering during therapeutic temperature modulation: The bedside shivering assessment scale. *Stroke.* (2008) 39:3242–7. doi: 10.1161/STROKEAHA.108.523654
35. Halloran OJ. Warming our Cesarean section patients: why and how? *J Clin Anesth.* (2009) 21:239–41. doi: 10.1016/j.jclinane.2009.03.001
36. Jun J-H, Chung MH, Kim EM, Jun I-J, Kim JH, Hyeon J-S, et al. Effect of pre-warming on perioperative hypothermia during holmium laser enucleation of the prostate under spinal anesthesia: a prospective randomized controlled trial. *BMC Anesthesiol.* (2018) 18:201. doi: 10.1186/s12871-018-0668-4
37. Rajagopalan S, Mascha E, Na J, Sessler DI. The effects of mild perioperative hypothermia on blood loss and transfusion requirement. *Anesthesiology.* (2008) 108:71–7. doi: 10.1097/01.anes.0000296719.73450.52
38. Kander T, Schött U. Effect of hypothermia on haemostasis and bleeding risk: a narrative review. *J Int Med Res.* (2019) 47:3559–68. doi: 10.1177/0300060519861469
39. Modell JG, Katholi CR, Kumaramangalam SM, Hudson EC, Graham D. Unreliability of the infrared tympanic thermometer in clinical practice: a comparative study with oral mercury and oral electronic thermometers. *South Med J.* (1998) 91:649–54. doi: 10.1097/00007611-199807000-00008
40. Idei M, Nomura T. Accuracy of a new zero-heat-flux cutaneous thermometer (SpotOn^{TM}) in pediatric intensive care patients. *Tokyo Womens Med Univ J.* (2019) 3:51–7. doi: 10.1097/CCM.0000000000002317

16

Priorities Towards Fair Allocation of Ventilators During COVID-19 Pandemic: A Delphi Study

Seyyed-Hadi Ghamari†, Mohsen Abbasi-Kangevari†, Nasim Zamani, Hossein Hassanian-Moghaddam and Ali-Asghar Kolahi**

Social Determinants of Health Research Center, Shahid Beheshti University of Medical Sciences, Tehran, Iran

***Correspondence:**
Ali-Asghar Kolahi
a.kolahi@sbmu.ac.ir
Nasim Zamani
nasim.zamani@gmail.com

†These authors share first authorship

Background: COVID-19 pandemic has resulted in severe shortage in vital resources, including invasive mechanical ventilators. The current imbalance between demand and supply of mechanical ventilators has called for investigations on the fair allocation of mechanical ventilators.

Objective: To determine the priorities of the medical experts towards the fair allocation of ventilators during the COVID-19 pandemic.

Methods: This study was conducted from May 28 to Aug 20, 2020. The questionnaire was sent to 50 medical specialists as the Delphi panel. Participants were asked to rate each prioritising factor: "−1" for low priority, "+1" for high priority, and "Zero" for equal priority.

Results: Among 38 experts who responded to the email, the responses of 35 were analysed. 31 (88.6%) participants recommended that pregnant women be considered high priority in allocating ventilators, 27 (77.1%) mothers of children<5 years, 26 (74.3%) patients under 80-years, and 23 (65.7%) front-line-healthcare-workers. In contrast, 28 (80.0) participants recommended that patients who are terminally ill should be considered as a low priority, 27 (77.1%) patients with active-malignancy, 25 (71.4%) neurodegenerative diseases, and 16 (45.7%) patients aged >80. The panel did not reach a consensus regarding the role of patients' laboratory profiles, underlying diseases, or drug abuse in the prioritisation of ventilators.

Conclusions: The panel considered pregnant mothers, mothers of children under 5 years, age groups younger than 80, and front-line healthcare workers to have high priority in allocating mechanical ventilators.

Keywords: coronavirus infections, health care rationing, ethics, health policy, resource allocation, SARS-CoV-2, mechanical ventilators

INTRODUCTION

The coronavirus disease 2019 (COVID-19) pandemic is rapidly intensifying worldwide and continues to place an extraordinary burden on humankind (1). Since the early days of the pandemic, a severe shortage in vital resources, including invasive mechanical ventilators, has remained a significant concern of healthcare professionals (2, 3).

During the pandemic, of all patients diagnosed with COVID-19, 17–35% required hospitalisation at ICUs (4, 5) and 9–19% required invasive mechanical ventilation (4, 6). The estimated number of invasive mechanical ventilators in various countries would not be adequate to serve all clinically eligible patients during the current pandemic (3). Therefore, the current imbalance between demand and supply of mechanical ventilators has called for investigations on the fair allocation of mechanical ventilators. Although the research has been ongoing on the subject since the early days of the pandemic, significant concerns remain controversial (7–9).

Medical experts working at the COVID-19 care units interact with patients of different socioeconomic, clinical, paraclinical, and overall health statuses. Nevertheless, physicians should not be faced with situations where they would be obliged to decide which patient to treat due to the risk of human error and the life-long emotional toll (10). Therefore, prioritisation recommendations and guidelines are being developed in the hope of helping physicians, especially those less experienced, with the real-time decision-making process based on the resources and contexts (11, 12). Nevertheless, most studies on the subject have focused on experts' opinions from a single country or region, limiting their generalizability (7–9).

The objective of this study was to determine the priorities of the medical experts towards the fair allocation of ventilators during the COVID-19 pandemic via an international online Delphi survey.

MATERIALS AND METHODS

This online Delphi survey has been approved by the Ethical Committee of Shahid Beheshti University of Medical Sciences, Tehran, Iran, under the reference code IR.SBMU.RETECH.REC.1399.103. Participation was anonymous and upon the participant's own decision.

Review of Literature and Expert Selection

This study was conducted from May 28 to Aug 20, 2020. To design the Delphi questionnaire, an extensive literature review was conducted by the authors. The explored resources for data collection included the Centres for Disease Control (CDC), World Health Organisation (WHO), Infectious Diseases Society of America (IDSA), and European Centre for Disease Prevention and Control (ECDC). Electronic databases including PubMed, EMBASE, Medline, and Cochrane library were precisely investigated using the terms: COVID-19, SARS-CoV-2, mechanical ventilation, prioritisation, healthcare rationing, ethics, health policy, resource allocation, and invasive mechanical ventilators. After the initial preparation of the questionnaire, the Delphi survey was conducted in two phases.

Firstly, an expert panel of 10 individuals, two public health experts, two anesthesiologists, two emergency medicine specialists, two pulmonologists, and two infectious diseases specialists were asked to evaluate the questionnaire and provide other potential variables. The invitation link to participate was sent via email with a brief description of the aim of the study.

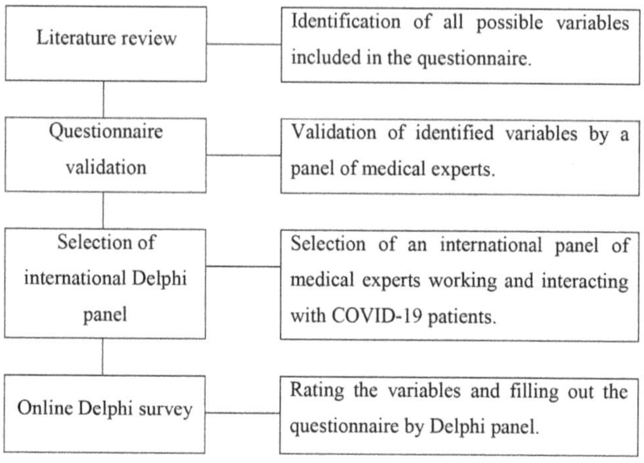

FIGURE 1 | Flowchart of Delphi survey.

Data were gathered through an online questionnaire via the Google Form platform.

Secondly, the revised version of the questionnaire based on the comments of the first-phase panellists was sent to a group of 50 medical specialists as our Delphi panel. All potential members were professionally involved in managing the patients with COVID-19 during the pandemic and were identified by investigating their professional academic curriculum vitae and the acquaintance of authors with them. Of them, 20 were intensive care experts, 10 were internal medicine specialists, 10 were emergency medicine specialists, 5 were forensic medicine experts, and 5 were infectious diseases specialists worldwide. Like the first phase, an email explaining the objective of the survey, their involvement in the study, how the Delphi study works, and the invitation link was sent to each potential participant. Among all participants who received the invitation email, 38 (76% response rate) agreed to participate in the study. Responses of three participants were incomplete, and therefore responses of 35 participants were analysed. Participants' responses in the second phase were considered as final responses. The authors of the article and the medical experts who contributed in the first phase were not included in the Delphi panel (**Figure 1**).

Variables and the Questionnaire

Variables included the personal information of the participants and the criteria for prioritising the ventilators during the pandemic. Personal information included participants' gender, age, area of study or speciality, affiliated institution, country, and the ventilator allocation experience in a setting of scarcity during the COVID-19 pandemic.

Among the criteria of prioritising the mechanical ventilators during the pandemic, all potential factors associated with the poor outcome of COVID-19 and the social responsibility of the patient were included and being divided into four sections: (1) non-medical determinants, (2) the underlying health conditions, (3) clinical, and (4) paraclinical presentation of COVID-19. It is worth mentioning that gender differences, religious beliefs, various nationalities, chronic disabilities, and being refugees or immigrants were not included among the criteria of prioritising the mechanical ventilators due to ethical considerations (12).

Among non-medical determinants, various age groups of the patients, being healthcare professionals, smoking status, drug abuse, and being the mother of a child under 5 years were included. Giving the significance of various age groups in COVID-19 prognosis, age groups of patients were considered in eight different groups including below 19, 20 to 49 years, 50–59 years, 60–69 years, 70–74 years, 75–79 years, 80–84 years and above 85 years (13).

The underlying health conditions section included 12 health conditions, which would exacerbate the COVID-19 status of the patient. Obesity, pregnancy, uncontrolled hypertension, ischemic heart disease, poorly controlled diabetes mellitus, chronic kidney disease, neurodegenerative diseases, chronic respiratory failure, organ transplantation, hepatic failure, active malignancy, receiving immunosuppressive therapy, and being infected by Human Immunodeficiency Virus (HIV) were significant factors.

In the third and fourth sections, all clinical and paraclinical presentations of COVID-19 associated with the poor prognosis of the COVID-19 were included. Clinical presentations included clinicians' overall assessment of the COVID-19 prognosis based on the frailty scale (14), hypoxia based on disparate levels of oxygen saturation (SpO_2), hypotension and organ failure based on mean arterial pressure (MAP), the dosage of vasoactive agents required, having disseminated intravascular coagulation (DIC) and cardiac arrest. Paraclinical presentation of patients was included leukopenia, lymphopenia, low platelet counts, high bilirubin, creatinine, lactate-dehydrogenase (LDH), troponin, erythrocyte sedimentation rate (ESR), C-reactive protein (CPR), ferritin, and D-dimer.

Data Analysis

To quantify the opinions of the Delphi panel, we asked the participants to rate each prioritising factor based on three scores; "−1" was considered as low priority, "+1" high priority, and "Zero" which indicated that the factor should not be deciding at all and was considered "equal priority." The central tendency statistics, including mean, median, and mode, in addition to 95% confidence intervals (95% CI), standard deviation (SD), interquartile ranges (IQR), and skewness, were reported. The Mann-Whitney U test and Kruskal-Wallis one-way analysis of variance tests were applied to define the differences between the means of two groups and three groups or more, respectively. Statistical analyses were performed using IBM SPSS Statistics 21. A probability level of <0.05 was considered significant.

RESULTS

Of 38 participants, responses of 35 (92.1%) participants were analysed. The mean (SD) age of participants was 50.1 (9.0), range 39–78, being 51.2 (9.8) among men and 47.2 (5.4) among women. Among participants, 22 (64.7%) declared that they had not encountered the situation of deciding to allocate invasive mechanical ventilators in the setting of scarcity during the COVID-19 pandemic. Other sociodemographic characteristics of participants are presented in **Table 1**.

TABLE 1 | Sociodemographic characteristics of participants.

Variable	*n* (%)
Sex	
Female	9 (25.7)
Male	26 (74.3)
Country	
Iran	14 (40.0)
Belgium	3 (8.6)
United States of America	3 (8.6)
United Kingdom	2 (5.7)
India	2 (5.7)
Norway	2 (5.7)
Other	9 (25.7)
Specialty	
Intensive care medicine	15 (42.9)
Internal medicine	7 (20.0)
Emergency medicine	7 (20.0)
Infectious diseases	4 (11.4)
Forensic medicine	2 (5.7)

Among various non-medical prioritising determinants, most participants believed that younger ages, healthcare workers, and the mothers of children under 5 years should be considered a high priority in allocating mechanical ventilators. As many as 26 (74.3%) participants reported high priority for patients under 80 years of age; however, 16 (45.7%) participants said they would give lower priority to patients aged 80 or more. There was no consensus regarding the prioritisation of ventilator allocation for patients' smoking and drug abuse status (**Table 2**).

When the Delphi panel was asked to prioritise patients regarding their underlying health condition, 31 (88.6%) participants recommended that pregnant women take high priority. Among underlying diseases, 27 (77.1%) and 25 (71.4%) participants reported low priority for active malignancy and neurodegenerative diseases, respectively. Although patients with BMI>40, diabetes mellitus, chronic kidney disease, and chronic respiratory failure received low priority, the number of participants reporting high or equal priority for the diseases was high as well. The participants' responses on prioritising ventilator allocation regarding underlying health conditions are presented in **Table 3**.

While the Delphi panel assigned a high priority for hypotensive and hypoxic patients, the end stages of hypotension, including DIC and cardiac arrest, received lower priority. Considering the clinician's judgment about the prognosis of COVID-19 based on the frailty scale, severely frail and terminally ill patients were given lower priority than very fit, well, and managing well patients (**Table 4**).

Considering the importance of paraclinical factors in anticipating the prognosis of COVID-19 among patients, we asked the panellists to rate every paraclinical factor, including blood cell counts, liver and kidney function tests, inflammatory

TABLE 2 | Responses on prioritising ventilator allocation regarding non-medical characteristics of patients.

Factor	Low priority (%)	Equal priority (%)	High priority (%)	Mean (SD)	95% CI	Median (IQR)	Skewness
Age							
<19 years	2 (5.7)	7 (20.0)	26 (74.3)	0.7 (0.6)	0.5, 0.9	1 (0, 1)	−1.7
20–49	1 (2.9)	6 (17.1)	28 (80.0)	0.8 (0.5)	0.6, 0.9	1 (1, 1)	−2.0
50–59	0 (0.0)	5 (14.3)	30 (85.7)	0.8 (0.4)	0.7, 1.0	1 (1, 1)	−2.0
60–69	0 (0.0)	6 (17.1)	29 (82.9)	0.8 (0.4)	0.6, 0.9	1 (1, 1)	−1.5
70–74	2 (5.7)	10 (28.7)	23 (65.6)	0.6 (0.6)	0.3, 0.7	1 (0, 1)	−1.2
75–79	8 (22.8)	10 (28.6)	17 (48.6)	0.3 (0.8)	0.0, 0.5	1 (0, 1)	−0.5
80–84	14 (40.0)	6 (17.1)	15 (42.9)	0.0 (0.9)	−0.4, 0.3	1 (−1, 1)	−0.1
≥85 years	17 (48.6)	5 (14.3)	13 (37.1)	−0.1 (0.9)	−0.4, 0.2	−1 (−1, 1)	0.2
Occupation							
Frontline HCW*	1 (2.9)	11 (31.4)	23 (65.7)	0.6 (0.5)	0.4, 0.8	1 (0, 1)	−1.0
Non-frontline HCW	1 (2.9)	14 (40.0)	20 (57.1)	0.5 (0.6)	0.3, 0.7	1 (0, 1)	−0.6
Smoking	10 (28.6)	15 (42.8)	10 (28.6)	0.3 (0.6)	−0.3, 0.3	0 (−1, 1)	−0.3
Drug abuse	14 (40.0)	16 (45.7)	5 (14.3)	−0.3 (0.7)	−0.5, 0.0	0 (−1, 0)	0.4
Mother of child under 5 years	1 (2.9)	7 (20.0)	27 (77.1)	0.6 (0.6)	0.5, 0.9	1 (0, 1)	−1.6

*Healthcare worker.

TABLE 3 | Responses on prioritising ventilator allocation regarding the underlying health condition of patients.

Factor	Low priority (%)	Equal priority (%)	High priority (%)	Mean (SD)	95% CI	Median (IQR)	Skewness
Obesity							
30< BMI ≤35	2 (5.7)	19 (54.3)	14 (40.0)	0.3 (0.6)	0.1, 0.6	0 (0, 1)	−0.3
35< BMI ≤40	8 (22.9)	18 (51.4)	9 (25.7)	0.0 (0.7)	−0.2, 0.3	0 (0, 1)	0.0
BMI >40	18 (51.4)	10 (28.6)	7 (20.0)	−0.3 (0.8)	−0.6, 0.0	−1 (−1, 0)	0.6
Pregnancy	0 (0.0)	4 (11.4)	31 (88.6)	0.9 (0.3)	0.7, 1.0	1 (1, 1)	−2.3
Uncontrolled hypertension	8 (22.9)	16 (45.7)	11 (31.4)	0.1 (0.7)	−0.3, 0.4	0 (−1, 1)	−0.1
Ischemic heart disease	10 (28.6)	15 (42.8)	10 (28.6)	0.0 (0.8)	−0.3, 0.3	0 (−1, 1)	0.0
Diabetes mellitus	13 (37.1)	9 (25.8)	13 (37.1)	0.0 (0.9)	−0.3, 0.3	0 (−1, 1)	0.0
Chronic kidney disease	13 (37.1)	12 (34.3)	10 (28.6)	−0.1 (0.8)	−0.4, 0.2	0 (−1, 1)	0.2
Neurodegenerative diseases	25 (71.4)	5 (14.3)	5 (14.3)	−0.5 (0.8)	−0.8, −0.3	−1 (−1, 0)	1.1
Chronic respiratory failure	20 (57.2)	4 (11.4)	11 (31.4)	−0.3 (0.9)	−0.6, 0.1	−1 (−1, 1)	0.6
Organ transplantation	6 (17.1)	14 (40.0)	15 (42.9)	0.3 (0.7)	0.0, 0.5	0 (0, 1)	−0.5
Immunosuppressive use	7 (20.0)	15 (42.9)	13 (37.1)	0.2 (0.8)	−0.1, 0.4	0 (0, 1)	−0.3
HIV/AIDS	10 (28.6)	19 (54.3)	6 (17.1)	−0.1 (0.7)	−0.4, 0.1	0 (−1, 0)	0.1
Hepatic failure	20 (57.2)	6 (17.1)	9 (25.7)	−0.3 (0.9)	−0.6, 0.0	−1 (−1, 1)	0.7
Active malignancy	27 (77.1)	3 (8.6)	5 (14.3)	−0.6 (0.7)	−0.9, −0.4	−1 (−1, −1)	1.7

factors, troponin, and D-dimer tests. The majority of paraclinical factors associated with the severity of COVID-19 were considered unimportant in resource allocation by panellists (**Table 5**).

No correlations were observed with participants' responses on resources allocation and their age, religion, country of residence, the field of study, and the dilemma of allocating invasive mechanical ventilators in the setting of scarcity during the COVID-19 pandemic.

DISCUSSION

The study showed that the panel considered younger age groups, healthcare workers, and mothers of children under 5 years for prioritising mechanical ventilators. While most participants reported high priority for patients under 80 years of age, almost half of participants said they would give lower priority to patients aged 80 or more. There was no consensus regarding the prioritisation of ventilator allocation for patients' smoking and drug abuse status.

Some 89% of participants recommended that pregnant women must take high priority. Many guidelines also prioritised pregnant women, younger age groups, and healthcare professionals to allocate ventilators (15). There is evidence that the mortality due to COVID-19 is lower among younger age groups. Nevertheless, young hospitalised patients with COVID-19 regularly require ventilators for extended periods (16). Thus, cohort and investigational studies could help healthcare professionals and experts.

TABLE 4 | Responses on prioritising ventilator allocation regarding clinical presentation of COVID-19.

Factor	Low priority (%)	Equal priority (%)	High priority (%)	Mean (SD)	95% CI	Median (IQR)	Skewness
Frailty scale							
Very fit	2 (5.7)	8 (22.9)	25 (71.4)	0.7 (0.6)	0.5, 0.9	1 (0, 1)	−1.6
Well	3 (8.6)	7 (20.0)	25 (71.4)	0.6 (0.6)	0.4, 0.9	1 (0, 1)	−1.6
Managing well	1 (2.9)	11 (31.4)	23 (65.7)	0.6 (0.5)	0.4, 0.8	1 (0, 1)	−1.1
Vulnerable	2 (5.7)	12 (34.3)	21 (60.0)	0.5 (0.6)	0.3, 0.8	1 (0, 1)	−1.0
Mildly frail	6 (17.1)	10 (28.6)	19 (54.3)	0.4 (0.8)	0.1, 0.6	1 (0, 1)	−0.8
Moderately frail	11 (31.4)	12 (34.3)	12 (34.3)	0.0 (0.8)	−0.3, 0.3	0 (−1, 1)	−0.1
Severely frail	22 (62.8)	3 (8.6)	10 (28.6)	−0.3 (0.9)	−0.7, 0.0	−1 (−1, 1)	0.8
Very severely frail	23 (65.7)	3 (8.6)	9 (25.7)	−0.4 (0.9)	−0.7, −0.1	−1 (−1, 1)	0.9
Terminally Ill	28 (80.0)	2 (5.7)	5 (14.3)	−0.7 (0.7)	−0.9, −0.4	−1 (−1, −1)	1.8
Hypoxia							
88<SpO2≤93%	4 (11.4)	9 (25.8)	22 (62.8)	0.5 (0.7)	0.3, 0.8	1 (0, 1)	−1.0
SpO2<88%	3 (8.6)	6 (17.1)	26 (74.3)	0.7 (0.6)	0.4, 0.9	1 (0, 1)	−1.7
Hypotension and organ failure							
MAP* <70 mmHg	2 (5.7)	12 (34.3)	21 (60.0)	0.5 (0.6)	0.3, 0.8	1 (0, 1)	−1.0
Dopamine ≤5 or Dobutamine (any dose)	2 (5.7)	13 (37.1)	20 (57.2)	0.5 (0.6)	0.3, 0.7	1 (0, 1)	−0.9
Dopamine >5, Epinephrine ≤0.1, or norepinephrine ≤0.1	4 (11.4)	12 (34.3)	19 (54.3)	0.4 (0.7)	0.2, 0.7	1 (0, 1)	−0.8
Dopamine >15, Epinephrine >0.1, or norepinephrine >0.1	7 (20.0)	11 (31.4)	17 (48.6)	0.3 (0.8)	0.0, 0.6	0 (0, 1)	−0.6
DIC**	13 (37.2)	11 (31.4)	11 (31.4)	0.0 (0.9)	−0.3, 0.3	0 (−1, 1)	0.7
Cardiac arrest	28 (80.0)	2 (5.7)	5 (14.3)	−0.7 (0.7)	−1, −0.4	−1 (−1, −1)	0.5

* *Mean Arterial Pressure.*
** *Disseminated intravascular coagulation.*

Although patients with BMI>40, diabetes mellitus, chronic kidney disease, and chronic respiratory failure received low priority, the number of participants reporting high or equal priority for the diseases was high as well. While the panel considered a high priority for hypotensive and hypoxic patients, the end stages of hypotension, including DIC and cardiac arrest, received lower priority.

More than two-thirds of participants considered patients with active malignancy and neurodegenerative diseases to have low priority. COVID-19 pandemic has disrupted the conventional care delivery for both malignancies and neurodegenerative diseases (17, 18). Patients with neurodegenerative diseases, which is more common among advanced age groups (19), often live in residential homes, which puts them at greater risk of COVID-19 transmission (20). Similar to considering these groups as low-priority in our study, many resource allocation guidelines have excluded these patients (21), which could put them at risk of systemic discrimination in the near future (22).

Among underlying diseases, COPD is reported to be an independent risk factor for all-cause mortality among patients with COVID-19 (23). Hypertension and uncontrolled hypertension were the most common comorbidity among hospitalised patients with COVID-19 infection (24).

The majority of paraclinical factors associated with the severity of COVID-19 were considered unimportant in resource allocation. There is evidence that LDH and CRP independently predicted ventilation requirements among COVID-19 patients (16).

Considering the clinician's judgment about the prognosis of COVID-19 based on the frailty scale, severely frail and terminally ill patients were given lower priority than very fit, well, and managing well patients. Evidence shows that the frailty scale is linearly associated with increased mortality due to COVID-19 (25). Although some studies proposed using Sequential Organ Failure Assessment (SOFA) score for prioritising ventilator allocation in the early days of the pandemic (26), the SOFA score has been shown to have inadequate accuracy for ventilator triage of patients with COVID-19 (27). The combination of the frailty scale with the SOFA score did not improve the performance of the SOFA score either (28). Thus, better alternatives are needed for prognostic prediction of patients with COVID-19 pneumonia requiring mechanical ventilation.

Unresolved ethical dilemmas regarding the fair allocation of ventilators threaten the success of the response to a public health emergency. Nevertheless, not all healthcare systems have developed allocation guidelines (26, 29, 30). Some studies challenge the "save the most lives" strategy. A study proposes that the following considerations be taken into account, when necessary while allocating scarce resources: maximising survival to hospital discharge, maximising the number of life-years saved,

TABLE 5 | Responses on prioritising ventilator allocation regarding laboratory presentation of COVID-19.

Factor	Low priority (%)	Equal priority (%)	High priority (%)	Mean (SD)	95% CI	Median (IQR)	Skewness
Leukopenia	5 (14.2)	20 (57.2)	10 (28.6)	0.2 (0.7)	0.0, 0.5	0 (0, 1)	−0.3
Lymphopenia	4 (11.4)	16 (45.7)	15 (42.9)	0.3 (0.7)	0.1, 0.6	0 (0, 1)	−0.5
Low platelet count							
100< PLT ≤149	1 (2.9)	27 (77.1)	7 (20.0)	0.2 (0.5)	0.1, 0.4	0 (0, 1)	0.6
50< PLT ≤99	2 (5.7)	20 (57.2)	13 (37.1)	0.3 (0.6)	0.1, 0.5	0 (0, 1)	−0.2
20< PLT ≤49	9 (25.7)	15 (42.9)	11 (31.4)	0.1 (0.8)	−0.2, 0.3	0 (−1, 1)	−0.1
PLT <20	11 (31.4)	15 (42.9)	9 (25.7)	−0.1 (0.8)	−0.3, 0.2	0 (−1, 1)	0.1
High LDH	3 (8.6)	21 (60.0)	11 (31.4)	0.3 (0.6)	0.1, 0.5	0 (0, 1)	−0.2
High troponin	6 (17.1)	16 (45.7)	13 (37.2)	0.2 (0.7)	0.0, 0.5	0 (0, 1)	−0.4
High bilirubin							
1.2–1.9 mg/dL	4 (11.4)	25 (71.5)	6 (17.1)	0.1 (0.6)	0.0, 0.3	0 (0, 0)	0.0
2.0–5.9 mg/dL	4 (11.4)	22 (62.9)	9 (25.7)	0.1 (0.6)	−0.1, 0.4	0 (0, 1)	−0.1
6.0–11.9 mg/dL	14 (40.0)	13 (37.1)	8 (22.9)	−0.2 (0.8)	−0.5, 0.1	0 (−1, 0)	0.3
≥12.0 mg/dL	16 (45.7)	10 (28.6)	9 (25.7)	−0.2 (0.8)	−0.5, 0.1	0 (−1, 1)	0.4
High creatinine							
1.2–1.9 mg/dL	0 (0.0)	24 (68.6)	11 (31.4)	0.3 (0.5)	0.2, 0.5	0 (0, 1)	0.6
2.0–3.4 mg/dL	3 (8.6)	21 (60.0)	11 (31.4)	0.2 (0.6)	0.0, 0.4	0 (0, 1)	−0.1
3.5–4.9 mg/dL	7 (20.0)	18 (51.4)	10 (28.6)	0.1 (0.7)	−0.2, 0.3	0 (0, 1)	−0.1
≥5.0 mg/dL	10 (28.6)	14 (40.0)	11 (31.4)	0.0 (0.8)	−0.2, 0.3	0 (−1, 1)	−0.1
High ESR	2 (5.7)	24 (68.6)	9 (25.7)	0.2 (0.5)	0.0, 0.4	0 (0, 1)	0.2
High CRP	2 (5.7)	20 (57.2)	13 (37.1)	0.3 (0.6)	0.1, 0.5	0 (0, 1)	−1.5
High D-dimer	1 (2.9)	21 (60.0)	13 (37.1)	0.3 (0.5)	0.2, 0.5	0 (0, 1)	0.1
High ferritin	2 (5.7)	25 (71.4)	8 (22.9)	0.2 (0.5)	0.0, 0.4	0 (0, 0)	0.3

maximising individuals' chances to live through each of life's stages, the severity of impairment, and patients' instrumental value into prioritisation considerations. In this sense, the public also needs to participate in choosing among ethically permissible allocation strategies (7, 31). Some studies have investigated people's opinions on the fair allocation of ventilators (32). A community-based survey reported that people considered age, expected ventilation effectiveness, smoking status, having dependents, being a healthcare worker, and having disabilities to be of importance in resource allocation (33).

STRENGTHS AND LIMITATIONS

This is among the few studies investigating the experts' opinions on priorities towards fair allocation of mechanical ventilators during the COVID-19 pandemic. Findings could empower public health authorities better to understand experts' opinions to be considered in future guidelines. It is worth mentioning that the COVID-19 pandemic disrupted the supply chain of medical resources, which was only successful when demand was predictable (34). Focusing on the fair allocation of ventilators during this crisis should not distract the authorities from optimising the supply chain.

We realise the limitations of the study. The number of participants was limited; however, the pandemic disrupted people's daily schedule worldwide, and experts were no exception (35). Nevertheless, given the response rate, the generalisation of results could be limited. Considering that the panel was approached based on the acquaintance of authors, our sample was over-representative of colleagues in the authors' network. Using the authors' network would increase the chance of the panel's participation in the study, given that experts would be too busy during the pandemic and would probably ignore emails from unfamiliar senders. While the study had a poor representation of some regions, especially considering different social, religious and healthcare systems approaches, the findings could be used as a basis for a broader represented experts' panel.

CONCLUSION

The panel considered younger age groups, healthcare workers, pregnant mothers, and mothers of children under 5 years for prioritising mechanical ventilators. There was no general consensus regarding the prioritisation of ventilator allocation based on the patient's laboratory profile, underlying diseases, or drug abuse. It could be suggested that more research is essential to develop comprehensive resource allocation strategies which are easy to apply, objective, accurate, reproducible, and would not discriminate against vulnerable populations.

ETHICS STATEMENT

The studies involving human participants were reviewed and approved by Ethical Committee of Shahid Beheshti University of Medical Sciences, Tehran, Iran under the reference code IR.SBMU.RETECH.REC.1399.103. Written informed consent for participation was not required for this study in accordance with the national legislation and the institutional requirements.

AUTHOR CONTRIBUTIONS

A-AK, NZ, HH-M, S-HG, and MA-K: study conception and design. A-AK, S-HG, and MA-K: acquisition, analysis, or interpretation of data. S-HG and MA-K: drafting of the manuscript. A-AK, HH-M, and NZ: critical revision of the manuscript for important intellectual content. A-AK: study supervision. The corresponding authors attests that all listed authors meet the authorship criteria and that no others meeting the criteria have been omitted. All authors contributed to the article and approved the submitted version.

ACKNOWLEDGMENTS

The authors would like to express their profound gratitude to all 38 medical experts for participating in this Delphi survey and for sharing their precious knowledge and experience. Special thanks to: Cynthia Aaron (Emergency Medicine Department, Michigan Poison Center, Detroit, USA); Kurt Anseeuw (Emergency Medicine Department, Ziekenhuis Netwerk Antwerpen (ZNA), Antwerp, Belgium); Mahdi Balali-Mood (Clinical Toxicology Department, Mashhad University of Medical Sciences, Mashhad, Iran); Shabnam Bazmi (Medical Ethics Department, Shahid Beheshti University of Medical Sciences, Tehran, Iran); Ashish Bhalla (Internal Medicine Department, PGIMER, Chandigarh, India.); Jeffrey Brent (School of Medicine, University of Colorado, Denver, USA); Ilad Alavi Darazam (Infectious Diseases Department, Shahid Beheshti University of Medical Sciences, Tehran, Iran); Paul I Dargan (Clinical Toxicology Department, Guy's and St Thomas' NHS Foundation Trust, London, UK); Dylan W De Lange (Intensive Care Unit, UMC Utrecht, Utrecht, Netherlands); Peter De Paepe (Emergency Department, Ghent University Hospital, Ghent, Belgium); Hamideh Esalati (Ghaem Hospital, Mashhad University of Medical Sciences, Mashhad, Iran); Florian Eyer (Department of Clinical Toxicology Poisons Control Centre Munich, TUM School of Medicine, Klinikum rechts der Isar, Technical University of Munich, Munich, Germany); Marc Ghannoum (Nephrology Department, University of Montreal, Montreal, Canada); Mohammadreza Hajiesmaeili (Anesthesiology Department, Shahid Beheshti University of Medical Science, Tehran, Iran); Philippe Hantson (Intensive Care Unit, Cliniques St-Luc, Université catholique de Louvain, Brussels, Belgium); Fridtjof Heyerdahl (Air Ambulance Department, Oslo University Hospital, Oslo, Norway); Knut Erik Hovda (Department of Acute Medicine, Oslo University Hospital, Oslo, Norway); Mehrzad Kiani (Medical Ethics Department, Shahid Beheshti University of Medical Sciences, Tehran, Iran); Ata Mahmoodpoor (Anesthesiology Department, Tabriz University of Medical Sciences, Tehran, Iran); Alex Manini (Emergency Medicine Department, Icahn School of Medicine at Mount Sinai, New York, USA); Bruno Megarbane (Medical and Toxicological Critical Care Department, Lariboisiere Hospital, Paris, France); Amirhossein Mirafzal (Emergency Medicine Department, Kerman University of Medical Sciences, Kerman, Iran); Majid Mokhtari (Department of Pulmonary and Critical Care Medicine, Loghman Hakim Hospital, Shahid Beheshti University of Medical Sciences, Tehran, Iran); Viorela Nitescu (Toxicology Intensive Care, Emergency Clinical Hospital for Children "Grigore Alexandrescu", Bucharest, Romania); Marlies Ostermann (Clinical Toxicology Department, Guy's and St Thomas' NHS Foundation Trust, London, UK); Raido Paasma (Department of Anesthesia and ICU, Foundation Pärnu Hospital, Pärnu, Estonia); Darren Roberts (Renal Medicine and Transplantation, and Clinical Pharmacology and Toxicology, St Vincent's Hospital, Sydney, Australia); Emilio Salgado (Emergency Department, Hospital Clinic Barcelona, Barcelona, Spain); Mohsen Savaie (Anesthesiology and Critical Care, Ahvaz Jundishapur University of Medical Sciences, Ahvaz, Iran); Bhavesh Seerubhai Jarwani (Emergency Medicine Department, Smt. NHLM Medical College, SVP hospital, Ahmedabad, India); Kamran Shadvar (Anesthesiology Department, Tabriz University of Medical Sciences, Tabriz, Iran); Seyedpouzhia Shojaei (Department of Critical Care Medicine, Imam Hossein Medical and Educational Center, Shahid Beheshti University of Medical Sciences, Tehran, Iran); Shervin Shokouhi (Infectious Diseases Department, Loghman Hakim Hospital, Shahid Beheshti University of Medical Sciences, Tehran, Iran); Roberto Zoppellari (Anesthesiology Department, S. Anna Hospital, Ferrara, Italy).

REFERENCES

1. Mehta S, Machado F, Kwizera A, Papazian L, Moss M, Azoulay É, et al. COVID-19: a heavy toll on healthcare workers. *Lancet Respir Med.* (2021) 9:226–8. doi: 10.1016/S2213-2600(21)00068-0
2. Zhou W, Wang A, Wang X, Cheke RA, Xiao Y, Tang S. Impact of hospital bed shortages on the containment of covid-19 in wuhan. *Int J Environ Res Public Health.* (2020) 17:1–18. doi: 10.3390/ijerph17228560
3. Dos Santos MJ, Martins MS, Santana FLP, Furtado MCSPC, Miname FCBR, Pimentel RRDS, et al. COVID-19: Instruments for the allocation

of mechanical ventilators- a narrative review. *Crit Care.* (2020) 24:582. doi: 10.1186/s13054-020-03298-3

4. Potere N, Valeriani E, Candeloro M, Tana M, Porreca E, Abbate A, et al. Acute complications and mortality in hospitalised patients with coronavirus disease 2019: a systematic review and meta-analysis. *Crit Care.* (2020) 24:389. doi: 10.1186/s13054-020-03022-1
5. Docherty AB, Harrison EM, Green CA, Hardwick HE, Pius R, Norman L, et al. Features of 20 133 UK patients in hospital with covid-19 using the ISARIC WHO Clinical Characterisation Protocol: Prospective observational cohort study. *BMJ.* (2020) 369:m1985. doi: 10.1136/bmj.m1985
6. Grant MC, Geoghegan L, Arbyn M, Mohammed Z, McGuinness L, Clarke EL, et al. The prevalence of symptoms in 24,410 adults infected by the novel coronavirus (SARS-CoV-2; COVID-19): a systematic review and meta-analysis of 148 studies from 9 countries. *PLoS ONE.* (2020) 15:e0234765. doi: 10.2139/ssrn.3582819
7. White DB, Katz MH, Luce JM, Lo B. Who should receive life support during a public health emergency? Using ethical principles to improve allocation decisions. *Ann Intern Med.* (2009) 150:132–8. doi: 10.7326/0003-4819-150-2-200901200-00011
8. Peterson A, Largent EA, Karlawish J. Ethics of reallocating ventilators in the covid-19 pandemic. *BMJ.* (2020) 369:m1828. doi: 10.1136/bmj.m1828
9. Wicclair M. Allocating ventilators during the COVID-19 pandemic and conscientious objection. *Am J Bioeth.* (2020) 20:204–7. doi: 10.1080/15265161.2020.1777347
10. The Lancet. COVID-19: protecting healthcare workers. *Lancet.* (2020) 395:922. doi: 10.1016/S0140-6736(20)30644-9
11. Emanuel EJ, Persad G, Upshur R, Thome B, Parker M, Glickman A, et al. Fair allocation of scarce medical resources in the time of Covid-19. *N Engl J Med.* (2020) 382:2049–55. doi: 10.1056/NEJMsb2005114
12. Swiss Academy Of Medical Sciences. COVID-19 pandemic: triage for intensive-care treatment under resource scarcity. *Swiss Med Wkly.* (2020) 150:w20229. doi: 10.4414/smw.2020.20229
13. Undurraga EA, Chowell G, Mizumoto K. COVID-19 case fatality risk by age and gender in a high testing setting in Latin America: Chile, March–August 2020. *Infect Dis Poverty.* (2021) 10:11. doi: 10.1186/s40249-020-00785-1
14. Sablerolles RSG, Lafeber M, van Kempen JAL, van de Loo BPA, Boersma E, Rietdijk WJR, et al. Association between Clinical Frailty Scale score and hospital mortality in adult patients with COVID-19 (COMET): an international, multicentre, retrospective, observational cohort study. *Lancet Heal Longev.* (2021) 2:e163–70. doi: 10.1016/S2666-7568(21)00006-4
15. Wunsch H, Hill AD, Bosch N, Adhikari NKJ, Rubenfeld G, Walkey A, et al. Comparison of 2 triage scoring guidelines for allocation of mechanical ventilators. *JAMA Netw open.* (2020) 3:e2029250. doi: 10.1001/jamanetworkopen.2020.29250
16. Nicholson CJ, Wooster L, Sigurslid HH, Li RH, Jiang W, Tian W, et al. Estimating risk of mechanical ventilation and in-hospital mortality among adult COVID-19 patients admitted to Mass General Brigham: the VICE and DICE scores. *EClinicalMedicine.* (2021) 33:100765. doi: 10.1016/j.eclinm.2021.100765
17. Berardelli A, Silani V, Barone P, Calabresi P, Girlanda P, Lopiano L, et al. Neurology and the COVID-19 emergency. *Neurol Sci.* (2020) 41:1343–4. doi: 10.1007/s10072-020-04465-8
18. Neal RD, Nekhlyudov L, Wheatstone P, Koczwara B. Cancer care during and after the pandemic. *BMJ.* (2020) 370:m2622. doi: 10.1136/bmj.m2622
19. Hou Y, Dan X, Babbar M, Wei Y, Hasselbalch SG, Croteau DL, et al. Ageing as a risk factor for neurodegenerative disease. *Nat Rev Neurol.* (2019) 15:565–81. doi: 10.1038/s41582-019-0244-7
20. Kim SYH, Grady C. Ethics in the time of COVID: What remains the same and what is different. *Neurology.* (2020) 94:1007–8. doi: 10.1212/WNL.0000000000009520
21. Hensel W, Wolf L. Playing god: the legality of plans denying scarce resources to people with disabilities in public health emergencies. *Fla Law Rev.* (2013) 63:719. doi: 10.1525/9780520967731
22. Richards CT, Crawley LM, Magnus D. Use of neurodevelopmental delay in pediatric solid organ transplant listing decisions: Inconsistencies in standards across major pediatric transplant centers. *Pediatr Transplant.* (2009) 13:843–50. doi: 10.1111/j.1399-3046.2008.01072.x
23. Lee SC, Son KJ, Han CH, Park SC, Jung JY. Impact of COPD on COVID-19 prognosis: a nationwide population-based study in South Korea. *Sci Rep.* (2021) 11:3735. doi: 10.1038/s41598-021-83226-9
24. Ran J, Song Y, Zhuang Z, Han L, Zhao S, Cao P, et al. Blood pressure control and adverse outcomes of COVID-19 infection in patients with concomitant hypertension in Wuhan, China. *Hypertens Res.* (2020) 43:1267–76. doi: 10.1038/s41440-020-00541-w
25. Pranata R, Henrina J, Lim MA, Lawrensia S, Yonas E, Vania R, et al. Clinical frailty scale and mortality in COVID-19: A systematic review and dose-response meta-analysis: Clinical Frailty Scale in COVID-19. *Arch Gerontol Geriatr.* (2021) 93:104324. doi: 10.1016/j.archger.2020.104324
26. Piscitello GM, Kapania EM, Miller WD, Rojas JC, Siegler M, Parker WF. Variation in ventilator allocation guidelines by us state during the coronavirus disease 2019 pandemic: a systematic review. *JAMA Netw Open.* (2020) 3:e2012606. doi: 10.1001/jamanetworkopen.2020.12606
27. Raschke RA, Agarwal S, Rangan P, Heise CW, Curry SC. Discriminant accuracy of the SOFA score for determining the probable mortality of patients with COVID-19 pneumonia requiring mechanical ventilation. *JAMA - J Am Med Assoc.* (2021) 325:1469–70. doi: 10.1001/jama.2021.1545
28. Langlais E, Nesseler N, Le Pabic E, Frasca D, Launey Y, Seguin P. Does the clinical frailty score improve the accuracy of the SOFA score in predicting hospital mortality in elderly critically ill patients? A prospective observational study. *J Crit Care.* (2018) 46:67–72. doi: 10.1016/j.jcrc.2018.04.012
29. Malekpour MR, Abbasi-Kangevari M, Azadnajafabad S, Ghamari SH, Rezaei N, Rezazadeh-Khadem S, et al. How the scientific community responded to the COVID-19 pandemic: a subject-level time-trend bibliometric analysis. *PLoS ONE.* (2021) 16:e0258064. doi: 10.1371/journal.pone.0258064
30. Riccioni L, Ingravallo F, Grasselli G, Mazzon D, Cingolani E, Forti G, et al. The Italian document: decisions for intensive care when there is an imbalance between care needs and resources during the COVID-19 pandemic. *Ann Intensive Care.* (2021) 11:100. doi: 10.1186/s13613-021-00888-4
31. Hick JL, Rubinson L, O'Laughlin DT, Christopher JC. Clinical review: allocating ventilators during large-scale disasters - problems, planning, and process. *Crit Care.* (2007) 11:217. doi: 10.1186/cc5929
32. Abbasi-Kangevari M, Arshi S, Hassanian-Moghaddam H, Kolahi AA. Public opinion on priorities toward fair allocation of ventilators during COVID-19 pandemic: a nationwide survey. *Front Public Health.* (2021) 9:753048. doi: 10.3389/fpubh.2021.753048
33. Norman R, Robinson S, Dickinson H, Williams I, Meshcheriakova E, Manipis K, et al. Public preferences for allocating ventilators in an intensive care unit: a discrete choice experiment. *Patient.* (2021) 14:319–30. doi: 10.1007/s40271-021-00498-z
34. Okeagu CN, Reed DS, Sun L, Colontonio MM, Rezayev A, Ghaffar YA, et al. Principles of supply chain management in the time of crisis. *Best Pract Res Clin Anaesthesiol.* (2021) 35:369. doi: 10.1016/j.bpa.2020.11.007
35. Nasa P, Azoulay E, Khanna AK, Jain R, Gupta S, Javeri Y, et al. Expert consensus statements for the management of COVID-19-related acute respiratory failure using a Delphi method. *Crit Care.* (2021) 25:1–17. doi: 10.1186/s13054-021-03491-y

17

Effect of Serum Phosphate on the Prognosis of Septic Patients: A Retrospective Study Based on MIMIC-IV Database

Zhaoyang Li[1†], Tingwen Shen[2†] and Yi Han[3]*

[1] Department of Intensive Care Medicine, The First Affiliated Hospital of Nanjing Medical University, Nanjing, China, [2] The Health Management Center, The First Affiliated Hospital of Nanjing Medical University, Nanjing, China, [3] Department of Geriatric Intensive Care Medicine, The First Affiliated Hospital of Nanjing Medical University, Nanjing, China

***Correspondence:**
Yi Han
hanyi@jsph.org.cn

† These authors have contributed equally to this work

Objective: To assess the effect of serum inorganic phosphate (Pi) on the prognosis of patients with sepsis.

Methods: A retrospective analysis of patients with sepsis selected from the Medical Information Mart for Intensive Care (MIMIC)-IV database was performed. Sepsis was diagnosed according to the Third International Consensus Definition for sepsis and septic shock (Sepsis-3). The time-weighted values of the serum Pi measurements within the first 24 h of sepsis were analyzed. The association between serum Pi and in-hospital mortality was evaluated with a generalized linear model (log-binomial model).

Results: The analysis of 11,658 patients from six intensive care units (ICUs) showed a nearly linear correlation between serum Pi and in-hospital mortality in all patients with sepsis, especially in those with acute kidney injury (AKI). The increase of serum Pi was related to a higher risk of AKI, higher norepinephrine doses, ICU mortality, and in-hospital mortality. The generalized linear model showed that serum Pi was an independent predictor for in-hospital mortality in all patients with sepsis even within the normal range. The adjusted risk ratios (RRs) were also significant in subgroup analyses according to kidney function, gender, respiratory infection, vasopressor use, and Sequential Organ Failure Assessment (SOFA) score.

Conclusion: Higher levels of serum Pi, even within the normal range, were significantly associated with a higher risk of in-hospital mortality in patients with sepsis regardless of kidney function, gender, respiratory infection, vasopressor use, and SOFA score.

Keywords: sepsis-3, phosphate levels, prognosis, MIMIC-IV, septic shock

INTRODUCTION

Sepsis is a complex condition that remains the major cause of morbidity and mortality worldwide, and the true global burdens of sepsis are likely much higher than reported (1, 2).

A better understanding of sepsis has been researched in the past three decades (3). In 2016, the Third International Consensus Definition for Sepsis and Septic Shock (Sepsis-3) defined sepsis as life-threatening organ dysfunction resulting from dysregulated host responses to infection, which offers greater consistency for epidemiologic studies and clinical trials (4). The hour-1-bundle proposed by Surviving Sepsis Campaign in 2018 encourages clinicians to act as quickly as possible to make an accurate diagnosis and start appropriate treatment if clinically indicated (5).

Although great progress has been made into the pathobiology, management, and epidemiology of the disease, the high mortality is still unacceptable (2). The early identification of patients with sepsis at high risk of death allows clinicians to administer treatment in time. Inorganic phosphate (Pi) plays crucial roles in several aspects of physiological processes including energy metabolism, cellular signal transduction, and membrane transport (6, 7). Serum Pi disorders are common in critically ill patients, which can be attributed to several factors including gastrointestinal dysfunction, acute kidney dysfunction, and redistribution of Pi from the extracellular space into the cells (8, 9).

The predictive value of serum Pi has been studied in several specific patient populations. It was reported that even a minor increase in serum Pi was associated with a higher risk of several adverse outcomes including worsened heart failure and all-cause mortality in patients with heart failure (10–12). Numerous studies have confirmed the association between higher serum Pi and adverse outcomes in patients with chronic kidney disease (CKD) with or without kidney transplantation (13, 14). In the general population, it was also reported that a minor increase in phosphate at the base level was associated with a significant increase in all-cause mortality (15, 16).

Though serum Pi was considered to be a good predictor of adverse outcomes for several diseases, its prognostic value for patients with sepsis has not been well investigated yet, and the conclusions are mixed. For instance, in Shor et al's study, severe hypophosphatemia in sepsis increased the risk of death by nearly 8-fold (8). In contrast, in Miller et al.'s study, they concluded that patients with hyperphosphatemia had higher 28-day in-hospital mortality while those with hypophosphatemia did not (17).

Moreover, the heterogeneity of disease severity and classification are great in intensive care units (ICUs). Thus, it is of vital importance to re-evaluate the association between serum Pi and mortality in patients with sepsis and different septic subgroups. We aimed to assess the effect of serum Pi within the first day of sepsis on the prognosis of patients with sepsis. In particular, the subgroup analyses were performed according to the presence or absence of acute kidney injury (AKI) or CKD, gender, respiratory infection, vasopressor use, and Sequential Organ Failure Assessment (SOFA) score in this study.

MATERIALS AND METHODS

Study Design and Participants

The Medical Information Mart for Intensive Care (MIMIC)-III database provided critical care data for over 40,000 patients admitted to ICUs at the Beth Israel Deaconess Medical Center (BIDMC) from 2001 to 2012. Importantly, patient identifiers were removed according to the Health Insurance Portability and Accountability Act (HIPAA) Safe Harbor provision. MIMIC-IV, an update to MIMIC-III, incorporates contemporary data and improves on numerous aspects of MIMIC-III. The project was approved by the Institutional Review Boards of BIDMC (Boston, MA, United States) and the Massachusetts Institute of Technology (Cambridge, MA, United States). The latest version of MIMIC-IV was available on the PhysioNet, an online forum for the dissemination and exchange of recorded biomedical signals and open-source software for analyzing them (Johnson, Alistair, et al. "MIMIC-IV" (version 1.0), PhysioNet (2021), https://doi.org/10.13026/s6n6-xd98) (18).

The database is accessible to researchers who have completed a 'protecting human subjects' training. The data presented in this study were extracted by author Li, who completed the online training course of Data or Specimens Only Research (certification number: 38455531). Data extraction was performed using PostgreSQL tools V 12.4.

Patients meeting the diagnostic criteria of Sepsis-3 and older than 18 years old were enrolled in the study. For clinical operationalization, organ dysfunction associated with sepsis can be represented by an increase [Sepsis-related] in the SOFA score of 2 points or more, which is associated with an in-hospital mortality greater than 10%, and patients with septic shock can be clinically identified by a vasopressor requirement to maintain a mean arterial pressure of 65 mmHg or greater and serum lactate level greater than 2 mmol/L (>18 mg/dl) in the absence of hypovolemia(4, 19).

Data Collection

The following information was extracted: age, gender, weight, pre-ICU comorbidities [hypertension, diabetes, CKD, coronary artery disease (CAD)], AKI, hospital and ICU length of stay (HLOS and ILOS), in-hospital mortality, ICU mortality, SOFA score, vasopressor use, white blood cell count, Serum Pi, serum creatinine, and blood lactate, infection sites. The definition of vasopressor use was any use of the following vasopressors, including norepinephrine, epinephrine, dopamine, and dobutamine, within the first 24 h of sepsis. The diagnosis and staging of AKI were according to the criteria of the Kidney Disease: Improving Global Outcomes (KDIGO) AKI Guideline Work Group (20).

The measurements of serum Pi and blood lactate within 24 h after the diagnosis of sepsis were extracted, and the time-weighted mean (TWM) values were calculated to represent the serum Pi and blood lactate level over the course by taking the area under the time-value curve divided by the time between the first and the last measurement assuming a linear trend between measurements (17). The serum levels of creatinine and the white blood cell count at the diagnosis of sepsis were extracted. The normal range of serum Pi is 2.7–4.5 mg/dl in MIMIC IV. Thus, crude outcomes were compared among the three groups based on the TWM values of the serum Pi measurements: hypophosphatemia (<2.7 mg/dl), normophosphatemia (2.7–4.5 mg/dl), and hyperphosphatemia (>4.5mg/dl).

Primary Exposure and the Primary Outcome

The primary exposure was serum Pi level and the primary endpoint was in-hospital mortality. The secondary endpoints included ICU mortality, development of AKI, HLOS, ILOS, SOFA scores at diagnosis of sepsis, and norepinephrine doses.

Statistical Analysis

The data were analyzed using the software Stata V.12.1. Continuous variables are presented as mean ± SD or median with interquartile ranges (IQR) and compared by the Student's *t*-test and the Wilcoxon rank-sum test as appropriate. Categorical variables are reported as numbers and percentages and the comparisons were analyzed by Chi-squared and Fisher's exact tests. One-way ANOVA or the Kruskal–Wallis test was performed for comparisons of crude outcomes between the three groups. Locally weighted scatterplot smoothing (LOWESS) regression and logistic regression were used to explore the crude relationship between serum Pi and in-hospital mortality. It has been studied that the odd ratio always overstates the relative risk when the outcome incidence is common (>10%). A generalized linear model (log-binomial model) utilized to determine the adjusted RRs is statistically appropriate in this situation. This model is applied because the overall in-hospital mortality in this study was not rare (21.3%) (21).

The subgroup analyses were based on the diagnosis of CKD or AKI for the kidney is the main regulator of extracellular fluid Pi concentration by virtue of having a tubular maximum reabsorptive capacity for Pi (22). Also, subgroup analyses based on gender, respiratory infection, vasopressor use, and SOFA score were performed. In the subgroup analysis, according to SOFA score, the patients were divided into two groups according to the median of the SOFA score (3 in this study).

RESULTS

Demographic Data and General Clinical Characteristics

The MIMIC-IV contains records for 524,520 admissions, of which 69,619 were admitted to ICUs. Of these, 54,177 admissions without suspicious infections were excluded for no antibiotic

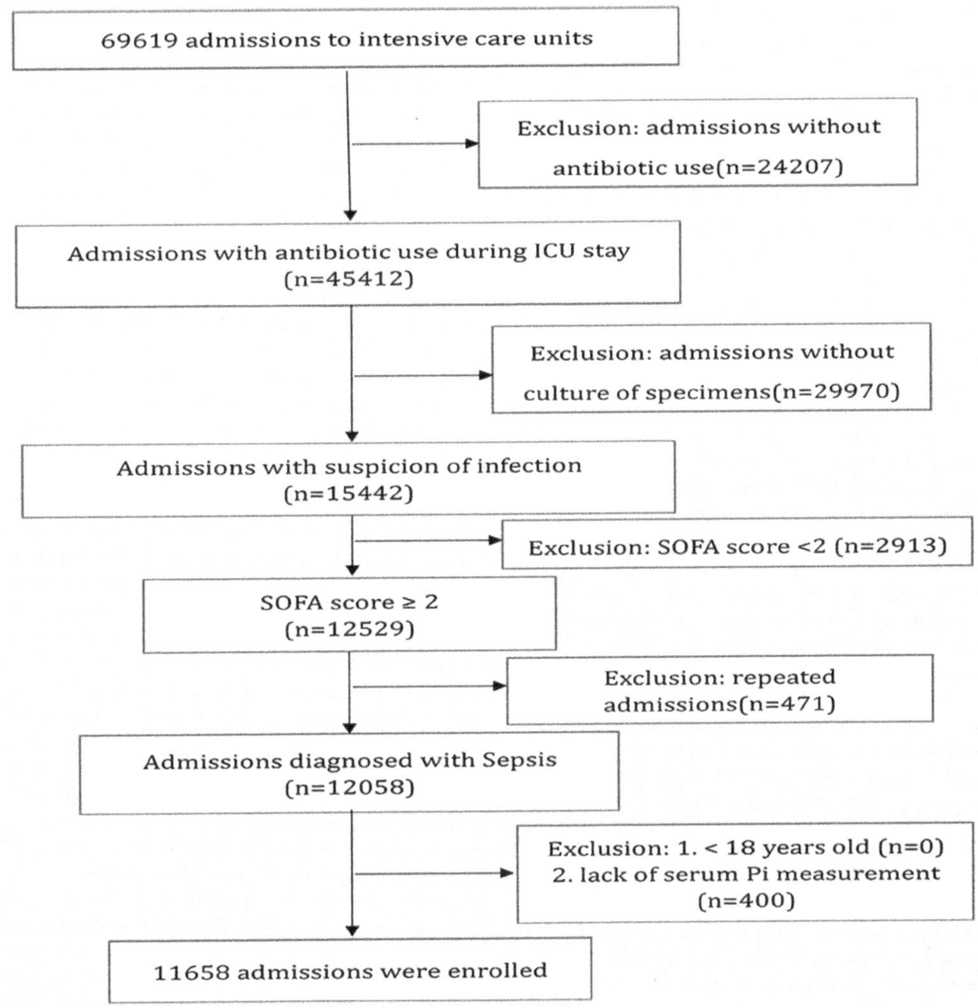

FIGURE 1 | Study flowchart. ICU, intensive care unit.

TABLE 1 | Comparisons of demographics between survivors and non-survivors.

	Survivors (n = 9179)	Non-survivors (n = 2479)	P value
Age (years)	66.7 ± 16.2	70.2 ± 14.9	< 0.01
Female(n%)	4427(48.2%)	1169(47.2%)	0.34
Weight (kilograms)	81.8 ± 26.9	80.2 ± 24.7	0.01
SOFA score	3(2-4)	4(3-6)	< 0.01
Vasopressor use[n (%)]	2130(32.2%)	1132(45.7%)	< 0.01
Hypertension [n (%)]	1962(21.4%)	479(19.3%)	0.03
Diabetes [n (%)]	2470(26.9%)	637(25.7%)	0.23
CKD [n (%)]	2251(24.5%)	694(28.0%)	< 0.01
CAD [n (%)]	1387(15.1%)	429(17.3%)	0.01
WBC (*10^9/l)	13.4 ± 10.9	15.3 ± 13.6	< 0.01
Creatinine (mg/dl)	1.77 ± 1.79	2.04 ± 1.66	< 0.01
Blood lactate (mmol/l)	1.92 ± 1.15	3.42 ± 3.06	< 0.01
Serum Pi (mg/dl)	3.96 ± 1.23	4.22 + 1.74	< 0.01
AKI [n (%)]	958(10.4%)	454(18.3%)	< 0.01
Infection site [n (%)]			
Respiratory system [n (%)]	2744(29.9%)	979(39.5%)	< 0.01
Digestive system [n (%)]	983(10.7%)	261(10.5%)	0.80
Urinary system [n (%)]	3057(33.3%)	621(25.1%)	< 0.01
Blood system [n (%)]	659(7.18%)	128(5.16%)	< 0.01
Other sites [n (%)]	3586(39.1%)	982(39.6%)	0.62

BMI, body mass index; SOFA score, the Sequential Organ Failure Assessment; CKD, chronic kidney disease; CAD, coronary artery disease; WBC, white blood cell; Pi, inorganic phosphate; AKI, acute kidney disease.

administration or culture of specimens during ICU stays. A total of 2,913 admissions were excluded for the SOFA scores were less than 2. A total of 12,529 admissions were considered to be patients with sepsis according to the definition of Sepsis-3. A total of 471 repeated admissions were excluded for we only take the patient's first admission to ICUs. In total, 400 admissions were excluded due to the lack of serum Pi measurement. Finally, 11,658 admissions (9,179 survivors and 2,479 non-survivors) from 6 ICUs, including trauma surgical ICU, neurosurgical ICU, medical ICU, postanesthesia care unit, coronary care unit, and cardiac vascular ICU were analyzed. All enrolled patients were older than 18 years old (**Figure 1**).

The baseline characteristics of the survivors and non-survivors are presented in **Table 1**. The overall in-hospital mortality was 21.3%. The non-survivors were older ($p < 0.01$) and had lower weight ($p = 0.01$), higher SOFA scores ($p < 0.01$), higher white blood cell count ($p < 0.01$), higher serum creatinine levels ($p < 0.01$), higher blood lactate levels ($p < 0.01$), and higher serum Pi levels ($p < 0.01$). A higher percentage of patients had hypertension ($p = 0.03$), CKD ($p < 0.01$), CAD ($p = 0.01$), AKI ($p < 0.01$), and vasopressor use ($p < 0.01$) in the non-survivor group than in the survivor group. Respiratory infection seemed to be associated with higher in-hospital mortality compared with urinary system infection and blood system infection.

Serum Pi and Outcome of Patients With or Without Kidney Dysfunction

The results for crude outcomes are listed in **Table 2**. These results revealed that hyperphosphatemia was associated with a longer duration of ICU stay ($p < 0.01$) and higher SOFA scores ($p < 0.01$). And the increase of serum Pi, even in the normal range, was related to higher risks of AKI ($p = 0.01$, $p < 0.01$), higher norepinephrine doses ($p < 0.01$, all), ICU death ($p < 0.01$, all), and hospital death ($p < 0.01$, all). **Figure 2** shows the unadjusted relationship between serum Pi and in-hospital mortality using LOWESS smoothing technique in different kidney function subgroups. A nearly linear relationship was found in all patients with sepsis, especially those with AKI (**Figures 2A,C**). This relationship was less clear for patients with sepsis with CKD and those without AKI and CKD (**Figures 2B,D**).

Serum Pi and In-Hospital Mortality of Patients With or Without Kidney Dysfunction

A logistic regression model with Pi < 1.5 mg/dl as the reference group was used to evaluate the unadjusted relationship between serum Pi and the risk of in-hospital mortality. The results were shown in **Figure 3**. It showed that the increase of Pi was related to higher odds ratios (ORs) of in-hospital mortality even in the normal range. But it was only significant for the extremely high values in the CKD and AKI subgroups (**Figures 3B,C**). Also, the OR of in-hospital mortality was higher among those with a serum Pi level less than 1.5 mg/dl compared with those with a serum Pi level between 1.5 and 2.5 mg/dl in the overall septic population and patients with sepsis without CKD and AKI though they are not statistically significant (**Figures 3A,D**).

Predictive Value of Serum Pi for In-Hospital Mortality

In order to eliminate the influences of possible confounding factors, an adjusted risk ratio was used to confirm the relationship between the Pi and in-hospital mortality. The results were shown in **Table 3**. Variables considered to be associated with in-hospital mortality and serum Pi homeostasis, i.e., variables with a p-value less than0.1 in **Table 1** and gender in this study, were included in the analysis. After adjusting for other confounders, including age, gender, SOFA scores, weight, vasopressor use, hypertension, CAD, CKD, AKI, white blood cell (WBC) count, serum creatinine level, blood lactate level, respiratory infection, urinary infection, and bloodstream infection, the log-binomial model indicated that Pi was an independent predictor of in-hospital mortality (RR 1.11, 95%CI 1.08–1.23, $p < 0.01$). It means that a 1 mg/dl increase in Pi was associated with an incremental increase of 11% in in-hospital mortality. Older age, higher SOFA scores, lower weight, more vasopressor use, more AKI, lower serum creatinine levels, and respiratory infection were also significantly associated with an increased risk of in-hospital mortality. The same model was built for the subgroup analyses. The results showed that Pi performed well in these subgroups too (RR 1.13, 95%CI 1.08–1.18, $p < 0.01$ for patients with sepsis with CKD; RR 1.08, 95%CI 1.03–1.13, $p < 0.01$ for patients with sepsis with AKI; RR 1.09, 95%CI 1.05–1.13, $p < 0.01$ for patients with sepsis without CKD and AKI; RR 1.09, 95%CI 1.05–1.13, $p < 0.01$ for male patients; RR 1.11, 95%CI 1.07–1.16, $p < 0.01$ for female patients; RR 1.13, 95%CI 1.08–1.18, $p < 0.01$ for patients with

TABLE 2 | Unadjusted relationships between serum inorganic phosphate (Pi) groups and crude outcomes.

Serum Pi [mg/dl, (*n*)]	**<2.7(2749)**	**2.7-4.5(6486)**	**> 4.5(2423)**	**P_1P_2 value**
ICU stay [day, median (IQR)]	4.58(1.96–12.1)	4.57(2.0–11.8)	5.16(2.19-12.7)	0.42 <0.01
Hospital stay [day, median (IQR)]	10.7(6.09–19.4)	10.8(6.06–19.8)	11.7(5.98-21.8)	0.78 0.14
SOFA score [median (IQR)]	3(2–4)	3(2–4)	4(3-6)	0.11 <0.01
Norepinephrine rate [mcg/kg/min, median (IQR)]	0.12(0.06–0.24)	0.15(0.08–0.29)	0.25(0.10–0.42)	<0.01 <0.01
AKI [*n* (%)]	235(8.55%)	674(10.4%)	502(20.7%)	0.01 <0.01
ICU mortality [*n* (%)]	312(11.3%)	931(14.4%)	713(29.4%)	<0.01 <0.01
In-hospital mortality [*n* (%)]	415(15.1%)	1221(18.8%)	843(34.8%)	<0.01 <0.01

P1 represents the p-value of comparisons between the hypophosphatemia group and the normophosphatemia group and p2 represents the p-value of comparisons between the normophosphatemia group and the hyperphosphatemia group; Pi, inorganic phosphate; SOFA score, the Sequential Organ Failure Assessment; AKI, acute kidney disease.

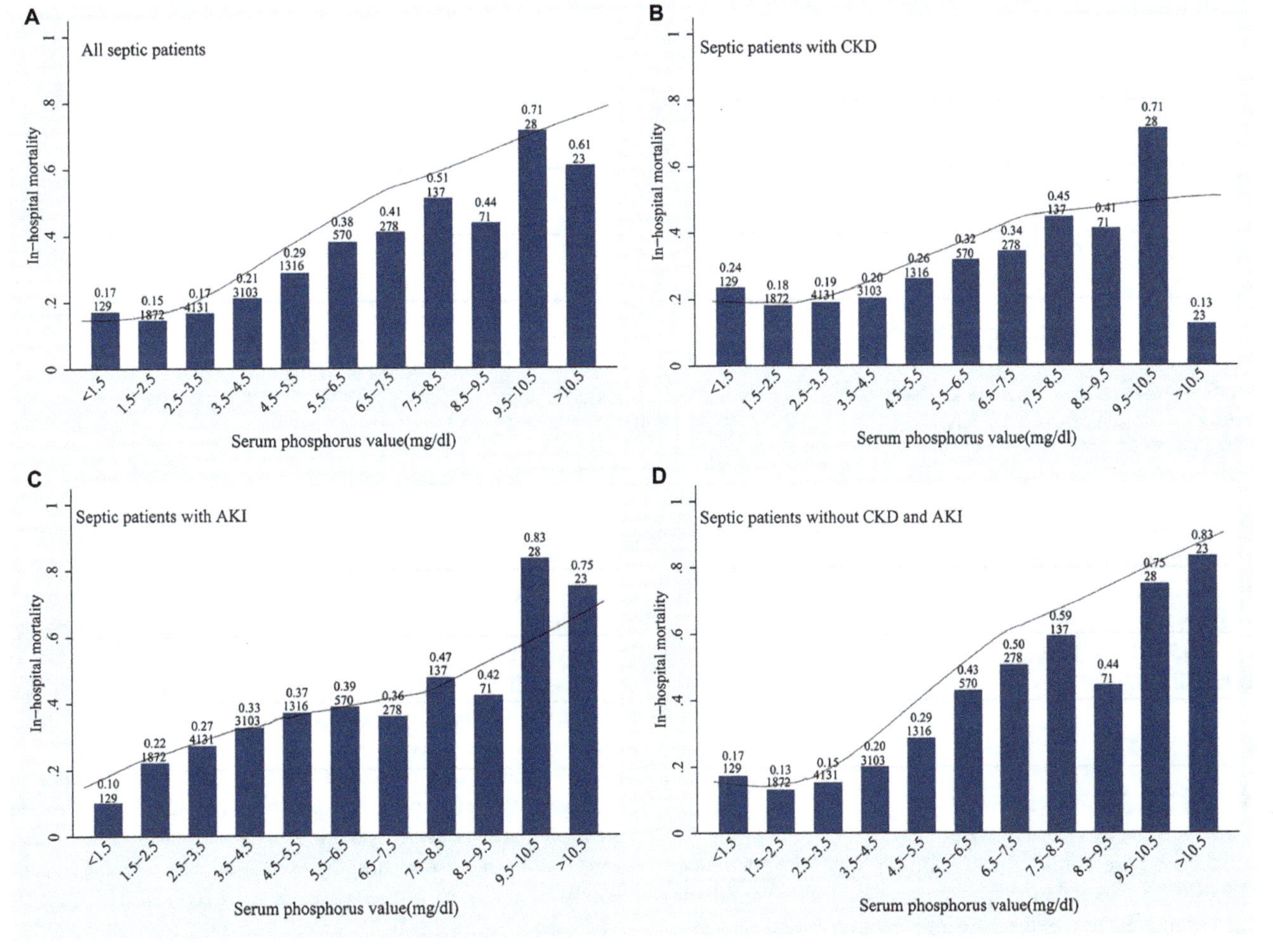

FIGURE 2 | Association between serum inorganic phosphate (Pi) and the in-hospital mortality of patients with sepsis with **(A–C)** or without **(D)** chronic kidney disease (CKD) and acute kidney injury (AKI). A nearly linear relationship was found in this figure, especially in the overall population **(A)** and the AKI subgroup **(C)**. Pi, inorganic phosphate; CKD, chronic kidney disease; AKI, acute kidney injury. The legends on the top of each bar mean the in-hospital mortality and number of admissions in each serum Pi group.

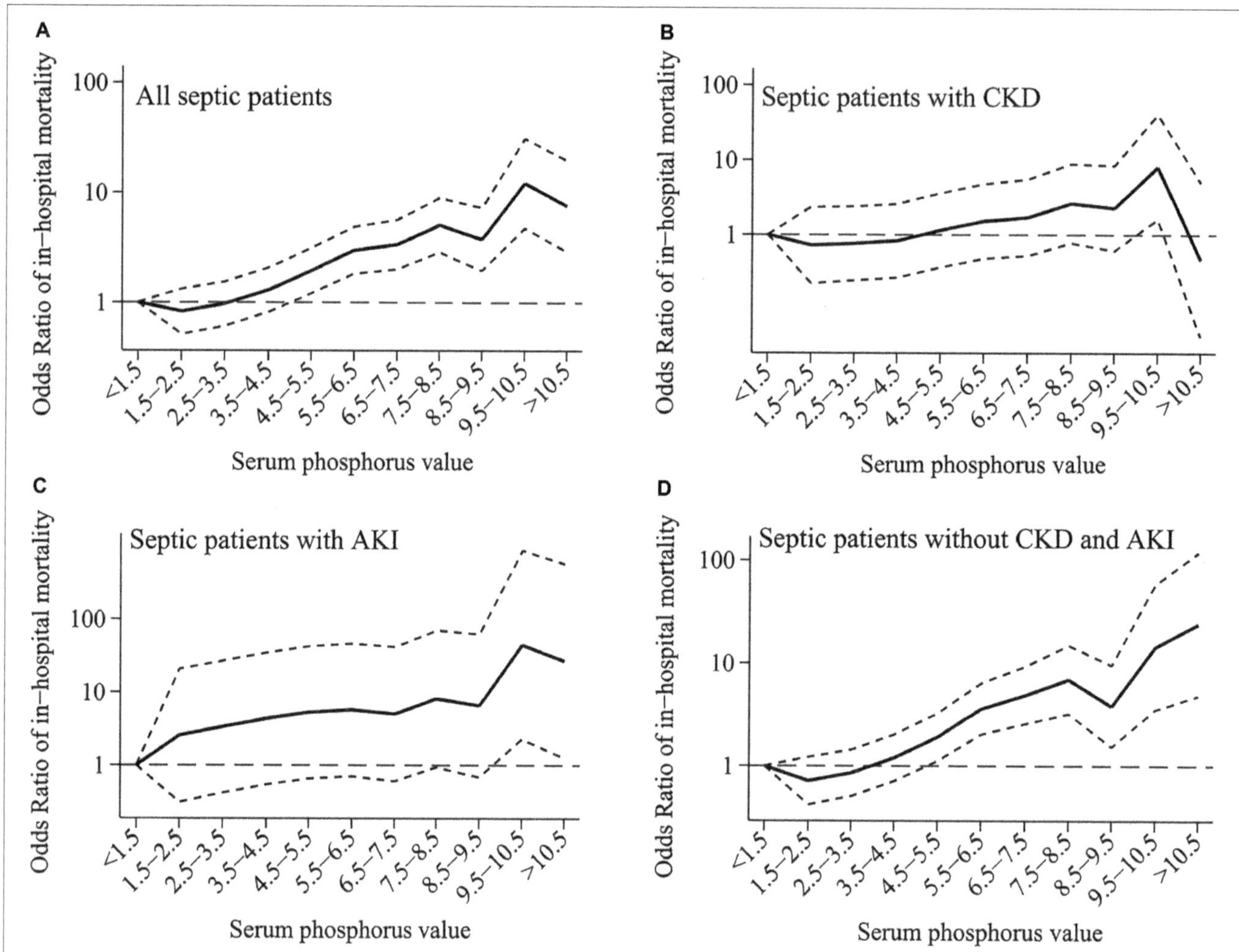

FIGURE 3 | (A–D) Unadjusted odds ratios (Ors) of in-hospital mortality with <1.5 mg/dl as the reference group in patients with sepsis with CKD and AKI or not. The figure shows higher Pi was related to a higher risk of in-hospital mortality even in the normal range though it was only significant for extremely high value in the CKD and AKI subgroups. CKD, chronic kidney disease; AKI, acute kidney injury.

respiratory infection; RR 1.10, 95%CI 1.06–1.13, $p < 0.01$ for patients without respiratory infection; RR 1.10, 95%CI 1.07–1.13, $p < 0.01$ for patients with vasopressor use; RR 1.09, 95%CI 1.05–1.14, $p < 0.01$ for patients without vasopressor use; RR 1.11, 95%CI 1.05–1.18, $p < 0.01$ for patients with SOFA score ≤ 3; RR 1.10 95%CI 1.07–1.13, $p < 0.01$ for patients with SOFA score >3. **Figure 4**).

DISCUSSION

In this study, we found that serum Pi was an independent predictor of in-hospital mortality in the overall septic population and subgroups categorized according to kidney function, gender, respiratory infection, vasopressor use, and SOFA score. Even in the normal range, a minor increase of Pi was also associated with a higher risk of in-hospital mortality. However, this study did not reveal hypophosphatemia as a risk factor for mortality. To our best knowledge, this is the first research studying the relationship between serum Pi and in-hospital mortality in patients with sepsis with a large sample size.

The prognostic values of serum Pi were well studied in many diseases, while published studies in critically ill patients mainly focused on hypophosphatemia (8, 23–25). Most of the studies either included too few cases or were single-centered. The conclusions about the relationships between serum Pi abnormalities and ICU outcomes were inconsistent. In Shor et al.'s study, they reported that severe hypophosphatemia increased the risk of death by nearly 8-fold (8). However, only 55 patients were included. The algorithm for selecting and calculating the serum Pi levels was not clear. A recently published study including patients with bloodstream infection (BSI) from different ICUs concluded that hypophosphatemia was independently associated with a two-fold increase in 90-day mortality in ICU patients with BSI (24). However, the serum Pi level was assessed by only a single measurement obtained during ICU admission. Similarly, the conclusion of a large, multicenter retrospective study that hypophosphatemia at admission was

TABLE 3 | Results of log-binomial model analysis.

Variables	B	SE	Z	Adjusted RRs	*P* value
Age (years)	0.02	0.00	10.36	1.02(1.01–1.02)	< 0.01
Gender (Female)	−0.00	0.04	−0.07	1.00(0.92–1.08)	0.92
SOFA score	0.07	0.01	10.11	1.07(1.06–1.09)	< 0.01
Weight (kilograms)	−0.00	0.00	−2.38	1.00(1.00–1.00)	0.02
Vasopressor use	0.41	0.07	9.45	1.51(1.38–1.64)	< 0.01
Hypertension	−0.08	0.05	−1.54	0.92(0.83–1.02)	0.12
CAD	−0.04	0.05	−0.67	0.97(0.87–1.07)	0.50
CKD	−0.01	0.05	−0.17	0.99(0.90–1.10)	0.86
AKI	0.23	0.07	4.48	1.26(1.14–1.40)	< 0.01
WBC(*10^9/l)	0.00	0.00	1.35	1.00(1.00–1.00)	0.18
Creatinine(mg/dl)	−0.05	0.01	−3.59	0.95(0.92–0.98)	< 0.01
Blood lactate(mmol/l)	0.09	0.01	13.16	1.10(1.08–1.11)	< 0.01
Respiratory infection	0.27	0.05	6.49	1.31(1.21–1.42)	< 0.01
Urinary infection	−0.27	0.03	−5.63	0.76(0.69–0.84)	< 0.01
Bloodstream infection	−0.18	0.07	−1.89	0.84(0.69–1.00)	0.06
Serum Pi(mg/dl)	0.10	0.01	7.68	1.11(1.08–1.23)	< 0.01

SOFA score, sequential organ failure assessment score; BMI, body mass index; CAD, coronary artery disease; CKD, chronic kidney disease; AKI, acute kidney injury; WBC, white blood cell; Pi, inorganic phosphate.

independently associated with increased risk of death was questionable for hypophosphatemia was defined as at least one measurement meeting the criteria of hypophosphatemia and no measurement of hyperphosphatemia (26). In contrast, using a similar definition of hypo- and hyperphosphatemia, Broman et al. did not find any difference between the hypophosphatemic group and the control group (27). In our study, the TWM values of serum Pi were calculated. We think this algorism could reflect the level of serum Pi more accurately. Similar to another study by Suzuki et al. (28), we found that the OR of in-hospital mortality of severe hypophosphatemia (<1.5mg/dl in this study) was higher but not statistically significant in the overall septic population and patients with sepsis without CKD and AKI. Although conclusions regarding the effect of hypophosphatemia on the prognosis of critically ill patients were different, these studies agreed that hyperphosphatemia was an independent predictor of poor prognosis (26, 27). Several other studies also confirmed the association between hyperphosphatemia and adverse outcomes in critically ill patients (17, 29, 30). In these studies, the higher risk of hyperphosphatemia for unfavorable outcomes was all compared to the normophosphatemia group. Many studies have shown that even a slight increase in serum Pi within the normal range was associated with a higher risk of adverse outcomes significantly in the non-critically ill population. However, this relationship in patients with sepsis has never been studied. In our study, the serum Pi was evaluated as a continuous variable. It showed that minor elevation was independently associated with a higher risk of in-hospital mortality whether in the normal range or not in septic patients.

The mechanism is still unclear. Possible explanations include low muscle strength, subclinical vascular disease, vascular calcification, cardiovascular disorders, etc. (12, 17, 31–34). Several studies have shown that an increase of serum phosphate within the normal range can independently predict a greater likelihood of vascular calcification or increased arterial stiffness in CKD and the general population (32). In Ginsberg et al.'s study, they reported that higher serum phosphate levels, even within the normal range, are associated with microvascular dysfunction in community-living individuals (33). In this study, we found that the higher serum Pi level was associated with a higher

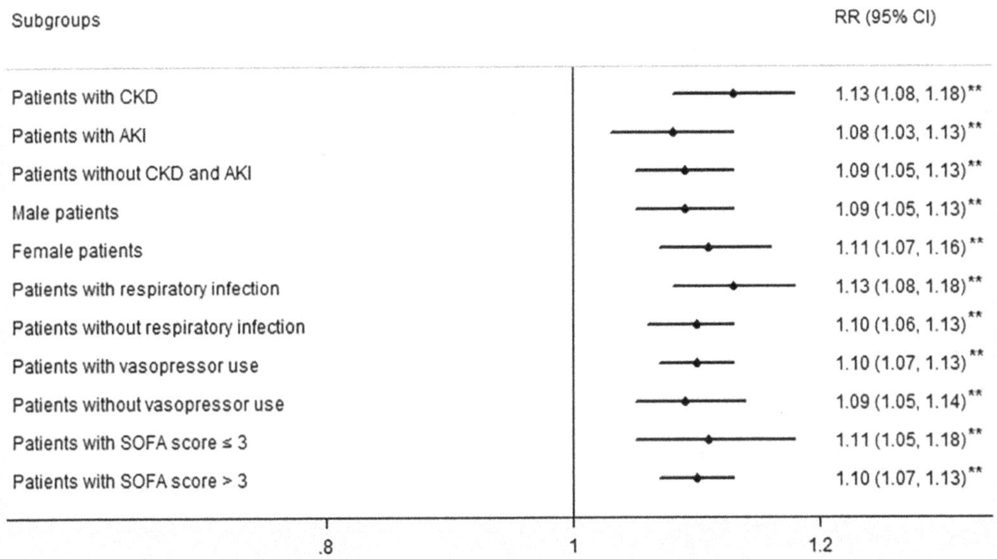

FIGURE 4 | Adjusted risk ratio (RR) of serum Pi for in-hospital mortality in different septic subgroups. **$p < 0.01$; CKD, chronic kidney disease; AKI, acute kidney injury. SOFA score, sequential organ failure assessment score.

norepinephrine infusion rate. This may be attributed to vascular disorders associated with increased serum Pi as described above.

Also, higher quartiles of serum phosphate were found to have a significant association with lower muscle strength and a higher risk of dynapenia (31). This may explain the longer ICU stay associated with hyperphosphatemia in our study.

Whether higher Pi was a direct cause of increased mortality or a marker of disease severity is still unclear. More research studying the potential mechanisms and assessing the potential benefits of lowering serum Pi are needed.

The present investigation had several limitations. First, this study only used serum Pi measurements within the first 24 h of sepsis and did not study the effects of all measurements obtained during ICU stay and the changes in serum Pi on the prognosis of septic patients. Second, the baseline SOFA score was assumed to be zero, as we did not know if the patient has preexisting organ dysfunction before the onset of infection.

CONCLUSION

A minor increase of serum Pi, even in the normal range, could be closely associated with a higher risk of in-hospital mortality significantly in septic patients regardless of kidney function, gender, respiratory infection, vasopressor use, and SOFA score.

AUTHOR CONTRIBUTIONS

ZL, TS, and YH conceived the idea. ZL completed the online training course of data or specimens only research and extracted the date. ZL and TS performed the analysis and drafted the manuscript. YH interpreted the results and helped revise the manuscript. All authors contributed to the article and approved the submitted version.

REFERENCES

1. Chiu C, Legrand M. Epidemiology of sepsis and septic shock. *Curr Opin Anaesthesiol.* (2021) 34:71–6. doi: 10.1097/ACO.0000000000000958
2. Cecconi M, Evans L, Levy M, Rhodes A. Sepsis and septic shock. *Lancet.* (2018) 392:75–87. doi: 10.1016/s0140-6736(18
3. Salomo R, Ferreira BL, Salomo MC, Santos SS, Azevedo LCP, Brunialti MKC. Sepsis: evolving concepts and challenges. *Braz J Med Biol Res.* (2019) 52:e8595. doi: 10.1590/1414-431X20198595
4. Singer M, Deutschman CS, Seymour CW, Shankar-Hari M, Annane D, Bauer M, et al. The Third international consensus definitions for sepsis and septic shock (Sepsis-3). *JAMA.* (2016) 315:775–87. doi: 10.1001/jama.2016.0287
5. Lehman KD. Update: surviving sepsis campaign recommends hour-1 bundle use. *Nurse Pract.* (2019) 44:10. doi: 10.1097/01.NPR.0000554123.08252.ae
6. Jung YH, Lee BK, Jeung KW, Youn CS, Lee DH, Lee SM, et al. Prognostic value of serum phosphate level in adult patients resuscitated from cardiac arrest. *Resuscitation.* (2018) 128:56–62. doi: 10.1016/j.resuscitation.2018.04.026
7. Cheungpasitporn W, Thongprayoon C. Admission serum phosphate levels predict hospital mortality. *Hosp Pract (1995).* (2018) 46:121–7. doi: 10.1080/21548331.2018.1483172
8. Shor R, Halabe A, Rishver S, Tilis Y, Matas Z, Fux A, et al. Severe hypophosphatemia in sepsis as a mortality predictor. *Ann Clin Lab Sci.* (2006) 36:67–72.
9. Geerse DA, Bindels AJ, Kuiper MA, Roos AN, Spronk PE, Schultz MJ. Treatment of hypophosphatemia in the intensive care unit: a review. *Crit Care.* (2010) 14:R147. doi: 10.1186/cc9215
10. Ess M, Heitmair-Wietzorrek K, Frick M, Umlauf N, Ulmer H, Poelzl G. Serum phosphate and long-term outcome among patients with stable heart failure. *J Card Fail.* (2013) 19:25–30. doi: 10.1016/j.cardfail.2012.11.008
11. Plischke M, Neuhold S, Adlbrecht C, Bielesz B, Shayganfar S, Bieglmayer C, et al. Inorganic phosphate and FGF-23 predict outcome in stable systolic heart failure. *Eur J Clin Invest.* (2012) 42:649–56. doi: 10.1111/j.1365-2362.2011.02631.x
12. Poudel K, Shah AM, Michos ED, Folsom AR, Konety S, Lutsey PL. Association of serum calcium and phosphorus with measures of left ventricular structure and function: the ARIC study. *Nutr Metab Cardiovasc Dis.* (2020) 30:758–67. doi: 10.1016/j.numecd.2020.01.003
13. Schaeffner ES, Födinger M, Kramar R, Sunder-Plassmann G, Winkelmayer WC. Prognostic associations of serum calcium, phosphate and calcium phosphate concentration product with outcomes in kidney transplant recipients. *Transpl Int.* (2007) 20:247–55. doi: 10.1111/j.1432-2277.2006.00436.x
14. Sueta D, Tabata N, Tanaka M, Hanatani S, Arima Y, Sakamoto K, et al. Associations between corrected serum calcium and phosphorus levels and outcome in dialysis patients in the Kumamoto Prefecture. *Hemodial Int.* (2020) 24:202–11. doi: 10.1111/hdi.12824
15. Larsson TE, Olauson H, Hagström E, Ingelsson E, Arnlöv J, Lind L, et al. Conjoint effects of serum calcium and phosphate on risk of total, cardiovascular, and noncardiovascular mortality in the community. *Arterioscler Thromb Vasc Biol.* (2010) 30:333–9. doi: 10.1161/atvbaha.109.196675
16. Campos-Obando N, Lahousse L, Brusselle G, Stricker BH, Hofman A, Franco OH, et al. Serum phosphate levels are related to all-cause, cardiovascular and COPD mortality in men. *Eur J Epidemiol.* (2018) 33:859–71. doi: 10.1007/s10654-018-0407-7
17. Miller CJ, Doepker BA, Springer AN, Exline MC, Phillips G, Murphy CV. Impact of serum phosphate in mechanically ventilated patients with severe sepsis and septic shock. *J Intensive Care Med.* (2020) 35:485–93. doi: 10.1177/0885066618762753
18. Goldberger AL, Amaral LA, Glass L, Hausdorff JM, Ivanov PC, Mark RG, et al. PhysioBank, PhysioToolkit, and PhysioNet: components of a new research resource for complex physiologic signals. *Circulation.* (2000) 101:E215–20. doi: 10.1161/01.cir.101.23.e215
19. Vincent JL, Moreno R, Takala J, Willatts S, De Mendonça A, Bruining H, et al. The SOFA (Sepsis-related Organ Failure Assessment) score to describe organ dysfunction/failure. On behalf of the working group on sepsis-related problems of the european society of intensive care medicine. *Intensive Care Med.* (1996) 22:707–10. doi: 10.1007/bf01709751
20. Kellum JA, Lameire N. Diagnosis, evaluation, and management of acute kidney injury: a KDIGO summary (Part 1). *Crit Care.* (2013) 17:204. doi: 10.1186/cc11454
21. McNutt L-A, Wu C, Xue X, Hafner JP. Estimating the relative risk in cohort studies and clinical trials of common outcomes. *Am J Epidemiol.* (2003) 157:940–3. doi: 10.1093/aje/kwg074

22. Peacock M. Phosphate metabolism in health and disease. *Calcif Tissue Int.* (2021) 108:3–15. doi: 10.1007/s00223-020-00686-3
23. Schwartz A, Gurman G, Cohen G, Gilutz H, Brill S, Schily M, et al. Association between hypophosphatemia and cardiac arrhythmias in the early stages of sepsis. *Eur J Intern Med.* (2002) 13:434. doi: 10.1016/s0953-6205(02)00130-9
24. Padelli M, Aubron C, Huet O, Héry-Arnaud G, Vermeersch V, Hoffmann C, et al. Is hypophosphataemia an independent predictor of mortality in critically ill patients with bloodstream infection? A multicenter retrospective cohort study. *Aust Crit Care.* (2021) 34:47–54. doi: 10.1016/j.aucc.2020.05.001
25. Brotfain E, Schwartz A, Boniel A, Koyfman L, Boyko M, Kutz R, et al. Clinical outcome of critically ill patients with thrombocytopenia and hypophosphatemia in the early stage of sepsis. *Anaesthesiol Intensive Ther.* (2016) 48:294–9. doi: 10.5603/AIT.a2016.0053
26. Sin JCK, Laupland KB, Ramanan M, Tabah A. Phosphate abnormalities and outcomes among admissions to the intensive care unit: a retrospective multicentre cohort study. *J Crit Care.* (2021) 64:154–9. doi: 10.1016/j.jcrc.2021.03.012
27. Broman M, Wilsson AMJ, Hansson F, Klarin B. Analysis of hypo- and hyperphosphatemia in an intensive care unit cohort. *Anesth Analg.* (2017) 124:1897–905. doi: 10.1213/ANE.0000000000002077
28. Suzuki S, Egi M, Schneider AG, Bellomo R, Hart GK, Hegarty C. Hypophosphatemia in critically ill patients. *J Crit Care.* (2013) 28:536.e9–19. doi: 10.1016/j.jcrc.2012.10.011
29. Kuo G, Lee CC, Yang SY, Hsiao YC, Chuang SS, Chang SW, et al. Hyperphosphatemia is associated with high mortality in severe burns. *PLoS One.* (2018) 13:e0190978. doi: 10.1371/journal.pone.0190978
30. Jang DH, Jo YH. Moderate to severe hyperphosphataemia as an independent prognostic factor for 28-day mortality in adult patients with sepsis. *Emerg Med J.* (2020) 37:355–61. doi: 10.1136/emermed-2019-208976
31. Chen YY, Kao TW, Chou CW, Wu CJ, Yang HF, Lai CH, et al. Exploring the link between serum phosphate levels and low muscle strength, dynapenia, and sarcopenia. *Sci Rep.* (2018) 8:3573. doi: 10.1038/s41598-018-21784-1
32. Gutiérrez OM. Increased serum phosphate and adverse clinical outcomes: unraveling mechanisms of disease. *Curr Opin Nephrol Hypertens.* (2011) 20:224–8. doi: 10.1097/MNH.0b013e328343ea70
33. Ginsberg C, Houben A, Malhotra R, Berendschot T, Dagnelie PC, Kooman JP, et al. Serum phosphate and microvascular function in a population-based cohort. *Clin J Am Soc Nephrol.* (2019) 14:1626–33. doi: 10.2215/cjn.02610319
34. Cozzolino M, Ciceri P, Galassi A, Mangano M, Carugo S, Capelli I, et al. The key role of phosphate on vascular calcification. *Toxins (Basel).* (2019) 11:213. doi: 10.3390/toxins11040213

18

The Prognostic Capacity of the Radiographic Assessment for Lung Edema Score in Patients with COVID-19 Acute Respiratory Distress Syndrome—An International Multicenter Observational Study

Christel M. A. Valk[1*†], *Claudio Zimatore*[1,2†], *Guido Mazzinari*[3,4], *Charalampos Pierrakos*[1,5], *Chaisith Sivakorn*[6], *Jutamas Dechsanga*[7], *Salvatore Grasso*[2], *Ludo Beenen*[8], *Lieuwe D. J. Bos*[1,9], *Frederique Paulus*[1,10], *Marcus J. Schultz*[1,11,12] and *Luigi Pisani*[1,11,13]

[1] Department of Intensive Care and Laboratory of Experimental Intensive Care and Anesthesiology (L·E·I·C·A), Amsterdam UMC, Amsterdam, Netherlands, [2] Department of Emergency and Organ Transplantation, University of Bari Aldo Moro, Bari, Italy, [3] Department of Anaesthesiology and Critical Care, Hospital Universitario y Politecnico la Fe, Valencia, Spain, [4] Perioperative Medicine Research Group, Instituto de Investigación Sanitaria la Fe, Valencia, Spain, [5] Department of Intensive Care, Centre Hospitalier Universitaire Brussels, Brussels, Belgium, [6] Department of Clinical Tropical Medicine, Mahidol University, Bangkok, Thailand, [7] Division of Pulmonary and Critical Care, Department of Medicine, Chonburi Hospital, Chonburi, Thailand, [8] Department of Radiology, Amsterdam UMC, Amsterdam, Netherlands, [9] Department of Pulmonology, Amsterdam UMC, Amsterdam, Netherlands, [10] Center of Expertise Urban Vitality, Faculty of Health, Amsterdam University of Applied Sciences, Amsterdam, Netherlands, [11] Mahidol-Oxford Tropical Medicine Research Unit (MORU), Mahidol University, Bangkok, Thailand, [12] Nuffield Department of Medicine, University of Oxford, Oxford, United Kingdom, [13] Anaesthesia and Intensive Care Unit, Miulli Regional Hospital, Acquaviva delle Fonti, Italy

***Correspondence:**
Christel M. A. Valk
c.m.valk@amsterdamumc.nl

† These authors have contributed equally to this work

Background: The radiographic assessment for lung edema (RALE) score has an association with mortality in patients with acute respiratory distress syndrome (ARDS). It is uncertain whether the RALE scores at the start of invasive ventilation or changes thereof in the next days have prognostic capacities in patients with COVID-19 ARDS.

Aims and Objectives: To determine the prognostic capacity of the RALE score for mortality and duration of invasive ventilation in patients with COVID-19 ARDS.

Methods: An international multicenter observational study included consecutive patients from 6 ICUs. Trained observers scored the first available chest X-ray (CXR) obtained within 48 h after the start of invasive ventilation ("baseline CXR") and each CXRs thereafter up to day 14 ("follow-up CXR"). The primary endpoint was mortality at day 90. The secondary endpoint was the number of days free from the ventilator and alive at day 28 (VFD-28).

Results: A total of 350 CXRs were scored in 139 patients with COVID-19 ARDS. The RALE score of the baseline CXR was high and was not different between survivors and non-survivors (33 [24–38] vs. 30 [25–38], $P = 0.602$). The RALE score of the baseline CXR had no association with mortality (hazard ratio [HR], 1.24 [95% CI 0.88–1.76]; $P = 0.222$; area under the receiver operating characteristic curve (AUROC) 0.50 [0.40–0.60]). A change in the RALE score over the first 14 days of invasive ventilation, however, had an independent association with mortality (HR, 1.03 [95% CI 1.01–1.05]; $P < 0.001$). When the event of death was considered, there was no significant association between the RALE score of the baseline CXR and the probability of being liberated from the ventilator (HR 1.02 [95% CI 0.99–1.04]; $P = 0.08$).

Conclusion: In this cohort of patients with COVID-19 ARDS, with high RALE scores of the baseline CXR, the RALE score of the baseline CXR had no prognostic capacity, but an increase in the RALE score in the next days had an association with higher mortality.

Keywords: intensive and critical care, ARDS, corona virus (COVID-19), mechanical ventilated, chest X-ray (CXR), RALE score, prognostication, radiograph (X-ray)

INTRODUCTION

Patients with coronavirus disease 2019 (COVID-19) frequently develop acute respiratory distress syndrome (ARDS), mandating intensive care unit (ICU) admission, usually for invasive ventilation (1, 2). Outcome prediction in these patients could use the classification based on the severity of oxygenation problems (3), albeit that this approach has been shown to be not so successful, at least not in patients with ARDS due to another cause (4). The chest radiograph (CXR) is a routine imaging tool for critically ill patients that receive invasive ventilation (5, 6) and could contribute to defining severity, progression, and complications and maybe also predict outcomes from COVID-19 (7, 8). One important drawback of the CXR, however, is the poor interobserver reliability in qualitative visual scoring of pulmonary opacifications (9).

The radiographic assessment for lung edema (RALE) score is a numeric scoring system, recently introduced in an attempt to improve the quantification of pulmonary abnormalities on the CXR. For this score, each quadrant of the chest at the CXR is scored for the extent of consolidations and density of opacities to define the extent and severity of lung parenchymal abnormalities. The RALE score has not only been found to have excellent diagnostic accuracy (10–12) but also to have the prognostic capacity in patients with ARDS due to COVID-19 (13, 14).

We hypothesized that the RALE score has the prognostic capacity in patients with COVID-19 ARDS (15, 16). In this international study, we determined the prognostic capacity of the RALE score of the first available CXRs that was obtained under invasive ventilation for COVID-19 ARDS. We also wished to determine the prognostic capacity of changes in the RALE score over the first 14 days after initiation of invasive ventilation.

METHODS

Study Design

This is an international, multicenter, retrospective observational study in invasively ventilated patients with COVID-19 admitted to participating ICUs between December 1, 2019, and May 31, 2020. The study enrolled ICU patients in the Amsterdam UMC, location AMC, Amsterdam, The Netherlands; University of Bari Policlinic Hospital, Bari, Italy; Miulli Regional Hospital, Acquaviva Delle Fonti, Italy; Centre Hospitalier Universitaire Brussels, Brussels, Belgium; Mahidol University Hospital in Bangkok, Thailand; and Chonburi Hospital, Chonburi, Thailand. The study protocol was initially approved by the institutional review board of the Amsterdam UMC, location AMC, Amsterdam, The Netherlands (approval letter W20_311 # 20.346). Thereafter, the protocol was approved in other hospitals. The need for individual patient informed consent was waived because of the observational nature of the study. The study is registered at clinicaltrials.gov (trial identification number NCT 04485338).

Inclusion and Exclusion Criteria

Consecutive patients were included if (1) admitted to one of the participating ICUs, (2) received invasive ventilation; and (3) with ARDS due to COVID-19 that was confirmed by reverse transcriptase-PCR. Patients were excluded if aged <18 years of age, when COVID-19 was not the reason for invasive ventilation, or if there was no CXR within 48 h after starting intubation.

Data Collection

An online case report form (www.castoredc.com) was used to collect and store the study data. Baseline and demographic characteristics included age, gender, body mass index (BMI); severity indexes, such as the acute physiology and chronic health evaluation (APACHE) II and IV score and the Sequential Organ Failure Assessment (SOFA); and ventilation characteristics at the moment of the CXR, such as FiO_2, positive end-expiratory pressure (PEEP), maximum airway pressure (Pmax), respiratory rate, tidal volume, and the nearest blood gas analysis results.

We collected all CXRs that were taken within the first 14 days after the start of invasive ventilation from each electronic imaging system and uploaded de-identified CXRs in JPEG format into the database.

RALE Scoring

The RALE score was calculated as described before (11, 13). In short, the chest at the CXR was divided into 4 quadrants by a vertical line over the spine and a horizontal line at the level of the first branch of the left main bronchus; each quadrant was then scored for the extent of alveolar opacities (*consolidation* score, from 0 to 4) and the corresponding density of alveolar opacities (*density* score, from 1 to 3) (**Supplementary Figure 1**). In case no consolidations were visible, the consolidation score was "0," and density was not scored. The final score is the sum of the product of the consolidation and density scores for each quadrant. The RALE score ranges from 0 (no abnormalities) to 48 (maximum abnormalities), where in a recent study, patients with ARDS have

RALE scores that range from 15 to as high as 26 (16). Among patients with ARDS, the baseline RALE score is not associated with the ARDS severity groups by P/F ratio (16).

Every CXR was scored by at least two independent scorers that were extensively educated in calculating RALE scores. For this, each scorer was trained in the RALE score by one of the investigators (CZ), who was trained during a 1-month focused period by the team that developed the RALE score (11). An interclass correlation coefficient (ICC) > 0.8 between the trainer and other scorers on a training sample of 22 CXRs from another set of CXRs of patients with ARDS was a prerequisite for scoring CXRs in the study dataset. A third scorer was involved only if the difference in numeric RALE score between two scorers was >25%, to reach a final consensus.

Endpoints

The primary endpoint was 90-day mortality; the secondary endpoint was the number of days free from the ventilator and alive at day 28 (VFD-28).

The ventilator and alive at day 28 was calculated as the number of days that a patient was alive and free of invasive ventilation if the period of unassisted breathing lasted > 24 consecutive hours. Patients who died or received invasive ventilation for more than 28 days had the lowest number of VFD-28, i.e., 0 days.

Statistical Analysis

We did not perform a formal sample size calculation—instead, the available patients served as the sample size for this study.

Demographic data and outcomes are summarized as mean (SD) or medians (interquartile range) for continuous variables and as frequencies (percentage) for categorical variables. In the case of normally distributed, continuous variables were compared between groups with a *t*-test or ANOVA. When not considered normally distributed, continuous variables were compared between groups with Mann–Whitney U test or Kruskal–Wallis test, as appropriate. Categorical variables were compared between groups by chi-square analysis. Missing data imputations were performed by random forest whenever any variable included in the analysis showed a missing data percentage of >10%.

Interobserver variability was assessed using ICC with a two-way mixed agreement model. Bland–Altman plots were used to visualize the aggregate agreement between the two scorers initially assessing a CXR.

The first CXR was labeled "baseline CXR." The association between the RALE score of the baseline CXR with mortality as a time-to-event was analyzed with a Cox regression model, reporting the hazard ratio (HR) with a 95% CI. Herein, baseline RALE score was used as a continuous numerical variable, while age, gender, pH, and lactate were entered as covariates. In an additional Cox model, the RALE score was categorized into quartiles. Herein, proportionality assumptions were checked by Schoenfeld and martingale residuals and influential observations. The predictive accuracy of the RALE score of the baseline CXR for 90-day mortality was also described by the area under the receiver operating characteristics curve (AUROC) with 95% CI.

The association of the baseline RALE score with VFDs was tested using a competing risk model with extubation and death as the events of interest. The results are described with the use of cumulative incidence function and reported as sub-distribution HR with 95% CI estimated from a Fine–Gray model (12).

To assess the association of changes in the RALE score overtime in the first 14 days from onset of mechanical ventilation of consecutive CXRs with mortality, we use a joint model fitting repeated RALE scores with a mixed model and mortality as a time-to-event variable using the same covariates specified in the previous models. The joint model combines Cox regression and linear mixed-effects (LME) models, where the LME part of the models estimates the linear change pattern of the RALE score over follow-up time.

All analyses were performed using a two-sided superiority hypothesis test, with a significance level of 0.05, and presented with a two-sided 95% CI. No corrections were performed for multiple comparisons across secondary clinical outcomes, thus, these findings should be considered exploratory. Analyses were performed using software R (version 4.0.2, R Core Team, 2016, Vienna, Austria).

RESULTS

Patients

From December 1, 2019, to May 31, 2020, 178 patients were screened in 6 ICUs. We excluded 36 patients from the analysis because a baseline CXR was missing and 3 other patients because of incomplete data (**Supplementary Figure 2**). In the remaining 139 patients, 350 CXRs were available within the first 14 days of invasive ventilation.

Baseline characteristics, ventilation characteristics, and outcomes are presented in **Tables 1, 2**. The median age was 65 [59–74] years; the most common comorbidities were hypertension and diabetes. The majority of patients had moderate-to-severe ARDS with low lung compliance. Patients who did not survive had no improvement in lung compliance nor the RALE score compared to survivors during the first 14 days (**Supplementary Figure 3**). Non-survivors did receive a higher FiO_2, PEEP, and peak pressure than survivors. The crude 90-day mortality was high, 61.2%.

RALE Scoring

The interobserver agreement was high (ICC, 0.95 [95% CI 0.93–0.96]). In 14 of 350 (4%) CXRs, a third scorer was needed to reach the final consensus. Bland–Altman plots are shown in **Supplementary Figure 4.** The RALE scores of baseline CXRs were high, with a median RALE score of 32 [24–38], but comparable between survivors and non-survivors (**Figure 1A**). The RALE score of the baseline CXR was increased with worsening of ARDS severity (**Figure 1B**). Linear regression analysis showed how the RALE had no significant association with the dynamic compliance, with an R^2 of 0.0001.

TABLE 1 | Baseline characteristics of the patients.

	Overall (n = 139)	Alive* (n = 54)	Dead (n = 85)	P-value	SMD
Demographics					
Age, years (median [IQR])	65 [59–74]	61.0 [55–71]	69 [60–75]	0.002	0.505
Male gender—no (%)	65 (46.8)	27 (50.0)	38 (44.7)	0.663	0.106
Body mass index, kg·m^2 (median [IQR])	27.3 [24.7–30.0]	26.9 [24.2–29.4]	27.5 [25.4–30.0]	0.595	0.086
Comorbidities and severity					
Co-existing disorders—no (%)					
Hypertension—no (%)	70 (50.4)	25 (46.3)	45 (52.9)	0.555	0.133
Diabetes—no (%)	41 (29.5)	13 (24.1)	28 (32.9)	0.354	0.197
Chronic obstructive pulmonary disease—no (%)	23 (16.5)	7 (13.0)	16 (18.8)	0.502	0.161
Cardiovascular disease—no (%)	17 (12.2)	3 (5.6)	14 (16.5)	0.099	0.354
None—no (%)	17 (12.2)	9 (16.7)	8 (9.4)	0.314	0.217
Other—no (%)	60 (43.2)	14 (25.9)	46 (54.1)	0.002	0.601
APACHE II (median [IQR])	15 [12–20]	15 [12–18]	15 [12–20]	0.132	0.318
SOFA score (median [IQR])	6 [4–8]	6 [4–8]	5 [4–8]	0.481	0.033
Outcomes					
Survival time, days (median [IQR])	26 [19–90]	90 [90–90]	11 [7–21]	<0.001	4.525
ICU length of stay, days (median [IQR])	12 [70–20]	12 [6–21]	11 [7–20]	0.416	0.285
Hospital length of stay, days (median [IQR])	15 [8–29]	26 [15 –38]	11 [7–21]	<0.001	0.214

Data are median (quartile 25%–quartile 75%), mean (±SD) or No (%). Percentages may not total 100 because of rounding.
ICU, intensive care unit; APACHE, acute physiology and chronic health evaluation; SOFA, sequential organ failure assessment.
**At day 90.*

TABLE 2 | Ventilation parameters measured with the baseline chest radiography.

	Overall (n = 139)	Alive* (n = 54)	Dead (n = 85)	P-value	SMD
Ventilatory parameters					
Ventilation mode—*n* (%)				0.252	0.413
Pressure controlled	36 (28.1%)	11 (21.6%)	25 (32.5%)		
Pressure support	7 (5.5%)	5 (9.8%)	2 (2.6%)		
Volume controlled	53 (41.4%)	20 (39.2%)	33 (42.9%)		
ASV/Intellivent	8 (6.2)	3 (5.9%)	5 (6.5%)		
Spontaneous	24 (18.8)	12 (23.5%)	12 (15.6%)		
FiO_2, % (median [IQR])	70 [50–90]	55 [40–80]	80 [60–100]	0.001	0.663
PaO_2/FiO_2 (median [IQR])	130 [88–175]	138 [96–184]	112 [86–152]	0.082	0.294
Tidal volume set, ml (median [IQR])	450 [410–500]	475 [403–500]	450 [415–495]	0.532	0.236
Tidal volume measured, ml (median [IQR])	450 [400–500]	458 [378–512]	450 [408–500]	0.852	0.069
Tidal volume, ml/kg PBW (median [IQR])	7.0 [6.3–7.5]	6.6 [6.0–7.6]	7.2 [6.5–7.6]	0.065	0.298
Respiratory rate, breaths/min (median [IQR])	20 [17–26]	24 [18–26]	20 [16–25]	0.134	0.225
Peak pressure, cmH_2O (median [IQR])	25 [18–29]	23 [17–26]	26 [21–30]	0.017	0.464
PEEP, cmH_2O (median [IQR])	10 [8–12]	9 [8–10]	10 [8–12]	0.013	0.378
Plateau pressure, cmH_2O (median [IQR])	25 [23–28]	25 [21–26]	26 [24–30]	0.281	0.578
Dynamic compliance, ml/cmH_2O (median [IQR])	29 [21–51]	34 [23–47]	26 [20–61]	0.491	0.113

Data are median (quartile 25%–quartile 75%), mean (±SD) or No (%). Percentages may not total 100 because of rounding.
PEEP, positive end-expiratory pressure; ASV, adaptive support ventilation; FiO_2, fraction of inspired oxygen; PaO_2, partial pressure of oxygen.
**At day 90.*

The Prognostic Capacity of the RALE Score of the Baseline CXR

The RALE score of the baseline CXR had no association with mortality (HR, 1.24 [95% CI 0.88–1.76]; P = 0.222). Estimates of 90 days survival in patients stratified by quartiles of the baseline RALE score is shown in **Figure 2**. There was no difference in survival between the quartiles after adjusting for age, gender, arterial pH, and plasma lactate. The baseline RALE score had no prognostic capacity for mortality (**Figure 3**).

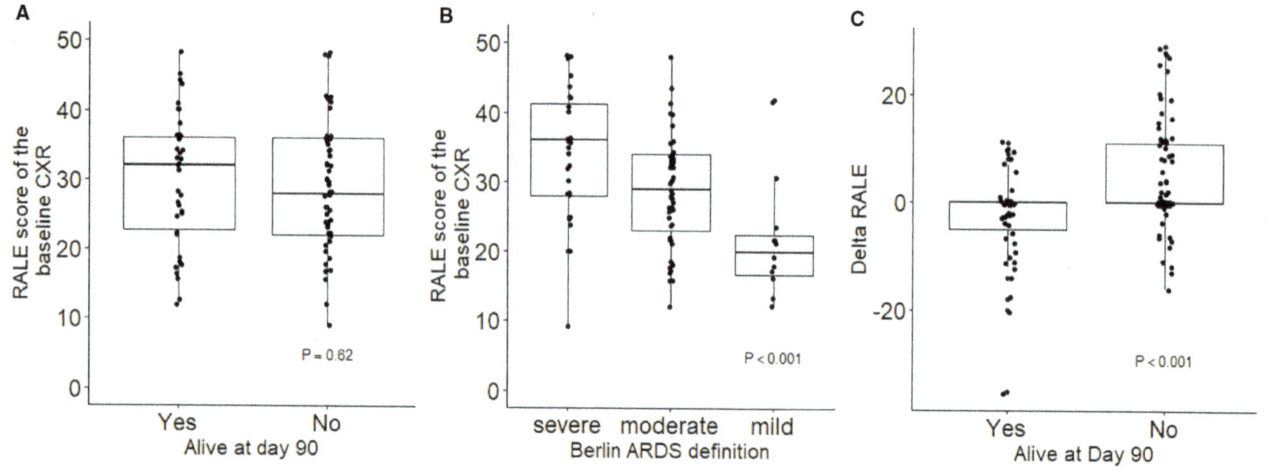

FIGURE 1 | Baseline RALE scores in survivors vs. non-survivors **(A)** and patients with different ARDS severity **(B)**. Changes in RALE score across the first 14 days after onset of invasive ventilation in survivors vs. non-survivors **(C)**. RALE, radiographic assessment for lung edema; ARDS, acute respiratory distress syndrome.

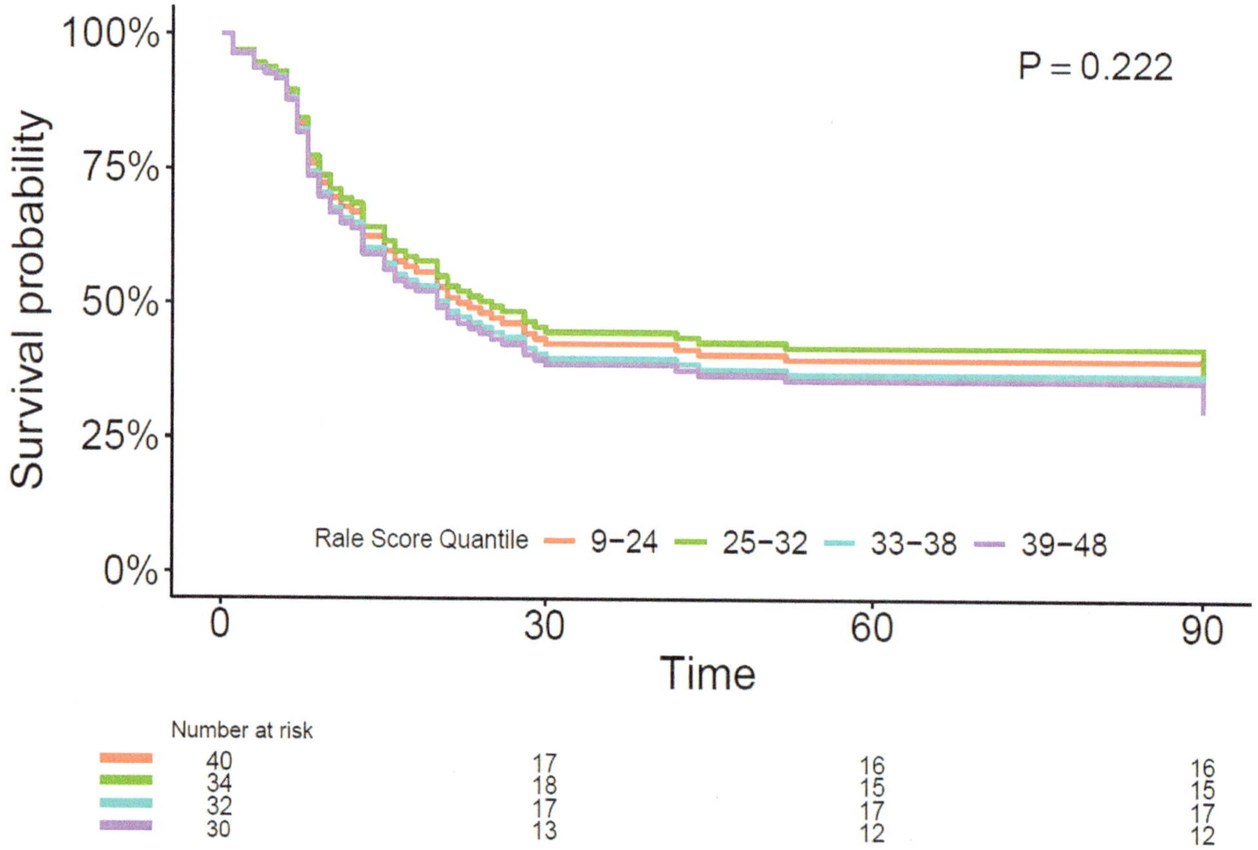

FIGURE 2 | Multivariable Cox model with survival estimates during the 90-day follow-up period in patients stratified by baseline RALE score quartiles. RALE, radiographic assessment for lung edema.

The Prognostic Capacity of Changes in RALE Score

The change in the RALE score over time was different between survivors and non-survivors (**Figure 1C**). An increase in the RALE score until day 14 had an independent association with mortality (HR, 1.03 [95% CI 1.01–1.05]; $P < 0.001$). In other words, for every point increase in the RALE score over time the risk of death increased by 3% [95% CI 1–5%].

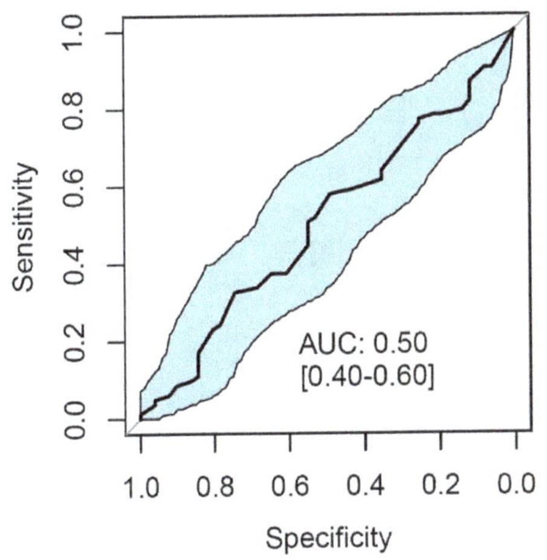

FIGURE 3 | Discriminative capacity of the baseline RALE score for 90-day mortality. AUC, area under the curve; RALE, radiographic assessment for lung edema.

Supplementary Figure 5 shows how the gradual worsening in RALE score over time increases the probability of death at 28 days.

Association Between the RALE Score and VFD-28

Overall patients had 0 [0–14] VFD-28, where survivors had 18 [11–23] VFD-28 and a duration of invasive mechanical ventilation of 10 [6–16] days. When the event of death was considered, there was no significant association between the RALE score of the baseline CXR and the probability of being liberated from the ventilator (HR 1.02 [95% CI 0.99–1.04]; $P = 0.08$).

DISCUSSION

The findings of this international multicenter study in patients with COVID-19 ARDS can be summarized as follows: (i) the extent and severity of parenchymal damage quantified by the RALE score were very high in survivors and non-survivors; (ii) the RALE score of the baseline CXR was neither associated with mortality in the first 90 days nor with successful liberation from invasive ventilation; and (iii) a worsening of the RALE score over the first 14 days of invasive ventilation was associated with an increased risk of death.

This study has several strengths. The study was designed to minimize bias by strictly adhering to a predefined statistical analysis plan and training of scorers. There was a minimal loss to follow-up. We had a low interobserver variability between the scorers, confirming the feasibility and reliability of the RALE score (11, 12, 16, 17). Finally, patients were enrolled in 6 hospitals in 4 different countries and included patients in university hospitals, teaching and non-teaching hospitals, contributing to the generalizability of the findings.

Counter to our hypothesis, we did not find an association of the RALE score of the baseline CXR with mortality or liberation from mechanical ventilation. We could even not find an association with mortality in the quartile with the highest RALE scores. The findings of our study are in line with those from a recent study that could not establish an association between RALE and mortality in ICU patients with COVID-19 (18). Contrasting, the baseline RALE score in patients with COVID-19 presenting to the emergency department did predict adverse outcomes (19) and also in patients with less severe COVID-19 ARDS located outside of an ICU (15). However, another study with a lower median RALE score in both survivors and non-survivors confirmed the capacity of the RALE score to predict adverse outcomes, defined as death or need for invasive ventilation (10). Our findings ultimately suggest that, when baseline RALE scores are high, the RALE score may not be helpful in predicting mortality and the chance of liberation from the ventilator.

Studies that assessed the prognostic capacity of the RALE score in patients with ARDS due to another cause than COVID-19 had conflicting results. The baseline RALE score did not predict outcome in these patients (16). Another study did find an association of baseline RALE with mortality (14). However, patients in this latter study showed very similar baseline RALE between survivors and non-survivors, just as in our cohort. In another RALE study, there was an association between the baseline RALE score and 28-day mortality, but without an association with VFDs (13). The median RALE score in our cohort of patients with COVID-19 ARDS was much higher than the RALE score reported in patients with ARDS due to another cause (12, 14–16, 20). For instance—in patients with ARDS included in the original study that reported on the RALE score, the RALE score was 27 [18–35] (13). Moreover, patients with a RALE score >30, frequently seen in our cohort, were in the highest quartile in a recent secondary analysis of another non-COVID ARDS trial (14). Whether COVID-19 ARDS is characterized by important pathophysiological differences compared to classical ARDS is still debated (21–24). In our cohort, median values of compliance were consistently low and in line with findings in previous studies (25, 26). Furthermore, our study confirmed the association between the change in RALE score over time and outcome, already identified in a recent study conducted on ARDS patients due to other etiologies (14). The change of RALE score over time was independently associated with outcome. This confirms recent findings in patients with COVID-19 in which the RALE score predicted mortality and the need for invasive ventilation (10). Furthermore, an increase in the RALE score was found to be associated with a prolonged need for invasive ventilation and with a lower number of VFDs in ICU patients with ARDS (16). In addition, the prognostic effect of early changes in RALE score in moderate-to-severe ARDS has been confirmed by another study in 135 ICU patients (14). The consistency of these findings, added to the feasibility of repeated bedside CXRs in patients with COVID-19, allows for the changes in RALE score to be used as an increasingly established prediction tool.

The RALE score is an easy reproducible tool that can be easily computed after a CXR is made. The interobserver variability we found is comparable to one of the original studies (11) and subsequent investigations (12–14, 16). Although dedicated CXR apparatuses are still not ubiquitous in ICUs in some low- and middle-income countries (27), it is considered a routine imaging tool for patients who receive invasive ventilation (5, 6). Conversely, CT is a more costly and less available imaging technique, with feasibility issues in patients with COVID-19 and with a radiation load that is much higher than that of a CXR (28). The findings of this and previous studies suggest that the RALE score is an attractive visual metric, especially in settings with low resources.

This study has several limitations. The retrospective design limits the inclusion of all potential confounders. The sample size of this study was relatively small. However, the narrow CI suggests that repeating the study on a larger sample is unlikely to change the result of a significant association between change in RALE score and outcome. Similarly, due to the retrospective collection of study CXRs, time points for CXRs could not be strictly predefined. The third scorer was not blinded for the previous scores, and this could have generated scoring bias. However, high interobserver variability between first and second scorers was only found in <5% of CXRs.

CONCLUSIONS

In this cohort of patients with COVID-19 ARDS, the RALE score of the baseline CXR was neither associated with 90-day mortality nor with the probability of being liberated from the ventilator. However, an increase in the RALE score over the next days had an association with higher mortality.

ETHICS STATEMENT

The studies involving human participants were reviewed and approved by Medical Ethical Board AMC. Written informed consent for participation was not required for this study in accordance with the national legislation and the institutional requirements.

AUTHOR CONTRIBUTIONS

All authors listed have made a substantial, direct, and intellectual contribution to the work and approved it for publication.

REFERENCES

1. Grasselli G, Zangrillo A, Zanella A, Antonelli M, Cabrini L, Castelli A, et al. Baseline Characteristics and Outcomes of 1591. patients infected with SARS-CoV-2 admitted to ICUs of the Lombardy Region, Italy. *JAMA.* (2020) 20:5394. doi: 10.1001/jama.2020.5394
2. Guan WJ, Ni ZY, Hu Y, Liang WH, Ou CQ, He JX, et al. Clinical characteristics of coronavirus disease 2019 in China. *N Engl J Med.* (2020) 9:1404–12. doi: 10.1056/NEJMoa2002032
3. Ranieri VM, Rubenfeld GD, Thompson BT, Ferguson ND, Caldwell E, Fan E, et al. Acute respiratory distress syndrome: the Berlin Definition. *JAMA.* (2012) 307:2526–33. doi: 10.1001/jama.2012.5669
4. Ferguson ND, Fan E, Camporota L, Antonelli M, Anzueto A, Beale R, et al. The Berlin definition of ARDS: an expanded rationale, justification, and supplementary material. *Intensive Care Med.* (2012) 38:1573–82. doi: 10.1007/s00134-012-2682-1
5. Trotman-Dickenson B. Radiology in the intensive care unit (Part I). *J Intens Care Med.* (2003) 18:198–210. doi: 10.1177/0885066603251897
6. Graat ME, Hendrikse KA, Spronk PE, Korevaar JC, Stoker J, Schultz MJ. Chest radiography practice in critically ill patients: a postal survey in the Netherlands. *BMC Med Imaging.* (2006) 6:8. doi: 10.1186/1471-2342-6-8
7. Lomoro P, Verde F, Zerboni F, Simonetti I, Borghi C, Fachinetti C, et al. COVID-19 pneumonia manifestations at the admission on chest ultrasound, radiographs, and CT: single-center study and comprehensive radiologic literature review. *Eur J Radiol Open.* (2020) 7:100231. doi: 10.1016/j.ejro.2020.100231
8. Prokop M, van Everdingen W, van Rees Vellinga T, Quarles van Ufford H, Stoger L, Beenen L, et al. CO-RADS: A Categorical CT assessment scheme for patients suspected of having Covid-19-definition and evaluation. *Radiology.* (2020) 296:E97–E104. doi: 10.1148/radiol.2020201473
9. Rubenfeld GD, Caldwell E, Granton J, Hudson LD, Matthay MA. Interobserver variability in applying a radiographic definition for ARDS. *Chest.* (1999) 116:1347–53. doi: 10.1378/chest.116.5.1347
10. Ebrahimian S, Homayounieh F, Rockenbach M, Putha P, Raj T, Dayan I, et al. Artificial intelligence matches subjective severity assessment of pneumonia for prediction of patient outcome and need for mechanical ventilation: a cohort study. *Sci Rep.* (2021) 11:858. doi: 10.1038/s41598-020-79470-0
11. Zimatore C, Pisani L, Lippolis V, Calfee CS, Ware LB, Algera AG, et al. The radiographic assessment of lung edema (RALE) score has excellent diagnostic accuracy for ARDS. *Euro Respirat J.* (2019) 54:OA3299. doi: 10.1183/13993003.congress-2019.OA3299
12. Zimatore C, Pisani L, Lippolis V, Warren MA, Calfee CS, Ware LB, et al. Accuracy of the radiographic assessment of lung edema score for the diagnosis of ARDS. *Front Physiol.* (2021) 12:731. doi: 10.3389/fphys.2021.672823
13. Warren MA, Zhao Z, Koyama T, Bastarache JA, Shaver CM, Semler MW, et al. Severity scoring of lung oedema on the chest radiograph is associated with clinical outcomes in ARDS. *Thorax.* (2018) 73:840–6. doi: 10.1136/thoraxjnl-2017-211280
14. Jabaudon M, Audard J, Pereira B, Jaber S, Lefrant JY, Blondonnet R, et al. Early changes over time in the radiographic assessment of lung edema score are associated with survival in ARDS. *Chest.* (2020) 158:2394–403. doi: 10.1016/j.chest.2020.06.070

15. Sensusiati AD, Amin M, Nasronudin N, Rosyid AN, Ramadhan NA, Lathifah R, et al. Age, neutrophil lymphocyte ratio, and radiographic assessment of the quantity of lung edema (RALE) score to predict in-hospital mortality in COVID-19 patients: a retrospective study. *F1000Res.* (2020) 9:1286. doi: 10.12688/f1000research.26723.1
16. Kotok D, Yang L, Evankovich JW, Bain W, Dunlap DG, Shah F, et al. The evolution of radiographic edema in ARDS and its association with clinical outcomes: a prospective cohort study in adult patients. *J Crit Care.* (2020) 56:222–8. doi: 10.1016/j.jcrc.2020.01.012
17. Cozzi D, Albanesi M, Cavigli E, Moroni C, Bindi A, Luvarà S, et al. Chest X-ray in new Coronavirus Disease (2019). (COVID-19) infection: findings and correlation with clinical outcome. *Radiol Med.* (2020). 125:730–7. doi: 10.1007/s11547-020-01232-9
18. Herrmann J, Adam EH, Notz Q, Helmer P, Sonntagbauer M, Ungemach-Papenberg P, et al. COVID-19 induced acute respiratory distress syndrome—a multicenter observational study. *Front Med.* (2020) 7:995. doi: 10.3389/fmed.2020.599533
19. Mushtaq J, Pennella R, Lavalle S, Colarieti A, Steidler S, Martinenghi CMA, et al. Initial chest radiographs and artificial intelligence (AI) predict clinical outcomes in COVID-19 patients: analysis of 697 Italian patients. *Eur Radiol.* (2021) 31:1770–9. doi: 10.1007/s00330-020-07269-8
20. Todur P, Srikant N, Prakash P. Correlation of oxygenation and radiographic assessment of lung edema (RALE) score to lung ultrasound score (lus) in acute respiratory distress syndrome (ARDS) patients in the intensive care unit. *Can J Respir Ther.* (2021) 57:53–9. doi: 10.29390/cjrt-2020-063
21. Narayan A, Garg P, Arora U, Ray A, Wig N. Pathophysiology of COVID-19-associated acute respiratory distress syndrome. *Lancet Respir Med.* (2021) 9:e3. doi: 10.1016/S2213-2600(20)30509-9
22. Azoulay E, Zafrani L, Mirouse A, Lengliné E, Darmon M, Chevret S. Clinical phenotypes of critically ill COVID-19 patients. *Intens Care Med.* (2020) 46:1651–2. doi: 10.1007/s00134-020-06120-4
23. Tobin MJ. Pondering the atypicality of ARDS in COVID-19 is a distraction for the bedside doctor. *Intens Care Med.* (2021) 47:361–2. doi: 10.1007/s00134-020-06340-8
24. Goligher EC, Ranieri VM, Slutsky AS. Is severe COVID-19 pneumonia a typical or atypical form of ARDS? and does it matter? *Intens Care Med.* (2021) 47:83–5. doi: 10.1007/s00134-020-06320-y
25. Grasselli G, Cattaneo E, Florio G, Ippolito M, Zanella A, Cortegiani A, et al. Mechanical ventilation parameters in critically ill COVID-19 patients: a scoping review. *Crit Care.* (2021) 25:115. doi: 10.1186/s13054-021-03536-2
26. Grasselli G, Tonetti T, Protti A, Langer T, Girardis M, Bellani G, et al. Pathophysiology of COVID-19-associated acute respiratory distress syndrome: a multicentre prospective observational study. *Lancet Respirat Med.* (2020) 8:1201–8. doi: 10.1016/S2213-2600(20)30370-2
27. Pisani L, Algera AG, Serpa Neto A, Ahsan A, Beane A, Chittawatanarat K, et al. Epidemiological characteristics, ventilator management, and clinical outcome in patients receiving invasive ventilation in intensive care units from 10 asian middle-income countries (PRoVENT-iMiC): an international, multicenter, prospective study. *Am J Trop Med Hyg.* (2021) 104:1022–33. doi: 10.4269/ajtmh.20-1177
28. U.S. Food & Drugs administration (FDA). Available online at: https://www.fda.gov/radiation-emitting-products/medical-x-ray-imaging/what-are-radiation-risks-ct#:$\sim$:text=The%20effective%20doses%20from%20diagnostic,survivors%20of%20the%20atomic%20bombs (accessed May 12, 2017).

19

The Application of a SaCoVLM™ Visual Intubation Laryngeal Mask for the Management of Difficult Airways in Morbidly Obese Patients

Yongtao Sun [1], *Linlin Huang* [1], *Lingling Xu* [1], *Min Zhang* [1], *Yongle Guo* [2] *and Yuelan Wang* [1,2*]

[1] *Department of Anesthesiology, The First Affiliated Hospital of Shandong First Medical University & Shandong Provincial Qianfoshan Hospital, Shandong Institute of Anesthesia and Respiratory Critical Medicine, Jinan, China,* [2] *Department of Anesthesiology, Shandong First Medical University, Jinan, China*

Correspondence:
Yuelan Wang
wyldgf@163.com

We report insertion of the SaCoVLM™ in three awake morbidly obese patients (BMI 46. 7–52.1 kg/m^2). The patients were given intravenous atropine and midazolam injections after entering the operating room and then inhaled an anesthetic with 2% lidocaine atomization. After SaCoVLM™ insertion while patients were awake, when the vocal cords were visualized, controlled anesthetic induction commenced with spontaneous ventilation. The entire anesthesia induction and intubation process was completed under visualization, and no adverse events such as hypoxemia occurred. No patient had an unpleasant recall of the procedure. We conclude that the SaCoVLM™ is easy to use, well tolerated and suitable for awake orotracheal intubation in patients with known difficult airways.

Keywords: SaCoVLM™, visual intubation laryngeal mask, difficult airways, morbidly obese patients, laryngeal mask airway

INTRODUCTION

Awake tracheal intubation is recommended in patients with known or predicted difficult airways (1). The most widely used technique for awake intubation is the fibreoptic bronchoscope (FOB). New optical intubation devices have been developed and are currently being used as an alternative method for this purpose, but only a few cases of awake intubation have been reported (2–4). The SaCoVLM™ visible intubation laryngeal mask was independently developed in China. It is a three-cavity laryngeal mask that provides ventilation with a visual interpolation cavity and gastric duct cavity (**Figure 1**). Through the visual appliance external display screen, the laryngeal housing and tracheal intubation can be visualized, and the position of the laryngeal mask can be continuously monitored during the perioperative period. The intubating laryngeal mask airway (ILMA) is a supraglottic airway that facilitates ventilation and blind tracheal intubation (5). When using the ILMA, however, anesthesiologists must blindly try to optimize the position of the throat mask to meet the appropriate intubation conditions. Using SaCoVLM™, we can directly observe the impact of standard reset operations (e.g., Chandy and "UP-Down" operations (6, 7)) and visually insert the tracheal intubation device. We report the first case series utilizing the SaCoVLM™ LMA

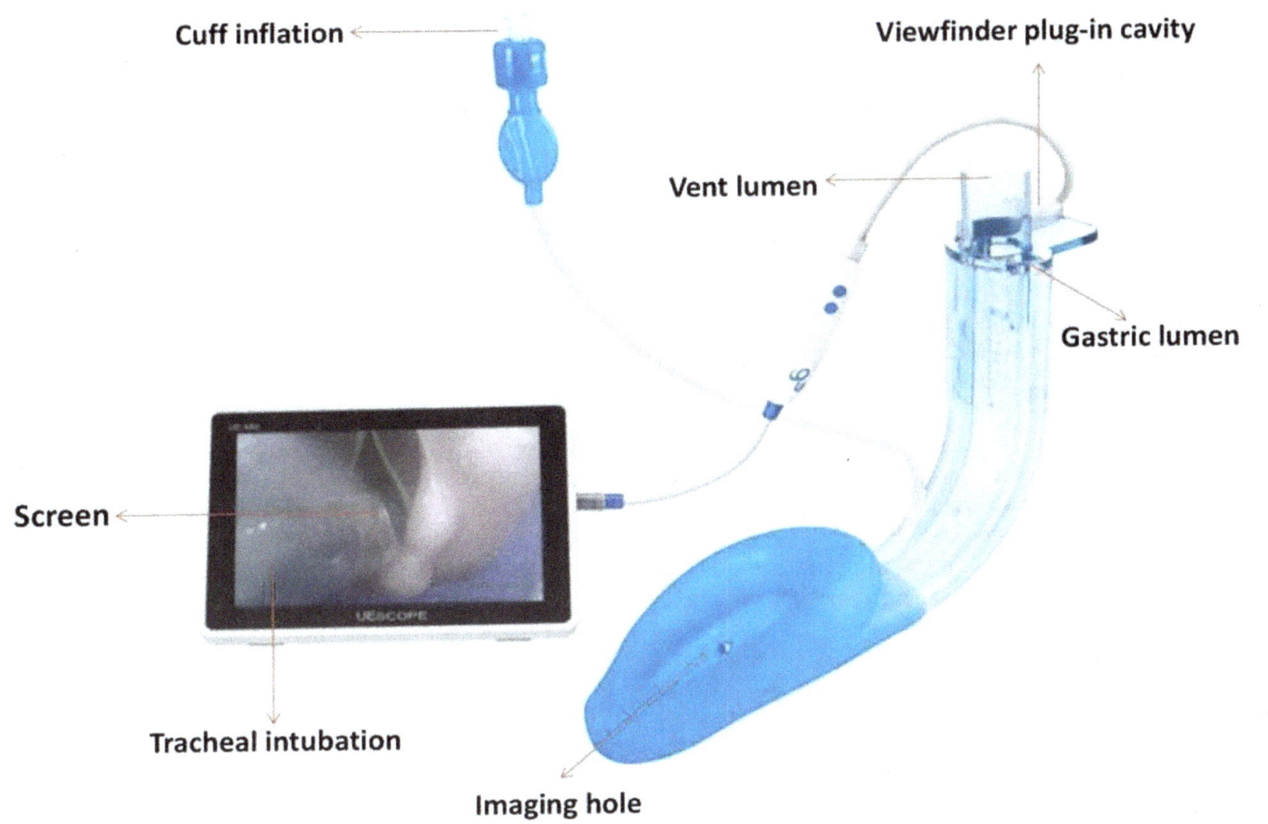

FIGURE 1 | SaCoVLM™ visible intubation laryngeal mask,photo courtesy of Youyi Medical Instrument Co. Ltd. (HangZhou, China).

(Youyi Medical Instrument Co. Ltd., HangZhou, China) as an awake tracheal intubating device in patients with an anticipated difficult airway management.

CASE PRESENTATION

With Institutional Review Board approval and written informed consent from all patients, we collected SaCoVLM™ insertion data on three morbidly obese patients who then received robot-assisted laparoscopic sleeve gastrectomies under general anesthesia. All three patients denied any history of gastric reflux, and all had been fasting for a minimum of 10 h.

Patient One

A 38-years-old, 124 kg, 163 cm, BMI 46.7 kg/ m^2, American Society of Anesthesiologists Classification (ASA) III level female. She had a history of 5 years hyperthyroidism (propylthiouracil 300 mg qd.) and Obstructive sleep apnea (OSA) for over 10 years, abdominal hernia for over 2 years, habitual mandibular dislocation, thyroidectomy and two cesarean deliveries without any significant personal or familial past history. Long-term high calorie diet and eating habits led her to gain weight gradually. Preoperative airway assessment included a Mallampati class III, a 7.5 cm thyromental distance, a 5 cm interincisor distance and a 46 cm neck circumference. Physical examination showed nutritional obesity, abdominal distension, two old transverse scars in the lower abdomen, and a transverse scar of about 5 cm in the neck. Admission diagnosis: Morbidly obese, Obstructive sleep apnea, Abdominal hernia, Hyperthyroidism, After thyroidectomy, After cesarean section.

Patient Two

A 48-years-old, 140 kg, 164 cm, BMI 52.1 kg/m^2, ASA III female. She was hospitalized for symptomatic angina. Owing to a gigantic appetite mainly on rice and pasta, her weight gradually increased in the past 20 years. Both her parents and sibling 3 were over obese. She had a history of hypertension (Bisoprolol 5 mg, Amlodipine 10 mg, and Olmesartan 40 mg), OSA, Diabetes, fatty liver and umbilical hernia, aortic stenosis and hypercholesterolemia. Preoperative airway assessment included a Mallampati class III, a 7.0 cm thyromental distance, a 5 cm interincisor distance and a 41 cm neck circumference. Physical examination showed nutritional obesity and mild cyanosis of the lips. Hematologic tests shows: WBC 10.93 × 10^9 /L, NEU% 0.798, CRP 11.7 mg/mL. CT showed fatty liver, umbilical hernia and dilatation of surrounding intestine. Admission diagnosis: Morbid obesity, Umbilical hernia, Hypertension, Fatty liver.

Patient Three

A 29-years-old, 145 kg, 172 cm, BMI 49.0 kg/m^2, ASA III male. His past medical history include liposuction surgery 3 years ago, hypertension, OSA and diabetes. progressive weight gain over 20 years, sleep snoring and gasping suppression for 5 years. By restricted diet, exercises he didn't get a good weight control and at home for Intermittently ventilator assisted breathing therapy at present. Preoperative airway assessment included a Mallampati class III, a 7.0 cm thyromental distance, a 5 cm interincisor distance and a 45 cm neck circumference. Physical examination showed nutritional obesity, abdominal distension, generalized fat accumulation. Hematologic tests shows: AST 52.10 U/L, UA 559.0 μmol/L, INS μIU/mL, UCP 5.25 ng/mL, $SpO_2$70.00 mmHg, GLU 6.40 mmol/L. Admission diagnosis: Morbid obesity, Obstructive sleep apnea.

All three patients were managed using the same protocol. The patients underwent routine monitoring and were given 2 mg of midazolam and 0.4 mg of atropine intravenously after being transferred to the operating room (OR). Aerosolized inhalation of 2% lidocaine was performed in the semisitting position on the transfer bed for 15–20 min without subglottic anesthesia. Each patient was placed in a slope position, the radial artery was punctured and catheterization under local anesthesia was performed to monitor invasive arterial blood pressure, and an intravenous micropump infusion of dexmedetomidine was given (load 1 $\mu g \cdot kg^{-1} \cdot 10\ min^{-1}$, maintenance amount 0.5 $\mu g \cdot kg^{-1} \cdot h^{-1}$ until 40 min before the end of the operation).

A laryngeal tube was used to test the sensation in the back of the oropharynx. If there was a pharyngeal reflex, 2 mL of 2% lidocaine was sprayed. The laryngeal mask model was chosen according to the patient's lean body mass. The SaCoVLM^{TM} No. 4 was used for patients one and two and the SaCoVLM^{TM} No. 5 was used for patient three chooses. All patients tolerated the procedure well, were connected to the anesthesia circuit, and received 100% oxygen. The glottis was directly observed in 2 patients, and the epiglottis was folded down in 1 patient. Through the "UP-Down" operation (slowly withdrawing the cuff from the pharynx 5-6 cm to aid in unfurling the epiglottis, and then re-inserting), a glottis view was obtained (**Figure 2A**). Once we observed the glottis, we observed the waveform of end-breathing carbon dioxide.

For the induction of anesthesia, 2.5 $mg \cdot kg^{-1}$ of propofol, 0.6 $mg \cdot kg^{-1}$ of rocuronium and 0.3 $\mu g \cdot kg^{-1}$ of sufentanil were immediately injected. When the BIS value reached 40–60, visual descending tracheal intubation was performed, and the 3 patients successfully completed tracheal intubation (**Figure 2B**). The tracheal intubation and the entrance of the LMA was fixed with the infusion paster, the laryngeal mask was kept to evacuate the cuff gas, and tracheal intubation was used to maintain anesthesia during the operation (**Figure 2C**). Forty milliliters of 0.375% ropivacaine was chosen, and bilateral transversus abdominis nerve blocks were conducted under ultrasound guidance. An intraoperative pump injection of propofol 4–12 $mg \cdot kg^{-1} \cdot h^{-1}$ and remifentanil 0.2–0.5$\mu g \cdot kg^{-1} \cdot min^{-1}$ was used to maintain anesthesia; after the operation, tracheal intubation was removed under deep anesthesia. The laryngeal mask was kept and transferred to the post-anesthesia care unit (PACU). During the resuscitation period, sugammadex sodium was used to antagonize muscle relaxation at a dose of 2–4 $mg \cdot kg^{-1}$. After the patients were awake, the laryngeal mask was well tolerated. After 1 h of observation, the laryngeal mask was removed. All 3 patients had no adverse reactions. They were safely transferred to the ward after continued observation for 1 h. The dosage of the above patients was calculated based on their lean body mass, the anesthesia management timeline are depicted on **Figure 3**.

On the first postoperative day, an interview was conducted with each patient on their induction and intubation experience. All 3 patients could recall being pushed to the operating room and had memories of procedures such as indwelling intravenous needles and aerosol inhalation. One patient had no memory of SaCoVLM^{TM} implantation, and two patients described it as if they had swallowed a very large object. After midazolam was given, all patients clearly denied fear or discomfort. All patients were willing to experience the same anesthesia again, and their satisfaction with anesthesia was high. The postoperative VAS scores were all below 3, and no complications, such as hypoxemia, nausea or vomiting, occurred.

DISCUSSION

This is the first reported series of awake insertion of the SaCoVLM^{TM} in morbidly obese patients. SaCoVLM^{TM} has shown advantages in clinical applications since its creation in 2018. Visualization of laryngeal mask placement and endotracheal intubation and Airway patency as well as 100% oxygen delivery was achieved. we can continuous monitoring the LMA location during Perioperative period. SaCoVLM^{TM} is comparable in price to a common LMA that can easily clinical promoted, nevertheless, it's easy to use, well tolerated and safe (with a 30 cm H_2O expected seal pressure). However, SaCoVLM^{TM} has some limitations. Its imaging was not sufficiently sharp and the only way to improve imaging quality by adjusting the LMA position was not flexible enough. Supplementary intubation instruments such as fibrobronchoscopy and bougie are sometimes required. Susceptibility to airway secretions makes suppressive secreting drugs (e.g., atropine, pentylenetrin) a reliance which is limited to exceptional patients (Glaucoma patients). At present, clinical research to confirm the application of SaCoVLM^{TM} is still needed.

Studies have shown that ILMA can be successfully placed in conscious patients (5). Combes et al., for example, reported the effectiveness of ILMA in morbidly obese patients (8). LMA CTrach^{TM} is the world's first visual intubation laryngeal mask and was applied in clinical practice in 2004. In 2006, Liu et al. (9) first reported the use of the LMA CTrach^{TM} in 84 normal volunteers. The first intubation success rate was 100% when the glottis could be seen in the center of the monitor. A number of studies have shown that LMA CTrach^{TM} has greater advantages in the treatment of difficult airways, including in morbidly obese patients, and for airway resuscitation, abnormal head and neck

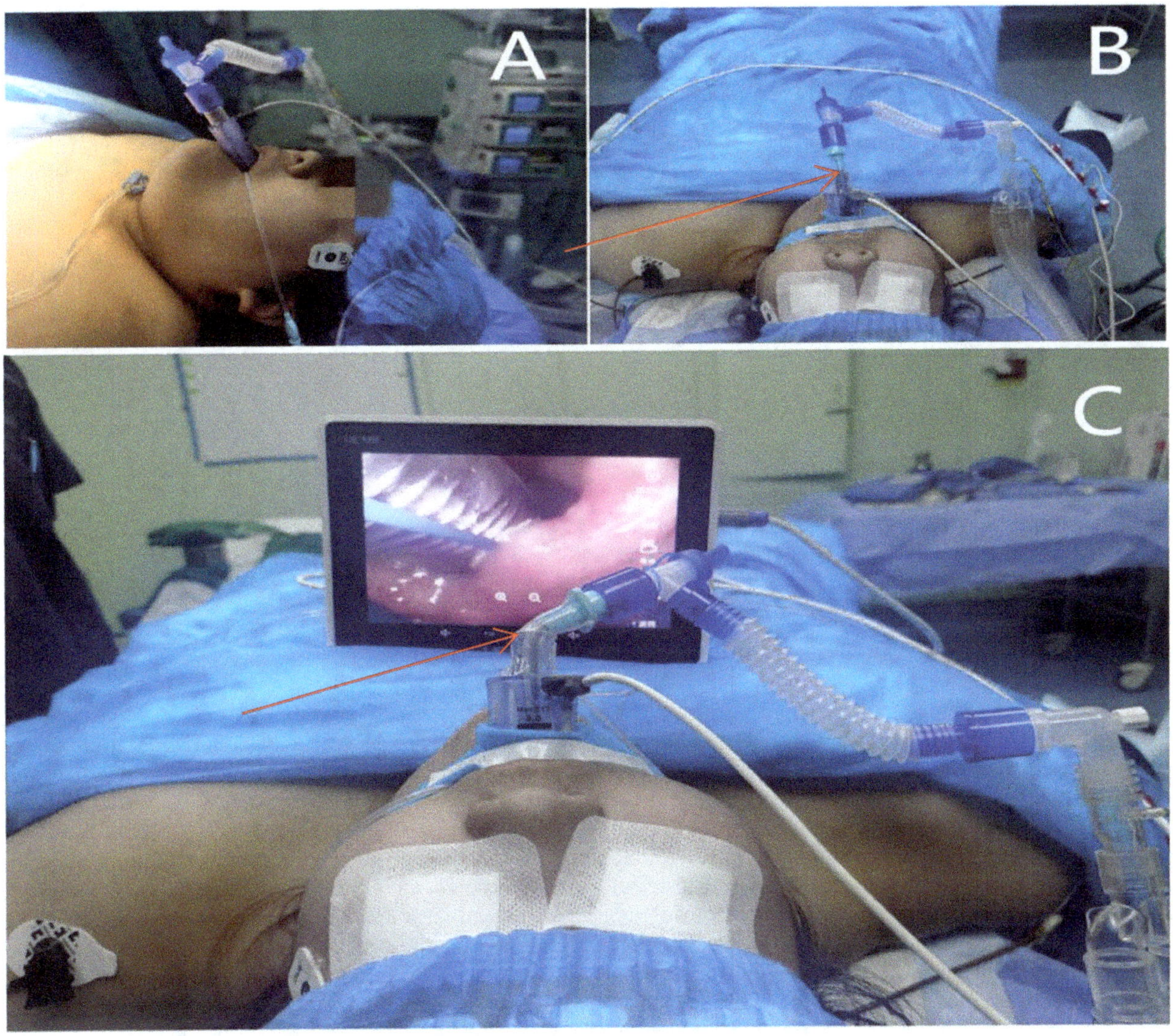

FIGURE 2 | Airway management, Fixed place of infusion paster (Ventilation lumen entrance and tracheal intubation).

movements and other difficult airway treatment problems (10). In addition, LMA CTrach^{TM} was not well clinically promoted due to its exorbitant price. The usage of the SaCoVLM^{TM} has overcome such difficulties. Although it does not provide a clear image like other fiber optic devices, the glottis can usually be seen and centered on the monitor, which is enough to successfully complete the first tracheal intubation.

Video-guided insertion can better locate the glottis, provide a more unobstructed airway, and improve the first success rate of tracheal intubation and gastric drainage tube insertion. Blind probe insertion into the supraglottic airway leads to poor positioning, downward folding of the epiglottis, and the use of more auxiliary devices, so the incidence of complications is higher (11). In fact, the Difficult Airway Society (DAS) guidelines state that "blind" airway management techniques are unreliable and are related to the high incidence of airway trauma (12, 13). Unlike traditional video laryngoscopes, the SaCoVLM^{TM} reduces the need for assistive devices. It can control the airway within a few seconds and establish the best ventilation for tracheal intubation, reducing the time of apnea, which is suitable for patients with poor physiological reserve. The SaCoVLM^{TM} is especially beneficial for certain patients such as morbidly obese patients or pregnant women.

The main cause of anesthesia-related injuries is respiratory safety, which cannot be ensured (12, 13). Actually, the most critical anesthetic skill for such patients is safe airway management, and a key component of this skill is the mastery of multiple techniques for securing the airway. When faced with a known or anticipated difficult-to-manage airway, although awake fiberoptic bronchoscopy may constitute "plan A" for intubation, a "plan B" is required, as fiberoptic bronchoscopy may fail to lead to successful tracheal intubation (e.g., due to airway secretions

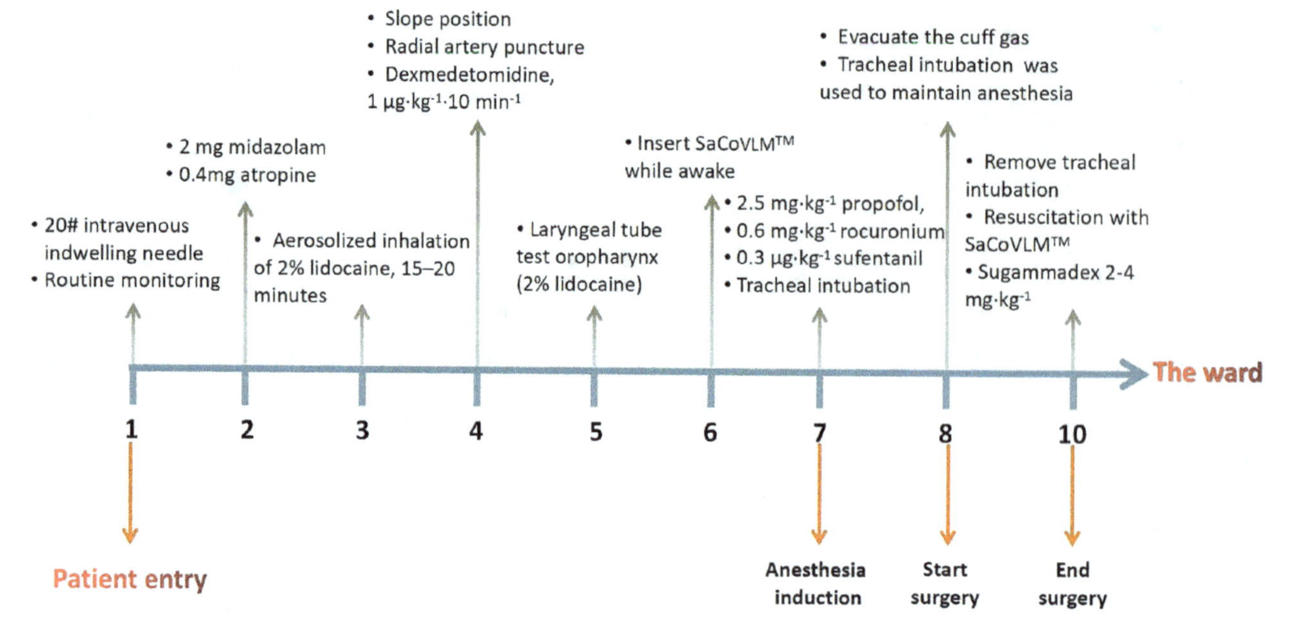

FIGURE 3 | Anesthesia management timeline.

or blood). All our patients had both a high Mallampati score and a thick neck circumference, a combination that is known to be a strong predictor of difficult airway (14). The use of the SaCoVLM^{TM} helped achieve safe, successful intubation while maintaining spontaneous respiration. As the vocal cords were always kept in view, we did not need to be concerned about the displacement of laryngeal structures that may occur with the induction of anesthesia. Awake SaCoVLM^{TM} insertion requires only that patients have adequate topical anesthetic applied to the oropharynx, whereas awake tracheal intubation using fiberoptic bronchoscopy requires that the infraglottic structures be anesthetized as well. The issue of infraglottic anesthesia is important in considering a patient's ability to protect his or her airway in the event of reflux or frank vomiting. Although none of the patients in our series reported having gastric reflux, a strong history of reflux may be an indication for rapid-sequence or awake intubation. When vocal cords and the immediate infraglottic areas are anesthetized, as is necessary for awake fiberoptic intubation, the cough reflex is suppressed, and it may become more difficult for patients to manage secretions. The use of rapid-sequence induction in patients who fasted with no risk factors for aspiration other than obesity is debatable.

Airway management in morbidly obese patients is extremely challenging and can result in serious adverse events and even death if mishandled. Poor satisfaction rates have been recorded despite fiberoptic bronchoscopy-guided awake intubation being the best choice for obese patients. The advantage of oxygenating morbidly obese patients with 100% oxygen cannot be overestimated, given the low functional residual capacity and rapid desaturation rates in this population. Thus, the ability to deliver high oxygen rates while using the CTrach^{TM} to secure a view of the vocal cords is a significant feature of the SaCoVLM^{TM}. Furthermore, it has been observed that ILMA is actually placed better in obese patients than in patients with a normal body habitus (8, 15).

Anatomical and /or physiological compromise can result in morbidity and mortality, which were common problems for Obesity and obstructive sleep apnea patients in the extubation time. Based on the management guideline for adult perioperative extubation issued by DAS in 2012 and the practical guide for difficult airway management issued by ASA in 2013 (1, 16), LMA as a replacement of tracheal intubation is superior to either awake or deep extubation (17, 18). However, it is inappropriate in patients in whom re-intubation would be difficult or if there is a risk of regurgitation. If SaCoVLM^{TM} can effectively ensure ventilation after implantation, we choose to remove tracheal intubation under deep anesthesia. Resuscitation with SaCoVLM^{TM} can be monitored visually while avoiding the risk of re-intubation. All 3 patients recovered well. This is the first time to report on this method. Of course, we will continue to study it in depth to support this view.

CONCLUSION

In summary, this is the first reported series of awake insertions of the SaCoVLM^{TM} LMA in morbidly obese patients with difficult airways. Intubation with the SaCoVLM^{TM} LMA can provide oxygen for patients at any time. Its simple operation, well tolerated, and high success rate makes it a better airway management implementation tool in our practical work.

ETHICS STATEMENT

The studies involving human participants were reviewed and approved by Ethics Committee of the First Affiliated Hospital of Shandong First Medical University. The patients/participants provided their written informed consent to participate in this study. Written informed consent was obtained from the individual(s) for the publication of any potentially identifiable images or data included in this article.

AUTHOR CONTRIBUTIONS

YS and YW conceived and wrote the manuscript. LH, LX, and YG collected patient's clinical information. YS and MZ analyzed and evaluated the treatment and curative effects. YW guided the entire process in terms of theory and practice and revised the manuscript. All other authors contributed to the analysis, reviewed results, and reviewed the manuscript.

REFERENCES

1. Apfelbaum JL, Hagberg CA, Caplan RA, Blitt CD, Connis RT, Nickinovich DG, et al. Practice guidelines for management of the difficult airway: an updated report by the american society of anesthesiologists task force on management of the difficult airway. *Anesthesiology.* (2013) 118:251–70. doi: 10.1097/ALN.0b013e31827773b2
2. López A M, Valero R, Pons M, Anglada T. Awake intubation using the LMA-CTrach in patients with difficult airways. *Anaesthesia.* (2009) 64:387–91. doi: 10.1111/j.1365-2044.2008.05797.x
3. Gómez-Ríos M, Freire-Vila E, Casans-Francés R, Pita-Fernández S. The Totaltrack(TM) video laryngeal mask:an evaluation in 300 patients. *Anaesthesia.* (2019) 74:751–7. doi: 10.1111/anae.14637
4. Gómez-Ríos M, Freire-Vila E, Abad-Gurumeta A, Barreto-Calvo P, Calvo-Vecino J M. Use of Totaltrack VLM as a rescue device after failed ventilation and tracheal intubation with LMA Fastrach in emergent difficult airways. *J Clin Anesth.* (2019) 52:29–30. doi: 10.1016/j.jclinane.2018.08.020
5. Hanna S F, Mikat-Stevens M, Loo J, Uppal R, Jellish W S, Adams M. Awake tracheal intubation in anticipated difficult airways: LMA Fastrach vs flexible bronchoscope: a pilot study. *J Clin Anesth.* (2017) 37:31–7. doi: 10.1016/j.jclinane.2016.10.040
6. Gerstein N S, Braude D A, Hung O, Sanders J C, Murphy M F. The fastrach intubating laryngeal mask airway: an overview and update. *Can J Anaesth.* (2010) 57:588–601. doi: 10.1007/s12630-010-9272-x
7. Wender R, Goldman A J. Awake insertion of the fibreoptic intubating LMA CTrach in three morbidly obese patients with potentially difficult airways. *Anaesthesia.* (2007) 62:948–51. doi: 10.1111/j.1365-2044.2007.05127.x
8. Combes X, Sauvat S, Leroux B, Dumerat M, Sherrer E, Motamed C, et al. Intubating laryngeal mask airway in morbidly obese and lean patients: a comparative study. *Anesthesiology.* (2005) 102:1106–9. doi: 10.1097/00000542-200506000-00008
9. Liu E H, Goy R W, Chen F G. The LMA CTrach, a new laryngeal mask airway for endotracheal intubation under vision: evaluation in 100 patients. *Br J Anaesth.* (2006) 96:396–400. doi: 10.1093/bja/ael001
10. Abdi W, Ndoko S, Amathieu R, Dhonneur G. Evidence of pulmonary aspiration during difficult airway management of a morbidly obese patient with the LMA CTrach. *Br J Anaesth.* (2008) 100:275–7. doi: 10.1093/bja/aem367
11. Van Zundert A A J, Gatt S P, Kumar C M, Van Zundert T, Pandit J J. 'Failed supraglottic airway': an algorithm for suboptimally placed supraglottic airway devices based on videolaryngoscopy. *Br J Anaesth.* (2017) 118:645–9. doi: 10.1093/bja/aex093
12. Frerk C, Mitchell V S, McNarry A F, Mendonca C, Bhagrath R, Patel A, et al. Difficult Airway Society 2015 guidelines for management of unanticipated difficult intubation in adults. *Br J Anaesth.* (2015) 115:827–48. doi: 10.1093/bja/aev371
13. Higgs A, McGrath B A, Goddard C, Rangasami J, Suntharalingam G, Gale R, et al. Guidelines for the management of tracheal intubation in critically ill adults. *Br J Anaesth.* (2018) 120:323–52. doi: 10.1016/j.bja.2017.10.021
14. Detsky M E, Jivraj N, Adhikari N K, Friedrich J O, Pinto R, Simel D. L. et al. Will this patient be difficult to intubate?: the rational clinical examination systematic review. *Jama.* (2019) 321:493–503. doi: 10.1001/jama.2018.21413
15. Arslan Z I, Özdamar D, Yildiz T S, Solak Z M, Toker K. Tracheal intubation in morbidly obese patients: a comparison of the Intubating Laryngeal Mask Airway^{TM} and Laryngeal Mask Airway CTrach^{TM}. *Anaesthesia.* (2012) 67:261–5. doi: 10.1111/j.1365-2044.2011.06991.x
16. Popat M, Mitchell V, Dravid R, Patel A, Swampillai C, Higgs A. Difficult airway society guidelines for the management of tracheal extubation. *Anaesthesia* 67 (2012) 318-40. doi: 10.1111/j.1365-2044.2012.07075.x
17. Koga K, Asai T, Vaughan R S, Latto I P. Respiratory complications associated with tracheal extubation. timing of tracheal extubation and use of the laryngeal mask during emergence from anaesthesia. *Anaesthesia.* (1998) 53:540–4. doi: 10.1046/j.1365-2044.1998.00397.x
18. Stix M S, Borromeo C J, Sciortino G J, Teague P D. Learning to exchange an endotracheal tube for a laryngeal mask prior to emergence. *Can J Anaesth.* (2001) 48:795–9. doi: 10.1007/BF03016697

20

A Positive Fluid Balance in the First Week was Associated with Increased Long-Term Mortality in Critically Ill Patients

Tsai-Jung Wang[1,2], *Kai-Chih Pai*[3,4], *Chun-Te Huang*[1,2], *Li-Ting Wong*[5], *Minn-Shyan Wang*[1,6], *Chun-Ming Lai*[3], *Cheng-Hsu Chen*[2], *Chieh-Liang Wu*[1,6,7,8†] and *Wen-Cheng Chao*[1,5,7,8,9*†]

[1] Department of Critical Care Medicine, Taichung Veterans General Hospital, Taichung, Taiwan, [2] Division of Nephrology, Department of Internal Medicine, Taichung Veterans General Hospital, Taichung, Taiwan, [3] College of Engineering, Tunghai University, Taichung, Taiwan, [4] Cloud Innovation School, Tunghai University, Taichung, Taiwan, [5] Department of Medical Research, Taichung Veterans General Hospital, Taichung, Taiwan, [6] Artificial Intelligence Workshop, Taichung Veterans General Hospital, Taichung, Taiwan, [7] Department of Computer Science, Tunghai University, Taichung, Taiwan, [8] Department of Automatic Control Engineering, Feng Chia University, Taichung, Taiwan, [9] Big Data Center, Chung Hsing University, Taichung, Taiwan

***Correspondence:**
Wen-Cheng Chao
cwc081@hotmail.com

† These authors have contributed equally to this work

Introduction: Early fluid balance has been found to affect short-term mortality in critically ill patients; however, there is little knowledge regarding the association between early cumulative fluid balance (CFB) and long-term mortality. This study aims to determine the distinct association between CFB day 1–3 (CFB 1–3) and day 4–7 (CFB 4–7) and long-term mortality in critically ill patients.

Patients and Methods: This study was conducted at Taichung Veterans General Hospital, a tertiary care referral center in central Taiwan, by linking the hospital critical care data warehouse 2015–2019 and death registry data of the Taiwanese National Health Research Database. The patients followed up until deceased or the end of the study on 31 December 2019. We use the log-rank test to examine the association between CFB 1–3 and CFB 4–7 with long-term mortality and multivariable Cox regression to identify independent predictors during index admission for long-term mortality in critically ill patients.

Results: A total of 4,610 patients were evaluated. The mean age was 66.4 ± 16.4 years, where 63.8% were men. In patients without shock, a positive CFB 4–7, but not CFB 1–3, was associated with 1-year mortality, while a positive CFB 1–3 and CFB 4–7 had a consistent and excess hazard of 1-year mortality among critically ill patients with shock. The multivariate Cox proportional hazard regression model identified that CFB 1–3 and CFB 4–7 (with per 1-liter increment, HR: 1.047 and 1.094; 95% CI 1.037–1.058 and 1.080–1.108, respectively) were independently associated with high long-term mortality in critically ill patients after adjustment of relevant covariates, including disease severity and the presence of shock.

Conclusions: We found that the fluid balance in the first week, especially on days 4–7, appears to be an early predictor for long-term mortality in critically ill patients. More studies are needed to validate our findings and elucidate underlying mechanisms.

Keywords: acute kidney injury, critical care, cumulative fluid balance, fluid balance, long-term outcome, mortality, shock

INTRODUCTION

Fluid homeostasis is frequently altered in critical illness, and fluid balance has been attributed as one of the fundamental managements in patients admitted to the intensive care unit (ICU) (1). Fluid resuscitation is necessary to maintain tissue perfusion and improve cardiac output (2); however, excessive fluid accumulation may lead to detrimental effects, including prolonged tissue edema, impaired oxygen transport, reduced metabolite diffusion, and damaged cell–cell interactions (3). Increasing evidence has suggested that a positive fluid balance in the early stage of ICU admission might deteriorate outcomes in critically ill patients (4–7). One recent meta-analysis found that a positive cumulative fluid balance (CFB) in the first 3 days of ICU stay was associated with high hospital mortality [Relative Risk 2.15 (95% CI, 1.51–3.07)] (8). However, the optimal management of post-resuscitation fluid management, such as the day 4–7 fluid balance, remains unclear. Moreover, few studies have explored the association between early fluid balance and long-term survival (9).

Despite steady improvements in short-term mortality among critically ill patients, post-discharge mortality remains high (10). Among the ICU survivors, 15%–21% may die within the following year (11, 12), with ~6–8% mortality per year in the subsequent 5 years (12). Therefore, long-term outcomes in critical medical illnesses, have become more important as more patients survive acute illness. Thus, the research priorities of critical care medicine have expanded to not only save lives while patients are in the ICU but also toward a goal of understanding and improving long-term outcomes. Nevertheless, outcome ascertainment of CFB in the meta-analysis was somehow restricted to short-term outcomes consisting of ICU mortality, hospital mortality, and 3-month mortality (8); data regarding the long-term effects of fluid balance on survival in medical ICU was sparse.

We linked data from the National Health Insurance Research Database (NHIRD) in Taiwan and Electronic Medical Records at Taichung Veterans General Hospital (TCVGH) to establish a critical care database. This database enabled us to test the hypothesis that a higher CFB at day 1-3 and day 4-7 might be associated with an increased risk of long-term mortality in patients admitted to the ICU.

Abbreviations: AKI, Acute kidney injury; APACHE, Acute Physiology and Chronic Health Evaluation; CCI, Charlson Comorbidity Index; CFB, Cumulative fluid balance; CFB 1-3, Cumulative fluid balance Day 1-3; CFB 4-7, Cumulative fluid balance Day 4-7; CI, Confident interval; HR, Hazard ratio; ICU, Intensive care unit; KDIGO, Kidney Disease: Improving Global Outcomes; NHIRD, National Health Insurance Research Database; RRT, Renal replacement therapy; TCVGH, Taichung Veterans General Hospital.

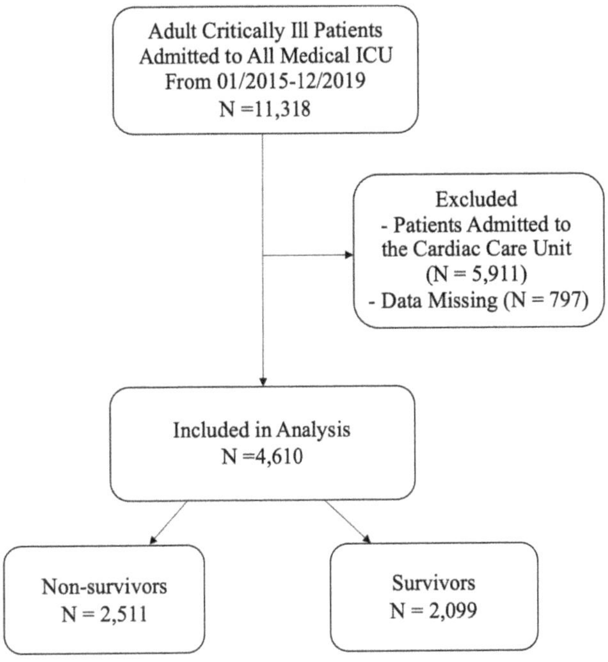

FIGURE 1 | Flowchart of enrollment of subjects eligible for analyses. ICU, intensive care unit.

MATERIALS AND METHODS

Study Population and Ethics Approval

This retrospective cohort study was conducted at TCVGH, a tertiary care teaching hospital in central Taiwan with 1,500 beds. The TCVGH Institutional Review Board approved this study with a waiver of informed consent since this was a retrospective analysis of anonymous data (number: CE20249B). All adult patients admitted to the medical ICU from January 2015 to December 2019 were included. We used the first ICU admission as the index admission. Of the available 11,318 patients admitted to medical ICU, we excluded patients in the Cardiac Care Unit ($N = 5,911$) and patients with missing data ($N = 797$); a total of 4,610 critically ill patients were eligible for analyses (**Figure 1**).

Data Source

We used two databases for this study: the clinical data warehouse at TCVGH and the cause-of-death data of the NHIRD in Taiwan. Demographic characteristics, comorbidities including Charlson Comorbidity Index (CCI), ICU admission, discharge diagnoses, daily fluid input and output, Acute Physiology and Chronic

Health Evaluation (APACHE) II score, mechanical ventilation usage, renal replacement therapy (RRT) commencement, use of vasopressors, serum creatinine, and hospital length of stay were obtained from the TCVGH clinical data warehouse. The presence of shock was defined as the requirement of vasopressors for more than 1 day. Acute kidney injury (AKI) was diagnosis, and the stage was determined according to the Kidney Disease: Improving Global Outcomes (KDIGO) clinical practice guidelines for AKI (13). A patient was diagnosed with AKI if they met the criteria for AKI stage 1 or higher within the 1 week of ICU admission. The encrypted TCVGH patient identification numbers were then linked to the cause-of-death data of the NHIRD to determine their date of death up to 2019.

Fluid Status and Study Outcome

The main exposure of interest in this study was daily fluid input, output, and balance. An intravenous or enteral fluid of any type was considered input. Output included urine, ultrafiltrate from RRT, all body fluid from drains, stool, and emesis. Fluid status was represented daily throughout the first week of ICU stay. We calculated the fluid balance for each patient as total fluid input minus total fluid output in each period. CFB of the first week was divided into two parts, the first 3 days from ICU admission and from admission day 4 to day 7 presented as CFB 1–3 and CFB 4–7, respectively. The primary outcome was the long-term all-cause mortality from the index ICU admission. The patients followed up until the ending date of NHIRD coverage or the end of the study on 31 December 2019, whichever came first. Given that National Health Insurance is a single-payer and mandatory program with a 99.9% coverage of Taiwanese population in 2019, the date of death and overall mortality in the present study should be accurate.

Statistical Analyses

Data for categorical variables are presented as numbers and percentages; data for continuous variables are shown as means ± standard deviation. We compared the baseline characteristics of the survivors vs. non-survivors by either Student's t-test or the chi-squared test. Kaplan–Meier analysis was used to analyze the association between long-term mortality and the day 1–3 or 4–7 CFB status, the Kaplan–Meier curve were presented up to 1-year. A Cox proportional hazards regression model was performed to identify independent variables that predicted long-term mortality. The adjusted hazard ratio (HR) and the corresponding 95% confidence interval (CI) for each variable were presented. We used the Wald test to determine the significance of modification effect by covariates, including age, sex, shock, and presence of sepsis. Additionally, we conducted a sensitivity analysis using a subset of our cohort consisting of 3,065 patients whose AKI stage could be determined. Moreover, we investigated the interaction of shock or AKI with CFB and long-term mortality by Kaplan–Meier analysis. All reported p-values were two-sided and considered significant if they are <0.05. Data cleaning and analysis were performed using SAS version 9.4 (SAS Institute Inc., Cary, NC, USA).

RESULTS

Baseline Characteristics of the Participants

Table 1 summarizes the baseline characteristics and clinical parameters of the participants. The mean age was 66.4 ± 16.4 years, and 2,943 patients (63.8%) were men. The reasons for ICU admission were sepsis ($n = 2{,}235$, 48.5%) followed by acute neurological disorder ($n = 444$, 9.6%) and respiratory disorder ($n = 420$, 9.1%). Among the total 4,610 patients, 1,291 (28%) passed away during the index admission, 1,741 (37.8%) died within 90 days, and 2,151 (46.7%) expired within 1 year after ICU admission. The patients were stratified into two groups, namely, survivors and non-survivors. The mean duration of follow-up among survivors was 2.1 ± 1.3 years. Compared with survivors, non-survivors were more likely to be older, male, with active cancer, and admitted due to sepsis or a respiratory disorder. Non-survivors compared with survivors had a significantly lower body mass index, a higher CCI, a higher APACHE II score, more mechanical ventilation, and a higher percent of shock. Besides, survivors had significantly less RRT initiated during admission compared with non-survivors. Collectively, there was high mortality among patients who survived after the index ICU admission.

Daily and CFB in the First Week

Table 2 presents the breakdown of fluid balance throughout the first week of ICU stay, categorized by survival status. The fluid balance was positive on day 1 in both survivors (1473.7 ± 2985.6 ml) and non-survivors (395.7 ± 2090.1 ml). The positive to negative fluid balance transition was earlier in survivors than non-survivors, which took place on day 2 and day 3, respectively. After day 3 from admission, daily fluid balance in either group was negative. Cumulative fluid positivity was common in our cohort, with a proportion of 49.6 and 23.9% positivity in CFB 1–3 and CFB 4–7, respectively. We further evaluated the CFB 1–3 and CFB 4–7 of the survivors and non-survivors. Notably, the survivors had a negative CFB 1–3, while the non-survivors had a positive CFB 1–3. Compared with the non-survivor group, a more negative CFB 4–7 was found in the survivor group (−580 ± 2995.6 vs. −910.7 ± 2664.5, $p < 0.01$). Together, **Table 2** shows that patients who survived presented a significantly lower daily fluid balance, CFB 1–3, and CFB 4–7, compared with those who died during long-term follow-up.

Both Day 1–3 and Day 4–7 Cumulative Fluid Positivity Are Correlated With Higher Long-Term Mortality

We further used CFB 1–3 and CFB 4–7 as a continuum to predict mortality. On univariate analysis, older age, male, lower BMI, CCI, APACHE II, shock, use of mechanical ventilation, active cancer, RRT initiated during ICU admission, CFB 1–3, and CFB 4–7 were significantly associated with an increased mortality risk. A multivariable model was done after adjusting for all these significant preexisting conditions and illness severity in the univariate model. Both CFB 1–3 and CFB 4–7 were independently associated with mortality (with per one liter

TABLE 1 | Patient characteristics by overall mortality ($N = 4{,}610$).

	All (N = 4,610)	Non-survivor (N = 2,511)	Survivor (N = 2,099)	*p*-value
Basic characteristics				
Age, years	66.4 ± 16.4	69.7 ± 15.5	62.5 ± 16.5	<0.01
Follow-up duration, years	1.2 ± 1.3	0.4 ± 0.7	2.1 ± 1.3	<0.01
Male	2,943 (63.8%)	1,658 (66.0%)	1,285 (61.2%)	<0.01
BMI	24.4 ± 4.7	24.0 ± 4.7	24.9 ± 4.7	<0.01
Charlson comorbidity index	2.4 ± 1.6	2.7 ± 1.6	1.9 ± 1.5	<0.01
Active cancer	627 (13.6%)	523 (20.8%)	104 (5.0%)	<0.01
Severity and managements				
APACHE II score	25.1 ± 7.5	27.8 ± 7.1	21.9 ± 6.7	<0.01
Shock	2,134 (46.3%)	1,500 (59.7%)	634 (30.2%)	<0.01
Ventilator	3,391 (73.6%)	2,074 (82.6%)	1,317 (62.7%)	<0.01
Renal replacement therapy (RRT)				
RRT initiated during ICU admission	738 (16%)	546 (21.7%)	192 (9.2%)	<0.01
RRT for end-stage renal disease	130 (2.8%)	69 (2.8%)	61 (2.9%)	0.75
Reasons for ICU admission				
Acute cardiac disorder	221 (4.8%)	42 (2.6%)	156 (7.4%)	<0.01
Acute gastrointestinal disorder	287 (6.2%)	146 (5.8%)	141 (6.7%)	0.22
Acute neurological disorder	444 (9.6%)	171 (6.8%)	273 (13.0%)	<0.01
Acute renal disorder	124 (2.7%)	57 (2.3%)	67 (3.2%)	0.06
Respiratory disorder	420 (9.1%)	289 (11.5%)	131 (6.2%)	<0.01
Sepsis	2,235 (48.5%)	1,402 (55.8%)	833 (39.7%)	<0.01
Others	879 (19.1%)	381 (15.2%)	498 (23.7%)	<0.01
Outcomes				
ICU-stay, days	9.9 ± 8.4	11.3 ± 8.8	8.3 ± 7.6	<0.01
Hospital-stay, days	24.2 ± 19.0	26.3 ± 19.7	21.8 ± 17.9	<0.01
Ventilator-day, days	9.7 ± 9.1	10.8 ± 9.6	8.1 ± 8.0	<0.01
In-hospital mortality	1,291 (28%)	1,291 (28%)	NA	
90-day mortality	1,741 (37.8%)	1,741 (37.8%)	NA	
1-year mortality	2,151 (46.7%)	2,151 (46.7%)	NA	

BMI, body mass index; APACHE II, acute physiology and chronic health evaluation; RRT, renal replacement therapy; ICU, intensive care unit; NA, not applicable.

increment, HR: 1.047 and 1.094; 95% CI 1.037–1.058 and 1.080–1.108, respectively) on multivariable analysis. Based on our results, the HR of mortality was even higher in per one liter increment of CFB 4–7 than CFB 1–3 (9.4 vs. 4.7%) in patients admitted to the medical ICU.

A Kaplan–Meier analysis for 1-year survival was completed using CFB positivity or negativity as a categorical variable. We disclosed that both CFB 1–3 and CFB 4–7 positivity were associated with a higher mortality risk (**Figure 2**). Considering that shock status may be an important confounder of survival, we constructed Kaplan–Meier survival curves for negative and positive CFB stratified by the presence of shock (**Figure 3**). Shock patients with a positive CFB 1–3 were more likely to die during long-term follow-up than patients with a negative CFB 1–3. However, CFB 1–3 was not a significant predictor of mortality in non-shock patients. Compared with CFB 1–3, CFB 4–7 positivity, an indicator of post-acute stage fluid balance, correlates with higher long-term mortality in either the shock or non-shock group.

Sensitivity Analysis

Sensitivity analysis limited the original cohort ($N = 4{,}610$) to a population without maintenance RRT for end-stage renal disease, stage 3 AKI at presentation in the medical ICU, or patients who stayed in the ICU <24 h, for a total analytic data set of 3,065 patients. The analysis produced robust results similar to those of the primary analysis (**Supplementary Table 1** and **Supplementary Figure 1** in the **Supplementary Material**).

Subgroup Analysis Stratified by AKI

The population in the subset was eligible for accessing in-hospital AKI status and stages. The multivariable model in **Table 3** reports that patients receiving new RRT during ICU admission were more likely to die during long-term follow-up than those without RRT (HR = 1.504; 95% CI 1.356–1.668, $p < 0.001$). Based on these results, we further explored the association of long-term outcomes and CFB in patients with different AKI status (**Supplementary Figure 2** in the **Supplementary Material**). Likewise, patients with a positive CFB 1–3 were more likely to die than those with a negative CFB 1–3,

TABLE 2 | Daily and cumulative fluid status in critically ill patients categorized by long-term mortality.

	All (*N* = 4,610)			Non-survivors (*N* = 2,511)			Survivors (*N* = 2,099)			*p*-value[a]
	Input (I)	Output (O)	IO balance	Input (I)	Output (O)	IO balance	Input (I)	Output (O)	IO balance	
Daily fluid status										
Day 1	3287.6 ± 2690.9	2196.9 ± 1715.5	982.9 ± 2670.4	3745.3 ± 3056.9	2036.2 ± 1763.3	1473.7 ± 2985.6	2782.8 ± 2106.9	2371.3 ± 1644.8	395.7 ± 2090.1	<0.01
Day 2	1710.7 ± 1221.1	1841.6 ± 1376.5	−61.4 ± 1388.4	1742.3 ± 1274.2	1708.4 ± 1269.5	65.5 ± 1417.5	1674.3 ± 1156.1	1993.8 ± 1475.1	−213.2 ± 1337.3	<0.01
Day 3	1641.5 ± 970.0	2013.4 ± 1384.2	−215.7 ± 1236.4	1634.4 ± 989.7	1903.6 ± 1369.1	−136.1 ± 1301.6	1650.2 ± 945.5	2145.7 ± 1391.2	−310.9 ± 1146.6	<0.01
Day 4	1632.2 ± 1035.7	2040.5 ± 1356.7	−228.0 ± 1172.4	1619.8 ± 1048.6	1951.4 ± 1337.0	−182.3 ± 1231.7	1648.1 ± 1019	2154.3 ± 1373.5	−282.7 ± 1094.9	<0.01
Day 5	1596.0 ± 935.7	2041.3 ± 1367.4	−216.6 ± 1070.5	1595.7 ± 966.5	1957.9 ± 1351.8	−177.6 ± 1130.5	1596.4 ± 892.3	2154.5 ± 1380.8	−263.3 ± 992.2	0.01
Day 6	1619.0 ± 911.7	1979.2 ± 1285.5	−159.5 ± 985.5	1606.3 ± 942.6	1926.0 ± 1246.2	−144.2 ± 1050.0	1637.4 ± 865.3	2054.6 ± 1336.1	−177.8 ± 902.3	0.25
Day 7	1610.5 ± 954	1939.9 ± 1271.4	−126.4 ± 897.9	1624.1 ± 1014.6	1842.2 ± 1280.1	−75.9 ± 969.1	1590.1 ± 855.0	2083.5 ± 1245.3	−186.9 ± 800.4	<0.01
Cumulative fluid status										
Day 1–3	6070.0 ± 3971.6	5328.4 ± 3484.3	705.8 ± 3710.0	6654.6 ± 4153.4	5075.6 ± 3409.5	1403.2 ± 4096	5427.2 ± 3656.2	5603.3 ± 3544.4	−128.4 ± 2981.3	<0.01
Day 4–7	4086.0 ± 3771.3	4993.3 ± 4711.1	−730.6 ± 2854.1	4523.5 ± 3761.8	5308.0 ± 4498.8	−580 ± 2995.6	3604.4 ± 3723.7	4650.3 ± 4910.4	−910.7 ± 2664.5	<0.01

[a]*Comparison of IO balance between the survivors and non-survivors. Data are presented as mean ± standard deviation.*

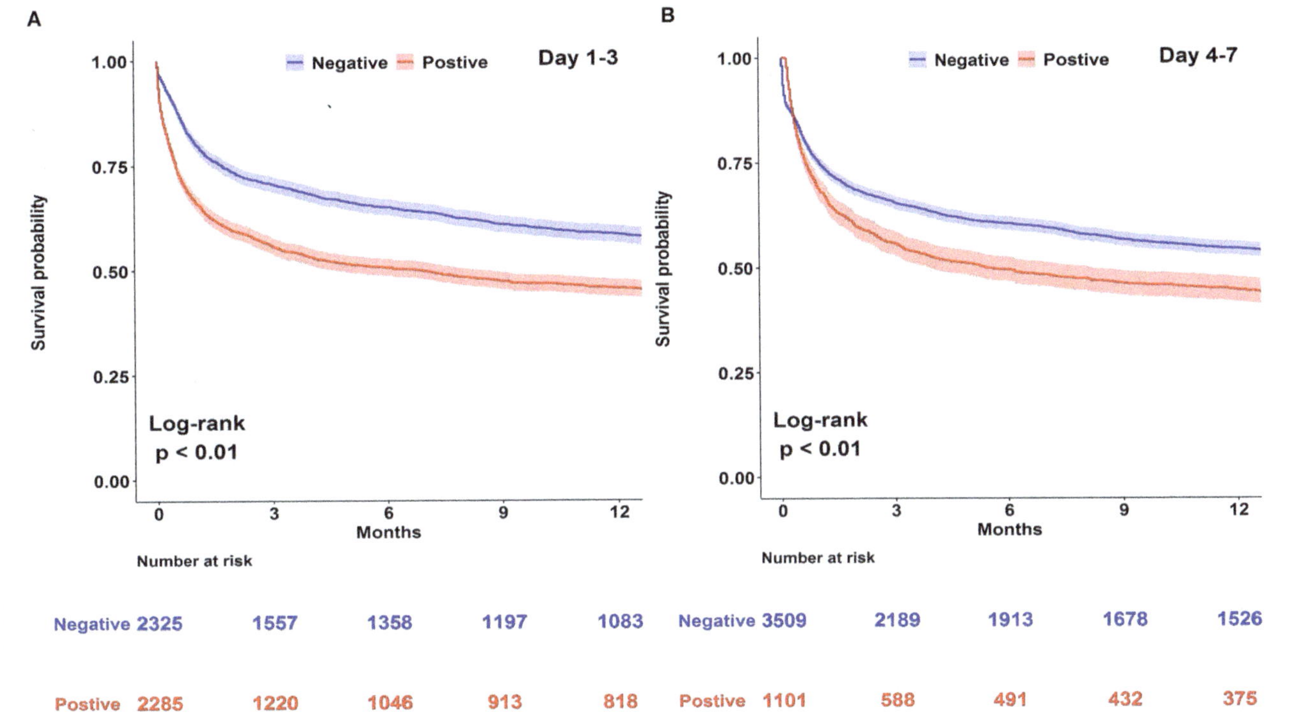

FIGURE 2 | Kaplan–Meier survival curves stratified by day 1–3 or day 4–7 cumulative fluid balance (CFB). Kaplan–Meier curves for long-term survival stratified by day 1–3 or day 4–7 CFB with log-rank test model among 4,610 patients admitted to medical intensive care units. **(A)** Day 1–3 CFB: negative vs. positive. **(B)** Day 4–7 CFB: negative vs. positive.

despite their AKI status. The analysis of CFB 4–7 and long-term mortality in patients with severe AKI (KDIGO stage 2 and 3) also produced similar results. Notably, in patients without AKI or mild AKI (KDIGO stage 1), those with a positive CFB 4–7 tended to have a higher likelihood of death. However, the difference was not significant. To conclude, CFB 1–3 and CFB 4–7 may have distinct impacts on long-term survival in patients with AKI. Despite these different risks, the results point in the risk of long-term survival of severe AKI patients in favor of the negative fluid balance group.

DISCUSSION

We addressed the association between early fluid balance and long-term mortality in critically ill patients and found that CFB 1–3 and CFB 4–7 positivity was independently associated with long-term mortality in patients with shock. Moreover, a positive CFB 4–7 was consistently associated with long-term mortality in critically ill patients without shock. These findings identify insights into the potential hazard of long-term mortality associated with positive fluid balance in critically ill patients and indicate future practical measures aiming a fluid status toward negative.

There is growing evidence that excess fluid administration may be detrimental to organ function (14). The FACCT trial addressed the 60-day mortality impact of liberal fluid management versus conservative therapy in patients with acute lung injury. They found no difference in mortality, but patients who received conservative fluid therapy had a shorter ventilator-day and ICU length of stay compared with those who underwent liberal fluid therapy (15). Messmer et al. performed a meta-analysis of 31 observational studies focusing on mortality association with fluid overload and found that a positive CFB 1–3 was associated with increased hospital mortality in critically ill patients (8). Several studies have further shown the clinical relevance of fluid balance in the first week among critically ill patients (5, 6, 16). Acheampong and Vincent (17) reported a positive association between the persistence of a positive fluid balance in the first week of ICU admission and high hospital mortality in 173 critically ill patients with sepsis. Similarly, Dhondup et al. (18), using a cohort comprised of 633 critically ill septic patients, reported that 61.1% of patients achieved a negative fluid balance during ICU admission, and a negative fluid balance tended to be associated with a lower 90-day mortality rate (36 vs. 44%; $p = 0.048$). In the present study, CFB 1–3 and CFB 4–7 positivity was common and highly associated with increased mortality. Collectively, this evidence indicates that a persistent positive fluid balance within the first week of ICU admission is relatively prevalent and associated with adverse outcomes among critically ill patients.

In this study, hospital mortality and 1-year mortality were 28.0% (1,291/4,610) and 46.7% (2,151/4,610), respectively. In other words, the post-acute 1-year mortality was 25.9%

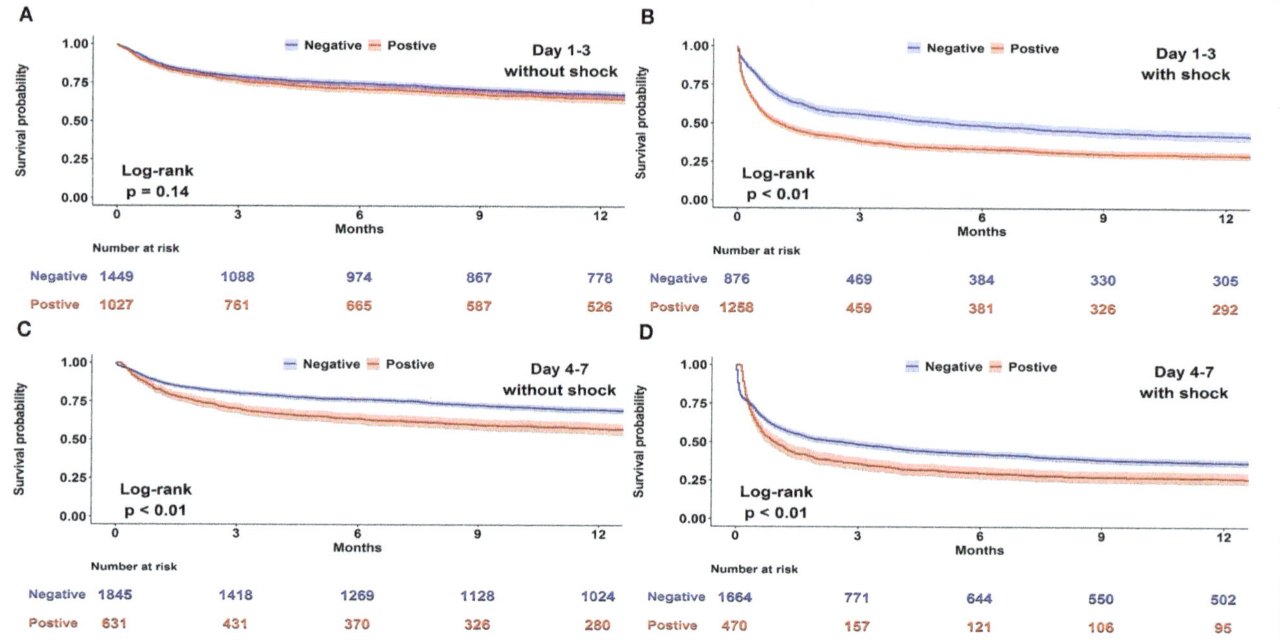

FIGURE 3 | Association between positive and negative cumulative fluid balance (CFB) and long-term survival stratified by shock status. Kaplan–Meier survival curves for negative and positive CFB among 4,610 patients admitted to medical intensive care units stratified by the presence of shock. **(A)** Day 1–3 CFB in patients without shock. **(B)** Day 1–3 CFB in patients with shock. **(C)** Day 4–7 CFB in patients without shock. **(D)** Day 4–7 CFB in patients with shock.

TABLE 3 | Cox proportional hazard regression analysis for long-term mortality.

Characteristics	Univariable		Multivariable**	
	HR (95% CI)	*P*-value	HR (95% CI)	*P*-value
Age, per year increment	1.017 (1.014–1.019)	<0.001	1.008 (1.006–1.011)	<0.001
Sex (male)	1.140 (1.049–1.238)	0.002	1.152 (1.060–1.252)	0.001
BMI, per 1 kg/m^2 increment	0.976 (0.967–0.984)	<0.001	0.963 (0.955–0.972)	<0.001
CCI, per 1 score increment	1.190 (1.164–1.217)	<0.001	1.093 (1.066–1.121)	<0.001
APACHE II score, per 1 increment	1.096 (1.089–1.102)	<0.001	1.063 (1.055–1.070)	<0.001
Presence of shock	2.564 (2.367–2.778)	<0.001	1.732 (1.582–1.897)	<0.001
Use of mechanical ventilation	2.096 (1.890–2.325)	<0.001	1.199 (1.072–1.340)	0.001
Active cancer	2.907 (2.637–3.206)	<0.001	2.633 (2.380–2.912)	<0.001
RRT initiated during ICU admission	2.305 (2.095–2.536)	<0.001	1.504 (1.356–1.668)	<0.001
RRT for end-stage renal disease	0.981 (0.772–1.246)	0.875	0.938 (0.735–1.197)	0.607
CFB of day 1–3*	1.096 (1.085–1.106)	<0.001	1.047 (1.037–1.058)	<0.001
CFB of day 4–7*	1.048 (1.033–1.064)	<0.001	1.094 (1.080–1.108)	<0.001

HR, hazard ratio; CI, confidence interval; BMI, body mass index; CCI, Charlson comorbidity index; APACHE II, acute physiology and chronic health evaluation II; RRT, renal replacement therapy; ICU, intensive care unit; CFB, cumulative fluid balance.

Per 1 liter increment.

**Additionally adjusted for age, sex, BMI, CCI, APACHE II score, presence of shock, use of mechanical ventilation, active cancer, RRT initiated during ICU admission, CFB of day 1–3, and CFB of day 4–7.*

(860/3,319), and the prolonged mortality hazard tended to be prominent within the first 3 months. This finding was consistent with previous studies (10, 12, 19). For example, Mohr et al. recently investigated the short- and long-term outcomes of 830,721 patients with sepsis in Medicare claim database (10). They reported that hospital mortality and 90-day mortality were 20 and 48%, respectively. The long-term survival of our study coincides with prior research (**Figure 2**). Several studies have attempted to explore early determinants of long-term mortality in critically ill patients (12), but few studies have focused on fluid balance and long-term survival. Balakumar et al. conducted a retrospective single-center cohort study in which fluid balance during ICU stay was categorized as negative, even, or positive among critically ill patients (9). A positive fluid balance was associated with a higher 1-year mortality than an even fluid balance. Although the aforementioned finding was consistent with our data; however, the population addressed in the study conducted by Balakumar et al. was different from our cohort in the medical ICUs, such as a high proportion of surgical admissions (59.2%) rather than medical admissions, fewer patients admitted due to sepsis than our study (15 vs. 48.5%), and a lower 1-year mortality (24.4%) than in our cohort (46.7%) (9). Therefore, fluid overload tends to be a crucial issue in patients admitted to either medical or surgical ICUs.

We recognized a positive fluid balance at different stages from the first week in ICU, including CFB 1–3 and CFB 4–7, as predictors of long-term mortality (**Figure 2**). Differences in survival between positive and negative fluid balance were most pronounced during the first 3 months. Similarly, 3-month is currently a critical time window to define the late recovery of organ failure after critical illness, such as AKI by the Acute Disease Quality Initiative (20). We hence postulate that the recovery of organ function in survivors may potentially mitigate the initial insults related to fluid balance. Aligned with our finding, van Mourik et al. found that a positive fluid balance after reversal of septic shock was associated with high long-term mortality (21). In detail, among the 636 patients with septic shock, a higher fluid balance in the ICU stay after reversal of shock correlated with an increased 30-day and 1-year mortality. Given that most patients achieved a reversal of shock within 2–3 days, the fluid balance in the study conducted by Mourik et al. appears to be comparable with the CFB 4–7 in our study. Indeed, the post-acute fluid balance might be overlooked after recovery from critical illness. Mitchell et al. explored fluid status on ICU-discharge in 247 patients who recovered from septic shock. They found that 35% (86/247) of patients had fluid overload, defined by an increase of body weight equal or higher than 10% of body weight on ICU admission (22). They reported that patients with a fluid overload on ICU discharge were less likely to ambulate on hospital discharge and tended to be discharged to a healthcare facility instead of home (22). Taken together, patient outcomes are not only dependent on early resuscitation but also potentially affected by the fluid status after resuscitation.

Indeed, fluid management may require different approaches depending on the time course of the disease (i.e., acute vs. post-acute period). We divided early fluid balance into CFB 1–3 and CFB 4–7 to address the different roles in distinct patient groups, such as patients without shock and with shock. In shock patients, the importance of early fluid balance and the achievement of a negative fluid balance in the de-escalation phase have been extensively studied (6, 23). However, evidence gaps exist regarding CFB and long-term mortality in non-shock patients. In patients without shock, accounting for 53.7% patients in our cohort, we found that CFB 4–7, instead of CFB 1–3, was associated with long-term survival. The long-term hazard of death of positive CFB 4–7 was not affected by age, sex, shock, or presence of sepsis (**Supplementary Table 2** in the **Supplementary Material**). Our finding highlights the importance of achieving a negative CFB in the post-acute phase even in patients without shock, which is potentially a modifiable target aimed at improved long-term outcomes.

We further point out the crucial role of fluid balance in patients with AKI. Owing to the fear that AKI might result from untreated hypovolemia, aggressive fluid administration is common in treating AKI patients. However, this practice is neither supported nor refuted by convincing clinical trials (1). The available knowledge about a higher CFB during AKI derives from observational studies focusing on short-term survival (24, 25). Thus, we specifically studied the role and the interaction of CFB with AKI and long-term survival. We found that negative CFB 1–3 had an inverse association with long-term mortality across all AKI stages (**Supplementary Figure 2**). In contrast, the significant survival importance of CFB 4–7 merely existed in AKI stage 2 and 3 patients, whose negative fluid balance was not easy to maintain without aggressive intervention. In a national sample of US veterans comprising 104,764 hospitalized patients (26), AKI developed in 16.3%. Most stage 1 AKI patients recovered within 2 days (71%), while slower AKI recovery was observed in patients with stage 2 and 3 AKI. The rapid restoration of renal function in less severe AKI echoes the lack of prognostic importance of CFB 4–7 in patients without AKI or mild AKI in our study. On the other hand, optimizing fluid balance in the post-acute phase among patients with severe and persistent AKI is of paramount importance and may be associated with long-term outcomes.

In the present study, the early fluid balance tended to be neutral in critically ill patients. For example, the mean CFB 1–3 was 1,403 ml and −128 ml among non-survivors and survivors, respectively. Therefore, we speculated less than half (48.5%) of enrolled patients had sepsis might account for the less requirement for aggressive fluid resuscitation. However, the enrollment of both septic and non-septic should reflect the nature of this real-world study. Moreover, the relative neutral fluid balance among patients enrolled during 2015–2019 aligns with a shift toward more restrictive fluid management in critically ill patients reported in recent trials (27).

A number of mechanistic studies have found prolonged fluid overload-associated deleterious effects, including microvascular abnormalities resulting from congestion within an encapsulated organ such as the kidney, impaired intestinal motility and nutrient absorption due to edema, dysregulated immunity possibly attributed to altered gut microbiota, and shedding of endothelial glycocalyx resulting in endothelial dysfunction (28–30). Furthermore, fluid overload may be alleviated by several measures, such as early vasopressor, higher dose of vasopressor, cautions for non-resuscitated fluid, fluid resuscitation guided by dynamic fluid responsiveness, early administration of diuretic, and protocolized diuresis (27, 31–34). Our data provides clinical evidence of a detrimental long-term impact of fluid overload and highlights that fluid balance during day 4–7 might potentially be an actionable target to alleviate fluid overload in critically ill patients.

There are limitations to be acknowledged. First, the observational design of the study does not allow the cause-and-effect relationship between CFB and outcomes to be inferred.

Second, this is a single-center study and the results may not be generalizable to other populations. Nevertheless, the main cause of ICU admission and the long-term mortality rate were consistent with previous studies (11, 35). Third, the confounders, such as diuretics prescription and the dose of vasopressors, cannot be assessed in this retrospective study although we have included variables such as RRT and the presence of shock in the regression model. Besides, we defined shock as a binomial variable although the presence of shock is not an on and off phenomenon. Fourth, we could not ascertain cause-of-death and data was presented as overall mortality. Fifth, we calculated CFB during ICU stay and did not include fluid management prior to ICU admission since fluid balance charting in the ward or emergency department might not be reliable (36). Given that bias could have resulted in underestimating the value of fluid overload, such a misclassification is more likely to influence the results toward the null hypothesis. Additionally, the individual physician made the decision of fluid therapy that could lead to a confounding effect. However, with dedicated intensivists and fluid management in accordance with the guidelines, it might partly mitigate the concern.

CONCLUSIONS

We linked two databases to address the long-term mortality association of fluid balance with the first week in critically ill patients. We found that patients with a positive CFB were independently associated with higher long-term mortality than those with a negative CFB. Patients with per one-liter increment of CFB 1–3 and CFB 4–7 significantly bore 4.7 and 9.4% risk odds of long-term mortality. Notably, we identified the role of a positive CFB 4–7 on long-term mortality in patients without shock or in those with severe AKI, indicating that CFB 4–7 might be a potentially modifiable factor to improve long-term outcomes. Further prospective studies focusing on both early fluid balance and post-acute fluid balance are warranted to validate our findings.

ETHICS STATEMENT

The studies involving human participants were reviewed and approved by the Institutional Review Board of Taichung Veterans General Hospital (TCVGH: SE20249B). The Ethics Committee waived the requirement of written informed consen for participation.

AUTHOR CONTRIBUTIONS

T-JW, C-HC, C-LW, and W-CC: study concept and design. C[t] LW: study coordination. T-JW, C-LW, K-CP, L-TW, M-SW, and W-CC: acquisition of data. K-CP, L-TW, C-ML, and W-CC: statistical analysis. T-JW, C-TH, C-HC, C-LW, and W-CC: interpretation of data. T-JW and W-CC: drafting the manuscript All authors read and approved the final manuscript.

REFERENCES

1. Finfer S, Myburgh J, Bellomo R. Intravenous fluid therapy in critically ill adults. *Nat Rev Nephrol.* (2018) 14:541–57. doi: 10.1038/s41581-018-0044-0
2. Hammond NE, Taylor C, Finfer SA-O, Machado FA-O, An Y, Billot LA-O, et al. Patterns of intravenous fluid resuscitation use in adult intensive care patients between 2007 and 2014: an international cross-sectional study. *PLoS ONE.* (2017) 12:e0176292. doi: 10.1371/journal.pone.0176292
3. Hatton GE, Du RE, Wei S, Harvin JA, Finkel KW, Wade CE, et al. Positive fluid balance and association with post-traumatic acute kidney injury. *J Am Coll Surg.* (2020) 230:190–9.e1. doi: 10.1016/j.jamcollsurg.2019.10.009
4. Boyd JH, Forbes J, Nakada TA, Walley KR, Russell JA. Fluid resuscitation in septic shock: a positive fluid balance and elevated central venous pressure are associated with increased mortality. *Crit Care Med.* (2011) 39:259–65. doi: 10.1097/CCM.0b013e3181feeb15
5. Wang M, Zhu B, Jiang L, Wen Y, Du B, Li W, et al. Dose-response association between fluid overload and in-hospital mortality in critically ill patients: a multicentre, prospective, observational cohort study. *BMJ Open.* (2020) 10:e039875. doi: 10.1136/bmjopen-2020-039875
6. Sakr Y, Rubatto Birri PN, Kotfis K, Nanchal R, Shah B, Kluge S, et al. Higher fluid balance increases the risk of death from sepsis: results from a large international audit. *Crit Care Med.* (2017) 45:386–94. doi: 10.1097/CCM.0000000000002189
7. Chao WC, Tseng CH, Chien YC, Sheu CC, Tsai MJ, Fang WF, et al. Association of day 4 cumulative fluid balance with mortality in critically ill patients with influenza: a multicenter retrospective cohort study in Taiwan. *PLoS ONE.* (2018) 13:e0190952. doi: 10.1371/journal.pone.0190952
8. Messmer AS, Zingg C, Muller M, Gerber JL, Schefold JC, Pfortmueller CA. Fluid Overload and mortality in adult critical care patients-a systematic review and meta-analysis of observational studies. *Crit Care Med.* (2020) 48:1862–70. doi: 10.1097/CCM.0000000000004617
9. Balakumar V, Murugan R, Sileanu FE, Palevsky P, Clermont G, Kellum JA. Both positive and negative fluid balance may be associated with reduced long-term survival in the critically ill. *Crit Care Med.* (2017) 45:e749–e57. doi: 10.1097/CCM.0000000000002372
10. Mohr NM, Zebrowski AM, Gaieski DF, Buckler DG, Carr BG. Inpatient hospital performance is associated with post-discharge sepsis mortality. *Crit Care.* (2020) 24:626. doi: 10.1186/s13054-020-03341-3
11. Gayat E, Cariou A, Deye N, Vieillard-Baron A, Jaber S, Damoisel C, et al. Determinants of long-term outcome in ICU survivors: results from the FROG-ICU study. *Crit Care.* (2018) 22:8. doi: 10.1186/s13054-017-1922-8
12. Shankar-Hari M, Harrison DA, Ferrando-Vivas P, Rubenfeld GD, Rowan K. Risk factors at index hospitalization associated with longer-term mortality in adult sepsis survivors. *JAMA Netw Open.* (2019) 2:e194900. doi: 10.1001/jamanetworkopen.2019.4900
13. Khwaja A. KDIGO clinical practice guidelines for acute kidney injury. *Nephron Clin Pract.* (2012) 120:c179–84. doi: 10.1159/000339789
14. Vincent JL, De Backer D. Circulatory shock. *N Engl J Med.* (2013) 369:1726–34. doi: 10.1056/NEJMra1208943
15. Wiedemann HP, Wheeler AP, Bernard GR, Thompson BT, Hayden D, deBoisblanc B, et al. Comparison of two fluid-management strategies in acute lung injury. *N Engl J Med.* (2006) 354:2564–75. doi: 10.1056/NEJMoa062200
16. Tigabu BM, Davari M, Kebriaeezadeh A, Mojtahedzadeh M. Fluid volume, fluid balance and patient outcome in severe sepsis and septic shock: a systematic review. *J Crit Care.* (2018) 48:153–9. doi: 10.1016/j.jcrc.2018.08.018
17. Acheampong A, Vincent JL. A positive fluid balance is an independent prognostic factor in patients with sepsis. *Crit Care.* (2015) 19:251. doi: 10.1186/s13054-015-0970-1

18. Dhondup T, Tien JC, Marquez A, Kennedy CC, Gajic O, Kashani KB. Association of negative fluid balance during the de-escalation phase of sepsis management with mortality: a cohort study. *J Crit Care.* (2020) 55:16–21. doi: 10.1016/j.jcrc.2019.09.025
19. Shankar-Hari M, Rubenfeld GD. Understanding long-term outcomes following sepsis: implications and challenges. *Curr Infect Dis Rep.* (2016) 18:37. doi: 10.1007/s11908-016-0544-7
20. Chawla LS, Bellomo R, Bihorac A, Goldstein SL, Siew ED, Bagshaw SM, et al. Acute kidney disease and renal recovery: consensus report of the acute disease quality initiative (ADQI) 16 workgroup. *Nat Rev Nephrol.* (2017) 13:241–57. doi: 10.1038/nrneph.2017.2
21. van Mourik N, Geerts BF, Binnekade JM, Veelo DP, Bos LDJ, Wiersinga WJ, et al. A higher fluid balance in the days after septic shock reversal is associated with increased mortality: an observational cohort study. *Crit Care Explor.* (2020) 2:e0219. doi: 10.1097/CCE.0000000000000219
22. Mitchell KH, Carlbom D, Caldwell E, Leary PJ, Himmelfarb J, Hough CL. Volume overload: prevalence, risk factors, and functional outcome in survivors of septic shock. *Ann Am Thorac Soc.* (2015) 12:1837–44. doi: 10.1513/AnnalsATS.201504-187OC
23. Huang AC, Lee TY, Ko MC, Huang CH, Wang TY, Lin TY, et al. Fluid balance correlates with clinical course of multiple organ dysfunction syndrome and mortality in patients with septic shock. *PLoS ONE.* (2019) 14:e0225423. doi: 10.1371/journal.pone.0225423
24. Wang N, Jiang L, Wen Y, Xi XM, Beijing Acute Kidney Injury Trial (BAKIT) Workgroup. Fluid balance and mortality in critically ill patients with acute kidney injury : a multicenter prospective epidemiological study. *Crit Care.* 19:371. doi: 10.1186/s13054-015-1085-4
25. Murugan R, Bellomo R, Palevsky PM, Kellum JA. Ultrafiltration in critically ill patients treated with kidney replacement therapy. *Nat Rev Nephrol.* (2021) 17:262–76. doi: 10.1038/s41581-020-00358-3
26. Heung M, Steffick DE, Zivin K, Gillespie BW, Banerjee T, Hsu C-y, et al. Acute kidney injury recovery pattern and subsequent risk of CKD: an analysis of veterans health administration data. *Am J Kidney Dis.* (2016) 67:742–52. doi: 10.1053/j.ajkd.2015.10.019
27. Vaara ST, Ostermann M, Bitker L, Schneider A, Poli E, Hoste E, et al. Restrictive fluid management versus usual care in acute kidney injury (REVERSE-AKI): a pilot randomized controlled feasibility trial. *Intensive Care Med.* (2021) 47:665–73. doi: 10.1007/s00134-021-06401-6
28. Bellomo R, Kellum JA, Ronco C, Wald R, Martensson J, Maiden M, et al. Acute kidney injury in sepsis. *Intensive Care Med.* (2017) 43:816–28. doi: 10.1007/s00134-017-4755-7
29. Jaffee W, Hodgins S, McGee WT. Tissue edema, fluid balance, and patient outcomes in severe sepsis: an organ systems review. *J Intensive Care Med.* (2018) 33:502–9. doi: 10.1177/0885066617742832
30. Juffermans NP, van den Brom CE, Kleinveld DJB. Targeting endothelial dysfunction in acute critical illness to reduce organ failure. *Anesth Analg.* (2020) 131:1708–20. doi: 10.1213/ANE.0000000000005023
31. Vignon P, Evrard B, Asfar P, Busana M, Calfee CS, Coppola S, et al. Fluid administration and monitoring in ARDS: which management? *Intensive Care Med.* (2020) 46:2252–64. doi: 10.1007/s00134-020-06310-0
32. Shen Y, Zhang W, Shen Y. Early diuretic use and mortality in critically ill patients with vasopressor support: a propensity score-matching analysis. *Crit Care.* (2019) 23:9. doi: 10.1186/s13054-019-2309-9
33. Bissell BD, Laine ME, Thompson Bastin ML, Flannery AH, Kelly A, Riser J, et al. Impact of protocolized diuresis for de-resuscitation in the intensive care unit. *Crit Care.* (2020) 24:70. doi: 10.1186/s13054-020-2795-9
34. Linden-Sonderso A, Jungner M, Spangfors M, Jan M, Oscarson A, Choi S, et al. Survey of non-resuscitation fluids administered during septic shock: a multicenter prospective observational study. *Ann Intensive Care.* (2019) 9:132. doi: 10.1186/s13613-019-0607-7
35. Mira JC, Gentile LF, Mathias BJ, Efron PA, Brakenridge SC, Mohr AM, et al. Sepsis pathophysiology, chronic critical illness, and persistent inflammation-immunosuppression and catabolism syndrome. *Crit Care Med.* (2017) 45:253–62. doi: 10.1097/CCM.0000000000002074
36. Wise LC, Mersch J, Racioppi J, Crosier J, Thompson C. Evaluating the reliability and utility of cumulative intake and output. *J Nurs Care Qual.* (2000) 14:37–42. doi: 10.1097/00001786-200004000-00005

21

Tools are Needed to Promote Sedation Practices for Mechanically Ventilated Patients

*Tao Wang [1], Dongxu Zhou [1], Zhongheng Zhang [2] and Penglin Ma [1]**

[1] Critical Care Medicine Department, Guiqian International General Hospital, Guiyang, China, [2] Department of Emergency Medicine, Sir Run Run Shaw Hospital, Zhejiang University School of Medicine, Hangzhou, China

***Correspondence:**
Penglin Ma
mapenglin1@163.com

Suboptimal sedation practices continue to be frequent, although the updated guidelines for management of pain, agitation, and delirium in mechanically ventilated (MV) patients have been published for several years. Causes of low adherence to the recommended minimal sedation protocol are multifactorial. However, the barriers to translation of these protocols into standard care for MV patients have yet to be analyzed. In our view, it is necessary to develop fresh insights into the interaction between the patients' responses to nociceptive stimuli and individualized regulation of patients' tolerance when using analgesics and sedatives. By better understanding this interaction, development of novel tools to assess patient pain tolerance and to define and predict oversedation or delirium may promote better sedation practices in the future.

Keywords: mechanical ventilation, suboptimal sedation, patient tolerability, assessment tools, sedation depth

INTRODUCTION

Mechanically ventilated (MV) patients can have a wide variety of discomforts resulting from multiple sources, including pathophysiological abnormalities (such as fever, hypoxia, and shock), emotional alterations (anxiety or fear), and intensive care procedures as well (such as non-physical ventilation, immobilization, frequent puncturing, and turning over, etc.) (1–4). Analgesics and sedatives are often used to maintain MV patients' comfort (5). In the last two decades, it has been observed that MV patients were deeply sedated very frequently in intensive care units (ICU) (6–8). Significantly, this behavior has been associated with poor outcomes, including prolonged duration of mechanical ventilation, increased incidence of ventilator associated pneumonia decline in cognitive ability, and even increased long-term mortality (6–10). Therefore, it has been strongly recommended to optimize sedation practices, such as implementing a light sedation protocol and the eCASH concept (early Comfort using Analgesia, minimal Sedatives and maximal Humane care) in MV patients (11, 12). Recently, more days without occurrence of coma or delirium were demonstrated in the patients receiving no sedation protocol than in those who were maintained at even light levels of sedation during the stay in the ICUs (13). These findings indicated that the lighter the level of sedation, the better outcomes would be for MV patients.

However, the frequency of deep sedation remains high in clinical practice based on recently published data from various studies (13–15), although a strong recommendation of minimizing sedation for MV patients has been published in the updated guidelines for several years. For instance, the mean depth of sedation was below RASS−2 (mean RASS = −2.3) on day 1 in the sedation group (i.e., the usual care arm) of Olsen's randomized control trial in ICUs where no sedation strategy was initiated 10 years ago (13, 16). It was previously recognized that the low adherence to a minimal sedation protocol was multifactorial, including inadequate assessments because of shortage of nurses, lack of multidisciplinary cooperation, and even misperception as well (17–20). However, the barriers to translating a minimal sedation protocol into standard care for MV patients are not well-defined. It is necessary to reveal fresh insight into the fact that the outcome favored minimal sedation protocol was poorly implemented in MV patients.

LIGHTLY SEDATED PATIENTS' TOLERANCE TO MECHANICAL VENTILATION

Lack of knowledge on patient intolerance to MV has been an important barrier to implementing a minimal sedation protocol in MV patients. Among the common signs of patient intolerance, agitation affected nearly half of ICU MV patients in previous reports (21, 22). Moreover, accumulating evidence has demonstrated that the risks of agitation or agitation-associated events were significantly increased while maintaining MV patients at light levels of sedation (usually defined as at levels of RASS from −2 to 1) (16, 23, 24). Notably, severe agitation has been associated with unplanned self-extubation, removal of important intralumenal tubes and vascular catheters, poor patient–ventilator synchrony, and increased morbidity, including PTSD (25–28). Accordingly, agitation or agitated adverse events have been of serious concern in most ICU nurses and physicians, which in turn has affected their willingness to implement light sedation practices in their routine clinical care (18, 29). In a nationwide cross-sectional survey, we also found that ICU physicians' perception of patients' tolerance to the support levels of ventilation with light sedation was highly varied across institutions. Importantly, their perceptions were largely translated into clinical practices (14). In addition, bolus administration of sedatives was usually given as a rescue intervention for agitation, which often led to unjustified deep sedation (18).

Actually, measurement of MV patients' tolerance (who are unable to communicate) remains problematic. Tools to evaluate patient tolerance or sedation depth in mechanical ventilation have evolved since the Ramsay sedation scale first used in 1974 as shown on **Table 1**. RASS offers broader discrimination in the mild-to-moderate sedation range. It is the most commonly used tool in clinical practice (41), and has demonstrated greater inter-rater reliability between clinical staff (37, 38, 42, 44). Therefore, frequent assessment of RASS has been strongly recommended to optimize the depth of sedation for MV patients and has been associated with improvement in outcomes (56). However, RASS, like other tools, is actually a transient result of patient tolerance to nociceptive stimuli as regulated by the infused analgesics and sedatives in MV. It is not a scale to directly assess the intensity of stimuli that patients experience instantaneously. Being complementary to RASS, the pain assessment tools such as Behavioral Pain Score (BPS) or Clinical Pain Observation Tool (CPOT) were suggested to improve the overall assessment of comfort of critically ill patients. However, the intensity of nociceptive stimuli might change over time because of occurrence of fever, thirst, drainage tube pain, or intestinal colic, etc., that would raise the risk of patient intolerance to MV (or vice versa). No matter how frequent the RASS assessment is, titration of analgesics and sedatives always lags behind patient intolerance (or oversedation), which partially at least accounts for frequent and unpredictable agitation. In fact, there is a lack of reliable criteria to scale responses to the stimuli that patients experience during MV. Accordingly, it is difficult for ICU physicians to properly estimate the intensity of patients' responses as well as their tolerance when patients are lightly sedated, which might be an important source of suboptimal sedation practices.

Burk et al. (26) previously reported several predictors of agitation within 24 h in adult critically ill patients, including Sequential Organ Failure Assessment score, $PaO_2/FiO_2 < 200$ mmHg, receiving MV, using restraints, etc. Based on the variables relating to fever, ventilator settings, alterations in respiratory physiology, and dosage of sedatives and analgesics, our study group recently developed an ensemble model for the prediction of agitation in invasive MV patients under light sedation (57). The model showed good calibration and discrimination in an independent dataset. However, the effectiveness of interventions based on the prediction model need to be investigated in further experimental trials. These findings indicate that agitation (i.e., severe patient intolerance in MV) is predictable by evaluating variables related to nocioceptive stimuli. Thus, development of a tool for evaluating the balance between the intensity of stimuli and patient tolerance when analgesics and sedatives are used is needed to implement a minimal sedation protocol in the future.

RECOGNITION, ESTIMATION, AND PREVENTION OF OVERSEDATION IN MV PATIENTS

Suboptimal sedation practices include both oversedation and undersedation. In the literature, numerous studies have shown that deep sedation continues to be common in the ICU (8, 9, 13–15). Generally, it has been recognized that deep sedation (below RASS−2) remains relevant only for the management of some situations in MV patients, such as severe acute respiratory distress syndrome with ventilator–patient asynchrony or with use of neuromuscular blocking agents, severe brain injury with intracranial hypertension, status epilepticus, etc. (58–61). For the vast majority of ICU MV patients, deep sedation is unnecessary and should be avoided (62). Oversedation is therefore suspected when MV patients are sedated at the depths below RASS−2. However, this concept is mainly based on expert opinions rather than empirical evidence, which is misleading for appropriate sedation practices. For instance, sedatives could be overused while maintaining the level of sedation at RASS−2 for MV patients ready for weaning. On the other hand, the sedation depth at RASS−3 (or even the deeper levels) might be necessary for acute critically ill patients with multiple organ dysfunction caused by aggressive inflammatory responses (63, 64). In fact, no consensus on the definitions of deep sedation and oversedation is available because of gaps in the evidence. There is a dearth of information regarding the interaction among sedative choice,

TABLE 1 | Tools for assessment of sedation depth or pain in mechanically ventilated patients.

Tools	Describe	Advantage	Disadvantage	Clinical studies	
				Comparator	**Findings**
RSS Dawson et al. (30)	The RSS is a single-item tool to measure consciousness across three levels in critically ill patients who are awake and three levels in patients who are judged to be asleep (31).	The earliest and the most widely used scale (32).	Use of a single item to assess two or more different aspects of sedation can lead to loss of clinically important information and systematic or random measurement error (33).	SAS (33)	No difference was found in validity between two scales
NICS Mirski et al. (34)	The NICS is a simpler, more intuitive sedation scale that is both easy to use and recall and favored by nurses as a sedation communication tool (34).	NICS ranked highest in nursing preference and ease of communication and may thus permit more effective and interactive management of sedation (34).	Subjective.	• RASS • RSS • SAS	NICS is a valid and reliable sedation scale for use in a mixed population of intensive care unit patients (34).
SAS Mirski et al. (34)	The SAS is a single-item seven point scale developed by Riker and colleagues and commonly used within ICU (35).	Both reliable and valid (36)	Not suitable for patients with hearing impairment, nerve damage, and hemiplegia (37)	RSS (33, 38)	• The SAS provides additional information by stratifying agitation into three categories without sacrificing validity or reliability (33). • The SAS showed the best correlation and the best agreement results in all professional categories (38).
ATIC De Jonghe et al. (39)	The ATICE consists of five items: Awakeness and Comprehension combined in a Consciousness domain, and Calmness, Ventilator Synchrony, and Face Relaxation combined in a Tolerance domain (39).	Evaluates sedation and tolerance; longitudinal validity demonstrated; explicit instructions provided (39).	Studied in medical patients; only properties may differ in surgical population; more complex scoring method-requires (39).	• RASS • RSS • SAS	Offers assessment of tolerance to the ICU environment;longitudinal validity demonstrated (39).
RASS Sessler et al. (40)	The RASS is a single-item scale that has 10 levels of response, which range from minus five to plus four.	Longitudinal validity demonstrated in diverse patient. It offers broader discrimination in the mild-to-moderate sedation range (41, 42).	If there are visual or auditory obstacles, it will affect the accuracy of the evaluation results (43) physical stimulation can increase anxiety of patient.	• RSS (34, 38, 41, 44, 45) • SAS (34, 37, 41) • MAAS (34)	• The RASS correlated more highly with BIS compared to RSS (39), and demonstrated greater inter-rater reliability between clinical staff compared to RSS and SAS (37, 38, 42, 44). • The RASS showed high levels of reliance and ease of use in scoring and communicating sedation, agitation and intuitiveness, compared to the RSS, MAAS, and SAS (34).
BIS Watson and Kane-Gill (46)	The BIS measures the level of sedation by integrating information from the electroencephalography and a mathematical technique referred to as bispectral analysis (46).	Offers objective monitoring; offers continuous monitoring; Continuous monitoring (47)	Variability; conflicting ICU validity results; muscle activity alters values; Unable to distinguish between natural sleep and drug-induced sleep (48).	• RASS • RSS • SAS • ATICE • MAAS	The BIS monitor has potential benefits in the ICU environment, although optimal use requires further investigation (46).
MAAS Devlin et al. (49)	The MAAS is also a single-item tool with seven response-defined categories of behavior, which originated from the SAS and is therefore structurally similar to the SAS (49).	The MAAS was superior to the LSS based upon the observation that MAAS scores were less variable (50).	There is insufficient evidence to warrant use of the MAAS as a new method of evaluating critically ill patients requiring sedation in the emergency department (50).	LSS (50)	The MAAS is a valid and reliable sedation scale for use with mechanically ventilated patients in the SICU (49).

(Continued)

TABLE 1 | Continued

Tools	Describe	Advantage	Disadvantage	Clinical studies	
				Comparator	**Findings**
BPS Payen et al. (51)	The BPS was based on a sum score of three items: facial expression, movements of upper limbs, and compliance with mechanical ventilation (51).	• Higher reliability shown for the muscular domain (52). Simplicity, easiness; Descriptors clear or precise (53).	• Discriminant validation seems less satisfactory in sedated or agitated patients (52). • Less specific (53).	CPOT	Both CPOT and the BPS showed good reliability and validity and were good options for assessing pain during painful procedures with intensive care unit patients unable to self-report on pain (54).
CPOT Gélinas et al. (55)	The CPOT scale includes four behavioral indicators:facial expression;body movements;muscle tension; and compliance with the ventilator (for intubated patients) or verbalization (for extubated patients) (55).	• Have particularly good reliability and validity in assessing pain during procedures (54). • Descriptors more detailed; Descriptors better described (53).	• Discriminant validation seems less satisfactory in sedated or agitated patients (52). • Descriptors less well-detailed or confusing (53).	BPS	Because of the discriminant validation, the CPOT is to be preferred (54).

SAS, Ramsay Sedation Scale; SAS, Riker Sedation-Agitation Scale; RASS, Richmond Agitation Sedation Scale; AITCE, Adaptation to the Intensive Care Environment; NICS, Nursing instrument for the communication of sedation; BIS, Bispectral index; LSS, Luer Sedation Scale; BPS, Behavioral Pain Scale.

sedation depth, and patient-specific factors that affect outcomes (65). Therefore, determining optimal sedation and oversedation in MV patients remains challenging.

Ambiguity in definition is an important barrier to the development of protocols to prevent oversedation in practice. Previously, the ABCDEF bundle (Assess, prevent, and manage pain; Both spontaneous awakening and breathing trials; Choice of analgesia and sedation; Delirium assess, prevent, and manage; Early mobility and exercise; Family engagement/empowerment) was developed to promote appropriate sedation practices by creating a safe and comfortable environment for MV patients (66). Although reduction in the rate of deep sedation and improvement in outcomes were demonstrated in patients who did receive more of the bundle elements each day, the major limitation was low adherence in clinical practice because of too many unresolved issues involved in this protocol (67). A novel sedation-monitoring technology (the Responsiveness Index, RI) based on facial electromyography was developed to provide an alert for possible deep sedation. Results showed that use of the monitor increased optimal sedation-analgesia quality but just by 7% (68). Results from the AWARE study (69) revealed that by decreasing use of intravenous hypnotics, the oversedation prevention protocol was feasible in clinical practice and resulted in a significantly earlier time to spontaneous breathing trial and reduced duration of mechanical ventilation (69). However, mortality was not significantly different between the study group and the control group. It should be interpreted with caution that the rate of oversedation or deep sedation was prevented in this study. Therefore, a precision definition is fundamental for development of a reliable scale for estimation as well as an effective protocol for prevention of oversedation in MV patients.

DELIRIUM PREDICTION

Delirium is a well-established syndrome in the ICU that is considered to be an acute onset of brain dysfunction (70). There are two motor subtypes of delirium that are categorized according to its clinical presentation, namely, the hyperactive and hypoactive subtypes (71, 72). The primary presentation of hyperactive delirium is agitation, which is reported to occur in many ICU patients (26). Although agitated delirium is found to be less harmful than the hypoactive type with respect to 12-month mortality (72, 73), potential serious consequences of agitation as opposed to its hypoactive counterpart, mentioned above included medical device removal (such as urinary catheter, venous or arterial line, or surgical drain), falling out of bed, immobilization device removal, or self-aggression or aggression toward medical staff (25–28, 74). Thus, the prediction and appropriate prevention of agitated delirium is of paramount importance in the management of MV patients.

The mechanism of delirium remains unclear (75). Risk factors for delirium include illness-related acute pathophysiological abnormalities (e.g., hypotension, acidosis, hypoxia, and sepsis), environmental factors (e.g., lighting, alarm sounds, and noise); and iatrogenic harm (e.g., frequent suctions, puncture, immobilization, and even use of analgesic and sedative drugs) (76–79). Among these, there are potentially modifiable risk factors, for example, minimizing sedation and benzodiazepine use (80). Significantly, numerous studies have reported that patients receiving deep sedation were more susceptible to post-traumatic stress disorder syndrome, ICU memory disorder, and delirium (81, 82). On the other hand, two recently published meta-analyses revealed that delirium occurred more frequently in the light than in the deep sedation group of MV patients (24, 83). Because of multiple etiologies, therefore, prediction and prevention of delirium remains problematic.

Some prediction models have been developed for delirium, but limitations remain. For example, the prediction model for delirium (PRE-DELIRIC) and early prediction model for delirium (E-PRE-DELIRIC) were initially developed in a single hospital and validated in four hospitals (84). However, the discriminatory ability of these models in an external dataset was less than satisfactory (area under curve: 0.68–0.79, respectively) (85–87). These studies are limited in several aspects. First, previous studies typically used variables collected on the day of ICU admission, and the delirium event may happen several days later. Some physiological variables change significantly in this interval. Second, there is no model to specifically predict hypoactive delirium. Third, previous models were usually developed in a single center, which partly explains the models' suboptimal performance in an external dataset. Foruth, the previous models were developed as generalized linear models that failed to capture higher- order and interaction terms between predictors. Therefore, a novel delirium prediction model is needed for MV patients.

CONCLUSION

Suboptimal sedation practices are common, which are largely attributable to the evidence gaps concerning the intensity of nociceptive stimuli that patients experience and patients' tolerance and its treatment by using analgesics and sedatives. Development of novel tools to assess patient tolerance and to define and predict oversedation or delirium are needed to implement better sedation practices in the future.

AUTHOR CONTRIBUTIONS

TW and PM were the major contributors in writing the manuscript. DZ and ZZ helped to revise the manuscript. PM critically reviewed the manuscript and agreed with the final version. All authors read and approved the submitted manuscript.

REFERENCES

1. Ma P, Liu J, Xi X, Du B, Yuan X, Lin H, et al. Practice of sedation and the perception of discomfort during mechanical ventilation in chinese intensive care units. *J Crit Care.* (2010) 3:451–7. doi: 10.1016/j.jcrc.2009.11.006
2. Puntillo KA, Max A, Timsit JF, Vignoud L, Chanques G, Robleda G, et al. Determinants of procedural pain intensity in the intensive care unit. the Europain® study. *Am J Respir Crit Care Med.* (2014) 189:39–47. doi: 10.1164/rccm
3. Samuelson KA, Lundberg D, Fridlund B. Stressful experiences in relation to depth of sedation in mechanically ventilated patients. *Nurs Crit Care.* (2007) 12:93–104. doi: 10.1111/j.1478-5153.2006.00199.x
4. Weinert CR, Calvin AD. Epidemiology of sedation and sedation adequacy for mechanically ventilated patients in a medical and surgical intensive care unit. *Crit Care Med.* (2007) 35:393–401. doi: 10.1097/01.CCM.0000254339.18639.1D
5. Jacobi J, Fraser GL, Coursin DB, Riker RR, Fontaine D, Wittbrodt ET, et al. Clinical practice guidelines for the sustained use of sedatives and analgesics in the critically ill adult. *Crit Care Med.* (2002) 30:119–41. doi: 10.1097/00003246-200201000-00020
6. Shehabi Y, Chan L, Kadiman S, Alias A, Ismail WN, Tan MA, et al. Sedation depth and long-term mortality in mechanically ventilated critically ill adults: a prospective longitudinal multicentre cohort study. *Intensive Care Med.* (2013) 39:910–8. doi: 10.1007/s00134-013-2830-2
7. Tanaka LM, Azevedo LC, Park M, Schettino G, Nassar AP, Réa-Neto A, et al. Early sedation and clinical outcomes of mv patients: a prospective multicenter cohort study. *Crit Care.* (2014) 18:R156. doi: 10.1186/cc13995
8. Balzer F, Weiß B, Kumpf O, Treskatsch S, Spies C, Wernecke KD, et al. Early deep sedation is associated with decreased in-hospital and two-year follow-up survival. *Crit Care.* (2015) 19:197. doi: 10.1186/s13054-015-0929-2
9. Shehabi Y, Bellomo R, Kadiman S, Ti LK, Howe B, Reade MC, et al. Sedation intensity in the first 48 hours of mechanical ventilation and 180-day mortality: a multinational prospective longitudinal cohort study. *Crit Care Med.* (2018) 46:850–9. 03071. doi: 10.1097/CCM.0000000000003071
10. Girard TD, Kress JP, Fuchs BD, Thomason JW, Schweickert WD, Pun BT. Efficacy and safety of a paired sedation and ventilator weaning protocol for MV patients in intensive care (awakening and breathing controlled trial): a randomised controlled trial. *Lancet.* (2008) 371:126–34. doi: 10.1016/S0140-6736(08)60105-1
11. Barr J, Fraser GL, Puntillo K, Ely EW, Gélinas C, Dasta JF, et al. Clinical practice guidelines for the management of pain, agitation, and delirium in adult patients in the intensive care unit. *Crit Care Med.* (2013) 41:263–306. doi: 10.1097/CCM.0b013e3182783b72
12. Vincent JL, Shehabi Y, Walsh TS, Pandharipande PP, Ball JA, Spronk P. Comfort and patient-centred care without excessive sedation: the ecash concept. *Intensive Care Med.* (2016) 42:962–71. doi: 10.1007/s00134-016-4297-4
13. Olsen HT, Nedergaard HK, Strøm T, Oxlund J, Wian KA, Ytrebø LM, et al. Nonsedation or light sedation in critically ill, mechanically ventilated patients. *N Engl J Med.* (2020) 382:1103–11. doi: 10.1056/NEJMoa1906759
14. Gong Y, Yang H, Xie J, Liu J, Zhou J, Ma P. ICU physicians' perception of patients' tolerance levels in light sedation impacts sedation practice for mechanically ventilated patients. *Front Med.* (2019) 6:226. doi: 10.3389/fmed.2019.00226
15. Fuller BM, Roberts BW, Mohr NM, Knight WA 4th, Adeoye O, Pappal RD, et al. The ED-SED study: a multicenter, prospective cohort study of practice patterns and clinical outcomes associated with emergency department sedation for mechanically ventilated patients. *Crit Care Med.* (2019) 47:1539–48. doi: 10.1097/CCM.0000000000003928
16. Strom T, Martnussen T, Toft P. A protocol of no sedation for critically ill patients receiving mechanical ventilation: a randomised trial. *Lancet.* (2010) 375:475–80. doi: 10.1016/S0140-6736(09)62072-9
17. Jackson DL, Proudfoot CW, Cann KF, Walsh TS. The incidence of sub-optimal sedation in the ICU: a systematic review. *Crit Care.* (2009) 13:R204. doi: 10.1186/cc8212
18. Mehta S, McCullagh, Burry L. Current sedation practices: lessons learned from international surveys. *Anesthesiol Clin.* (2011) 29:607–24. doi: 10.1016/j.anclin.2011.09.003

19. Peitz GJ, Balas MC, Olsen KM, Pun BT, Ely EW. Top 10 myths regarding sedation and delirium in the ICU. *Crit Care Med.* (2013) 41(Suppl. 1):S46–56. doi: 10.1097/CCM.0b013e3182a168f5
20. Sneyers B, Laterre PF, Perreault MM, Wouters D, Spinewine A. current practices and barriers impairing physicians' and nurses' adherence to analgo-sedation recommendations in the intensive care unit–a national survey. *Crit Care.* (2014) 18:655. doi: 10.1186/s13054-014-0655-1
21. Jaber S, Chanques G, Altairac C, Sebbane M, Vergne C, Perrigault PF, et al. A prospective study of agitation in a medical-surgical ICU: incidence, risk factors, and outcomes. *Chest.* (2005) 128:2749–57. doi: 10.1378/chest.128.4.2749
22. Woods JC, Mion LC, Connor JT, Viray F, Jahan L, Huber C, et al. Severe agitation among ventilated medical intensive care unit patients: frequency, characteristics and outcomes. *Intensive Care Med.* (2004) 30:1066–72. doi: 10.1007/s00134-004-2193-9
23. Long L, Ren S, Gong Y, Zhao H, He C, Shen L, et al. Different depths of sedation versus risk of delirium in adult mechanically ventilated patients: a systematic review and meta-analysis. *PLoS ONE.* (2020) 15:e0236014. doi: 10.1371/journal.pone.0236014
24. Shehabi Y, Bellomo R, Reade MC, Bailey M, Bass F, Howe B. Early goal-directed sedation versus standard sedation in MV critically Ill patients: a pilot study. *Crit Care Med.* (2013) 41:1983–91. doi: 10.1097/CCM.0b013e31828a437d
25. Carrión MI, Ayuso D, Marcos M, Paz Robles M, de la Cal MA, Alía I, et al. Accidental removal of endotracheal and nasogastric tubes and intravascular catheters. *Crit Care Med.* (2000) 28:63–6. doi: 10.1097/00003246-200001000-00010
26. Burk RS, Grap MJ, Munro CL, Schubert CM, Sessler CN. Predictors of agitation in critically ill adults. *Am J Crit Care.* (2014) 23:414–23. doi: 10.4037/ajcc2014714
27. Chevrolet JC, Jolliet P. Clinical review: agitation and delirium in the critically ill–significance and management. *Crit Care.* (2007) 11:214. doi: 10.1186/cc5787
28. De Bels D, Honore PM, Redant S. Nonsedation or light sedation in critically ill, mechanically ventilated patients. *N Engl J Med.* (2020) 382:e107. doi: 10.1056/NEJMc2011055
29. Rose L, Fitzgerald E, Cook D, Kim S, Steinberg M, Devlin JW, et al. Clinician perspectives on protocols designed to minimize sedation. *J Crit Care.* (2015) 30:348–52. doi: 10.1016/j.jcrc.2014.10.021
30. Dawson R, von Fintel N, Nairn S. Sedation assessment using the Ramsay scale. *Emerg Nurse.* (2010) 18:18–20. doi: 10.7748/en2010.06.18.3.18.c7825
31. Némethy M, Paroli L, Williams-Russo PG, Blanck T. Assessing sedation with regional anesthesia [sic]: inter-rater agreement on a modified Wilson Sedation Scale. *Anesth Analg.* (2002) 94:723–8. doi: 10.1097/00000539-200203000-00045
32. Peck M, Down J. Use of sedatives in the critically ill. *Anaesth Intensive Care Med.* (2010) 11:12–15. doi: 10.1016/j.mpaic.2009.10.007
33. De Jonghe B, Cook D, Appere-De-Vecchi C, Guyatt G, Meade M, Outin H. Using and understanding sedation scoring systems: a systematic review. *Intensive Care Med.* (2000) 26:275–85. doi: 10.1007/s001340051150
34. Mirski MA, LeDroux SN, Lewin JJ III, Thompson CB, Mirski KT, Griswold M. Validity and reliability of an intuitive conscious sedation scoring tool: the nursing instrument for the communication of sedation. *Crit Care Med.* (2010) 38:1674–84. doi: 10.1097/CCM.0b013e3181e7c73e
35. Riker R, Fraser G, Cox P. Continuous infusion of haloperidol controls agitation in critically ill patients. *Crit Care Med.* (1994) 22:433–40. doi: 10.1097/00003246-199403000-00013
36. Riker RR, Picard JT, Fraser GL. Prospective evaluation of the Sedation-Agitation Scale for adult critically ill patients. *Crit Care Med.* (1999) 27:1325–9. doi: 10.1097/00003246-199907000-00022
37. Ryder-Lewis M, Nelson K. Reliability of the Sedation-Agitation Scale between nurses and doctors. *Intensive Crit Care Nurs.* (2008) 24:211–7. doi: 10.1016/j.iccn.2007.11.004
38. Nassar Junior AP, Pires Neto RC, de Figueiredo WB, Park M. Validity, reliability and applicability of Portuguese versions of sedation-agitation scales among critically ill patients. *Sáo Paulo Med J.* (2008) 126:215–9. doi: 10.1590/S1516-31802008000400003
39. De Jonghe B, Cook D, Griffith L, Appere-de-Vecchi C, Guyatt G, Théron V, et al. Adaptation to the Intensive Care Environment (ATICE): development and validation of a new sedation assessment instrument. *Crit Care Med.* (2003) 31:2344–54. doi: 10.1097/01.CCM.0000084850.16444.94
40. Sessler CN, Grap MJ, Brophy GM. Multidisciplinary management of sedation and analgesia in critical care. *Semin Respir Crit Care Med.* (2001) 22:211–25. doi: 10.1055/s-2001-13834
41. Sessler CN, Gosnell MS, Grap MJ, Brophy GM, O'Neal PV, Keane KA, et al. The richmond agitation-sedation scale: validity and reliability in adult intensive care unit patients. *Am J Respir Crit Care Med.* (2002) 166:1338–44. doi: 10.1164/rccm.2107138
42. Ely EW, Truman B, Shintani A, Thomason JWW, Wheeler AP, Gordon S, et al. Monitoring sedation status over time in I.C.U. patients: reliability validity of the Richmond Agitation-Sedation Scale (RASS). *JAMA.* (2003) 289:2983–91. doi: 10.1001/jama.289.22.2983
43. Vincent JL, Takala J, Moreno RP, Sakr Y, Marshall JC. The Richmond Agitation-Sedation Scale should not be used to evaluate neurologic function. *Crit Care Med.* (2016) 44:e450. doi: 10.1097/CCM.0000000000001597
44. Brandl K, Langley K, Riker R, Dork L, Qualis C, Levy H. Confirming the reliability of the sedation-agitation scale administered by ICU nurses without experience in its use. *Pharmcotherapy.* (2001) 21:431–6. doi: 10.1592/phco.21.5.431.34487
45. Deogaonkar A, Gupta R, Degeorgia M, Sabharwal V, Gopakumaran B, Schubert A, et al. Bispectral Index monitoring correlates with sedation scales in brain-injure patients. *Crit Care Med.* (2004) 32:2403–6. doi: 10.1097/01.CCM.0000147442.14921.A5
46. Watson BD, Kane-Gill SL. Sedation assessment in critically ill adults: 2001–2004 update. *Ann Pharmacother.* (2004) 38:1898–906. doi: 10.1345/aph.1E167
47. Consales G, Chelazzi C, Rinaldi S, De Gaudio AR. Bispectral Index compared to Ramsay score for sedation monitoring in intensive care units. *Minerva Anestesiol.* (2006) 72:329–36. doi: 10.1111/mec.12739
48. Burjek NE, Wagner CE, Hollenbeck RD, Wang L, Yu C, McPherson JA, et al. Early bispectral index and sedation requirements during therapeutic hypothermia predict neurologic recovery following cardiac arrest. *Crit Care Med.* (2014) 42:1204–12. doi: 10.1097/CCM.0000000000000126
49. Devlin J, Boleski G, Mlynarek M, Narenz D, Peterson E, JankowskiM, et al. Motor activity assessment scale: a valid and reliable sedation scale for use with mechanically ventilated patients in an adult surgical intensive care unit. *Crit Care Med.* (1999) 27:1271–5. doi: 10.1097/00003246-199907000-00008
50. Varndell W, Elliott D, Fry M. The validity, reliability, responsiveness and applicability of observation sedation-scoring instruments for use with adult patients in the emergency department: a systematic literature review. *Australas Emerg Nurs J.* (2015) 18:1–23. doi: 10.1016/j.aenj.2014.07.001
51. Payen JF, Bru O, Bosson JL, Lagrasta A, Novel E, Deschaux I, et al. Assessing pain in critically ill sedated patients by using a behavioral pain scale. *Crit Care Med.* (2001) 29:2258–63. doi: 10.1097/00003246-200112000-00004
52. Rijkenberg S, Stilma W, Bosman RJ, van der Meer NJ, van der Voort PHJ. Pain measurement in mechanically ventilated patients after cardiac surgery: comparison of the Behavioral Pain Scale (BPS) and the Critical-Care Pain Observation Tool (CPOT). *J Cardiothorac Vasc Anesth.* (2017) 31:1227–34. doi: 10.1053/j.jvca.2017.03.013
53. Chanques G, Pohlman A, Kress JP, Molinari N, de Jong A, Jaber S, et al. Psychometric comparison of three behavioural scales for the assessment of pain in critically ill patients unable to self-report. *Crit Care.* (2014) 18:R160. doi: 10.1186/cc14000
54. Birkedal HC, Larsen MH, Steindal SA, Solberg MT. Comparison of two behavioural pain scales for the assessment of procedural pain: a systematic review. *Nurs Open.* (2021) 8:2050–60. doi: 10.1002/nop2.714
55. Gélinas C, Fillion L, Puntillo KA, Viens C, Fortier M. Validation of the critical-care pain observation tool in adult patients. *Am J Crit Care.* (2006) 15:420–7. doi: 10.4037/ajcc2006.15.4.420
56. Qi Z, Yang S, Qu J, Li M, Zheng J, Huang R, et al. Effect of nurse-led sedation protocols on mechanically ventilated intensive care adults: a systematic review and meta-analysis. *Aust Crit Care.* (2021) 34:278–86. doi: 10.1016/j.aucc.2020.07.013
57. Zhang Z, Liu J, Xi J, Gong Y, Zeng L, Ma P. Derivation and validation of an ensemble model for the prediction of agitation in mechanically ventilated

patients maintained under light sedation. *Crit Care Med.* (2021) 49:e279–90. doi: 10.1097/CCM.0000000000004821

58. Papazian L, Forel JM, Gacouin A, Penot-Ragon C, Perrin G, Loundou A, et al. Neuromuscular blockers in early acute respiratory distress syndrome. *N Engl J Med.* (2010) 363:1107–16. doi: 10.1056/NEJMoa1005372
59. Luauté J, Plantier D, Wiart L, Tell L, SOFMER group. Care management of the agitation or aggressiveness crisis in patients with TBI. Systematic review of the literature and practice recommendations. *Ann Phys Rehabil Med.* (2016) 59:58–67. doi: 10.1016/j.rehab.2015.11.001
60. Brophy GM, Bell R, Claassen J, Alldredge B, Bleck TP, Glauser T, et al. Guidelines for the evaluation and management of status epilepticus. *Neurocrit Care.* (2012) 17:3–23. doi: 10.1007/s12028-012-9695-z
61. Devlin JW, Skrobik Y, Gélinas C, Needham DM, Slooter AJC, Pandharipande PP, et al. Clinical practice guidelines for the prevention and management of pain, agitation/sedation, delirium, immobility, and sleep disruption in adult patients in the ICU. *Crit Care Med.* (2018) 46:e825–73. doi: 10.1097/CCM.0000000000003299
62. Temesgen N, Chekol B, Tamirie T, Eshetie D, Simeneh N, Feleke A. Adult sedation and analgesia in a resource limited intensive care unit– a systematic review and evidence based guideline. *Ann Med Surg.* (2021) 66:102356. doi: 10.1016/j.amsu.2021.102356
63. Qiu HB. [Disease-specific analgesia and sedation in critically ill patients]. *Zhonghua Nei Ke Za Zhi.* (2013) 52:279–81. doi: 10.1157/13063183
64. Page V, McKenzie C. Sedation in the intensive care unit. *Curr Anesthesiol Rep.* (2021) 11:92–100. doi: 10.1007/s40140-021-00446-5
65. Shehabi Y, Howe B, Bellomo R, Arabi YM, Bailey M, Bass FE, et al. Early sedation with dexmedetomidine in critically ill patients. *N Engl J Med.* (2019) 380:2506–17. doi: 10.1056/NEJMoa1904710
66. Marra A, Ely EW, Pandharipande PP, Patel MB. The ABCDEF bundle in critical care. *Crit Care Clin.* (2017) 2:225–43. doi: 10.1016/j.ccc.2016.12.005
67. Pun BT, Balas MC, Barnes-Daly MA, Thompson JL, Aldrich JM, Barr J, et al. Caring for critically ill patients with the ABCDEF bundle: results of the ICU liberation collaborative in over 15,000 adults. *Crit Care Med.* (2019) 47:3–14. doi: 10.1097/CCM.0000000000003482
68. Walsh TS, Kydonaki K, Antonelli J, Stephen J, Lee RJ, Everingham K, et al. Development and Evaluation of Strategies to Improve Sedation Practice in Intensive Care (DESIST) study investigators. staff education, regular sedation and analgesia quality feedback, and a sedation monitoring technology for improving sedation and analgesia quality for critically ill, mechanically ventilated patients: a cluster randomised trial. *Lancet Respir Med.* (2016) 4:807–17. doi: 10.1016/S2213-2600(16)30178-3
69. SRLF Trial Group. Impact of oversedation prevention in ventilated critically ill patients: a randomized trial-the AWARE study. *Ann Intensive Care.* (2018) 8:93. doi: 10.1186/s13613-018-0425-3
70. Salluh JI, Soares M, Teles JM, Ceraso D, Raimondi N, Nava VS, et al. Delirium Epidemiology in Critical Care (DECCA): an international study. *Crit Care.* (2010) 14:R210. doi: 10.1186/cc9333
71. Krewulak KD, Stelfox HT, Leigh JP, Ely EW, Fiest KM. Incidence and prevalence of delirium subtypes in an adult ICU: a systematic review and meta-analysis. *Crit Care Med.* (2018) 46:2029–35. doi: 10.1097/CCM.0000000000003402
72. Krewulak KD, Stelfox HT, Ely EW, Fiest KM. Risk factors and outcomes among delirium subtypes in adult ICUs: a systematic review. *J Crit Care.* (2020) 56:257–64. doi: 10.1016/j.jcrc.2020.01.017
73. Avelino-Silva TJ, Campora F, Curiati JAE, Jacob-Filho W. Prognostic effects of delirium motor subtypes in hospitalized older adults: a prospective cohort study. *PLoS ONE.* (2018) 13:e0191092. doi: 10.1371/journal.pone.0191092
74. Vourc'h M, Feuillet F, Mahe PJ, Sebille V, Asehnoune K, BACLOREA trial group. Baclofen to prevent agitation in alcohol-addicted patients in the ICU: study protocol for a randomised controlled trial. *Trials.* (2016) 17:415. doi: 10.1186/s13063-016-1539-2
75. Reade MC, Finfer S. Sedation and delirium in the intensive care unit. *N Engl J Med.* (2014) 370:444–54. doi: 10.1056/NEJMra1208705
76. Hsieh SJ, Ely EW, Gong MN. Can intensive care unit delirium be prevented and reduced? lessons learned and future directions. *Ann Am Thorac Soc.* (2013) 10:648–56. doi: 10.1513/AnnalsATS.201307-232FR
77. Van Rompaey B, Elseviers MM, Schuurmans MJ, Shortridge-Baggett LM, Truijen S, Bossaert L. Risk factors for delirium in intensive care patients: a prospective cohort study. *Crit Care.* (2009) 13:R77. doi: 10.1186/cc7892
78. Zaal IJ, Spruyt CF, Peelen LM, van Eijk MM, Wientjes R, Schneider MM, et al. Intensive care unit environment may affect the course of delirium. *Intensive Care Med.* (2013) 39:481–8. doi: 10.1007/s00134-012-2726-6
79. Girard TD, Ware LB, Bernard GR, Pandharipande PP, Thompson JL, Shintani AK, et al. Associations of markers of inflammation and coagulation with delirium during critical illness. *Intensive Care Med.* (2012) 38:1965–73. doi: 10.1007/s00134-012-2678-x
80. Zaal IJ, Devlin JW, Peelen LM, Slooter AJ. A systematic review of risk factors for delirium in the ICU. *Crit Care Med.* (2015) 43:40–7. doi: 10.1097/CCM.0000000000000625
81. Treggiari MM, Romand JA, Yanez ND, Deem SA, Goldberg J, Hudson L, et al. Randomized trial of light versus deep sedation on mental health after critical illness. *Crit Care Med.* (2009) 37:2527–34. doi: 10.1097/CCM.0b013e3181a5689f
82. Sieber FE, Zakriya KJ, Gottschalk A, Blute MR, Lee HB, Rosenberg PB, et al. Sedation depth during spinal anesthesia and the development of postoperative delirium in elderly patients undergoing hip fracture repair. *Mayo Clin Proc.* (2010) 85:18–26. doi: 10.4065/mcp.2009.0469
83. Stephens RJ, Dettmer MR, Roberts BW, Ablordeppey E, Fowler SA, Kollef MH, et al. Practice patterns and outcomes associated with early sedation depth in mechanically ventilated patients: a systematic review and meta-analysis. *Crit Care Med.* (2018) 46:471–9. doi: 10.1097/CCM.0000000000002885
84. van den Boogaard M, Pickkers P, Slooter AJ, Kuiper MA, Spronk PE, van der Voort PH, et al. Development and validation of PRE-DELIRIC (PREdiction of DELIRium in ICu patients) delirium prediction model for intensive care patients: observational multicentre study. *BMJ.* (2012) 344:e420. doi: 10.1136/bmj.e420
85. Wassenaar A, Schoonhoven L, Devlin JW, van Haren FMP, Slooter AJC, Jorens PG, et al. Delirium prediction in the intensive care unit: comparison of two delirium prediction models. *Crit Care.* (2018) 22:114. doi: 10.1186/s13054-018-2037-6
86. van den Boogaard M, Schoonhoven L, Maseda E, Plowright C, Jones C, Luetz A, et al. Recalibration of the delirium prediction model for ICU patients (PRE-DELIRIC): a multinational observational study. *Intensive Care Med.* (2014) 40:361–9. doi: 10.1007/s00134-013-3202-7
87. Linkaite G, Riauka M, Bunevičiute I, Vosylius S. Evaluation of PRE-DELIRIC (PREdiction of DELIRium in ICu patients) delirium prediction model for the patients in the intensive care unit. *Acta Med Litu.* (2018) 25:14–22. doi: 10.6001/actamedica.v25i1.3699

22

Pathophysiology of Coagulopathy Induced by Traumatic Brain Injury is Identical to that of Disseminated Intravascular Coagulation with Hyperfibrinolysis

Takeshi Wada [1], Atsushi Shiraishi [2], Satoshi Gando [1,3], Kazuma Yamakawa [4], Seitaro Fujishima [5], Daizoh Saitoh [6], Shigeki Kushimoto [7], Hiroshi Ogura [8], Toshikazu Abe [9,10], Toshihiko Mayumi [11], Junichi Sasaki [12], Joji Kotani [13], Naoshi Takeyama [14], Ryosuke Tsuruta [15], Kiyotsugu Takuma [16], Shin-ichiro Shiraishi [17], Yasukazu Shiino [18], Taka-aki Nakada [19], Kohji Okamoto [20], Yuichiro Sakamoto [21], Akiyoshi Hagiwara [22], Satoshi Fujimi [23], Yutaka Umemura [23] and Yasuhiro Otomo [24]*

[1] Division of Acute and Critical Care Medicine, Department of Anesthesiology and Critical Care Medicine, Hokkaido University Faculty of Medicine, Sapporo, Japan, [2] Emergency and Trauma Center, Kameda Medical Center, Kamogawa, Japan, [3] Department of Acute and Critical Care Medicine, Sapporo Higashi Tokushukai Hospital, Sapporo, Japan, [4] Department of Emergency Medicine, Osaka Medical and Pharmaceutical University, Takatsuki, Japan, [5] Center for General Medicine Education, Keio University School of Medicine, Tokyo, Japan, [6] Division of Traumatology, Research Institute, National Defense Medical College, Tokorozawa, Japan, [7] Division of Emergency and Critical Care Medicine, Tohoku University Graduate School of Medicine, Sendai, Japan, [8] Department of Traumatology and Acute Critical Medicine, Osaka University Graduate School of Medicine, Suita, Japan, [9] Department of Emergency and Critical Care Medicine, Tsukuba Memorial Hospital, Tsukuba, Japan, [10] Health Services Research and Development Center, University of Tsukuba, Tsukuba, Japan, [11] Department of Emergency Medicine, School of Medicine, University of Occupational and Environmental Health, Kitakyushu, Japan, [12] Department of Emergency and Critical Care Medicine, Keio University School of Medicine, Tokyo, Japan, [13] Division of Disaster and Emergency Medicine, Department of Surgery Related, Kobe University Graduate School of Medicine, Kobe, Japan, [14] Advanced Critical Care Center, Aichi Medical University Hospital, Nagakute, Japan, [15] Advanced Medical Emergency & Critical Care Center, Yamaguchi University Hospital, Ube, Japan, [16] Emergency & Critical Care Center, Kawasaki Municipal Hospital, Kawasaki, Japan, [17] Department of Emergency and Critical Care Medicine, Aizu Chuo Hospital, Aizu, Japan, [18] Department of Acute Medicine, Kawasaki Medical School, Kurashiki, Japan, [19] Department of Emergency and Critical Care Medicine, Chiba University Graduate School of Medicine, Chiba, Japan, [20] Department of Surgery, Center for Gastroenterology and Liver Disease, Kitakyushu City Yahata Hospital, Kitakyushu, Japan, [21] Emergency and Critical Care Medicine, Saga University Hospital, Saga, Japan, [22] Center Hospital of the National Center for Global Health and Medicine, Tokyo, Japan, [23] Division of Trauma and Surgical Critical Care, Osaka General Medical Center, Sumiyoshi, Japan, [24] Trauma and Acute Critical Care Center, Medical Hospital, Tokyo Medical and Dental University, Tokyo, Japan

***Correspondence:**
Takeshi Wada
twada1@med.hokudai.ac.jp*

Background: Traumatic brain injury (TBI)-associated coagulopathy is a widely recognized risk factor for secondary brain damage and contributes to poor clinical outcomes. Various theories, including disseminated intravascular coagulation (DIC), have been proposed regarding its pathomechanisms; no consensus has been reached thus far. This study aimed to elucidate the pathophysiology of TBI-induced coagulopathy by comparing coagulofibrinolytic changes in isolated TBI (iTBI) to those in non-TBI, to determine the associated factors, and identify the clinical significance of DIC diagnosis in patients with iTBI.

Methods: This secondary multicenter, prospective study assessed patients with severe trauma. iTBI was defined as Abbreviated Injury Scale (AIS) scores ≥4 in the head and neck, and ≤2 in other body parts. Non-TBI was defined as AIS scores ≥4 in single body parts other than the head and neck, and the absence of AIS scores ≥3 in any other trauma-affected parts. Specific biomarkers for thrombin and plasmin generation, anticoagulation, and fibrinolysis inhibition were measured at the presentation to the emergency department (0 h) and 3 h after arrival.

Results: We analyzed 34 iTBI and 40 non-TBI patients. Baseline characteristics, transfusion requirements and in-hospital mortality did not significantly differ between groups. The changes in coagulation/fibrinolysis-related biomarkers were similar. Lactate levels in the iTBI group positively correlated with DIC scores (rho = −0.441, $p = 0.017$), but not with blood pressure (rho = −0.098, $p = 0.614$). Multiple logistic regression analyses revealed that the injury severity score was an independent predictor of DIC development in patients with iTBI (odds ratio = 1.237, $p = 0.018$). Patients with iTBI were further subdivided into two groups: DIC ($n = 15$) and non-DIC ($n = 19$) groups. Marked thrombin and plasmin generation were observed in all patients with iTBI, especially those with DIC. Patients with iTBI and DIC had higher requirements for massive transfusion and emergency surgery, and higher in-hospital mortality than those without DIC. Furthermore, DIC development significantly correlated with poor hospital survival; DIC scores at 0 h were predictive of in-hospital mortality.

Conclusions: Coagulofibrinolytic changes in iTBI and non-TBI patients were identical, and consistent with the pathophysiology of DIC. DIC diagnosis in the early phase of TBI is key in predicting the outcomes of severe TBI.

Keywords: disseminated intravascular coagulation, fibrinolysis, shock, thrombin, trauma-induced coagulopathy, traumatic brain injury

INTRODUCTION

Traumatic brain injury (TBI) is one of the leading causes of death and disability, with more than 10 million people hospitalized for TBI every year (1). Although primary damage to the brain is inevitable, secondary injuries are potentially avoidable and can affect the therapeutic interventions and outcomes of patients with TBI. TBI-associated coagulopathy is widely recognized as a risk factor for secondary brain damage and contributes to poor clinical outcomes. Two meta-analyses reported that the overall prevalence of TBI-associated coagulopathy was 32.7–35.2%, and a strong association was confirmed between the incidence of coagulopathy and poor outcomes (2, 3). TBI-associated coagulopathy contributes to poor outcomes in both hypocoagulability, leading to the expansion of intracranial hemorrhage, and hypercoagulability, leading to secondary cerebral ischemia due to intravascular thrombosis in the injured brain (4–8). Therefore, elucidation of the pathophysiology of TBI-induced coagulopathy may contribute to improving the outcomes of TBI patients, but no consensus has been reached thus far.

Disseminated intravascular coagulation (DIC) is acknowledged as the primary pathophysiological mechanism of trauma-induced coagulopathy (TIC), which is caused by multiple factors, such as anemia, hemodilution, hypothermia, acidosis, hemorrhagic shock, and serious trauma itself (9). Coagulopathy that occurs in patients with TBI is consistent with the definition of DIC proposed by the International Society on Thrombosis and Haemostasis: the activation of coagulation with the loss of localization and damage to the microvasculature (10, 11). Previous studies have clearly demonstrated consumption coagulopathy and disseminated microvascular thrombosis formation in the brain and other organs, which is the pathophysiology of DIC itself (12, 13).

A recent consensus statement from the International Society on Thrombosis and Haemostasis described that TIC is driven by two distinct and synergic insults: hypovolemic shock due to blood loss and extensive tissue disruption (14). However, it is unclear whether this concept can be applied to patients with TBI, since these patients do not suffer substantial blood loss, indicating that they are less likely to develop hemorrhagic shock.

Therefore, this study aimed to elucidate the pathophysiology of TBI-induced coagulopathy by comparing the coagulofibrinolytic changes in isolated TBI (iTBI) with those in non-TBI trauma, and to determine the associated factors, particularly shock-related factors such as blood pressure and serum lactate levels. To gain a deeper insight into the pathomechanisms of TBI-induced coagulopathy, coagulofibrinolytic changes were compared between iTBI patients with and without DIC, and the clinical significance of DIC diagnosis in patients with iTBI was evaluated.

TABLE 1 | Demographics and parameters at the scene and admission to the emergency department in patients with isolated traumatic brain injury and non-traumatic brain injury.

	Non-TBI $n = 40$	iTBI $n = 34$	*p*-value
Demographics			
Age (years)	67 (55–79)	59 (48–76)	0.633
Male sex, *n* (%)	27 (67.5)	23 (67.6)	0.989
Charlson comorbidity index	0 (0–1)	0 (0–0)	0.711
ISS	20 (17–26)	17(16–25)	0.196
AIS			
Head	0 (0–0)	4 (4–5)	< 0.001
Face	0 (0–0)	0 (0–0)	0.814
Neck	0 (0–0)	0 (0–0)	0.357
Thorax	4 (0–4)	0 (0–0)	< 0.001
Abdomen	0 (0–2)	0 (0–0)	0.001
Spine			
Cervical	0 (0–0)	0 (0–0)	0.019
Thoracic	0 (0–0)	0 (0–0)	0.019
Lumber	0 (0–0)	0 (0–0)	0.105
Upper extremity	0 (0–0)	0 (0–0)	0.022
Lower extremity	0 (0–2)	0 (0–0)	< 0.001
External	0 (0–1)	0 (0–0)	0.048
DIC 0 h, *n* (%)	8 (20.0)	9 (26.5)	0.510
DIC score 0 h	3 (2–3)	3 (1–4)	0.920
DIC 3 h, *n* (%)	10 (28.6)	10 (38.4)	0.416
DIC score 3 h	3(1–4)	3(1–4)	0.875
DIC 24 h, *n* (%)	10 (26.3)	3 (11.1)	0.131
DIC score 24 h	3 (1–4)	3 (0–3)	0.042
SIRS criteria	2 (1–2)	2 (1–3)	0.205
Shock (ABP) at scene, *n* (%)	6 (15.4)	3 (8.8)	0.489
Shock (ABP) at ED, *n* (%)	8 (20.0)	1 (2.9)	0.033
Shock (lac), *n* (%)	21 (56.8)	20 (69.0)	0.310
Tranexamic acid, *n* (%)	8 (20.0)	14 (41.2)	0.047
At the scene			
Systolic blood pressure (mmHg)	119 (103–136)	150 (121–169)	0.004
Diastolic blood pressure (mmHg)	72 (63–87)	80 (65–104)	0.187
Heart rate (bpm)	83 (69–99)	84 (74–97)	0.747
Respiratory rate (breaths/min)	20 (18–24)	18 (18–20)	0.001
At the ED			
Systolic blood pressure (mmHg)	140 (107–151)	144 (131–161)	0.007
Diastolic blood pressure (mmHg)	77 (6,693)	84 (71–95)	0.110
Heart rate (bpm)	82 (65–93)	84 (72–97)	0.520
Respiratory rate (breaths/min)	20 (18–26)	18 (16–20)	< 0.001
Lactate (mmol/L)	1.7 (1.1–3.1)	3.1 (1.7–4.3)	0.372
Body temperature (°C)	36.4 (36.1–36.8)	36.3 (35.9–37.0)	0.853

Reported proportions (counts) for categorical variables and medians (interquartile ranges) for continuous variables. Shock (ABP) represents a systolic blood pressure of <90 mmHg. Shock (lac) represents lactate levels of >2 mmol/L in the emergency department (ED). AIS, Abbreviated Injury Scale; DIC, disseminated intravascular coagulation; ISS, Injury Severity Score; iTBI, isolated traumatic brain injury; SIRS, systemic inflammatory response syndrome; TBI, traumatic brain injury.

TABLE 2 | Requirement for transfusion and emergency surgery, and in-hospital mortality.

	Non-TBI $n = 40$	iTBI $n = 34$	*p*-value
Operation within 24 h after admission, *n* (%)	17 (42.5)	14 (42.4)	0.995
Massive transfusion, *n* (%)	2 (5.0)	4 (11.8)	0.404
3-h Transfusion			
Packed red blood cells (mL)	0 (0–0)	0 (0–0)	0.909
Fresh frozen plasma (mL)	0 (0–0)	0 (0–0)	0.636
Platelet concentrate (U)	0 (0–0)	0 (0–0)	1.000
Cryoprecipitate (U)	0 (0–0)	0 (0–0)	1.000
24-h Transfusion			
Packed red blood cells (mL)	0 (0–280)	0 (0–0)	0.772
Fresh frozen plasma (mL)	0 (0–0)	0 (0–480)	0.693
Platelet concentrate (U)	0 (0–0)	0 (0–0)	0.705
Cryoprecipitate (U)	0 (0–0)	0 (0–0)	1.000
In-hospital mortality, *n* (%)	1 (2.5)	4 (12.1)	0.169

Reported median (interquartile range) for continuous variables.
iTBI, isolated traumatic brain injury; TBI, traumatic brain injury.

MATERIALS AND METHODS

Study Design, Setting, and Ethical Approval

This descriptive study was performed as a secondary analysis of a multicenter prospective study conducted by the Japanese Association for Acute Medicine (JAAM) Focused Outcomes Research in Emergency Care in Acute Respiratory Distress Syndrome, Sepsis, and Trauma (FORECAST) study group (15). The JAAM FORECAST TRAUMA study recruited participants between April 1, 2016 and January 31, 2018, from 39 emergency departments (EDs) and intensive-care units (ICUs) in tertiary hospitals and was registered at the University Hospital Medical Information Network Clinical Trial Registry (UMIN-CTR ID: UMIN000019588). This study was approved under the condition that written informed consent was obtained from the patient or next of kin by the JAAM and the Ethics Committee of each hospital (JAAM, 2014-01; Hokkaido University Graduate School of Medicine, Head Institute of the FORECAST group, 014-0307) and was performed in accordance with the Declaration of Helsinki.

Participants

The JAAM FORECAST TRAUMA study enrolled adult trauma patients with severe trauma injury (aged ≥16 years old) with an Injury Severity Score (ISS) of ≥16 who were directly transported from the scene by emergency medical services. Patients with a history of cardiac arrest and resuscitation, who were receiving anticoagulants, who had hemorrhagic diathesis or coagulopathy due to any cause, or who had been transferred from other hospitals were excluded before registration. The size of the study population was dependent on the study period. All patients were followed up until discharge. Twenty-seven healthy volunteers who were not age- or sex-matched were enrolled to obtain the control values of the measured markers.

Definition and Diagnosis

Injury severity was assessed using the ISS. A DIC diagnosis was made based on the JAAM DIC diagnostic criteria (16) (**Supplementary Table 1**). The DIC scores were calculated at 0,

3, and 24 h, and the DIC group was defined as patients who met the DIC criteria at least once during the study period. In the present study, the prothrombin time international normalized ratio (PT-INR) was used as a substitute for the prothrombin time ratio for the diagnosis of DIC. Transfusion of packed red blood cells of more than the estimated circulating blood volume (7.5% of body weight) within 24 h after presentation to the ED met the definition of massive transfusion. Shock was defined as a systemic inflammatory response syndrome criteria were used to assess systemic inflammation (17). A systolic blood pressure of <90 mmHg at the scene or at the ED and lactate levels >2 mmol/L at the ED. The Charlson comorbidity index was used to assess comorbidities (18).

iTBI was defined as an Abbreviated Injury Scale (AIS) score of ≥4 in the head and neck and ≤2 in other body parts. To match the injury severity of iTBI, non-TBI was defined as an AIS score of ≥4 in one body part other than the head and neck and the absence of AIS score of ≥3 in any part affected by trauma.

Data Collection and Measurements

Immediately after arrival at the ED (0 h) and 3 h after admission (3 h), 15 mL of blood was collected in citrate containing tubes at each sampling point. The samples were immediately centrifuged at 4°C in the laboratories of each hospital, and the obtained plasma was stored at −80°C. All plasma samples were measured at the center laboratory of the LSI Medience Corporation (Tokyo, Japan). We measured the following molecular markers: (1) soluble fibrin (marker of direct thrombin generation) (LA, IATRO SFII; LSI Medience), (2) antithrombin (marker of anti-thrombin) (chromogenic assay, HemosIL Antithrombin LQ; Instrumental Laboratory), (3) protein C (marker of anticoagulation) (LPIA, LPIA-ACE PCII; LSI Medience), (4) plasmin antiplasmin complex (marker of plasmin generation) (LPIA, LPIA-ACE PPI II; LSI Medience), (5) plasminogen activator inhibitor-1 (PAI-1) (marker of inhibition of fibrinolysis) (LA, LPIA-tPAI test; LSI Medience), (6) D-dimer (marker of fibrinolysis) (LPIA, LPIA GENESIS D-dimer; LSI Medience),

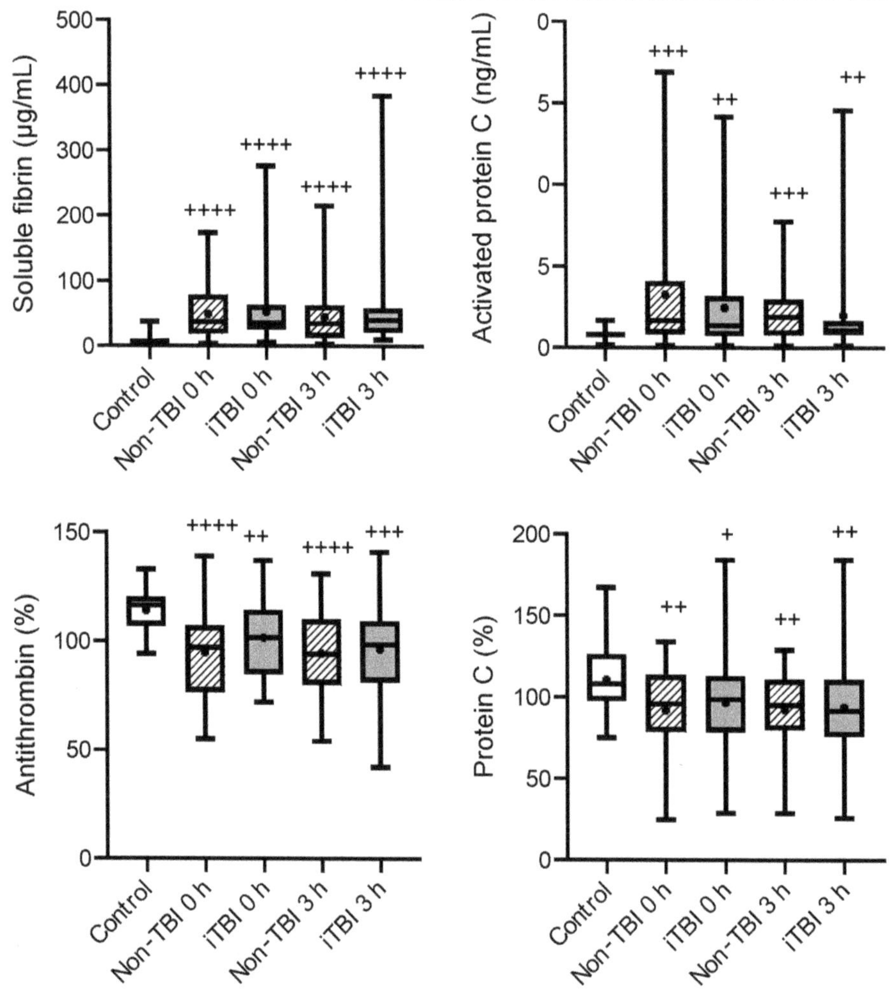

FIGURE 1 | Serial changes in the coagulation-related molecular markers. Healthy controls (white box), non-traumatic brain injury (TBI) (hatched boxes), and isolated TBI (iTBI) (gray boxes) at presentation to the emergency department (0 h) and 3 h after hospital arrival (3 h). The horizontal bars in the box indicate the median (middle) and interquartile ranges (upper 25% and lower 75%). Black boxes are mean values. $+p < 0.05$ vs. healthy controls; $++p < 0.01$ vs. healthy controls; $+++p < 0.001$ vs. healthy controls; $++++p < 0.0001$ vs. healthy controls. None of the markers significantly differed between the iTBI and non-TBI groups.

and (7) circulating activated protein C (APC) (marker of inhibition of thrombin) (EIA, EIA Kit For Activated Protein C Cloud-Clone Corp.). In addition to routine laboratory tests and blood gas analysis, measurements of platelet counts, PT-INR, activated partial thromboplastin time (APTT), fibrinogen, fibrin/fibrinogen degradation products (FDPs), and the FDP/D-dimer ratio, a surrogate marker of fibrin(ogen)olysis, were measured at 0, 3, and 24 h after arrival at the ED.

Statistical Analyses

Measurements are expressed as the median with the 25th–75th interquartile range or as numbers (percentages). Missing values were used without manipulation. Differences in demographics and measured parameters between the two groups were compared using the Mann–Whitney *U*-test for continuous variables and using either the chi-square test or Fisher's exact test for nominal variables when required. Platelet counts and global markers of coagulation and fibrinolysis were also evaluated using the Mann–Whitney *U*-test. Correlations were evaluated using Spearman's rank test when required. Survival probability curves with and without a DIC diagnosis in iTBI were constructed using the Kaplan–Meier method. The receiver operating characteristic (ROC) curve was constructed, and the area under the ROC curve (AUC) was used to assess the ability of DIC scores to predict in-hospital mortality. Differences were considered statistically significant at a two-tailed $p < 0.05$. SPSS software (version 26; IBM Japan, Tokyo, Japan) was used for all statistical analyses and calculations.

RESULTS

Baseline Characteristics, Transfusion, and In-Hospital Mortality

In total, 295 consecutive patients were registered during the study period in the FORECAST TRAUMA cohort. Ultimately,

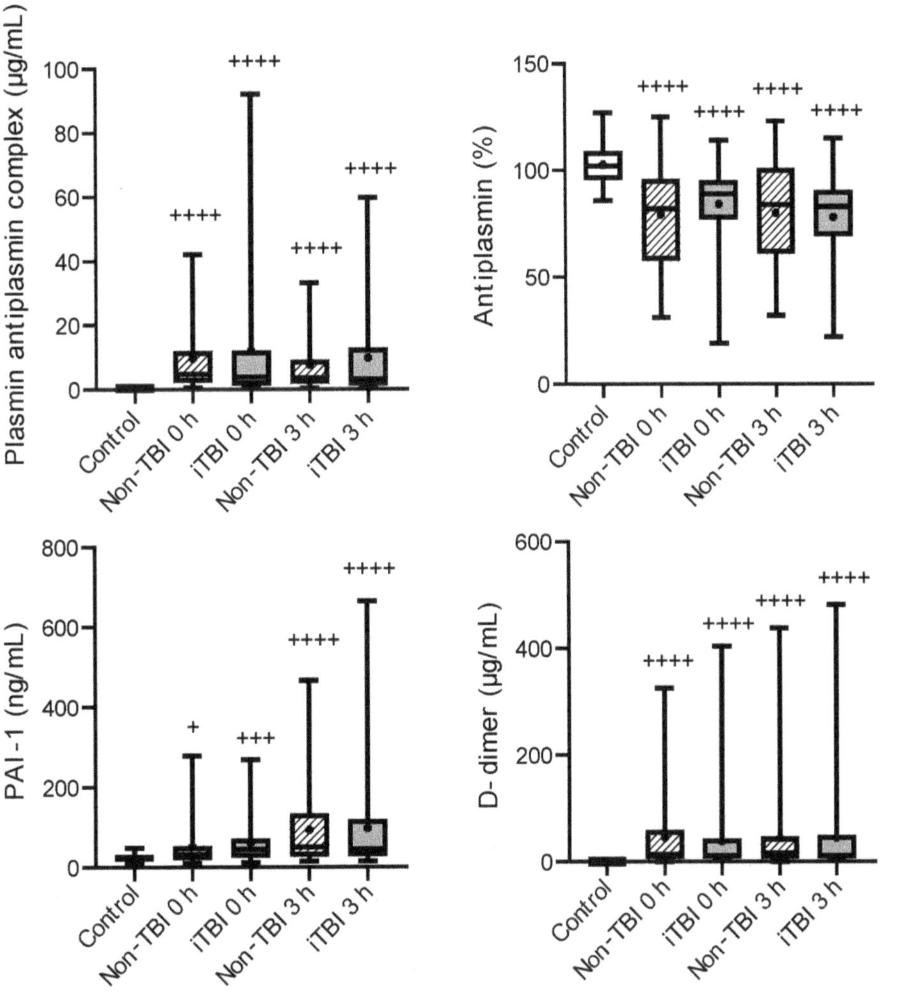

FIGURE 2 | Serial changes in the fibrinolysis-related molecular markers. Healthy controls (white box), non-traumatic brain injury (TBI) (hatched boxes), and isolated TBI (iTBI) (gray boxes) at presentation to the emergency department (0 h) and 3 h after hospital arrival (3 h). Horizontal bars in the box indicate the median (middle) and interquartile ranges (upper 25% and lower 75%). Black boxes are mean values. $+p < 0.05$ vs. healthy controls, $+++p < 0.001$ vs. healthy controls, $++++p < 0.0001$ vs. healthy controls. None of the markers significantly differed between the iTBI and non-TBI groups.

276 patients who met the eligibility criteria were divided into the iTBI (n = 34) and non-TBI (n = 40) groups (**Supplementary Figure 1**).

There were no significant differences in age, sex, comorbidities, or ISS between the groups. In addition, the DIC scores and prevalence at 0 and 3 h did not significantly differ between the groups (**Table 1**). The requirement for massive transfusion, transfusion volumes, and in-hospital mortality did not significantly differ between the two groups (**Table 2**).

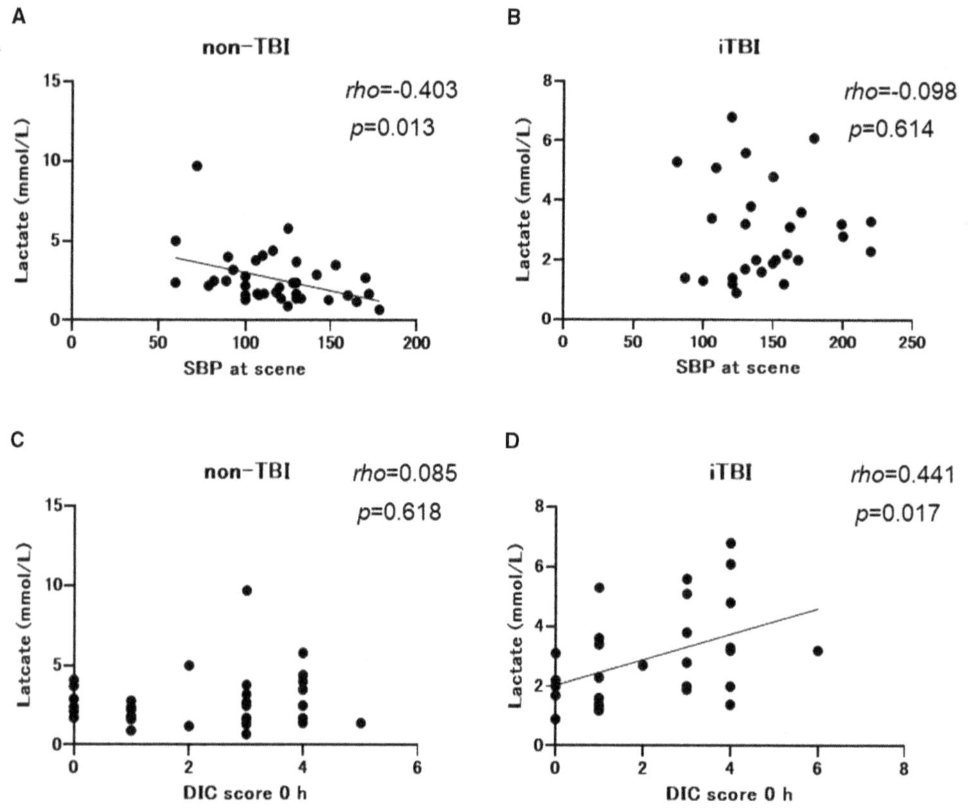

FIGURE 3 | Spearman's rank correlation coefficients between the lactate levels and systolic blood pressure (SBP) at scene and the disseminated intravascular coagulation (DIC) score at arrival to the emergency department. TBI, traumatic brain injury; iTBI, isolated traumatic brain injury.

TABLE 3 | Results of logistic regression analyses of variables predicting the development of disseminated intravascular coagulation in patients with isolated traumatic brain injury.

	Univariable			Multivariable		
	Odds ratio	***p*-value**	**95% CI**	**Odds ratio**	***p*-value**	**95% CI**
Age	1.027	0.202	0.986–1.070			
Sex	3.281	0.120	0.733–14.683			
ISS	1.220	0.018	1.034–1.439	1.237	0.018	1.034–1.439
SBP at scene	1.004	0.595	0.989–1.020			
Shock (ABP) at scene	2.769	0.425	0.226–33.879			
SBP at ED	1.025	0.078	0.997–1.053			
Shock (ABP) at ED, *n* (%)	0.000	1.000	0–0			
Lactate 0 h	1.403	0.177	0.858–2.295			
Shock (lac), *n* (%)	3.500	0.172	0.579–21.161			

Shock (ABP) represents a systolic blood pressure of <90 mmHg. Shock (lac) represents lactate levels of >2 mmol/L at the emergency department (ED).
CI, confidence interval; ED, emergency department; ISS, injury severity score; iTBI, isolated traumatic brain injury; SBP, systolic blood pressure; TBI, traumatic brain injury.

TABLE 4 | Demographics and parameters at the scene and admission to the emergency department in isolated traumatic brain injury patients with and without disseminated intravascular coagulation.

	Non-DIC $n = 19$	DIC $n = 15$	p-value
Demographics			
Age (years)	59 (51–73)	58 (49–74)	0.242
Male sex, n (%)	15 (78.9)	8 (53.3)	0.112
Charlson comorbidity index	0 (0–0)	0 (0–1)	0.190
Glasgow coma scale	14 (13–15)	7 (3–9)	0.004
ISS	17 (16–17)	25 (16–25)	0.120
AIS			
Head	4 (4–4)	5 (4–5)	0.004
Face	0 (0–0)	0 (0–0)	0.023
Neck	0 (0–0)	0 (0–0)	0.451
Thorax	0 (0–0)	0 (0–0)	1.000
Abdomen	0 (0–0)	0 (0–0)	0.811
Spine			
Cervical	0 (0–0)	0 (0–0)	1.000
Thoracic	0 (0–0)	0 (0–0)	1.000
Lumber	0 (0–0)	0 (0–0)	1.000
Upper extremity	0 (0–0)	0 (0–0)	0.811
Lower extremity	0 (0–0)	0 (0–0)	1.000
External	0 (0–0)	0 (0–0)	0.918
SIRS criteria	1 (1–2)	3 (1–3)	0.116
Shock (ABP) at scene, n (%)	1 (5.3)	2 (13.3)	0.409
Shock (ABP) at ED, n (%)	1 (5.3)	0 (0)	0.559
Shock (lac), n (%)	10 (58.8)	10 (83.3)	0.160
At the scene			
Systolic blood pressure (mmHg)	138 (121–155)	144 (138–179)	0.537
Diastolic blood pressure (mmHg)	78 (60–86)	83 (70–109)	0.708
Heart rate (bpm)	84 (77–87)	80 (66–98)	0.421
Respiratory rate (breaths/min)	18 (18–21)	18 (16–18)	0.167
At the ED			
Systolic blood pressure (mmHg)	138 (128–155)	144 (138–179)	0.083
Diastolic blood pressure (mmHg)	82 (65–90)	84 (74–98)	0.202
Heart rate (bpm)	74 (70–86)	95 (81–98)	0.401
Respiratory rate (breaths/min)	18 (16–19)	17 (15–20)	0.319
Lactate (mmol/L)	2.0 (1.3–2.9)	4.3 (3.2–6.1)	0.152
Body temperature (°C)	36.8 (36.0–37.0)	36.0 (35.7–36.8)	0.132

Reported proportions (counts) for categorical variables and medians (interquartile ranges) for continuous variables. Shock (ABP) represents a systolic blood pressure of <90 mmHg. Shock (lac) represents lactate levels of >2 mmol/L in the emergency department (ED). AIS, Abbreviated Injury Scale; DIC, disseminated intravascular coagulation; ISS, Injury Severity Score; iTBI, isolated traumatic brain injury; SIRS, systemic inflammatory response syndrome.

TABLE 5 | Requirement for transfusion and emergency surgery, and in-hospital mortality in isolated traumatic brain injury patients with and without disseminated intravascular coagulation.

	Non-DIC $n = 19$	DIC $n = 15$	p-value
Operation for TBI within 24 h after admission, n (%)	4 (21.1)	9 (60.0)	0.024
Massive transfusion, n (%)	0 (0)	4 (26.7)	0.029
3-h transfusion			
Packed red blood cells (mL)	0 (0–0)	0 (0–0)	0.451
Fresh frozen plasma (mL)	0 (0–0)	0 (0–0)	0.681
Platelet concentrate (U)	0 (0–0)	0 (0–0)	1.000
Cryoprecipitate (U)	0 (0–0)	0 (0–0)	1.000
24-h transfusion			
Packed red blood cells (mL)	0 (0–0)	560 (0–5,880)	0.096
Fresh frozen plasma (mL)	0 (0–0)	1,080 (480–8,160)	0.077
Platelet concentrate (U)	0 (0–0)	0 (0–32)	0.202
Cryoprecipitate (U)	0 (0–0)	0 (0–0)	1.000
In-hospital mortality, n (%)	0 (0)	4 (26.7)	0.033

Reported median (interquartile range) for continuous variables.
TBI, traumatic brain injury; DIC, disseminated intravascular coagulation.

Comparison of Coagulofibrinolytic Changes Between the iTBI and Non-TBI Groups

Serial changes in the molecular markers of coagulation are shown in **Figure 1**. The levels of anticoagulation factors such as antithrombin and protein C were lower, while the levels of soluble fibrin and APC were significantly higher in the iTBI and non-TBI groups than in the healthy control group. These coagulation markers showed similar changes in patients with and without TBI. As shown in **Figure 2**, increased levels of plasmin-antiplasmin complex, D-dimer, and PAI-1 were observed in iTBI and non-TBI patients than in healthy controls. The levels of antiplasmin significantly decreased in the iTBI and non-TBI groups compared to those in the control group. These fibrinolysis-related molecular markers also underwent similar changes in the iTBI and non-TBI groups. In addition, serial changes in platelet counts and global markers of coagulation and fibrinolysis were similar between the groups (**Supplementary Table 2**).

Factors Associated With Lactate Levels

Non-TBI patients exhibited lower systolic blood pressure at the scene and at the ED with a higher incidence of shock defined as a systolic blood pressure of <90 mmHg at the ED than the iTBI group. However, the incidence of shock defined by lactate levels of >2 mmol/L was identical between the two groups (**Table 1**). There was a negative correlation between systolic blood pressure and lactate levels in the non-TBI group (Spearman's rho $= -0.403$, $p = 0.013$; **Figure 3A**), while no significant correlation was observed between these variables in the iTBI group (Spearman's rho $= 0.098$, $p = 0.614$; **Figure 3B**). By contrast, no correlation was observed between lactate levels and the DIC score at 0 h in the non-TBI group (Spearman's rho $= 0.085$, $p = 0.618$; **Figure 3C**), but a positive correlation was observed between these values in the iTBI group (Spearman's rho $= 0.441$, $p = 0.017$; **Figure 3D**).

Factors Associated With the Development of DIC in the iTBI Group

Logistic regression analysis was performed to evaluate the factors associated with the development of DIC. Multiple logistic regression analysis indicated that ISS was an independent

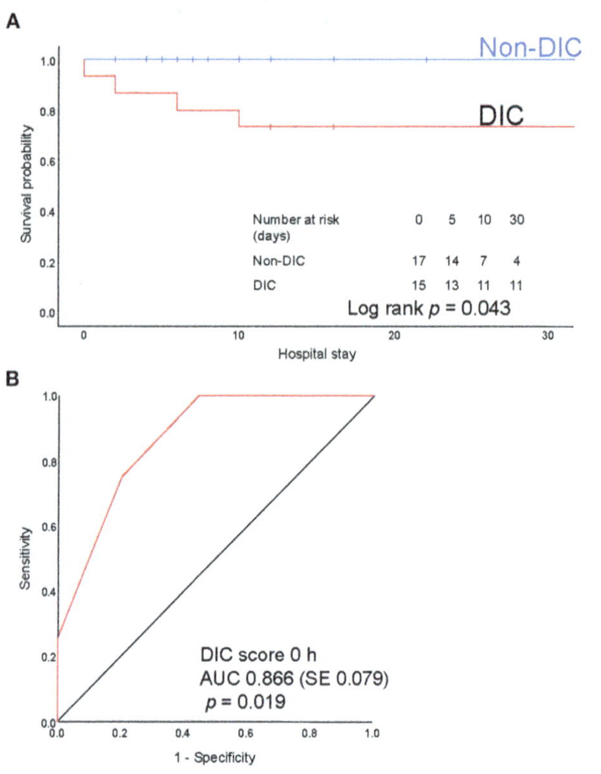

FIGURE 4 | (A) Kaplan-Meier survival provability curves for mortality during hospitalization. Numbers at risk represent the number of patients with isolated traumatic brain injury (iTBI) with or without disseminated intravascular coagulation (DIC) at risk of death on the indicated days. **(B)** Receiver operating characteristics (ROC) curves of the DIC score immediately after arrival at emergency department. AUC, area under the ROC curve; SE, standard error.

predictor of DIC development in patients with iTBI (odds ratio=1.237, p=0.018; **Table 3**).

Baseline Characteristics, Transfusion, and In-Hospital Mortality in iTBI Patients With and Without DIC

Next, we focused on iTBI patients and divided them into the DIC group (n = 15) and the non-DIC group (n = 19). The baseline characteristics of the patients are presented in **Table 4**. The median ISSs in the DIC and non-DIC groups were 25 and 17, respectively. DIC patients had a higher AIS score in the head and worse Glasgow Coma Scale scores than non-DIC patients. The physiological parameter values at the scene and ED did not differ between the groups. Only few patients had blood pressure-defined shock in both groups, whereas >50% of the patients had lactate-defined shock (DIC, 83.3%; non-DIC, 58.8%). The median lactate levels in the DIC and non-DIC groups were 4.3 and 2.0 mmol/L, respectively. The requirements for massive transfusion and emergency surgery for TBI were significantly higher, and in-hospital mortality was higher in the DIC group than in the non-DIC group (**Table 5**). The survival probability was significantly lower among iTBI patients diagnosed with DIC immediately after presentation to the ED than among patients without DIC (log rank p=0.043; **Figure 4A**). ROC curves indicated that the DIC scores immediately after arrival to the ED were a good predictor of in-hospital mortality in patients with iTBI (AUC 0.866, p=0.019; **Figure 4B**).

Comparison of Coagulofibrinolytic Changes Between iTBI Patients With and Without DIC

Higher levels of soluble fibrin and lower levels of antithrombin were confirmed in iTBI patients with DIC than in those without DIC (**Figure 5**). As shown in **Figure 6**, there were increased plasmin generation and fibrinolysis and lower levels of antiplasmin at 0 and 3 h in the iTBI with DIC group than in the iTBI without DIC group. The PAI-1 levels in iTBI patients with DIC at 3 h after hospital arrival tended to be higher than those in patients without DIC (p = 0.091). Higher levels of FDP at 0 h and lower platelet counts were observed in iTBI patients with DIC than in those without DIC (**Supplementary Table 3**).

DISCUSSION

This study aimed to elucidate the pathophysiology of TBI-induced coagulopathy by comparing the coagulofibrinolytic changes in iTBI patient with those in non-TBI trauma patients, to determine the associated factors, and to identify the clinical significance of DIC diagnosis in patients with iTBI. In the present study, similar requirements for massive transfusion and in-hospital mortality were observed between iTBI and non-TBI patients with a similar severity of trauma. The changes in the levels of coagulofibrinolytic biomarkers were also identical between the groups. The lactate levels in the iTBI group were positively correlated with DIC scores but not with blood pressure. Moreover, the ISS was an independent predictor of DIC development in patients with iTBI. iTBI patients with DIC showed a significantly higher requirement for emergency surgery for TBI, and a higher incidence of massive transfusion than did those without DIC. DIC development was significantly associated with poor hospital survival, and DIC scores at 0 h were predictive of in-hospital mortality. In patients with iTBI with DIC, marked thrombin and plasmin generation was confirmed.

Although numerous mechanisms that are potentially associated with coagulopathy after TBI have been suggested, we previously demonstrated that the main pathomechanism of TIC, with or without TBI, is DIC (19–21). DIC is characterized by increased thrombin generation and subsequent consumption coagulopathy due to damage-associated molecular patterns derived from injured cells and tissues (22). That is, DIC is caused by trauma itself (23). However, another theory advocates that TBI alone does not cause early coagulopathy (24) and that coagulopathy occurs only in patients with shock-induced profound acidosis and high lactate concentrations (25–27). The results of the present study indicated no correlation between lactate levels and systolic blood pressure (**Figure 3B**) in iTBI patients, but the positive correlation between lactate levels and DIC score (**Figure 3D**) in those patients implies that the increase

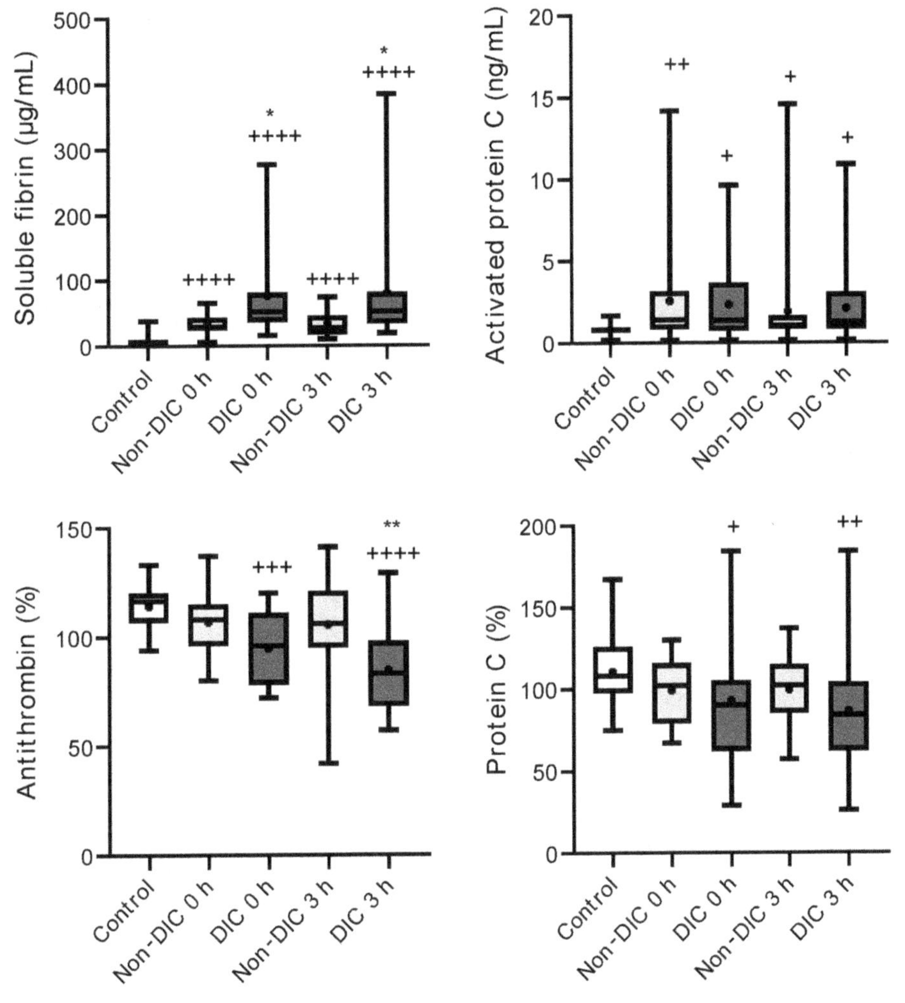

FIGURE 5 | Serial changes in the coagulation-related molecular markers in patients with isolated traumatic brain injury. Healthy controls (white box), non-disseminated intravascular coagulation (DIC) (light gray boxes), and DIC (dark gray boxes) at presentation to the emergency department (0 h) and 3 h after hospital arrival (3 h). Horizontal bars in the box indicate the median (middle) and interquartile ranges (upper 25% and lower 75%). Black boxes represent the mean values. $+p < 0.05$ vs. healthy controls, $++p < 0.01$ vs. healthy controls, $+++p < 0.001$ vs. healthy controls, $++++p < 0.0001$ vs. healthy controls, $^{*}p < 0.05$ vs. non-DIC, $^{**}p < 0.01$ vs. non-DIC.

in lactate levels in TBI patients is caused by DIC-mediated secondary tissue hypoperfusion rather than by hypotension due to hemorrhagic shock. The results demonstrated that ISS was an independent predictor of pathological coagulofibrinolytic changes, namely DIC, in iTBI patients (**Table 2**), which also supports the concept that TIC is caused by trauma itself, with or without shock (23). The current results revealed similar coagulofibrinolytic changes, characterized by DIC with hyperfibrinolysis, between iTBI and non-TBI (**Figures 1, 2**), which was in line with the findings of a previous study (28).

iTBI patients with DIC had a higher requirement for massive transfusion and emergency surgery and had a higher in-hospital mortality than did those without DIC (**Table 5**). In addition, the DIC score in the iTBI group immediately after arrival to the hospital was predictive of in-hospital mortality (**Figure 4B**). Similar results have been reported not only in the setting of iTBI (2, 3), but also in other trauma settings (29). These results suggest the importance of DIC diagnosis in severely injured patients with or without TBI.

The present study revealed marked thrombin generation with lower levels of antithrombin in iTBI patients, particularly those with DIC (**Figure 5**). Previous studies confirmed such thrombin generation after iTBI, as evaluated by the high levels of the thrombin–antithrombin complex, prothrombin fragment 1 + 2, fibrinopeptide A, and fibrin monomers (28, 30, 31). High levels of soluble tissue factors have also been found (30, 32). Injury to the blood–brain barrier, caused by direct cerebral vascular disruption, potentially releases brain tissue factors into systemic circulation (5, 33). Tissue factors exposed to blood bind extensively to factor VIIa, followed by the initiation of the extrinsic coagulation pathway and subsequent consumption coagulopathy (23). Massive thrombin generation due to the activation of coagulation may lead to the consumption of anticoagulant factors, such as antithrombin

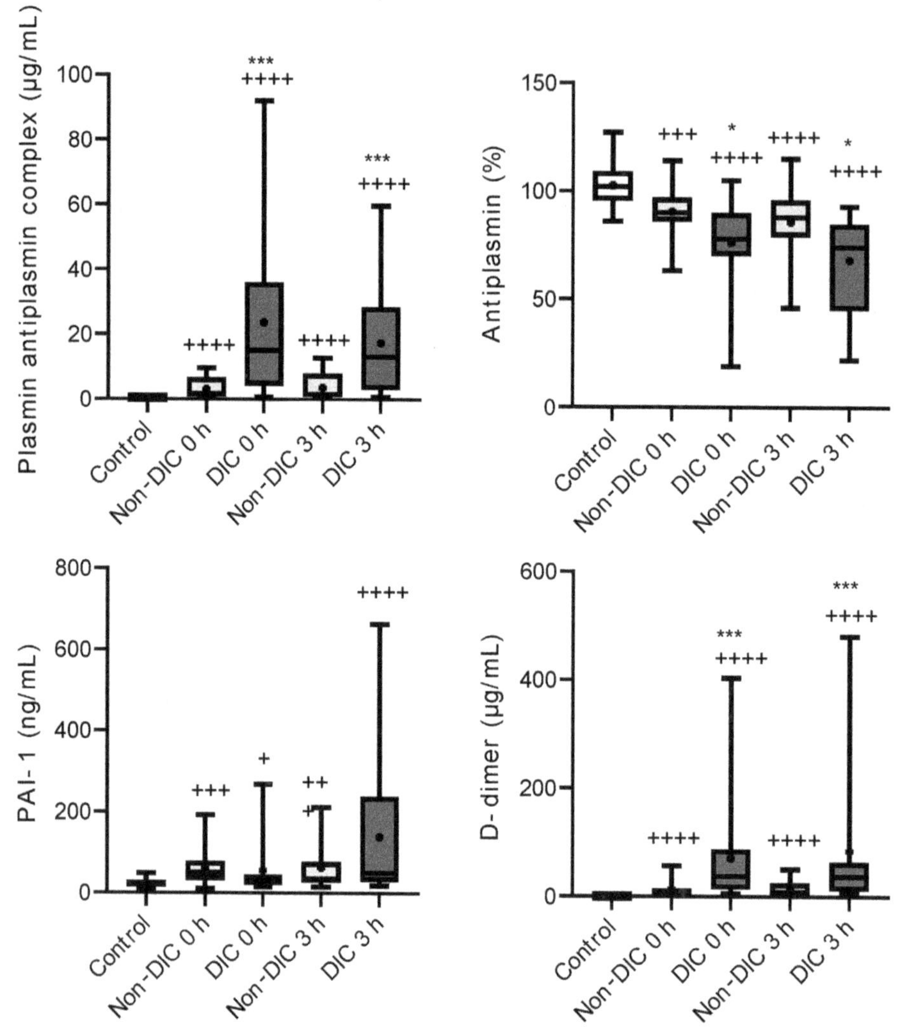

FIGURE 6 | Serial changes in the fibrinolysis-related molecular markers in patients with isolated traumatic brain injury. Healthy controls (white box), non-disseminated intravascular coagulation (DIC) (light gray boxes) and DIC (dark gray boxes) at presentation to the emergency department (0 h) and 3 h after hospital arrival (3 h). Horizontal bars in the box indicate the median (middle) and interquartile ranges (upper 25% and lower 75%). Black boxes represent the mean values. $+p < 0.005$ vs. healthy controls, $++p < 0.001$ vs. healthy controls, $+++p < 0.001$ vs. healthy controls, $++++p < 0.0001$ vs. healthy controls, $^{*}p < 0.05$ vs. non-DIC, $^{***}p < 0.001$ vs. non-DIC.

and protein C, followed by further activation of coagulation. These changes contribute to hypercoagulability inside the vessels, leading to intravascular microthrombosis in the brain and other organs, and hypocoagulability outside the vessels due to consumptive coagulopathy, leading to the progression of intracranial hemorrhage (34).

This study demonstrated marked plasmin generation with lower levels of antiplasmin in iTBI and these changes were prominent in iTBI patients with DIC (**Figure 6**). Hyperfibrinolysis after trauma is caused by the release of tissue-type plasminogen activator (t–PA) from the endothelial Weibel-Palade bodies due to traumatic shock-induced tissue hypoperfusion (22). However, patients with iTBI with high lactate levels had no low blood pressure (**Figure 3B**), and similar results were reported previously (35). These results indicate that increases in lactate levels are not caused by low blood pressure-related hypoperfusion, but by DIC-induced tissue-hypoperfusion. That is, high lactate levels in iTBI with coagulopathy are a result rather than a cause of TIC. Instead of traumatic shock-induced tissue hypoperfusion, the direct release of t-PA from injured brain tissue has been acknowledged as another explanation of hyperfibrinolysis in patients with iTBI (11). A previous study demonstrated that endogenous t-PA increases the lysis of plasma clots and contributes to intracerebral hemorrhage after TBI (36).

STUDY LIMITATIONS

Several limitations of our study need to be considered. First, although the present dataset was prospectively collected, causal relationships could not be defined because of the retrospective study design and missing values. Second, this study included a small number of patients. Third, we did not distinguish types of TBI (e.g., acute subdural hematoma, traumatic subarachnoid hemorrhage, and contusion), which may affect the pathology and severity of TBI-induced coagulopathy. Fourth, although more patients received tranexamic acid in the iTBI group than in the non-TBI group, the effects of tranexamic acid on the levels of coagulation and fibrinolysis-related markers were not determined. Fifth, bias may exist in trauma types in the non-TBI group, as suggested by the finding that many patients in this group had severe thoracic injury. Finally, this was a single nationwide study conducted in a developed country, which may have limited the global generalization of the results.

CONCLUSIONS

The present study demonstrated similar coagulofibrinolytic changes between iTBI and non-TBI patients, which are consistent with DIC. Marked generation of thrombin and plasmin was confirmed in iTBI patients, and these changes were more prominent in iTBI patients with DIC. The development of DIC in patients with iTBI was associated with a poor survival outcome, and DIC scores immediately after hospital arrival could predict in-hospital death. Therefore, the diagnosis of DIC in the early phase of trauma is important for predicting the outcome of severely injured patients, including those with iTBI.

ETHICS STATEMENT

This study was approved under the condition that written informed consent was obtained from the patient or next of kin by the JAAM and the Ethics Committee of each hospital (JAAM, 2014-01; Hokkaido University Graduate School of Medicine, Head institute of the FORECAST group, 014-0307). Written informed consent to participate in this study was provided by the participants' legal guardian/next of kin.

AUTHOR CONTRIBUTIONS

TW analyzed the study results, interpreted the data, and drafted the manuscript. AS checked the statistical methods and results. AS, SG, KY, SFujis, DS, SK, HO, TA, TM, JS, JK, NT, RT, KT, SS, YSh, TN, KO, YSa, AH, SFujim, YU, and YO planned the study, decided the methods, developed a web-based registration system, discussed the results, and critically revised the manuscript. All authors have read and approved the final version of the manuscript.

ACKNOWLEDGMENTS

We would like to thank Editage (www.editage.com) for English language editing. We wish to express our gratitude to all JAAM FORECAST Trauma investigators: Osaka City University Hospital (Yasumitsu Mizobata), National Hospital Organization Sendai Medical Center (Yasuo Yamada), Saitama Medical University Saitama Medical Center (Satoru Sugiyama), Fukui Prefectural Hospital (Hiroshi Ishida), Sapporo Medical University (Eichi Narimatsu), Fukuyama City Hospital (Koji Miyasho), Hiratsuka City Hospital (Toshio Kanai), Saiseikai Utsunomiya Hospital (Satoru Miyatake), Japanese Red Cross Society Kyoto Daini Hospital (Ryouji Iiduka), Shinsyu University School of Medicine (Hiroshi Imamura), Rinku General Medical Center (Yasuaki Mizushima), Subaru Health Insurance Society Ota Memorial Hospital (Yoshitake Sato), Saitama Medical University International Medical Center (Manabu Nemoto), Aomori Prefectural Central Hospital (Hiroyuki Hanada), National Hospital Organization Hokkaido Medical Center (Yasuo Shichinohe), Saga-ken Medical Center Koseikan (Kenji Hirahara), Hachinohe City Hospital (Akihide Kon), Juntendo University Nerima Hospital (Manabu Sugita), Kawaguchi Municipal Medical Center (Yasutaka Naoe), Kakogawa West City Hospital (Manabu Kirita), Osaka National Hospital (Daikai Sadamitsu), and Kouseiren Takaoka Hospital (Masahiro Yoshida). Additionally, the JAAM FORECST Study Group thanks Shuta Fukuda for his special assistance in completing the study.

REFERENCES

1. Iaccarino C, Carretta A, Nicolosi F, Morselli C. Epidemiology of severe traumatic brain injury. *J Neurosurg Sci.* (2018) 62:535–41. doi: 10.23736/S0390-5616.18.04532-0
2. Harhangi BS, Kompanje EJ, Leebeek FW, Maas AI. Coagulation disorders after traumatic brain injury. *Acta Neurochir.* (2008) 150:165–75; discussion 75. doi: 10.1007/s00701-007-1475-8
3. Epstein DS, Mitra B, O'Reilly G, Rosenfeld JV, Cameron PA. Acute traumatic coagulopathy in the setting of isolated traumatic brain injury: a systematic review and meta-analysis. *Injury.* (2014) 45:819–24. doi: 10.1016/j.injury.2014.01.011
4. Zou Z, Li L, Schäfer N, Huang Q, Maegele M, Gu Z. Endothelial glycocalyx in traumatic brain injury associated coagulopathy: potential mechanisms and impact. *J Neuroinflammation.* (2021) 18:134. doi: 10.1186/s12974-021-02192-1
5. Maegele M, Schöchl H, Menovsky T, Maréchal H, Marklund N, Buki A, et al. Coagulopathy and haemorrhagic progression in traumatic brain injury: advances in mechanisms, diagnosis, and management. *Lancet Neurol.* (2017) 16:630–47. doi: 10.1016/S1474-4422(17)30197-7

6. Stein SC, Young GS, Talucci RC, Greenbaum BH, Ross SE. Delayed brain injury after head trauma: significance of coagulopathy. *Neurosurgery.* (1992) 30:160–5. doi: 10.1097/00006123-199202000-00002
7. Stein SC, Chen XH, Sinson GP, Smith DH. Intravascular coagulation: a major secondary insult in nonfatal traumatic brain injury. *J Neurosurg.* (2002) 97:1373–7. doi: 10.3171/jns.2002.97.6.1373
8. Stein SC, Graham DI, Chen XH, Smith DH. Association between intravascular microthrombosis and cerebral ischemia in traumatic brain injury. *Neurosurgery.* (2004) 54:687–91; discussion 91. doi: 10.1227/01.NEU.0000108641.98845.88
9. Gando S, Sawamura A, Hayakawa M. Trauma, shock, and disseminated intravascular coagulation: lessons from the classical literature. *Ann Surg.* (2011) 254:10–9. doi: 10.1097/SLA.0b013e31821221b1
10. Taylor FB, Jr., Toh CH, Hoots WK, Wada H, Levi M. Towards definition, clinical and laboratory criteria, and a scoring system for disseminated intravascular coagulation. *Thromb Haemost.* (2001) 86:1327–30. doi: 10.1055/s-0037-1616068
11. Gando S. Hemostasis and thrombosis in trauma patients. *Semin Thromb Hemost.* (2015) 41:26–34. doi: 10.1055/s-0034-1398378
12. Kaufman HH, Hui KS, Mattson JC, Borit A, Childs TL, Hoots WK, et al. Clinicopathological correlations of disseminated intravascular coagulation in patients with head injury. *Neurosurgery.* (1984) 15:34–42. doi: 10.1097/00006123-198407000-00007
13. Stein SC, Smith DH. Coagulopathy in traumatic brain injury. *Neurocrit Care.* (2004) 1:479–88. doi: 10.1385/NCC:1:4:479
14. Moore HB, Gando S, Iba T, Kim PY, Yeh CH, Brohi K, et al. Defining trauma-induced coagulopathy with respect to future implications for patient management: communication from the SSC of the ISTH. *J Thromb Haemost.* (2020) 18:740–7. doi: 10.1111/jth.14690
15. Gando S, Shiraishi A, Wada T, Yamakawa K, Fujishima S, Saitoh D, et al. A multicenter prospective validation study on disseminated intravascular coagulation in trauma-induced coagulopathy. *J Thromb Haemost.* (2020) 18:2232–44. doi: 10.1111/jth.14931
16. Gando S, Saitoh D, Ogura H, Mayumi T, Koseki K, Ikeda T, et al. Natural history of disseminated intravascular coagulation diagnosed based on the newly established diagnostic criteria for critically ill patients: results of a multicenter, prospective survey. *Crit Care Med.* (2008) 36:145–50. doi: 10.1097/01.CCM.0000295317.97245.2D
17. American college of chest physicians/society of critical care medicine consensus conference: definitions for sepsis and organ failure and guidelines for the use of innovative therapies in sepsis. *Crit Care Med.* (1992) 20:864–74. doi: 10.1097/00003246-199206000-00025
18. Charlson ME, Pompei P, Ales KL, MacKenzie CR. A new method of classifying prognostic comorbidity in longitudinal studies: development and validation. *J Chronic Dis.* (1987) 40:373–83. doi: 10.1016/0021-9681(87)90171-8
19. Gando S, Nanzaki S, Kemmotsu O. Disseminated intravascular coagulation and sustained systemic inflammatory response syndrome predict organ dysfunctions after trauma: application of clinical decision analysis. *Ann Surg.* (1999) 229:121–7. doi: 10.1097/00000658-199901000-00016
20. Gando S. Disseminated intravascular coagulation in trauma patients. *Semin Thromb Hemost.* (2001) 27:585–92. doi: 10.1055/s-2001-18864
21. Gando S. Acute coagulopathy of trauma shock and coagulopathy of trauma: a rebuttal. You are now going down the wrong path. *J Trauma.* (2009) 67:381–3. doi: 10.1097/TA.0b013e3181a84f63
22. Gando S, Otomo Y. Local hemostasis, immunothrombosis, and systemic disseminated intravascular coagulation in trauma and traumatic shock. *Crit Care.* (2015) 19:72. doi: 10.1186/s13054-015-0735-x
23. Gando S, Hayakawa M. Pathophysiology of trauma-induced coagulopathy and management of critical bleeding requiring massive transfusion. *Semin Thromb Hemost.* (2016) 42:155–65. doi: 10.1055/s-0035-1564831
24. Cohen MJ, Brohi K, Ganter MT, Manley GT, Mackersie RC, Pittet JF. Early coagulopathy after traumatic brain injury: the role of hypoperfusion and the protein C pathway. *J Trauma.* (2007) 63:1254–61; discussion 61–2. doi: 10.1097/TA.0b013e318156ee4c
25. Brohi K, Cohen MJ, Ganter MT, Matthay MA, Mackersie RC, Pittet JF. Acute traumatic coagulopathy: initiated by hypoperfusion: modulated through the protein C pathway? *Ann Surg.* (2007) 245:812–8. doi: 10.1097/01.sla.0000256862.79374.31
26. Brohi K, Cohen MJ, Ganter MT, Schultz MJ, Levi M, Mackersie RC, et al. Acute coagulopathy of trauma: hypoperfusion induces systemic anticoagulation and hyperfibrinolysis. *J Trauma.* (2008) 64:1211–7; discussion 7. doi: 10.1097/TA.0b013e318169cd3c
27. Hess JR, Brohi K, Dutton RP, Hauser CJ, Holcomb JB, Kluger Y, et al. The coagulopathy of trauma: a review of mechanisms. *J Trauma.* (2008) 65:748–54. doi: 10.1097/TA.0b013e3181877a9c
28. Gando S, Nanzaki S, Kemmotsu O. Coagulofibrinolytic changes after isolated head injury are not different from those in trauma patients without head injury. *J Trauma.* (1999) 46:1070–6; discussion 6–7. doi: 10.1097/00005373-199906000-00018
29. Wada T, Shiraishi A, Gando S, Yamakawa K, Fujishima S, Saitoh D, et al. Disseminated intravascular coagulation immediately after trauma predicts a poor prognosis in severely injured patients. *Sci Rep.* (2021) 11:11031. doi: 10.21203/rs.3.rs-199070/v1
30. Di Battista AP, Rizoli SB, Lejnieks B, Min A, Shiu MY, Peng HT, et al. Sympathoadrenal activation is associated with acute traumatic coagulopathy and endotheliopathy in isolated brain injury. *Shock.* (2016) 46:96–103. doi: 10.1097/SHK.0000000000000642
31. Esnault P, Mathais Q, D'Aranda E, Montcriol A, Cardinale M, Cungi PJ, et al. Ability of fibrin monomers to predict progressive hemorrhagic injury in patients with severe traumatic brain injury. *Neurocrit Care.* (2020) 33:182–95. doi: 10.1007/s12028-019-00882-6
32. Rhind SG, Crnko NT, Baker AJ, Morrison LJ, Shek PN, Scarpelini S, et al. Prehospital resuscitation with hypertonic saline-dextran modulates inflammatory, coagulation and endothelial activation marker profiles in severe traumatic brain injured patients. *J Neuroinflammation.* (2010) 7:5. doi: 10.1186/1742-2094-7-5
33. Maegele M, Aversa J, Marsee MK, McCauley R, Chitta SH, Vyakaranam S, et al. Changes in coagulation following brain injury. *Semin Thromb Hemost.* (2020) 46:155–66. doi: 10.1055/s-0040-1702178
34. Wada T, Yamakawa K. Trauma-induced coagulopathy: the past, present, and future: a comment. *J Thromb Haemost.* (2019) 17:1571–4. doi: 10.1111/jth.14571
35. Wada T, Gando S, Maekaw K, Katabami K, Sageshima H, Hayakawa M, et al. Disseminated intravascular coagulation with increased fibrinolysis during the early phase of isolated traumatic brain injury. *Crit Care.* (2017) 21:219. doi: 10.1186/s13054-017-1808-9
36. Hijazi N, Abu Fanne R, Abramovitch R, Yarovoi S, Higazi M, Abdeen S, et al. Endogenous plasminogen activators mediate progressive intracerebral hemorrhage after traumatic brain injury in mice. *Blood.* (2015) 125:2558–67. doi: 10.1182/blood-2014-08-588442

23

Urine Output is Associated with In-hospital Mortality in Intensive Care Patients with Septic Shock: A Propensity Score Matching Analysis

Tianyang Hu[1†‡], *Zhao Qiao*[1†] *and Ying Mei*[2*]

[1] *Department of Cardiology, The Second Affiliated Hospital, Chongqing Medical University, Chongqing, China,* [2] *Health Management Center, The Second Affiliated Hospital, Chongqing Medical University, Chongqing, China*

***Correspondence:**
Ying Mei
meiying@cqmu.edu.cn

† *These authors have contributed equally to this work and share first authorship*

‡ORCID:
Tianyang Hu
orcid.org/0000-0001-6884-729X

Background: The relationship between urine output (UO) and in-hospital mortality in intensive care patients with septic shock is currently inconclusive.

Methods: The baseline data, UO, and in-hospital prognosis of intensive care patients with septic shock were retrieved from the Medical Information Mart for Intensive Care IV (MIMIC-IV) database. By drawing receiver operating characteristic (ROC) curves and comparing the areas under the ROC curves (AUC) to determine the predictive value of UO for in-hospital mortality, and by drawing the Kaplan-Meier curves to compare the difference in in-hospital mortality between different groups of UO.

Results: Before and after the propensity score matching (PSM) analysis, UO was always a risk factor for in-hospital mortality in patients with septic shock. The AUC of UO was comparable to the Sequential Organ Failure Assessment (SOFA) scoring system, while the AUC of combining UO and SOFA was greater than that of SOFA. The median survival time of the high-UO group (UO > 0.39 ml/kg/h, before PSM; UO > 0.38 ml/kg/h, after PSM) was longer than that of the low-UO group. Compared with the high-UO group, the hazard ratios (HR) of the low-UO group were 2.6857 (before PSM) and 1.7879 (after PSM).

Conclusions: UO is an independent risk factor for septic shock. Low levels of UO significantly increase the in-hospital mortality of intensive care patients with septic shock. The predictive value of UO is comparable to the SOFA scoring system, and the combined predictive value of the two surpasses SOFA alone.

Keywords: septic shock, urine output, MIMIC-IV, in-hospital mortality, propensity score matching

INTRODUCTION

Sepsis is a life-threatening organ dysfunction caused by a dysregulated host response to infection. Septic shock is the most severe form of sepsis, which is characterized by persisting hypotension requiring vasopressors to maintain mean arterial pressure ≥65 mmHg and having an increased serum lactate level >2 mmol/L despite adequate volume resuscitation (1, 2). The in-hospital mortality rate of sepsis exceeds 10%, and septic shock is even worse (1, 3). A meta-analysis of European and North American populations showed that the in-hospital mortality rate of septic shock was as high as 39% (95% CI: 34.4–43.9%) (4). It is of far-reaching significance to clarify the independent risk factors related to mortality, which can further guide nursing and treatment, so as to achieve the purpose of reducing mortality especially in the intensive care unit (ICU).

Daily urine output (UO) is measured routinely in the ICU, and its prognostic value has already emerged. In 2013, Oh et al. (5) found that UO was significantly associated with the prognosis in critically ill patients with acute kidney injury (AKI) requiring continuous renal replacement therapy (CRRT). When the timing of CRRT initiation was stratified by 6 h UO, 28-day all-cause mortality rates were significantly lower in the non-oliguric group compared with the oliguric group. Huang et al. (6) found that reduced initial 24 h UO was associated with an increased risk in 7- and 30-day all-cause mortality and major adverse cardiovascular events (MACE) in ST-segment elevation myocardial infarction (STEMI) patients admitted without cardiogenic shock and renal dysfunction. Zhang et al. (7) investigated the relationship between UO on the first day of admission to the ICU and the in-hospital mortality of unselected critically ill patients and found that UO was an independent risk factor of mortality regardless of whether diuretics were used or not. Oliguria is one of the important signs of hypoperfusion in septic shock (8). However, due to the complexity of the composition of patients admitted to the ICU, it is not known whether the conclusion of Zhang et al. is applicable to septic shock. To date, no researches have confirmed the relationship between UO and mortality of patients with septic shock. This study is based on a well-known public database, Medical Information Mart for Intensive Care IV (MIMIC-IV) database, to investigate the relationship between UO on the first day of admission and the in-hospital mortality of intensive care patients with septic shock.

METHODS

Database

MIMIC-IV (https://mimic.mit.edu/) builds upon the MIMIC-III database (9) and has made many improvements. MIMIC-IV contains comprehensive information (laboratory measurements, medications administered, vital signs documented, etc.) of patients admitted to a Tertiary Academic Medical Center in Boston, MA, USA between 2008 and 2019. The database is designed to support a wide variety of healthcare research. An individual who passed the "Protecting Human Research Participants" exam on the National Institutes of Health website can access the database (certification number 37474354 for author Tianyang Hu).

All patients in the database are anonymous and no informed consent is required.

Study Population and Data Extraction

The patients diagnosed with "septic shock" in the MIMIC-IV database are divided into two categories: "septic shock" with International Classification of Disease (ICD) code 78552 (9th revision), and "severe sepsis with septic shock" with ICD code (10th revision). The inclusion criteria were: (1) aged≥18 years; (2) UO (ml/day) assessed within 24 h from admission; (3) UO (ml/kg/h) could be calculated within 24 h from admission. Post-procedural septic shock was excluded. Since the same patient may have multiple admission records, we only included the first ICU stay for each patient.

The following data was extracted from the MIMIC-IV database (version 1.0) by Navicat Premium software (version 15.0): age, gender, length of ICU stay, length of hospital stay, Charlson comorbidity index, Sequential Organ Failure Assessment (SOFA) score/ hemoglobin/white blood cells/platelets/creatinine/blood urea nitrogen/total bilirubin/heart rate/mean arterial pressure/respiratory rate/weight/urine output/ whether complicated with AKI/whether to take diuretics/whether treated with renal replacement therapy (RRT) on the first day of admission and hospital expire flag (a binary flag which indicates whether the patient died in hospital). Charlson comorbidity index (10) is a scoring system to quantify comorbidities (including myocardial infarct, congestive heart failure, peripheral vascular disease, cerebrovascular disease, dementia, chronic pulmonary disease, rheumatic disease, peptic ulcer disease, liver disease, diabetes, paraplegia, renal disease, malignant cancer, metastatic solid tumor, and acquired immunodeficiency syndrome). Diuretics mainly include bumetanide, chlorothiazide, furosemide, hydrochlorothiazide, metolazone, and spironolactone. If a variable was assessed multiple times on the first day of admission, took the average value.

Statistical Analysis

Use the Kolmogorov-Smirnov test to evaluate whether the variables follow the normal distribution. If followed, then express the variable as mean ± standard deviation (M ± SD) and compare with independent sample *t*-test; if not follow, then express the variable as the median with interquartile range (IQR) and compare with Wilcoxon rank-sum test. Categorical variables were expressed as numbers and percentages, and compared by Chi-square test. Binomial Logistic regression analysis was conducted to evaluate the impact of UO on in-hospital mortality in patients with septic shock. Variables with a *P*-value <0.1 in the univariate analysis were included in the multivariate analysis. Z test was conducted following the method of Delong et al. (11) to compare the predictive value of UO, SOFA, and UO+SOFA by comparing the area under curves (AUC) of the receiver operating characteristic curves (ROC).

To reduce potential bias, propensity score matching (PSM) analysis was performed between the death group and survival

Abbreviations: UO, urine output; MIMIC-IV, Medical Information Mart for Intensive Care IV; AKI, acute kidney injury; CRRT, continuous renal replacement therapy; MACE, major adverse cardiovascular events; STEMI, ST-segment elevation myocardial infarction; ROC, receiver operating characteristic; AUC, areas under the receiver operating characteristic curves; PSM, propensity score matching; SOFA, Sequential Organ Failure Assessment; HR, hazard ratio; OR, Odds Ratio; CI, Confidence Interval; ICU, intensive care unit; ICD, International Classification of Disease; RRT, renal replacement therapy; M ± SD, mean ± standard deviation; IQR, interquartile range; LOS, Length of Stay; CCI, Charlson Comorbidity Index; Hb, Hemoglobin; WBC, White Blood Cells; PLT, Platelets; Cr, Creatinine; BUN, Blood Urea Nitrogen; TBil, Total Bilirubin; HR, Heart Rate; bpm, beat per minute; MAP, Mean Arterial Pressure; RR, Respiratory Rate; cpm, count per minute.

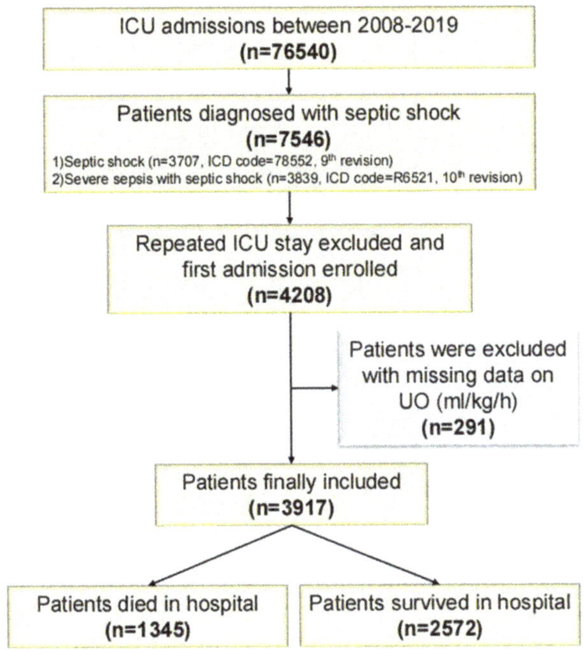

FIGURE 1 | Flowchart of study cohort. ICU, Intensive Care Unit; ICD, International Classification of Disease; UO, Urine Output.

group. All potential confounders were included in the PSM analysis: age, gender, Charlson comorbidity index, hemoglobin, white blood cells, platelets, creatinine, blood urea nitrogen, total bilirubin, heart rate, mean arterial pressure, respiratory rate on the first day of admission, whether complicated with AKI, whether to take diuretics, and whether treated with RRT on the first day of admission. The PSM analysis was performed by a 1:1 nearest neighbor matching algorithm (a caliper of 0.001) without replacement, and the propensity score was calculated by the logistic regression model.

In-hospital mortality is regarded as a time-to-event variable and the event is death during hospitalization. Patients were censored when they were discharged alive, and patients were followed during the hospital stay (7). UO was divided into high-UO group and low-UO group according to the optimal cut-off value indicated by the ROC curve, and Kaplan-Meier survival curves were drawn. The log-rank test was used to evaluate whether there was a difference in survival rate between the two groups.

All the analyses were performed using the software IBM SPSS Statistics (v26.0; IBM, Armonk, NY) and MedCalc (v19.6.1; MedCalc Software Ltd, Ostend, Belgium). A P-value < 0.05 was considered to be statistically significant.

RESULTS

Baseline Characteristics

MIMIC-IV database contains 76,540 ICU admissions. Finally, 3,917 patients were included in this study (of which 1,345 died and 2,572 survived in the hospital, **Figure 1**) and the in-hospital mortality rate was 34.34%. The length of hospital stay of the survival group was longer than that of the death group (P < 0.001). Age, Charlson Comorbidity Index, SOFA score, the level of creatinine, total bilirubin, blood urea nitrogen, heart rate and respiratory rate on the first day of admission in the death group were higher than in the survival group significantly (P < 0.001 for all). Mean arterial pressure, the level of hemoglobin and platelets in the survival group were higher than in the death group significantly (P < 0.001 for all). UO in the survival group was higher than in the death group significantly (P < 0.001). The proportions of complicated with AKI, treated with diuretics and RRT in the death group were higher than in the survival group (P < 0.001 for all). After PSM with age, gender, Charlson comorbidity index, the level of hemoglobin, white blood cells, platelets, creatinine, blood urea nitrogen, total bilirubin, heart rate, mean arterial pressure, respiratory rate, whether complicated with AKI, whether to take diuretics, and whether treated with RRT on the first day of admission, the matching variables were balanced and comparable between the two groups (of which 963 died and 963 survived, P > 0.05 for all, **Table 1**). After PSM, the length of hospital stay of the survival group was still longer than that of the death group (P < 0.001). SOFA score on the first day of admission in the death group was higher than in the survival group significantly (P < 0.001), and UO in the survival group was still significantly higher than in the death group (P < 0.001). The baseline characteristics were presented in **Table 1**.

Logistic Regression Analysis

Considering the collinearity between UO (ml/day) and UO (ml/kg/h), the latter was included in the binomial logistic regression analysis. UO was a risk factor for in-hospital mortality in patients with septic shock before (OR: 0.285, 95% CI: 0.247–0.330, P < 0.001) and after (OR: 0.507, 95% CI: 0.434–0.593, P < 0.001) adjustment (**Table 2**). After PSM, UO was still a risk factor for in-hospital mortality in patients with septic shock before (OR: 0.544, 95% CI: 0.465–0.638, P < 0.001) and after (OR: 0.678, 95% CI: 0.578–0.796, P < 0.001) adjustment (**Table 3**).

Comparison of ROC Curves

The ROC curves were drawn to clarify the predictive value of UO for in-hospital mortality of septic shock (**Figure 2**). Before PSM (**Figure 2A**), the AUCs of UO, SOFA, combining UO and SOFA (UO + SOFA) were 0.722, 0.725, and 0.753, respectively (**Table 4**). The AUC of UO was comparable to SOFA (Z = 0.237, P = 0.8127), while the AUC of UO+SOFA was greater than that of UO (Z = 5.079, P < 0.0001) and SOFA (Z = 6.264, P < 0.0001). UO+SOFA had the highest sensitivity (69.81%) and Youden's index (0.4007), while UO had the highest specificity (76.94%). After PSM (**Figure 2B**), the AUCs of UO, SOFA, and UO+SOFA were 0.637, 0.622, and 0.643, respectively (**Table 5**). The AUC of UO was still comparable to SOFA (Z = 1.090, P = 0.2756), while the AUC of UO + SOFA was also greater than that of SOFA (Z = 3.034, P = 0.0024), but comparable to UO (Z = 0.640, P = 0.5219). UO+SOFA had the Youden's index (0.2420), while UO

TABLE 1 | Demographic and clinical characteristics of the study population.

Characteristics	Before PSM			After PSM		
	Death (n = 2,572)	Survival (n = 1,345)	P	Death (n = 963)	Survival (n = 963)	P
*Age, year	71 (60–82)	68 (56–79)	0.000	72 (61–82)	72 (61–82)	0.961
*Gender, male	723 (53.8)	1398 (54.4)	0.720	521 (54.1)	512 (53.1)	0.681
LOS hospital, day	6.5 (2.0–14.5)	11.5 (6.6–20.6)	0.000	7.1 (2.5–14.6)	12.7 (7.1–21.6)	0.000
LOS ICU, day	3.7 (1.5–8.7)	3.4 (1.9–7.7)	0.243	3.9 (1.6–8.6)	3.8 (2.1–9.0)	0.005
*CCI	7 (5–9)	6 (4–8)	0.000	7 (5–9)	7 (5–9)	0.869
Laboratory tests						
*Hb, g/dL	9.8 (8.5–11.4)	10.3 (8.9–11.7)	0.000	9.9 (8.6–11.5)	10.2 (8.8–11.5)	0.147
*WBC, 10^9/L	14.0 (8.2–20.3)	13.8 (9.3–19.3)	0.854	14.1 (8.2–20.4)	13.7 (9.1–20.3)	0.776
*PLT, 10^9/L	156 (89–241)	183 (124–255)	0.000	169 (99–259)	163 (115–236)	0.668
*Cr, ng/dL	1.7 (1.2–2.7)	1.3 (0.9–2.0)	0.000	1.5 (1.1–2.5)	1.5 (1.0–2.4)	0.617
*BUN, mmol/L	36.0 (23.5–56.0)	26.0 (16.5–42.3)	0.000	33.5 (22.0–52.0)	32.5 (20.5–52.5)	0.318
*TBil, mg/dL	1.6 (0.6–2.9)	1.1 (0.5–2.7)	0.000	1.4 (0.6–2.7)	1.3 (0.6–2.7)	0.778
Vital signs						
*HR, bpm	96 (82–108)	90 (78–102)	0.000	94 (80–107)	94 (81–106)	0.899
*MAP, mmHg	71 (65–76)	72 (68–77)	0.000	71 (66–77)	72 (67–77)	0.207
*RR, cpm	22 (19–26)	21 (18–24)	0.000	22 (19–25)	22 (19–25)	0.519
SOFA score	12 (9–15)	8 (5–11)	0.000	11 (8–14)	8 (6–12)	0.000
Day 1 UO, ml/day	595 (186–1264)	1400 (825–2317)	0.000	715 (264–1400)	1170 (649–1950)	0.000
Day 1 UO, ml/kg/h	0.32 (0.10–0.67)	0.75 (0.41–1.25)	0.000	0.38 (0.13–0.73)	0.63 (0.33–1.05)	0.000
*Day 1 AKI	425 (31.6)	538 (20.9)	0.000	264 (27.4)	254 (26.3)	0.607
*Day 1 diuretic	269 (20.0)	318 (12.4)	0.000	166 (17.2)	161 (16.7)	0.762
*Day 1 RRT	366 (27.2)	271 (10.5)	0.000	181 (18.8)	182 (18.9)	0.954

Values are expressed as the median (IQR) or n (%).
PSM, Propensity Score Matching; LOS, Length of Stay; ICU, Intensive Care Unit; CCI, Charlson Comorbidity Index; Hb, Hemoglobin; WBC, White Blood Cells; PLT, Platelets; Cr, Creatinine; BUN, Blood Urea Nitrogen; TBil, Total Bilirubin; HR, Heart Rate; bpm, beat per minute; MAP, Mean Arterial Pressure; RR, Respiratory Rate; cpm, count per minute; SOFA, Sequential Organ Failure Assessment; UO, Urine Output; AKI, Acute Kidney Injury; RRT, Renal Replacement Therapy.
**Covariables included in the PSM.*

had the highest specificity (71.55%) and SOFA had the highest sensitivity (70.40%).

Comparison of Kaplan-Meier Curves

Before PSM, UO was divided into high-UO group and low-UO group with the optimal cut-off value of 0.39 ml/kg/h. The Kaplan-Meier curves are shown in **Figure 3**. The median survival time of the high-UO group was 42.097 days (95% CI: 37.842–52.060), while of the low-UO group was 14.470 days (95% CI: 12.726–16.674), and the difference was statistically significant (P < 0.0001). Compared with the high-UO group, the hazard ratio (HR) of the low-UO group was 2.6857 (95% CI: 2.3955–3.0112). After PSM, the optimal cut-off value was 0.38 ml/kg/h (**Figure 4**). The median survival time of the high-UO group was 23.632 days (95% CI: 21.448–27.116), while of the low-UO group was 11.449 days (95% CI: 9.955–12.926), and the difference was statistically significant (P < 0.0001). Compared with the high-UO group, the HR of the low-UO group was 1.7879 (95% CI: 1.5669–2.0401).

DISCUSSION

To the best of our knowledge, this study investigated the relationship between urine output on the first day of admission and in-hospital mortality of intensive care patients with septic shock for the first time. We confirmed that UO is an independent risk factor for septic shock. Before PSM, the optimal cut-off value determined by the ROC curve was 0.39 mg/kg/h. Compared with the high-UO group, the HR of the low-UO group was 2.6857, suggesting that the risk of in-hospital death in the low-UO group was 2.6857 times that of the high-UO group. The optimal cut-off value after PSM was 0.38 mg/kg/h, which was almost the same as before PSM. It was found that the risk of in-hospital death in the low-UO group was 1.7879 times that of the high-UO group. Therefore, the above results indicate that a low level of UO on the first day is significantly associated with an increase in in-hospital mortality.

The PSM is a "post-randomization" statistical analysis method, which reduces the influence of biases and confounding variables on the results in retrospective studies to a certain extent. AKI is the most frequent complication in septic shock and RRT is the standard of care for severe AKI (12). If patients with septic shock have oliguria or anuria on admission, they may progress to AKI at a later stage. A study showed that 3–5 h consecutive oliguria in patients with septic shock may be an indicator to measure the risk of AKI (13). Meanwhile, the most frequent indication for acute dialysis was oliguria (14). In

TABLE 2 | Binomial Logistic regression analysis of urine output for in-hospital mortality among intensive care patients with septic shock (before PSM).

Variable	Univariable		Multivariable	
	OR (95% CI)	***P***	**OR (95% CI)**	***P***
Age	1.014 (1.010–1.018)	0.000	1.009 (1.002–1.016)	0.007
Gender (male)	0.976 (0.855–1.114)	0.720		
LOS hospital	0.976 (0.971–0.982)	0.000	0.966 (0.960–0.973)	0.000
LOS ICU	1.004 (0.996–1.013)	0.282		
CCI	1.161 (1.133–1.188)	0.000	1.143 (1.107–1.181)	0.000
Hemoglobin	0.925 (0.894–0.956)	0.000	0.942 (0.904–0.982)	0.005
WBC	1.005 (0.999–1.010)	0.088	0.998 (0.992–1.004)	0.532
Platelets	0.998 (0.998–0.999)	0.000	1.001 (1.000–1.001)	0.095
Creatinine	1.182 (1.131–1.234)	0.000	0.719 (0.661–0.781)	0.000
BUN	1.015 (1.012–1.017)	0.000	1.009 (1.005–1.014)	0.000
Total bilirubin	1.182 (1.131–1.234)	0.000	1.035 (1.017–1.054)	0.000
Heart rate	1.016 (1.013–1.020)	0.000	1.017 (1.012–1.022)	0.000
MAP	0.967 (0.959–0.975)	0.000	0.988 (0.979–0.998)	0.016
Respiratory rate	1.086 (1.069–1.102)	0.000	1.045 (1.025–1.066)	0.000
SOFA score	1.015 (1.012–1.017)	0.000	1.175 (1.147–1.203)	0.000
Day 1 UO, mg/kg/h	0.285 (0.247–0.330)	0.000	0.507 (0.434–0.593)	0.000
Day 1 AKI	1.747 (1.505–2.027)	0.000	1.030 (0.854–1.240)	0.760
Day 1 diuretic	1.772 (1.483–2.117)	0.000	1.590 (1.284–1.968)	0.000
Day 1 RRT	3.174 (2.667–3.777)	0.000	2.285 (1.779–2.935)	0.000

PSM, Propensity Score Matching; OR, Odds Ratio; CI, Confidence Interval; LOS, Length of Stay; ICU, Intensive Care Unit; CCI, Charlson Comorbidity Index; WBC, White Blood Cells; BUN, Blood Urea Nitrogen; MAP, Mean Arterial Pressure; SOFA, Sequential Organ Failure Assessment; UO, Urine Output; AKI, Acute Kidney Injury; RRT, Renal Replacement Therapy.

TABLE 3 | Binomial Logistic regression analysis of urine output for in-hospital mortality among intensive care patients with septic shock (after PSM).

Variable	Univariable		Multivariable	
	OR (95% CI)	***P***	**OR (95% CI)**	***P***
Age	1.001 (0.995–1.007)	0.858		
Gender, male	1.038 (0.868–1.242)	0.681		
LOS hospital	0.981 (0.974–0.987)	0.000	0.979 (0.972–0.986)	0.000
LOS ICU	0.992 (0.982–1.002)	0.106		
CCI	1.006 (0.974–1.039)	0.715		
Hemoglobin	0.982 (0.939–1.027)	0.434		
WBC	0.999 (0.992–1.006)	0.792		
Platelets	1.001 (1.000–1.001)	0.099	1.002 (1.001–1.002)	0.000
Creatinine	1.005 (0.948–1.066)	0.871		
BUN	1.001 (0.998–1.004)	0.601		
Total bilirubin	0.999 (0.979–1.020)	0.913		
Heart rate	1.000 (0.994–1.005)	0.853		
MAP	0.999 (0.989–1.009)	0.801		
Respiratory Rate	0.993 (0.973–1.014)	0.513		
SOFA score	1.102 (1.078–1.127)	0.000	1.105 (1.079–1.133)	0.000
Day 1 UO, mg/kg/h	0.544 (0.465–0.638)	0.000	0.678 (0.578–0.796)	0.000
Day 1 AKI	1.054 (0.862–1.290)	0.607		
Day 1 diuretic	1.038 (0.818–1.316)	0.762		
Day 1 RRT	0.993 (0.790–1.248)	0.954		

PSM, Propensity Score Matching; OR, Odds Ratio; CI, Confidence Interval; LOS, Length of Stay; ICU, Intensive Care Unit; CCI, Charlson Comorbidity Index; WBC, White Blood Cells; BUN, Blood Urea Nitrogen; MAP, Mean Arterial Pressure; SOFA, Sequential Organ Failure Assessment; UO, Urine Output; AKI, Acute Kidney Injury; RRT, Renal Replacement Therapy.

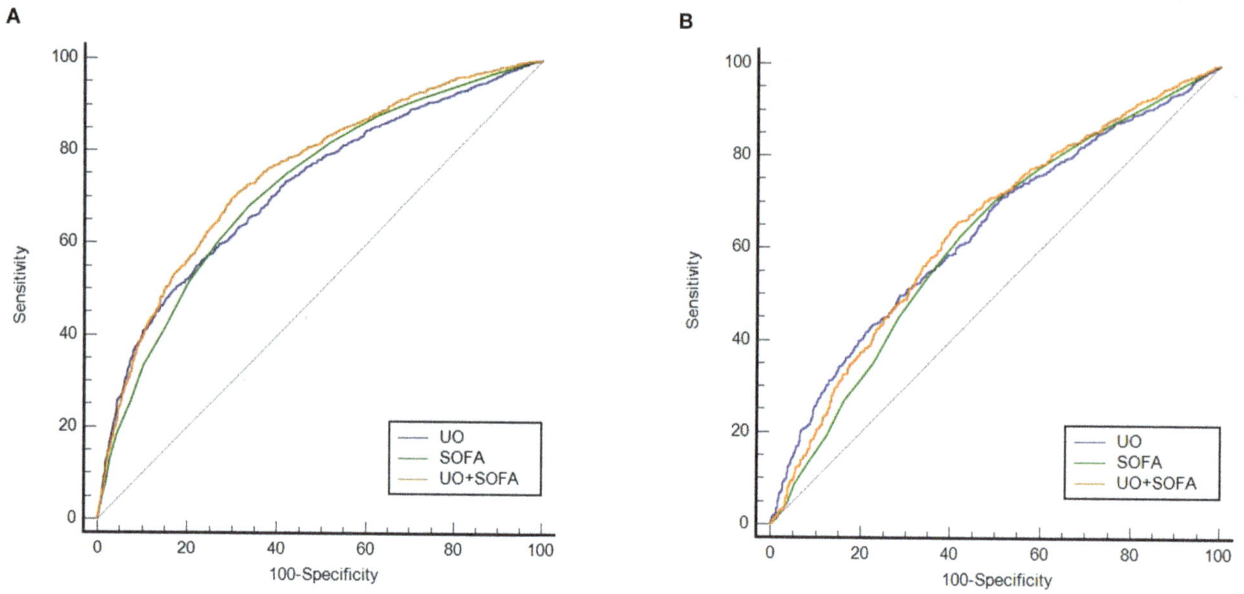

FIGURE 2 | (A) ROC curves of UO, SOFA, UO + SOFA (before propensity score matching); **(B)** ROC curves of UO, SOFA, UO + SOFA (after propensity score matching). UO, Urine Output (mg/kg/h); SOFA, Sequential Organ Failure Assessment.

TABLE 4 | Comparison of ROC curves (before PSM).

Factor	AUC	95%CI	Optimal cut-off	Sensitivity	Specificity	Youden's index
UO	0.722	0.708~0.736	0.39	56.21	76.94	0.3315
SOFA	0.725	0.710~0.739	9	68.18	66.45	0.3462
UO + SOFA	0.753	0.740~0.767	0.34265*	69.81	70.26	0.4007

UO, Urine Output (mg/kg/h); SOFA, Sequential Organ Failure Assessment.
**Prediction probability of logistic regression model for combining UO and SOFA, corresponding to UO = 0.94, SOFA = 11.*

TABLE 5 | Comparison of ROC curves (after PSM).

Factor	AUC	95%CI	Optimal cut-off	Sensitivity	Specificity	Youden's index
UO	0.637	0.615~0.659	0.38	49.64	71.55	0.2118
SOFA	0.622	0.600~0.644	8	70.40	50.36	0.2077
UO + SOFA	0.643	0.621~0.664	0.49034*	65.84	58.36	0.2420

UO, Urine Output (mg/kg/h); SOFA, Sequential Organ Failure Assessment.
**Prediction probability of logistic regression model for combining UO and SOFA, corresponding to UO = 0.58, SOFA = 9.*

general, whether patients are complicated with AKI and whether to undergo RRT or diuretic therapy are significantly related to UO theoretically. We have also balanced some important laboratory tests and vital signs. Among them, white blood cells count is related to infection and is often used to detect sepsis (15); creatinine and BUN can reflect renal function (16); platelets and total bilirubin can reflect coagulation function and liver function (17); respiratory rate is related to respiratory function; hemoglobin not only reflects the presence of anemia, but also is related to oxygenation (18). We were trying to evaluate indicators related to cardiac function, but the missing values of indicators such as troponin and BNP in the MIMIC-IV database are too many, and some even exceed 90%. Imaging data of cardiac function, such as ejection fraction, are currently not available in MIMIC-IV database. Thus, we finally used heart rate and mean arterial pressure as matching parameters to minimize the cardiac function bias between the two groups. After PSM, although the risk of in-hospital death in the low-UO group was lower than

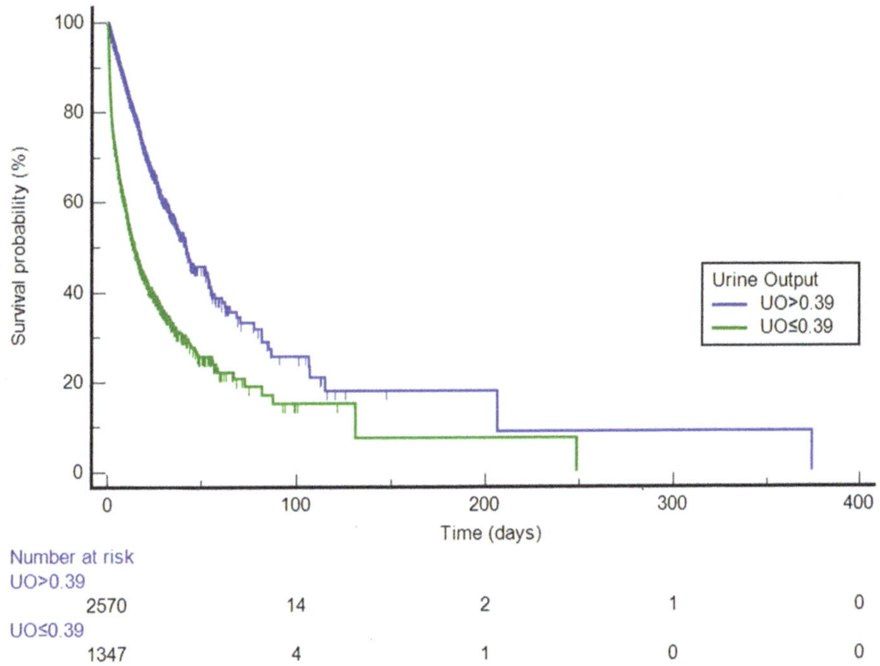

FIGURE 3 | Kaplan-Meier survival curves by urine output category (before propensity score matching, log-rank $P < 0.0001$). UO, Urine Output (mg/kg/h).

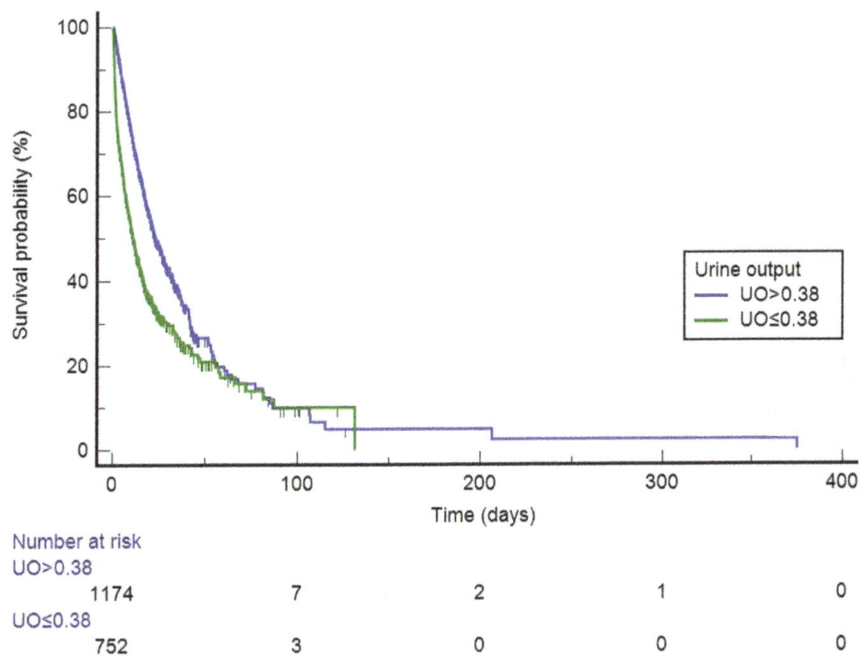

FIGURE 4 | Kaplan-Meier survival curves by urine output category (after propensity score matching, log-rank $P < 0.0001$). UO, Urine Output (mg/kg/h).

before, it still had approximately twice the risk of death (1.7879 times) compared to the high-UO group. It can be seen that the UO on the first day of admission does not depend on whether complicated with AKI and whether to undergo RRT or diuretic therapy, but is directly related to the prognosis of the patients, reflecting the independence of its predictive value.

Septic shock is a complex syndrome with severe hemodynamic changes, manifested by profound cardiovascular derangements, redistribution of blood flow between organs, and microcirculatory alterations (2). Cardiovascular derangements and the redistribution of blood flow can seriously affect splanchnic circulation, and if the kidney is compromised, it will correspondingly lead to a decrease in UO. Meanwhile, sepsis, especially in severe patients, is almost invariably related to altered coagulation, which can easily lead to disseminated intravascular coagulation (19) and microvascular thrombosis (20). Thrombus formation leads to insufficient tissue perfusion. Since the septic shock is a subtype and severe type of sepsis, which is more prone to progress to coagulation dysfunction and eventually leads to insufficient tissue perfusion, resulting a decrease in UO. In addition, septic shock can cause a vasodilatory state due to excessive NO production, vasopressin deficiency and resistance (21, 22), and further aggravate tissue hypoperfusion. The above reasons are independent of AKI and lead a decrease in UO, therefore, even after adjusting for confounding factors such as AKI, UO is still an independent risk factor for in-hospital mortality in patients with septic shock.

The essence of sepsis and septic shock is organ dysfunction, and the severity of organ dysfunction has been assessed through various scoring systems. Currently, SOFA is the predominant scoring system used for sepsis and septic shock, and it is also one of the definitions of sepsis recognized by Sepsis-3 (1). Several studies have confirmed the value of SOFA in predicting the mortality of septic shock (23–28), but its performance is not satisfactory. In our study, before PSM, the AUC of UO exceeded 0.7, which was of moderate predictive value. After PSM, AUC dropped to 0.637, suggesting that the predictive value was limited. However, the predictive value of UO was always comparable to the SOFA score system. Even so, the application of UO alone in the prediction of in-hospital mortality for septic shock still lacks practical significance. The combination of predictors may improve prediction performance. As the task force of Sepsis-3 pointed out, there are many novel biomarkers that can identify renal dysfunction or coagulopathy earlier than the elements used in SOFA, but they need to be more extensively verified before they are incorporated into the clinical criteria for sepsis (1). In this study, the combined prediction efficiency of UO and SOFA was higher than that of SOFA alone. However, since the respective weights were not given, the corresponding cut-off values of the two were not suitable for predicting in-hospital mortality directly. Thus, it may be a better choice to consider creating a new scoring system, such as incorporating UO into SOFA as a factor, similar to the "UO-corrected SOFA scoring system."

Our findings emphasize the importance of monitoring UO in clinical practice in order to identify high-risk patients with septic shock early and intervene as soon as possible to achieve the goal of reducing in-hospital mortality. UO monitoring is easy to perform and inexpensive, and is especially suitable for promotion in countries with limited resources. We recommend using the weight-corrected UO, namely UO (ml/kg/h). Moreover, we also emphasize the importance of UO in the hemodynamic management of septic shock. Hemodynamic support for patients with septic shock is crucial (29), including the use of large amounts of fluids in combination with vasopressors, and in some cases with inotropic agents. The hemodynamic targets for resuscitation of septic shock often rely on macro-hemodynamic parameters, including heart rate, mean arterial pressure, and central venous pressure. However, despite the restoration of macro-hemodynamic parameters, persistent alterations in microcirculatory blood flow can still lead to organ failure (2, 30, 31). This dissociation between the macrocirculation and microcirculation is the so-called "a loss of hemodynamic coherence" (32). UO reflects renal perfusion and is also an effective indicator of microcirculation perfusion. Thus, monitoring UO may play a positive role in hemodynamic management for septic shock.

We must point out the limitations of this study: (1) The patients in the MIMIC-IV database are mainly white, and a large number of patients cannot be identified by ethnicity. Therefore, the variable ethnicity was not included in the PSM analysis, which has a potential impact on the results; (2) At present, it is difficult to identify the exact sites of infection and causative organisms of the patients in the database. The predictive value of UO for septic shock caused by different reasons or in different sites of infection (such as kidney vs. other sites) may be significantly different; (3) The daily fluid intake (including drinking water) of the patients will also affect the UO, but since the exact values of these variables cannot be obtained, the influence of these confounding factors on the results cannot be ignored. It should be pointed out that a large part of the patients in this study may not have been diagnosed with septic shock at the time of admission. Therefore, our findings may also be applicable to intensive care patients with the potential to develop septic shock. The advantage of this study lies in the large sample size, which allows us to have enough space for the PSM analysis and makes our conclusions more reliable.

CONCLUSIONS

UO is an independent risk factor for septic shock. Low levels of UO significantly increase the in-hospital mortality of intensive care patients with septic shock. The predictive value of UO for patients with septic shock is comparable to the SOFA scoring system, and the combined predictive value of the two surpasses SOFA alone. Since the above results are based on this retrospective study, rigorous prospective clinical trials are still needed to confirm.

ETHICS STATEMENT

Ethical review and approval was not required for the study on human participants in accordance with the local legislation and institutional requirements. Written informed consent for participation was not required for this study in accordance with the national legislation and the institutional requirements.

AUTHOR CONTRIBUTIONS

TH and YM conceived and designed the study. TH and ZQ extracted the data, analyzed and interpreted the data, and drafted the work. YM participated in design of the study, assisted with revisions of the manuscript, and takes responsibility for the content of the manuscript including the data and analysis. All authors have approved the final version of the manuscript for submission and agree to be accountable for all aspects of the work.

ACKNOWLEDGMENTS

We would like to thank the Massachusetts Institute of Technology and the Beth Israel Deaconess Medical Center for the MIMIC-IV database.

REFERENCES

1. Singer M, Deutschman CS, Seymour CW, Shankar-Hari M, Annane D, Bauer M, et al. The third international consensus definitions for sepsis and septic shock (sepsis-3). *JAMA.* (2016) 315:801–10. doi: 10.1001/jama.2016.0287
2. De Backer D, Ricottilli F, Ospina-Tascón GA. Septic shock: a microcirculation disease. *Curr Opin Anaesthesiol.* (2021) 34:85–91. doi: 10.1097/ACO.0000000000000957
3. Font MD, Thyagarajan B, Khanna AK. Sepsis and Septic Shock - Basics of diagnosis, pathophysiology and clinical decision making. *Med Clin North Am.* (2020) 104:573–85. doi: 10.1016/j.mcna.2020.02.011
4. Vincent JL, Jones G, David S, Olariu E, Cadwell KK. Frequency and mortality of septic shock in Europe and North America: a systematic review and meta-analysis. *Crit Care.* (2019) 23:196. doi: 10.1186/s13054-019-2478-6
5. Oh HJ, Shin DH, Lee MJ, Ko KI, Kim CH, Koo HM, et al. Urine output is associated with prognosis in patients with acute kidney injury requiring continuous renal replacement therapy. *J Crit Care.* (2013) 28:379–88. doi: 10.1016/j.jcrc.2012.11.019
6. Huang B, Yang Y, Zhu J, Liang Y, Tan H, Yu L, et al. Impact of initial 24-h urine output on short-term outcomes in patients with ST-segment elevation myocardial infarction admitted without cardiogenic shock and renal dysfunction. *Atherosclerosis.* (2015) 240:137–43. doi: 10.1016/j.atherosclerosis.2015.03.005
7. Zhang Z, Xu X, Ni H, Deng H. Urine output on ICU entry is associated with hospital mortality in unselected critically ill patients. *J Nephrol.* (2014) 27:65–71. doi: 10.1007/s40620-013-0024-1
8. Seymour CW, Rosengart MR. Septic shock: advances in diagnosis and treatment. *JAMA.* (2015) 314:708–17. doi: 10.1001/jama.2015.7885
9. Johnson AE, Pollard TJ, Shen L, Lehman LW, Feng M, Ghassemi M, et al. MIMIC-III, a freely accessible critical care database. *Sci Data.* (2016) 3:160035. doi: 10.1038/sdata.2016.35
10. Charlson ME, Pompei P, Ales KL, MacKenzie CR. A new method of classifying prognostic comorbidity in longitudinal studies: development and validation. *J Chronic Dis.* (1987) 40:373–83. doi: 10.1016/0021-9681(87)90171-8
11. DeLong ER, DeLong DM, Clarke-Pearson DL. Comparing the areas under two or more correlated receiver operating characteristic curves: a nonparametric approach. *Biometrics.* (1988) 44:837–45. doi: 10.2307/2531595
12. Barbar SD, Clere-Jehl R, Bourredjem A, Hernu R, Montini F, Bruyère R, et al. Timing of renal-replacement therapy in patients with acute kidney injury and sepsis. *N Engl J Med.* (2018) 379:1431–42. doi: 10.1056/NEJMoa1803213
13. Leedahl DD, Frazee EN, Schramm GE, Dierkhising RA, Bergstralh EJ, Chawla LS, et al. Derivation of urine output thresholds that identify a very high risk of AKI in patients with septic shock. *Clin J Am Soc Nephrol.* (2014) 9:1168–74. doi: 10.2215/CJN.09360913
14. Wu VC, Chueh SJ, Chang JT, Hsu BG, Ostermann M, Chu TS. Acute kidney injury and septic shock-defined by updated sepsis-3 criteria in critically ill patients. *J Clin Med.* (2019) 8:1731. doi: 10.3390/jcm8101731
15. Crouser ED, Parrillo JE, Seymour C, Angus DC, Bicking K, Tejidor L, et al. Improved early detection of sepsis in the Ed with a novel monocyte distribution width biomarker. *Chest.* (2017) 152:518–26. doi: 10.1016/j.chest.2017.05.039
16. Kaiser R, Seiler S, Held M, Bals R, Wilkens H. Prognostic impact of renal function in precapillary pulmonary hypertension. *J Intern Med.* (2014) 275:116–26. doi: 10.1111/joim.12131
17. Peng J, He G, Chen H, Kuang X. Study on correlation between coagulation indexes and disease progression in patients with cirrhosis. *Am J Transl Res.* (2021) 13:4614–23.
18. Martin DS, Grocott MP. Oxygen therapy in critical illness: precise control of arterial oxygenation and permissive hypoxemia. *Crit Care Med.* (2013) 41:423–32. doi: 10.1097/CCM.0b013e31826a44f6
19. Levi M, van der Poll T. Inflammation and coagulation. *Crit Care Med.* (2010) 38(2 Suppl.):S26–34. doi: 10.1097/CCM.0b013e3181c98d21
20. Angus DC, van der Poll T. Severe sepsis and septic shock. *N Engl J Med.* (2013) 369:840–51. doi: 10.1056/NEJMra1208623
21. De Backer D. Hemodynamic management of septic shock. *Curr Infect Dis Rep.* (2006) 8:366–72. doi: 10.1007/s11908-006-0047-z
22. Sharshar T, Blanchard A, Paillard M, Raphael JC, Gajdos P, Annane D. Circulating vasopressin levels in septic shock. *Crit Care Med.* (2003) 31:1752–8. doi: 10.1097/01.CCM.0000063046.82359.4A
23. Vincent JL, de Mendonça A, Cantraine F, Moreno R, Takala J, Suter PM, et al. Use of the SOFA score to assess the incidence of organ dysfunction/failure in intensive care units: results of a multicenter, prospective study. Working group on "sepsis-related problems" of the European Society of Intensive Care Medicine. *Crit Care Med.* (1998) 26:1793–800. doi: 10.1097/00003246-199811000-00016
24. Macdonald SP, Arendts G, Fatovich DM, Brown SG. Comparison of PIRO, SOFA, and MEDS scores for predicting mortality in emergency department patients with severe sepsis and septic shock. *Acad Emerg Med.* (2014) 21:1257–63. doi: 10.1111/acem.12515
25. Baig MA, Sheikh S, Hussain E, Bakhtawar S, Subhan Khan M, Mujtaba S, et al. Comparison of qSOFA and SOFA score for predicting mortality in severe sepsis and septic shock patients in the emergency department of a low middle income country. *Turk J Emerg Med.* (2018) 18:148–51. doi: 10.1016/j.tjem.2018.08.002
26. Liu Z, Meng Z, Li Y, Zhao J, Wu S, Gou S, et al. Prognostic accuracy of the serum lactate level, the SOFA score and the qSOFA score for mortality among adults with Sepsis. *Scand J Trauma Resusc Emerg Med.* (2019) 27:51. doi: 10.1186/s13049-019-0609-3
27. Khwannimit B, Bhurayanontachai R, Vattanavanit V. Comparison of the accuracy of three early warning scores with SOFA score for predicting mortality in adult sepsis and septic shock patients admitted to intensive care unit. *Heart Lung.* (2019) 48:240–4. doi: 10.1016/j.hrtlng.2019.02.005
28. Bauer M, Gerlach H, Vogelmann T, Preissing F, Stiefel J, Adam D. Mortality in sepsis and septic shock in Europe, North America and Australia between 2009 and 2019- results from a systematic review and meta-analysis. *Crit Care.* (2020) 24:239. doi: 10.1186/s13054-020-02950-2
29. Cinel I, Kasapoglu US, Gul F, Dellinger RP. The initial resuscitation of septic shock. *J Crit Care.* (2020) 57:108–17. doi: 10.1016/j.jcrc.2020.02.004

30. Hariri G, Joffre J, Leblanc G, Bonsey M, Lavillegrand JR, Urbina T, et al. Narrative review: clinical assessment of peripheral tissue perfusion in septic shock. *Ann Intensive Care.* (2019) 9:37. doi: 10.1186/s13613-019-0511-1
31. Bakker J, Ince C. Monitoring coherence between the macro and microcirculation in septic shock. *Curr Opin Crit Care.* (2020) 26:267–72. doi: 10.1097/MCC.0000000000000729
32. Ince C. Hemodynamic coherence and the rationale for monitoring the microcirculation. *Crit Care.* (2015) 19 Suppl 3(Suppl. 3):S8. doi: 10.1186/cc14726

24

Extracorporeal Cytokine Removal in Critically Ill COVID-19 Patients

*Marcell Virág [1,2,3], Máté Rottler [1,2,3], Klementina Ocskay [1], Tamás Leiner [1,4], Balázs Horváth [1], Daniel Adam Blanco [5], Alexa Vasquez [5], László Bucsi [6], Ágnes Sárkány [2] and Zsolt Molnár [1,3,5,7,8]**

[1] Medical School, Institute for Translational Medicine, University of Pécs, Pécs, Hungary, [2] Department of Anesthesiology and Intensive Therapy, Szent György University Teaching Hospital of Fejér County, Székesfehérvár, Hungary, [3] Doctoral School of Clinical Medicine, University of Szeged, Szeged, Hungary, [4] Anaesthetic Department, Hinchingbrooke Hospital, North West Anglia National Health Service (NHS) Foundation Trust, Huntingdon, United Kingdom, [5] CytoSorbents Europe, Berlin, Germany, [6] Szent György University Teaching Hospital of Fejér County, Székesfehérvár, Hungary, [7] Department of Anesthesiology and Intensive Therapy, Poznan University of Medical Sciences, Poznan, Poland, [8] Department of Anesthesiology and Intensive Therapy, Semmelweis University, Budapest, Hungary

***Correspondence:**
Zsolt Molnár
zsoltmolna@gmail.com

Introduction: Extracorporeal hemoadsorption (HA) is a potential adjunctive therapy in severe cases of COVID-19 associated pneumonia. In this retrospective study we report data from critically ill patients treated with HA during the first and second wave of the pandemic.

Patients and Methods: All patients, who received HA therapy with CytoSorb within the first 96 h of intensive care unit (ICU) admission without hospital-acquired bacterial superinfection, were included. Clinical and laboratory data were collected: on admission, before (T_B) and after (T_A) HA therapy.

Results: Out of the 367 COVID-19 cases, 13 patients were treated with CytoSorb, also requiring mechanical ventilation and renal replacement therapy. All patients were alive at the end of HA, but only 3 survived hospital stay. From T_B-T_A there was a tendency of decreasing norepinephrine requirement: 193.7 [IQR: 34.8–270.4] to 50.2 [6.5–243.5] ug/kg/day and increasing PaO2/FiO2 ratio 127.8 (95% CI: 96.0–159.6) to 155.0 (115.3–194.6) mmHg but they did not reach statistical significance ($p = 0.14$ and 0.58, respectively). Treatment related adverse events were not reported.

Conclusion: The treatment was well-tolerated, and there was a tendency toward an improvement in vasopressor need and oxygenation during the course of HA. These observations render the need for prospective randomized trials.

Keywords: ARDS, cytokine storm, CRRT, COVID-19, hemoadsorption, Cytosorb

INTRODUCTION

Treating critically ill Coronavirus Disease 19 (COVID-19) patients has become the most significant challenge intensive care has ever faced. The vast number of patients requiring care simultaneously, and the novelty and unpredictability of the virus created an unprecedented environment for all involved. Hospitals were overwhelmed by the continuous influx of severely unwell patients, and intensive care units (ICUs) expanded beyond their original footprint. Critical care mortality of COVID-19 patients significantly exceeded the mortality of any other viral pneumonia (37.9 vs. 22.0%) (1).

Due to the early introduction of lockdown during the first wave of the pandemic, Hungary experienced significantly less pressure on its healthcare system compared to most of the Western European countries. However, it was hit very hard by the next consecutive waves during the autumn and winter of 2020–2021, which resulted in one of the, if not the highest rates of COVID-19 mortality per capita in the world (304.33 deaths/100,000) (2).

Early reports of observations indicated that cytokines might play a considerable role in the development of severe COVID-19. Patients who required critical care admission had higher levels of cytokines. Furthermore, tumour necrosis factor-alfa (TNFa) levels correlated with disease severity, and high interleukin 6 (IL-6), C-reactive protein (CRP), D-Dimer and ferritin levels were found to be predictors of mortality (3–5).

There is some evidence that with extracorporeal cytokine adsorption, substantial IL-6 removal is achievable in severely ill patients with septic shock, acute respiratory distress syndrome (ARDS), and multi-organ failure (6). In a Hungarian proof of concept randomised, controlled pilot study, a significant reduction in vasopressor need and serum pro-calcitonin levels were found (7). Moreover, in a retrospective study of patients with septic shock, cytokine removal was associated with a decreased observed vs. expected 28-day all-cause mortality (8).

In our tertiary intensive care unit (ICU) we have also used hemoadsorption (HA) as an adjuvant therapy in selected patients with septic shock since 2016. During the COVID-19 pandemic our institute served as one of the biggest referral centres in the country, with 120 dedicated COVID-19 ICU beds during the peak of the pandemic (un-published data). As the situation proved desperate, we also reached out for adjunctive therapies such as cytokine adsorption in the most severely ill COVID-19 patients.

The aim of the current retrospective study is to summarise our experience with extracorporeal cytokine adsorption in critically ill COVID-19 patients admitted to our ICU during the first and second wave of the pandemic.

PATIENTS AND METHODS

For this retrospective case-series we screened the records of all patients admitted to the ICU of the Department of Anaesthesia and Intensive Care Medicine at Fejér County St. György University Teaching Hospital, Székesfehérvár, Hungary, between March 1st 2020 and January 31st, 2021. Approval from the local ethics committee was obtained (No: 18/2021.05.11.). Due to the retrospective and anonymized data collection process, patients' informed consent was not deemed necessary.

We identified patients, who had severe, life-threatening COVID-19 confirmed with either polymerase chain reaction (PCR) or rapid antigen testing.

All patients had severe respiratory failure requiring mechanical ventilation and received standard intensive monitoring and therapy based on international guidelines and recommendations.

All patients, who received HA therapy within the first 96 h of ICU admission were considered eligible for the analysis. Hemadsorption treatment was applied as an additional adsorbent cartridge (CytoSorb/CytoSorbents Europe GmbH, Berlin, Germany) integrated into a continuous renal replacement (CRRT) circuit. Patients who received HA more, than up to a maximum of 96 h after ICU admission were presumed to have septic shock due to hospital acquired secondary infections, hence they were excluded. Those, who died within 48 h of the application of the first HA were excluded.

The indication to start CRRT was based on our local protocol: CRRT was commenced in patients with acute renal injury (AKI) stage II according to Kidney Disease Improving Global Outcomes (KDIGO) criteria or severe refractory fluid overload, furthermore in patients without renal indication in order to facilitate HA therapy in hemoperfusion mode only (9).

Executing CRRT with or without HA was at the discretion of the attending senior intensive care physician. Nevertheless, by-and-large the following indications were taken into account: suspicion of hyper-inflammatory state based on elevated inflammatory markers such as CRP and granulocyte count combined with considerable hemodynamic instability necessitating increasing doses of catecholamines and/or severe ARDS defined by the Berlin definition and/or multiple organ failure (10).

Integration of the adsorber into the CRRT circuit (Prismaflex System/Baxter International Inc., Deerfield, IL, USA) was handled by trained intensive care physicians following the manufacturer's instructions. The cartridge was placed in pre-dialyzer position. CRRT was performed in continuous hemodiafiltration mode (CVVHDF), as our standard practise, at a blood flow rate of 100–250 ml/min with systemic unfractionated heparin or regional citrate anticoagulant as recommended by the KDIGO 2012 recommendations (11). Based on the attending physician's decision the cartridges were changed every 12 or 24 h. According to our standard operating procedures, hemoadsorption was discontinued in cases of clinical improvement as indicated by a reduction in the required catecholamine dose, increase in the PaO2/FiO2 ratio, or due to deterioration in the patient's overall condition or no improvement after 2 treatment sessions.

Data collection was undertaken retrospectively by review of our electronic medical records. We gathered pertinent information on demographic data and past medical his-tory. For risk stratification the 4C and sequential organ failure assessment scores (SOFA) were calculated. Relevant clinical data were assessed at three different time points: (1) on admission, (2) at the onset of the adsorbent therapy ("before," TB), and 3) after the completion of adsorbent therapy ("after," TA). We measured inflammatory markers such as leukocyte and granulocyte count, CRP, procalcitonin (PCT), hemodynamic parameters such as catecholamine requirement, serum lactate levels; respiratory function as indicated by the PaO2/FiO2 ratio, PaCO2, and renal function assessed by blood urea nitrogen, creatinine and glomerular filtration rate. We analysed the association between the use of HA and changes in SOFA-score, in the PaO2/FiO2 ratio and in catecholamine dose, as well as days on mechanical ventilation, ICU length-of-stay and 28-day mortality.

Statistical Analysis

Data were collected in a preformatted, anonymized table, which had been used exclusively for all further analyses. All calculations were undertaken by means of descriptive statistics. Continuous variables were expressed as mean (confidence interval, CI) or median [interquartile range, IQR], as appropriate. Statistical analyses and graphs were performed with STATA 15 software using parametric and non-parametric methods for mean and median comparisons as appropriate.

RESULTS

Baseline Characteristics

Out of the 367 patients treated with COVID-19 in the ICU, invasive ventilation was necessary in 153 cases. Thirty-Seven patients were on CRRT, and 13 patients were included the current case series suffering from COVID-19 viral pneumonia, who received hemoadsorption therapy with CytoSorb. Three patients were admitted from a COVID-19 medical ward and one patient was transferred from another hospital's ICU. All four patients were admitted to our ICU within 24 h after the onset of symptoms, hence hospital acquired infection was highly unlikely.

Baseline characteristics, comorbidities and on-admission laboratory values of the included patients are presented in **Table 1**. All patients but one were male, with a mean age of 57 (±11) years. According to the 4C prognostic mortality score most patients (61.6%) had at high or very high risk on admission. Nine patients (69.2%) suffered from some sort of comorbidity, including hypertension, diabetes, or acute myocardial infarction. Regarding on-admission laboratory parameters, as indicated by the average values, granulocyte/lymphocyte ratio, CRP, lactate dehydrogenase, creatinine kinase, glutamic oxaloacetic transaminase, and gamma-glutamyl transferase, were elevated. The applied antiviral and adjunctive therapies are detailed in **Table 1**.

The mean time between the onset of symptoms and admission to the Emergency Department was 5.9 (95% CI: 4.11–7.55) days. The diagnosis of SARS-CoV2 infection was confirmed by PCR in ten and antigen testing in three cases. Two patients had chest computer tomography and eleven X-Ray, and except for one patient, bilateral pathology was observed. Nine patients were admitted from the Emergency Department to the ICU on the day of admission, three were transferred from the department of COVID-Internal Medicine and one from the ICU of another town.

TABLE 1 | Baseline characteristics.

	Patients (n = 13)
Age, years	62 [48–67]
Male	12 (92.3%)
Charlson comorbidity index	2.77 (1.1–4.4)
4C Mortality score for COVID-19	10.4 (7.6–13.2)
Low risk	1 (7.7%)
Intermediate risk	4 (30.8%)
High risk	5 (38.5%)
Very high risk	3 (23.1%)
Onset of symptoms before admission, days	5.8 (3.8–7.8)
Confirmed by COVID-19 antigen test	3 (23.1%)
Confirmed by PCR	10 (76.9%)
Comorbidities	
Hypertension	9 (69.2%)
Diabetes	6 (46.2%)
Gastroesophageal reflux disease	1 (7.7%)
Acute myocardial infarction	2 (15.4%)
Benign prostatic hyperplasia	2 (15.4%)
Other	6 (46.2%)
No comorbidities	4 (30.8%)
Laboratory values on admission	
Leukocytes, $\times 10^3/\mu L$	8.9 (6.6–11.2)
Lymphocytes, $\times 10^3/\mu L$	0.7 [0.58–1.04]
Granulocytes, $\times 10^3/\mu L$	7.4 (5.3–9.6)
Granulocyte/lymphocyte ratio	10.0 (6.9–13.1)*
C-reactive protein, mg/L	203 (116–290)*
Glutamic oxaloacetic transaminase, U/L	96 [42–113]*
Glutamate pyruvate transaminase, U/L	75 (40–109)*
Gamma-glutamyl transferase, U/L	131.1 (66.3–195.9)*
Alkaline phosphatase, U/L	100.1 (68.3–131.9)
Lactate dehydrogenase, U/L	1,164.8 (780.9–1,548.8)*
Blood urea nitrogen, mmol/L	6.4 [4.8–13.3]
Creatine kinase, U/L	160 [126–489]*
Initial antiviral therapy	**11 (84.6%)**
Oseltamivir	4 (30.8%)
Favipiravir	6 (46.2%)
Lopinavir	1 (7.7%)
Adjunctive therapy	
Dexamethasone	2 (15.4%)
Hydrocortisone	4 (30.8%)
Methyl-prednisolone	4 (30.8%)
Tocilizumab	4 (30.8%)
Anti-COVID-19 convalescent plasma	5 (38.5%)

*Data are presented as mean (95% CI), median [IQR], or n (%), unless otherwise specified. PCR, polymerase chain reaction. U/L, unit/litre; ICU, intensive care unit. *represents elevated values.*

Treatment Characteristics

In all cases, hemoadsorption was combined with CRRT. On average 1.6 days elapsed from admission to the application of the first adsorber. Regarding the number of treatments, 1 patient received only one treatment, 5 received two, 6 received three treatments and in 1 case hemoadsorption was repeated for four consecutive sessions.

All patients required mechanical ventilation due to acute hypoxemic respiratory failure. Vasopressor was also required in all patients. In the first 24 h the total dose of norepinephrine was

193.7 ug/kg/day [34.8–270.4] which decreased to 50.2 [6.5–243.5] ug/kg/day, by the end of the course of hemoadsorption, but did not reach statistical significance (**Figure 1A**). There was a similar tendency of an improvement in the PaO2/FiO2 ratio during the course of hemoadsorption from 127.8 (96.0–159.6) to 155.0 (115.3–194.6) mmHg (**Figure 1B**). Apart from the leukocyte count, all other recorded laboratory parameters and the SOFA score showed statistically non-significant changes from before to after the therapy (**Table 2**).

Fluid management and inotropic support are summarised in **Table 3**. The only significant change was a negative fluid balance (TB vs. TA) on the completion of hemoadsorption compared to the onset of implication of the first HA.

Overall Outcomes

All patients survived the course of hemoadsorption and were still alive 72 h after initiation of the treatment, hence therapy was not terminated due to deterioration and also no adverse

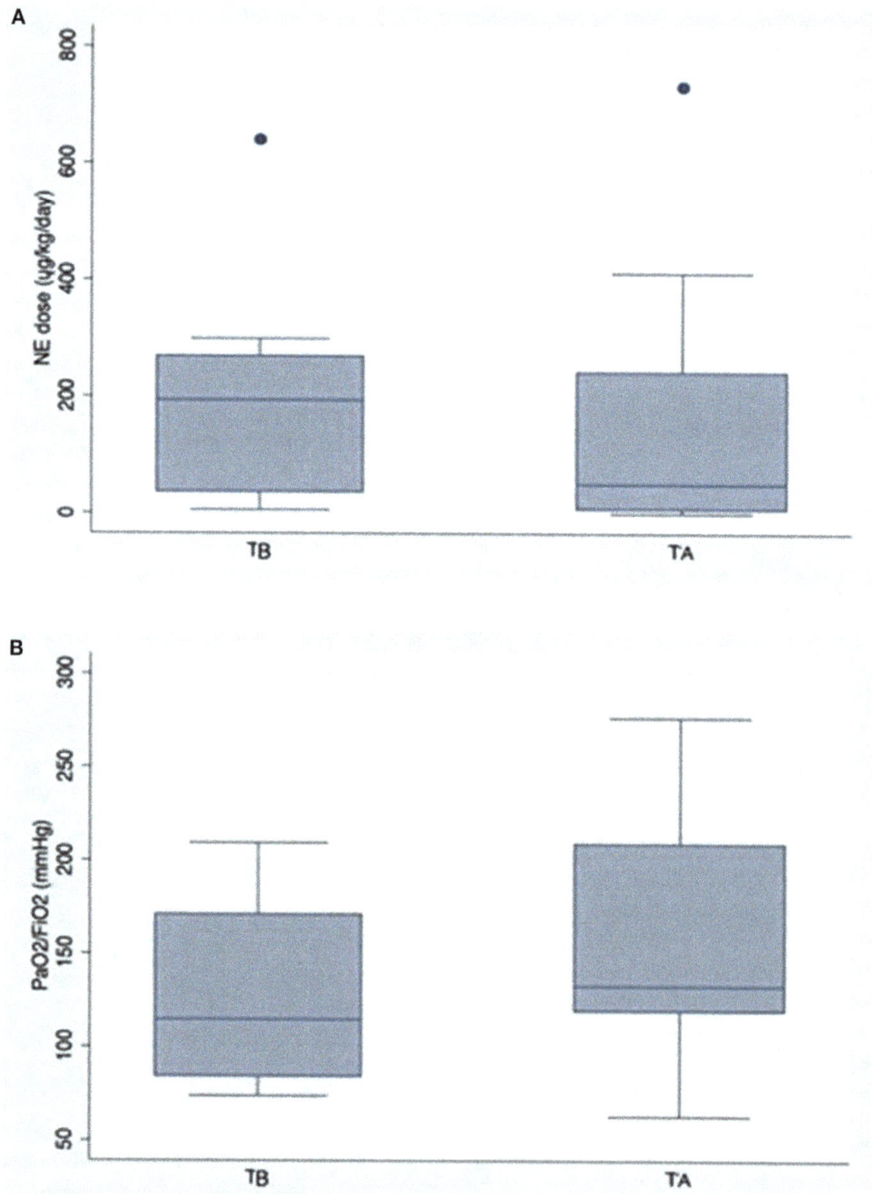

FIGURE 1 | (A) Change in norepinephrine requirement during hemoadsorption. NE, Norepinephrine; TB, data collected before the start of hemoadsorption; TA, data collected after the completion of hemoadsorption. Data are presented as box-plots. For statistical analysis Stata 15.1 was used. For explanation see main text. **(B)** Change in the PaO2/FiO2 ratio during hemoadsorption. TB, data collected before the start of hemoadsorption; TA, data collected after the completion of hemoadsorption. Data are presented as box-plots. For statistical analysis Stata 15.1 was used. For explanation see main text.

TABLE 2 | Before and after comparisons for all patients.

Laboratory values	T_B	T_A	*p*-value
Leukocytes, $\times 10^3/\mu L$	8.5 (6.5–10.4)	13.0 (9.0–16.9)	>0.01
Haemoglobin, g/L	119 (108–129)	115 (105–126)	0.33
Platelets, $\times 10^3/\mu L$	190 (140–241)	178 (130–225)	0.52
Creatinine, umol/L	109 [86–264]	104 [67–177]	0.05
Blood urea nitrogen, mmol/L	11.2 (6.9–15.6)	8.4 (5.7–11.2)	0.08
Glomerular filtration rate, mL/min/1.73 m^2	55.3 (34.1–76.5)	57.5 (38.4–76.6)	0.58
C-reactive protein, mg/L	266.1 (142.0–390.2)	206.4 (129.0–283.8)	0.28
Procalcitonin, ng/mL ($n = 5$)	0.64 [0.20–2.85]	0.49 [0.49–0.62]	0.59
Bilirubin, mmol/L ($n = 3$)	11.0 [10.0–333.0]	106.0 [30.0–182.0]	0.32
Arterial blood gases			
pH	7.35 (7.33–7.39)	7.31 (7.23–7.38)	0.28
PaO2, mm Hg	109 (82–135)	99 (85–112)	0.50
PaCO2, mm Hg	43 (37–48)	46 (37–55)	0.47
Plasma bicarbonate, mmol/L	23.3 (20.7–25.8)	22.6 (19.7–25.5)	0.65
Arterial lactate, mmol/L	1.68 [1.23–2.27]	1.58 [1.33–2.25]	0.74
SOFA score	15.0 [15.0–17.5]	14.5 [14.0–16.5]	0.03

Data are expressed as mean (95% CI) or median [IQR], unless otherwise specified. HA, hemoadsorption. n = number of patients when <13. PaO2, Partial pressure of oxygen. PaCO2, Partial pressure of carbon dioxide. PaO2/FiO2, Ratio of the partial pressure of oxygen and the fraction of inspired oxygen. SOFA, Sequential organ failure assessment.

TABLE 3 | Summary of daily changes in fluid balance and inotropic support requirement.

Fluid balance	T_B	T_A	*p*-value
Intake fluids per orally, ml	335 (141–529)	554 (150–958)	0.24
Intake fluids intravenously, ml	3,760 (3143–4377)	3,386 (2875–3897)	0.31
Spontaneous urinary output, ml	1,600 [750–2,300]	1,200 [0–3,850]	0.32
Other fluid loss, ml	200 [0–400]	0 [0–200]	0.24
Remove by continuous renal replacement, ml	0 [0–300]	953 [300–2,400]	0.20
Daily fluid balance, ml	1,947 (1,053–2,840)	−322 (−1,388–745)	>0.01
Vasopressor requirement			
Norepinephrine, μg/kg/day	193.7 [34.8–270.4]	50.2 [6.5–243.5]	0.48
Dobutamine, μg/kg/day ($n = 4$)	0.0 [0.0–1,005.7]	0.0 [0.0–5,437.5]	0.03

Data are expressed as mean (95% CI) or median [IQR], unless otherwise specified. HA, hemoadsorption.

events were detected. Four patients survived 28-days,, but overall, only 3 patients (23.1%) were discharged from the hospital alive. ICU length of stay was 14 [5–30] days while patients spent a median 17 [6–30] days in the hospital in total.

DISCUSSION

To the best of our knowledge, this is the first and largest comprehensive case series on COVID-19 patients treated with hemoadsorption from Eastern Europe—i.e.: from the former socialist block. Although the results showed some improvement in both haemodynamics and oxygenation, likely due to small sample size statistical significance was not achieved. Nevertheless, all patients were alive when treatment was decided to be terminated by the attending medical team, and treatment-related adverse events were not re-ported. Death occurred due to multiple organ failure at least 2 weeks later in most cases, suggesting that hemoadsorption started within 96 h after admission to ICU was well-tolerated and helped to stabilise and overcome the initial critical phase.

The purpose of hemoadsorption in the critically ill in general is to remove excessive inflammatory mediators and by doing so, to attenuate the host immune response. Whether a dysregulated immune response is present or not in COVID-19 patients at all, hence whether hemoadsorption is indicated or not, remains a controversial topic despite extensive publications in the field over the last year. There are several reports indicating elevated cytokine levels in the critically ill forms of COVID-19, some even observed the presence of cytokine storm (12, 13). However, there are also reports contradicting this hypothesis (14, 15). Nevertheless, as the clinical phenotype of COVID-19 is highly variable, ranging from asymptomatic cases to multi organ failure, one would expect a similar variability for the immune response (16). In recent correspondence by Rieder et al. on 8 patients with severe COVID-19 requiring veno-venous-extracorporeal membrane oxygenation (the CYCOV study), patients who received extracorporeal cytokine adsorption had lower IL-6 levels after 72 h of treatment compared to patients without cytokine adsorption (17). However, after completion of the study the difference was not significant (18).

In our patients there are some signals of increased inflammatory activity as indicated by the elevated granulocyte/lymphocyte ratio, and CRP and PCT levels, but these are certainly less pronounced as seen in septic shock or severe ARDS (14). Regardless of the measured inflammatory biomarker levels, the clinical picture of hemodynamic instability requiring vasopressor support, severe ARDS and renal failure indicates the presence of a dysregulated immune response of some sort. Therefore, which biomarkers are the most appropriate to be measured in COVID-19 patients remains to be elucidated (19).

Regarding the clinical effects of hemoadsorption with CytoSorb, there are several, consistent reports of hemodynamic stabilisation before and after the therapy from several fields of critical care including cardiac surgery, septic shock and also recent reports in COVID-19 patients (7, 20, 21). However, the amount of published data on hemoadsorption in COVID-19 patients remains very limited. The largest patient cohort on COVID-19 patients treated with hemoadsorption to date, was published by Alharthy et al. (22). Fifty patients with life threatening COVID-19 and acute kidney injury were treated with CytoSorb. Before and after treatment laboratory and clinical values were compared in the 35 survivors to 15 non-survivors. Most organ functions, including vasopressor need, PaO2/FiO2, and inflammatory biomarker levels improved significantly amongst survivors, while al-most all of these deteriorated in non-survivors. Due to the limited number of patients we could not compare the 10 non-survivors to the 3 survivors in our study. Nevertheless, the tendency was also similar in our cases, although the improvement did not reach statistical significance. This can be explained on the one hand by the small sample size, on the other hand there is some data suggesting the starting HA within 24 h as compared to the average 1.6 days found in our study, could have more profound effects (23).

Our patient cohort is similar to that presented in previous studies, as far as age, comorbidities and treatment modalities are concerned. However, the observed mortality was substantially higher (77%) than in other studies (22, 24, 25), apart from one recent randomised trial in patients requiring extracorporeal membrane oxygenation (ECMO) due to COVID-19 caused respiratory failure (18). In this study, Supady et al. (18) report a striking difference in 28-day survival of 18% in the cytokine adsorption treated vs. 76% in the controls. However, this was a small (17 vs. 17 patients) single centre study. There were also some baseline differences between the groups as far as baseline norepinephrine requirement, D-Dimer levels, and fluid balance were concerned, hence firm conclusions from this study cannot be drawn at present. Finally, this trial included patients on ECMO, which is different from our patient cohort. One most note, that the average 4C mortality score was 10.4, which indicates high risk and corresponds to 31.4–34.9% in-hospital mortality. Five patients were in the high risk and three in the very high risk category. However, these patients all required mechanical ventilation, therefore were of a selected subpopulation with even more severe conditions (26).

However, an important fact is that mortality rate during the 2nd and especially during the 3rd wave of COVID-19 was a lot higher in Eastern Europe in general than in West-ern Europe or in the United States (27–30). Unfortunately, we do not have detailed data on ICU/mechanical ventilation specific outcomes, hence we cannot give a clear explanation either for the differences between East and West Europe nor for the high mortality observed in our current case series.

However, it has long been reported by key opinion leaders of intensive care medicine in the region, that although we are more than 3 decades after the changing of the socialist system, several fundamental issues are still to be solved (31, 32). The most burning is the lack of human resources, including ICU nurses and doctors alike. Although our study did not focus on COVID-19 mortality in general, we cannot exclude that in the overall high ICU mortality, the low number of specialised ICU nurses and doctors and other logistic and organisational factors played a role. Unfortunately, we cannot refer to published data, but during the pandemic in our ICU, the specialised patient-to-nurse ratio often increased above 4:1. This is of utmost importance, as it has been shown by several studies that nurse/patient ratio has an exponential effect on mortality (33–35). In fact, if the patient-to-nurse ratio increases from 1:1 to >2.5:1 per shift, the adjusted risk ratio "shifts, with at least one death" increases from 1 to 3.5 (95% CI: 1.3–9.1) (31). In this region of Europe, we must take this opportunity to learn from the lessons of the pandemic that state-of-the art equipment and treatment strategies, such as CytoSorb, cannot make a difference if the human resources do not match the international/European standards.

Limitations

Our study has many more limitations than strengths. It is a retrospective, single centre, small sample size case series without a control group. However, there are very few studies in general available on this topic. Furthermore, our results are not negative as far as the treatment's immediate effects are concerned. Regarding long term outcomes, in comparison to international results, ours cannot be compared for the reasons detailed above. We could not present data on IL-6, and several other parameters.

Conclusions

In this small, singe centre cohort we present the results of COVID-19 patients treated with hemoadsorption during their life-threatening critical illness. The treatment was well-tolerated and there was a tendency toward improvement in both vasopressor need and oxygenation during the course of hemoadsorption. These observations render the need for prospective randomised trials.

ETHICS STATEMENT

The studies involving human participants were reviewed and approved by Ethics Committee of Fejér County St. György University Teaching Hospital, Székesfehérvár, Hungary (No: 18/2021.05.11). Written informed consent for participation was not required for this study in accordance with the national legislation and the institutional requirements. Written informed consent was not obtained from the individual(s) for the publication of any potentially identifiable images or data included in this article.

AUTHOR CONTRIBUTIONS

ZM: conceptualisation, supervision, project administration, and funding acquisition. MR and MV: methodology. MV and BH: software. KO and MR: validation. AV and DB: formal analysis. MV: investigation, resources, and data curation. TL, MR, MV, and KO: writing—original draft preparation. ZM, LB, and ÁS: writing—review and editing. BH: visualisation. All authors have read and agreed to the published version of the manuscript.

No. EFOP-3.6.2-16-2017-00006—LIVE LONGER is co-financed by the European Union (European Regional Development Fund) within the framework of Program Széchenyi 2020 and Hungarian National Research, Development and Innovation Office (Grant No. K 138816).

ACKNOWLEDGMENTS

Authors would like to thank Harriet Adamson for English language editing and Dr. Peter Recknagel for proofreading the manuscript.

REFERENCES

1. ICNARC. *Reports.* Available online at: https://www.icnarc.org/our-audit/audits/cmp/reports (accessed June 1, 2021).
2. John Hopkins University of Medicine Coronavirus Resource Center. *Mortality Analyses.* Available online at: https://coronavirus.jhu.edu/data/mortality (accessed June 2, 2021).
3. Qin C, Zhou L, Hu Z, Zhang S, Yang S, Tao Y, et al. Dysregulation of immune response in patients with coronavirus 2019 (COVID-19) in Wuhan, China. *Clin Infect Dis.* (2020) 71:762–8. doi: 10.1093/cid/ciaa248
4. Huang C, Wang Y, Li X, Ren L, Zhao J, Hu Y, et al. Clinical features of patients infected with 2019 novel coronavirus in Wuhan, China. *Lancet.* (2020) 395:497–506. doi: 10.1016/S0140-6736(20)30183-5
5. Ruan Q, Yang K, Wang W, Jiang L, Song J. Clinical predictors of mortality due to COVID-19 based on an analysis of data of 150 patients from Wuhan, China. *Intensive Care Med.* (2020) 46:846–8. doi: 10.1007/s00134-020-05991-x
6. Schädler D, Pausch C, Heise D, Meier-Hellmann A, Brederlau J, Weiler N, et al. The effect of a novel extracorporeal cytokine hemoadsorption device on IL-6 elimination in septic patients: a randomized controlled trial. *PLoS ONE.* (2017) 12:e0187015. doi: 10.1371/journal.pone.0187015
7. Hawchar F, László I, Öveges N, Trásy D, Ondrik Z, Molnar Z. Extracorporeal cytokine adsorption in septic shock: a proof of concept randomized, controlled pilot study. *J Crit Care.* (2019) 49:172–8. doi: 10.1016/j.jcrc.2018.11.003
8. Brouwer WAO, Duran S, Kuijper M, Ince C. Hemoadsorption with CytoSorb shows a decreased observed versus expected 28-day all-cause mortality in ICU patients with septic shock: a propensity-score-weighted retrospective study. *Crit Care.* (2019) 23:317. doi: 10.1186/s13054-019-2588-1
9. KDIGO AKI Work Group. KDIGO clinical practice guideline for acute kidney injury. *Kidney Int.* (2012) 2 (Suppl):1–138. doi: 10.1038/kisup.2012.1
10. ARDS Definition Task Force, Ranieri VM, Rubenfeld GD, Thompson BT, Ferguson ND, Caldwell E, et al. Acute respiratory distress syndrome: the Berlin definition. *JAMA.* (2012) 307:2526–33. doi: 10.1001/jama.2012.5669
11. Khwaja A. KDIGO clinical practice guidelines for acute kidney injury. *Nephron Clin Pract.* (2012) 120:c179–84. doi: 10.1159/000339789
12. Mustafa MI, Abdelmoneim AH, Mahmoud EM, Makhawi AM. Cytokine storm in COVID-19 patients, its impact on organs and potential treatment by QTY code-designed detergent-free chemokine receptors. *Mediators Inflamm.* (2020) 2020:8198963. doi: 10.1155/2020/8198963
13. Liu T, Zhang J, Yang Y, Ma H, Li Z, Zhang J, et al. The role of interleukin-6 in monitoring severe case of coronavirus disease 2019. *EMBO Mol Med.* (2020) 12:e12421. doi: 10.15252/emmm.202012421
14. Kox M, Waalders NJB, Kooistra EJ, Gerretsen J, Pickkers P. Cytokine levels in critically ill patients with COVID-19 and other conditions. *JAMA.* (2020) 324:1565–7. doi: 10.1001/jama.2020.17052
15. Leisman DE, Ronner L, Pinotti R, Taylor MD, Sinha P, Calfee CS, et al. Cytokine elevation in severe and critical COVID-19: a rapid systematic review, meta-analysis, and comparison with other inflammatory syndromes. *Lancet Respir Med.* (2020) 8:1233–44. doi: 10.1016/S2213-2600(20)30404-5
16. Rodríguez A, Ruiz-Botella M, Martín-Loeches I, Jimenez Herrera M, Solé-Violan J, Gómez J, et al. Deploying unsupervised clustering analysis to derive clinical phenotypes and risk factors associated with mortality risk in 2022 critically ill patients with COVID-19 in Spain. *Crit Care.* (2021) 25:63. doi: 10.1186/s13054-021-03487-8
17. Rieder M, Wengenmayer T, Staudacher D, Duerschmied D, Supady A. Cytokine adsorption in patients with severe COVID-19 pneumonia requiring extracorporeal membrane oxygenation. *Crit Care.* (2020) 24:435. doi: 10.1186/s13054-020-03130-y
18. Supady A, Weber E, Rieder M, Lother A, Niklaus T, Zahn T, et al. Cytokine adsorption in patients with severe COVID-19 pneumonia requiring extracorporeal membrane oxygenation (CYCOV): a single centre, open-label, randomised, controlled trial. *Lancet Respir Med.* (2021) 9:755–62. doi: 10.1016/S2213-2600(21)00177-6
19. Tang Y, Liu J, Zhang D, Xu Z, Ji J, Wen C. Cytokine storm in COVID-19: the current evidence and treatment strategies. *Front Immunol.* (2020) 11:1708. doi: 10.3389/fimmu.2020.01708
20. Boss K, Jahn M, Wendt D, Haidari Z, Demircioglu E, Thielmann M, et al. Extracorporeal cytokine adsorption: significant reduction of catecholamine requirement in patients with AKI and septic shock after cardiac surgery. *PLoS ONE.* (2021) 16:e0246299. doi: 10.1371/journal.pone.0246299
21. Poli EC, Alberio L, Bauer-Doerries A, Marcucci C, Roumy A, Kirsch M, et al. Cytokine clearance with CytoSorb® during cardiac surgery: a pilot randomized controlled trial. *Crit Care.* (2019) 23:108. doi: 10.1186/s13054-019-2399-4
22. Alharthy A, Faqihi F, Memish ZA, Balhamar A, Nasim N, Shahzad A, et al. Continuous renal replacement therapy with the addition of CytoSorb cartridge in critically ill patients with COVID-19 plus acute kidney injury: a case-series. *Artif Organs.* (2021) 45:E101–12. doi: 10.1111/aor.13864
23. Kogelmann K, Jarczak D, Scheller M, Drüner M. Hemoadsorption by CytoSorb in septic patients: a case series. *Crit Care.* (2017) 21:74. doi: 10.1186/s13054-017-1662-9
24. Rampino T, Gregorini M, Perotti L, Ferrari F, Pattonieri EF, Grignano MA, et al. Hemoperfusion with CytoSorb as adjuvant therapy in critically Ill patients with SARS-CoV2 pneumonia. *Blood Purif.* (2021) 50:566–71. doi: 10.1159/000511725
25. Lebreton G, Dorgham K, Quentric P, Combes A, Gorochov G, Schmidt M. Longitudinal cytokine profiling in patients with severe COVID-19 on extracorporeal membrane oxygenation and hemoadsorption. *Am J Respir Crit Care Med.* (2021) 203:1433–5. doi: 10.1164/rccm.202011-4140LE
26. Knight SR, Ho A, Pius R, Buchan I, Carson G, Drake TM, et al. Risk stratification of patients admitted to hospital with covid-19 using the ISARIC WHO clinical characterisation protocol: development and validation of the 4C mortality score. *BMJ.* (2020) 370:m3339. doi: 10.1136/bmj.m3339
27. Villani L, McKee M, Cascini F, Ricciardi W, Boccia S. Comparison of deaths rates for COVID-19 across Europe during the first wave of the COVID-19 pandemic. *Front Public Health.* (2020) 8:620416. doi: 10.3389/fpubh.2020.620416
28. *Comparisons of All-Cause Mortality Between European Countries and Regions.* (2020). Available online at: https://www.ons.gov.uk/peoplepopulationandcommunity/birthsdeathsandmarriages/deaths/articles/comparisonsofallcausemortalitybetweeneuropeancountriesandregions/2020 (accessed June 6, 2021).
29. James N, Menzies M, Radchenko P. COVID-19 second wave mortality in Europe and the United States. *Chaos.* (2021) 31:031105. doi: 10.1063/5.0041569
30. *Daily New Confirmed COVID-19 Deaths Per Million People.* Available online at: https://ourworldindata.org/covid-deaths (accessed June 6, 2021).
31. Molnar Z. SepsEast: bridging between east and west. *J Crit Care.* (2017) 40:323. doi: 10.1016/j.jcrc.2017.06.006
32. Lainscak M, Sustic A, Benes J, Czuczwar M, Jankovic R, Kirov M, et al. SepsEast and COVID-19: time to make a difference. *Signa Vitae.* (2020) 16:1–4. doi: 10.22514/sv.2020.16.0001
33. Chaudhry R, Dranitsaris G, Mubashir T, Bartoszko J, Riazi S. A country level analysis measuring the impact of government actions,

country preparedness and socioeconomic factors on COVID-19 mortality and related health outcomes. *EClinicalMedicine.* (2020) 25:100464. doi: 10.1016/j.eclinm.2020.100464

34. Neuraz A, Guérin C, Payet C, Polazzi S, Aubrun F, Dailler F, et al. Patient mortality is associated with staff resources and workload in the ICU: a multicenter observational study. *Crit Care Med.* (2015) 43:1587–94. doi: 10.1097/CCM.0000000000001015
35. Lucchini A, Giani M, Elli S, Villa S, Rona R, Foti G. Nursing activities score is increased in COVID-19 patients. *Intensive Crit Care Nurs.* (2020) 59:102876. doi: 10.1016%2Fj.iccn.2020.102876

The Effect of General Anesthesia vs. Regional Anesthesia on Postoperative Delirium

Xianlin Zhu [1], *Min Yang* [1], *Junying Mu* [1], *Zaiping Wang* [1], *Liang Zhang* [2*†], *Hongbai Wang* [3*†] *and Fuxia Yan* [3]

[1] Department of Anesthesiology, The Central Hospital of Enshi Tujia and Miao Autonomous Prefecture, Enshi City, China, [2] Department of Anesthesiology, Chongqing Hospital of Traditional Chinese Medicine, Chongqing, China, [3] Department of Anesthesiology, Fuwai Hospital, Chinese Academy of Medical Sciences and Peking Union Medical College, Beijing, China

***Correspondence:**
Liang Zhang
seamanzl@126.com
Hongbai Wang
jifeidanda66@163.com

† These authors have contributed equally to this work

Background: Postoperative delirium (POD) commonly occurs in patients following major surgeries and is associated with adverse prognosis. The modes of anesthesia may be associated with POD occurrence. General anesthesia (GA) causes loss of consciousness in the patient by altering the levels of some neurotransmitters as well as signaling pathways. We conducted this meta-analysis to investigate the effect of GA vs. regional anesthesia (RA) on POD incidence in surgical patients.

Methods: The databases of Pubmed, Embase, and Cochrane Library were searched till October 22, 2021. The eligible criteria were participants aged 18 years or older, patients undergoing surgery under GA and RA, and articles reporting the effect of GA vs. RA on POD incidence. RevMan 5.3 was used to perform statistical analyses.

Results: A total of 21 relevant trials with a total of 1,702,151 patients were included. The pooled result using random-effects model with OR demonstrated significant difference in POD incidence between patients with GA and RA (OR = 1.15, 95% CI: [1.02, 1.31], I^2 = 83%, p for effect = 0.02). We did not obtain the consistent pooled result after sensitivity analysis (OR = 0.95, 95% CI: [0.83, 1.08], I^2 =13%, p for effect = 0.44) and excluded the articles without the information on preoperative cognitive or neuropsychological assessment (OR = 1.12, 95% CI: [1.00, 1.25], I^2 =80%, p for effect = 0.05), respectively.

Conclusion: This meta-analysis could not identify that GA was significantly associated with POD occurrence in surgical patients compared with RA.

Keywords: general anesthesia, regional anesthesia, neuraxial anesthesia, peripheral nerve block, postoperative delirium, meta-analysis

INTRODUCTION

Postoperative delirium (POD) is a kind of acute complication characterized by brain dysfunction following surgery, and its main manifestations include inattention, disorganized thinking, and altered states of consciousness (1). Commonly, POD occurs in the first 3 days following surgery, and its higher incidence is in patients undergoing cardiac and major non-cardiac surgeries (2, 3).

Furthermore, POD is independently associated with other short- and long-term postoperative complications, adversely affecting prognosis (4–6). Given that there is no effective treatment for POD due to its unclear pathogenesis, identifying its risk factors is particularly important (7). Previous studies have identified some risk factors of POD, including major surgery, advanced age, lower educational level, preoperative anxiety, perioperative poor sleep quality, and imperfect postoperative analgesia (8).

Anesthesia is a critical intervention process for surgical patients. There are several methods of anesthesia, like general anesthesia (GA) and regional anesthesia (RA). RA includes neuraxial anesthesia (epidural anesthesia or spinal anesthesia) and peripheral nerve block (PNB). GA is the anesthesia method that keeps the patient in the state of unconsciousness, analgesia, and relaxed skeletal muscle through intravenous and/or inhaled general anesthetics during surgery. Some anesthetics act on the central nervous system to produce the effects of consciousness loss and analgesia by altering the levels of some neurotransmitters as well as signaling pathways (9, 10). However, the neuraxial anesthesia and PNB can contribute to analgesia and skeletal muscle relaxation without affecting the consciousness of the patient. Therefore, the patients undergoing GA are theoretically more likely to develop POD. Unexpectedly, the results of anesthesia mode associated with POD incidence are not consistent based on previous studies (11). Thus, we performed this systematic review and meta-analysis to clarify the effect of GA vs. RA on the incidence of delirium in adult patients undergoing surgery.

METHODS

This systematic review and meta-analysis were conducted according to the guidelines of the 2009 Preferred Reporting Items for Systematic Reviews and Meta-Analyses (PRISMA) (**Supplementary Table 1**) (12).

Search Strategy

Two authors independently searched the database of Pubmed, Embase, and Cochrane Library using the PICOS (Population, Intervention, Comparison, Outcome, and Study design) methods by the time of October 22, 2021. The entry terms included "general anesthesia" OR "general anesthesia" AND "local anesthesia" OR "local anesthesia" OR "regional anesthesia" OR "regional anesthesia" OR "spinal anesthesia" OR "spinal anesthesia" "epidural anesthesia" OR "epidural anesthesia" OR "neuraxial anesthesia" OR "neuraxial anesthesia" AND "delirium" OR "confusion" OR "agitation" OR "acute confusional state" OR "acute confusional syndrome," and the search field was "title and abstract." Since we sought to investigate all studies about the effect of GA vs. RA on POD incidence in adult patients undergoing surgery, we did not constrain the search terms for study designs.

Study Selection

Two authors were independently responsible for the screening process for titles and abstracts, while another two authors conducted the screening process for full text. The inclusion criteria were: (1) participants aged 18 years or older, (2) patients undergoing surgery under general and regional or local anesthesia, and (3) articles reporting the effect of GA vs. RA on POD incidence. The exclusion criteria were: (1) duplicate articles, (2) participants younger than 18 years old, (3) review or meta-analysis, (4) articles published as an abstract, letter, case report, basic research, editorial, note, method, or protocol, (5) articles presented in a non-English language; (6) studies without a specific number of patients with and/or without delirium, and (7) studies of all patients receiving GA or RA.

Quality Assessment of Included Studies

Two authors independently assessed the quality of included studies. For retrospective and prospective observational trials, the risk of bias was assessed using the Newcastle–Ottawa Quality Assessment Scale (NOS), which comprises the following three domains: selection, comparability, and outcome for cohort studies (13). There were four stars in the selection domain, two stars in the comparability domain, and three stars in the exposure domain. Trials with seven or more cumulative stars were considered to be of high quality, those with six stars of moderate quality, and those with <6 stars of low quality (13). For RCTs, risk of bias was assessed using the Cochrane Collaboration Risk of Bias Assessment tool, which included the following seven items: random sequence generation, allocation concealment, blinding of participants and personnel, blinding of outcome assessment, incomplete outcome data, selective reporting, and others (bias due to vested financial interest and academic bias) (14). If a trial was found to have one or more of the items associated with a high or unclear risk of bias, this trial was classified as high risk. If the two authors disagreed on their assessment, they consulted the third or fourth author. Eventually, we reached a consensus (14).

Data Extraction

Two authors were responsible for extracting the following information: (1) authors, (2) publication year, (3) study designs, (4) country of publication, (5) total number of participants in each study, (6) percentage of male, (7) mean age of all the participants, (8) procedures that the participants underwent, (9) the volatile anesthetic in patients underwent GA, (10) the anesthetic method of RA, (11) number of patients with and without POD, (12) methods of POD assessment, and (13) the follow-up time. Another three authors were responsible for adjusting data discrepancies.

Outcome Measures

The sole aim of this meta-analysis was to determine whether different anesthesia methods were associated with POD incidence in adult patients undergoing surgery.

Data Analysis

Review Manager version (RevMan) 5.3 (Cochrane collaboration, Oxford, UK) was used to perform statistical analyses. We assessed the heterogeneity of included studies using the values of I^2 and the Mantel–Haenszel chi-square test (p-value for heterogeneity). The values of $I^2 < 40\%$, $I^2 = 40–60\%$, and $I^2 > 60\%$ indicated

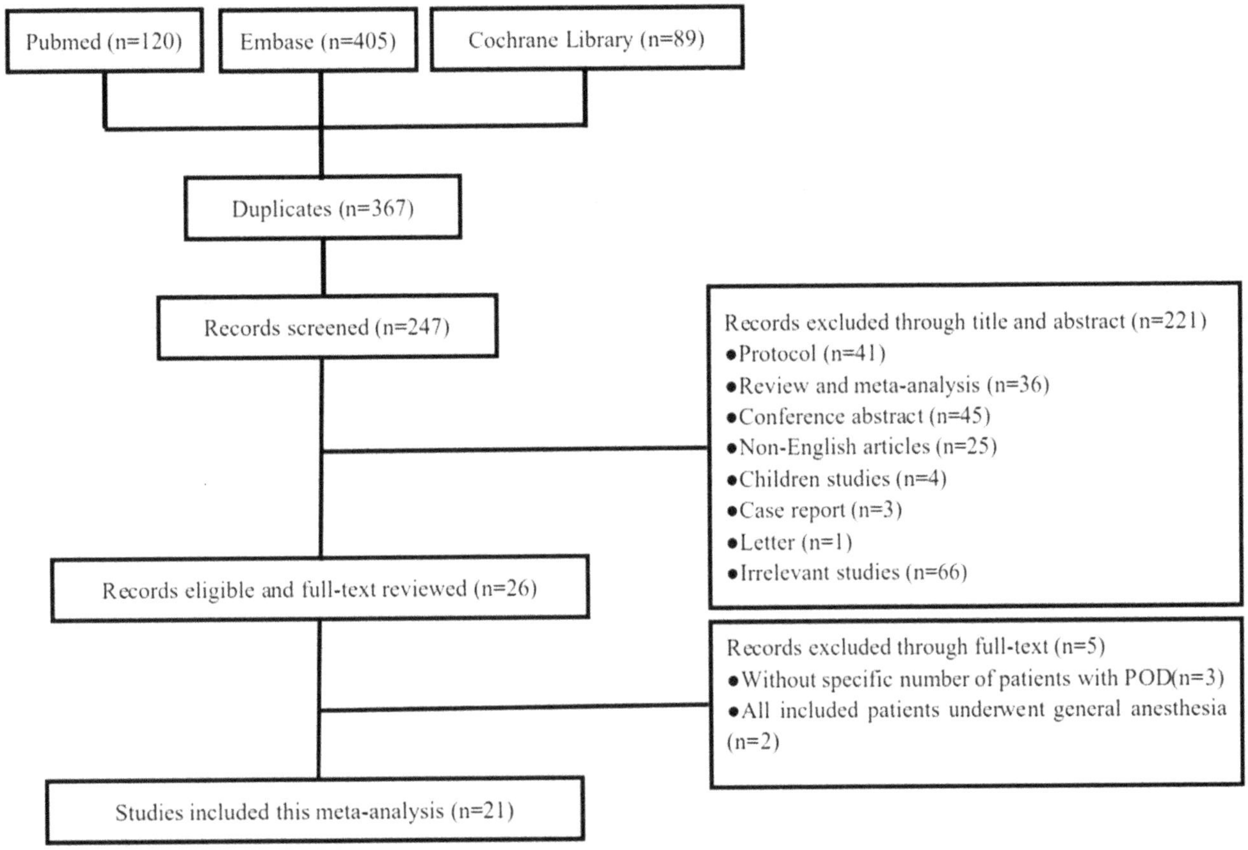

FIGURE 1 | The screening process of the eligible trials.

low, moderate, and high heterogeneity, respectively (15). If we identified $I^2 > 50\%$ or a p-value for heterogeneity <0.1, we used a random-effect model to analyze the data. Conversely, if we identified $I^2 < 50\%$ or a p-value for heterogeneity ≥ 0.1, we used a fixed-effect model to analyze the data (16). The dichotomous outcomes were presented as odds ratios (OR) with 95% confidence intervals (CI). The statistical tests were two-sided, and overall effects with a p-value for effect < 0.05 were considered to exhibit significant differences.

We conducted a sensitivity analysis to address high heterogeneity ($I^2 > 50\%$) through the methods of one-by-one article removal. Lastly, we performed the subgroup analyses according to study designs (retrospective and prospective), male percentage ($\geq$50 and <50%), age gaps ($\geq$80, 70–80, 60–70, and <60 years), and anesthesia methods (neuraxial anesthesia and PNB) in RA group to observe if these risk factors could affect the outcome.

RESULTS

Study Selection

Figure 1 shows the PRISMA flow chart for our screening process. We obtained 120 trials from Pubmed, 405 from Embase, and 89 from Cochrane Library. We removed 367 duplicate trials and excluded 221 trials at the title-and-abstract review stage based on our exclusion criteria. We excluded five trials at the full-text review stage, including three without a specific number of patients with POD, two with all included patients who underwent general anesthesia. Eventually, our search strategy yielded 21 relevant trials with a total of 1,702,151 patients (**Figure 1**) (17–37).

Study Characteristics

Tables 1, **2** present the basic characteristics of the included studies. There were nine retrospective (17, 18, 22, 25, 28–31, 35), and 12 prospective (19–24, 26, 27, 32–34, 36, 37) articles, including seven randomized and non-randomized controlled trials, in the prospective studies (20, 23, 24, 32–34, 37). Male accounted for 50% or more of all patients in 4 trials (17, 22, 23, 25). The mean or median age of all included patients was 80 years or older in five trials (20, 26, 31–33), 70–80 years in seven trials (21, 28, 29, 34–37), 60–70 years in seven trials (17, 18, 23–25, 27, 30), and younger than 60 years in two trials (19, 22). Except that the patients underwent lower limb vascular surgery in two articles (23, 25) and uncertain surgeries in one article (19), the patients underwent orthopedic surgery in the other trials. One trial included the patients undergoing simple urgent surgery (29), and five trials simple planned surgery (19, 21, 24, 27, 30). Three

TABLE 1 | The basic characteristics of included trials.

References	Study design	Country	Number of patients	Male (%)	Age (mean or median) (years)	Procedures	Urgent/ Planned	Preoperative cognition assessment	RA	POD assessment
Abe et al. (17)	Retrospective	Japan	11,796	69.1	69.2	Lower extremity amputation	Both	Yes	PNB	Based on newly prescribed antipsychotic drugs
Ahn et al. (18)	Retrospective	Korea	96,289	25.7	79	Hip surgery	Both	Yes	Neuraxial anesthesia	Based on administration of antipsychotic drugs
Bilge et al. (19)	Prospective	Turkey	250	43.2	59.7	Operation planned with general and regional anesthesia	Planned	Yes	Regional anesthesia	CAM-ICU
Casati et al. (20)	Prospective (RCT)	Italy	30	6.7	84	Hip surgery	Both	Yes	Neuraxial anesthesia	NA
Chew et al. (21)	Prospective	Singapore	462	29.9	72	Knee or hip surgery	Planned	Yes	Neuraxial anesthesia	CAM
Choi et al. (20)	Retrospective	Korea	24,379	61.0	52.9	Hip surgery	Both	Yes	Neuraxial anesthesia	Diagnosis codes or administration of antipsychotic drugs
Cook et al. (23)	Prospective (RCT)	Australia	101	70	66.8	Lower limb vascular surgery	Both	No	Neuraxial anesthesia	Based on change in mental state
Ehsani et al. (24)	Prospective (controlled trial)	Iran	94	47.9	67.12	Hip surgery	Planned	Yes	Neuraxial anesthesia	DSM-IV
Ellard et al. (25)	Retrospective	Canada	500	68.4	69	Vascular surgery	Both	Yes	Neuraxial anesthesia or PNB	NEECHAM confusion scale
Ilango et al. (26)	Prospective	Australia	318	30.0	81.6	Hip surgery	Both	Yes	Neuraxial anesthesia	Pittsburgh Agitation Scale
Krenk et al. (27)	Prospective	Denmark	225	49.3	69.4	Total knee or hip arthroplasty	Planned	Yes	Neuraxial anesthesia	DSM-IV
Li et al. (28)	Retrospective	China	89	48.3	76.8	Lower lumbar surgery	Both	No	Neuraxial anesthesia	NA
Liu et al. (29)	Retrospective	China	217	30.4	79.8	Hip surgery	Urgent	Yes	PNB	NA
Memtsoudis et al. (30)	Retrospective	USA	169,4795	39.7	67.3	Total knee or hip arthroplasty	Planned	Yes	Neuraxial anesthesia	ICD-9 codes and/or billing for antipsychotics
Nawi et al. (31)	Retrospective	Australia	154	33.1	83.1	Hip surgery	Both	Yes	Neuraxial anesthesia	NA
Parker et al. (32)	Prospective (RCT)	UK	322	29.2	82.95	Hip surgery	Both	Yes	Neuraxial anesthesia	NA
Shin et al. (33)	Prospective (RCT)	Korea	176	26.1	80.5	Hip surgery	Both	Yes	Neuraxial anesthesia	NA
Slor et al. (34)	Prospective (controlled trial)	Netherlands	526	22.1	77.45	Hip surgery	Both	Yes	Neuraxial anesthesia	DSM-IV and CAM
Song et al. (35)	Retrospective	Korea	3,611	49.4	>70	Orthopedic surgery	Both	No	Neuraxial anesthesia or PNB	NA
Song et al. (36)	Prospective	China	138	26.1	78.35	Hip surgery	Both	Yes	Neuraxial anesthesia	CAM
Tzimas et al. (37)	Prospective (RCT)	Greece	70	47.1	76	Hip surgery	Both	Yes	Neuraxial anesthesia	CAM

GA, general anesthesia; RA, regional anesthesia; POD, postoperative delirium; NA, not applicable; PNB, peripheral nerve block; CAM-ICU, the Confusion Assessment Method for Intensive Care Unit; RCT, randomized controlled trial; DSM-IV, the Diagnostic and Statistical Manual of Mental Disorders 4th Edition; ICD, International Classification of Diseases.

TABLE 2 | The follow-up time and number of patients with POD under different anesthesia modes.

Author and year	Assessment time	GA		RA	
		With POD	Without POD	With POD	Without POD
Abe et al. (17)	Within 30 days after surgery	1,017	10,032	69	678
Ahn et al. (18)	Hospital stay after surgery	5,828	19,765	12,733	57,963
Bilge et al. (19)	Postoperative 1 day	37	187	9	17
Casati et al. (20)	Postoperative 1–7 days	9	6	8	7
Chew et al. (21)	Postoperative 1–3 days	0	164	0	298
Choi et al. (22)	Hospital stay after surgery	142	9,779	209	14,249
Cook et al. (23)	1 year after surgery	6	45	9	41
Ehsani et al. (24)	Postoperative 1–3 days	14	33	2	45
Ellard et al. (25)	Hospital stay after surgery	73	323	24	80
Ilango et al. (26)	Hospital stay after surgery	84	83	88	63
Krenk et al. (27)	Hospital stay after surgery	0	22	0	203
Li et al. (28)	Hospital stay after surgery	4	38	0	47
Liu et al. (29)	Hospital stay after surgery	15	57	23	122
Memtsoudis et al. (30)	Hospital stay after surgery	28,933	974,263	13,579	545,573
Nawi et al. (31)	Hospital stay after surgery	46	112	10	42
Parker et al. (32)	Hospital stay after surgery	0	164	3	155
Shin et al. (33)	Hospital stay after surgery	17	101	8	50
Slor et al. (34)	Postoperative 1–5 days	18	42	171	295
Song et al. (35)	Hospital stay after surgery	165	2,373	7	1,066
Song et al. (36)	Hospital stay after surgery	24	57	12	45
Tzimas et al. (37)	Postoperative 1–4 days	4	29	10	27

articles did not provide information on preoperative cognitive or neuropsychological assessment (23, 28, 35). The patients in the RA group received the sole PNB in only two trials (17, 29), and underwent PNB or neuraxial anesthesia in another two trials (25, 35), while neuraxial anesthesia was the sole anesthesia in RA patients in the other 17 enrolled trials. The follow-up time was hospital stay after surgery in 13 trials (18, 22, 25–33, 35, 36), 1 year in one trial (23), 30 days in one trial (17), 1–7 days in one trial (20), 1–5 day in one trial (34), 1–4 days in one trial (37), 1–3 days in two trials (21, 24), and 1 day in one trial (19). The methods of POD identification included antipsychotic drug use (17, 18, 22, 30), Confusion Assessment Method for Intensive Care Unit (CAM-ICU) or CAM (19, 21, 36, 37), DSM-IV criteria (24, 27), NEECHAM confusion scale (25), change in mental state (23), and Pittsburgh Agitation Scale (26). Seven articles did not provide a specific diagnostic method of POD (20, 28, 29, 31–33, 35), and a combination of CAM with DSM-IV criteria (34).

Study Quality

We used NOS to assess the risk of bias in observational studies (retrospective and prospective), and all 14 trials obtained seven stars or more, indicating high quality (**Supplementary Table 2**) (17–19, 21, 22, 25–31, 35, 36). We used the Cochrane Collaboration Risk of Bias Assessment tool to assess the risk of bias in RCTs. Due to the considerable procedural difference in GA and neuraxial anesthesia or PNB, it is extremely difficult to conduct blindness in participants. Therefore, the performance bias was high risk in all included RCTs and non-RCTs. The included studies clearly assessed random sequence generation (three studies-42.9%), allocation concealment (four studies-57.1%), blinding of participants (0%), blinding of outcome assessment (seven studies-100%), incomplete outcome data (seven studies-100%), and selective outcome reporting (seven studies-100%), and the other bias (three-42.9%) (**Supplementary Figures 1, 2**) (20, 23, 24, 32–34, 37).

POD Incidence

The pooled result using random-effects model with OR demonstrated significant difference in POD incidence between patients with GA and RA (OR = 1.15, 95% CI: [1.02, 1.31], I^2 = 83%, p for effect = 0.02) (**Figure 2**). I^2 = 81% and the funnel plots demonstrated the considerable heterogeneity of included trials (**Figure 3A**). The sensitivity analysis was performed to solve the high heterogeneity by the method of one-by-one literature removal and found that six trials were the main sources of heterogeneity (**Figure 3B**) (18, 19, 24, 30, 35, 36). We conducted *post-hoc* meta-analysis for the remaining articles using a fixed-effects model with OR, and the pooled result was not consistent with that prior to sensitivity analysis (OR = 0.95, 95% CI: [0.83, 1.08], I^2 = 13%, p for effect = 0.44) (**Figure 4**). Additionally, we excluded the articles without the information on preoperative cognitive or neuropsychological assessment and did not obtain the statistical difference in POD incidence between patients with

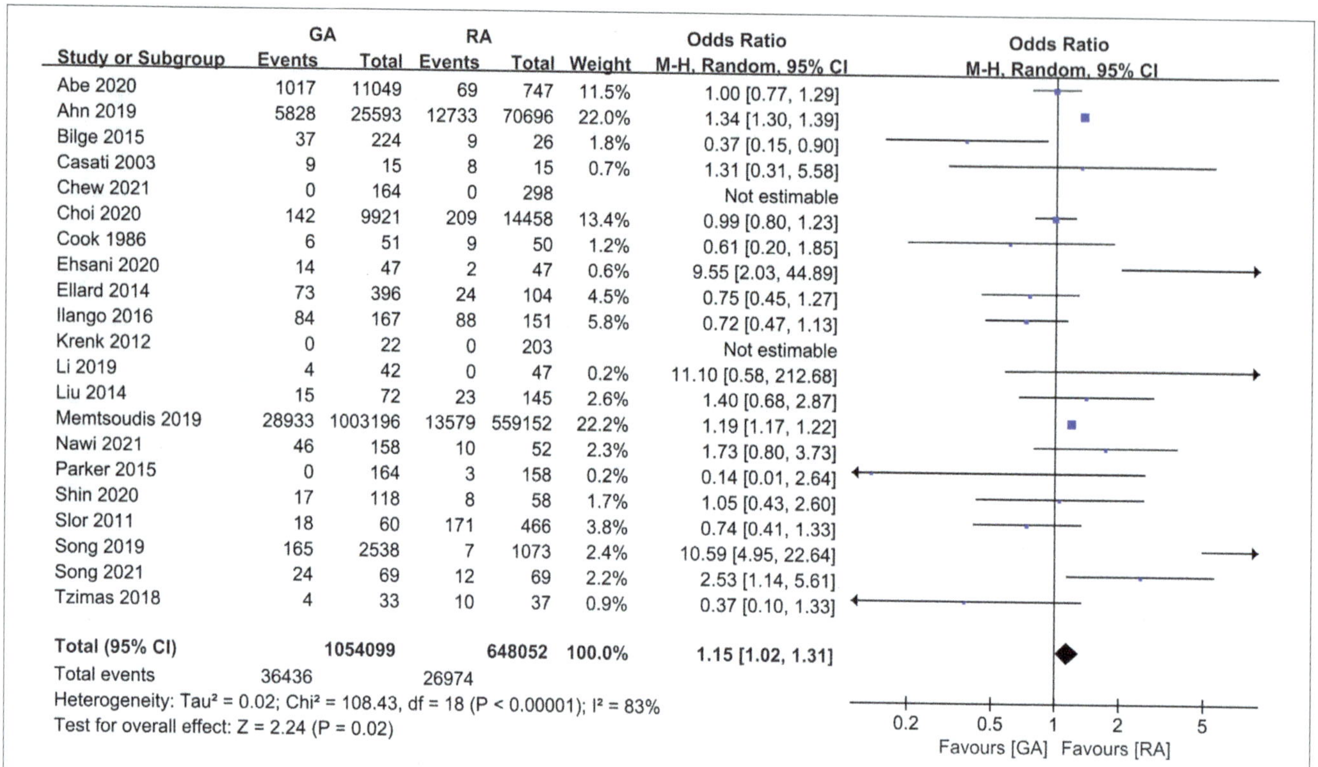

FIGURE 2 | The pooled results of POD incidence after surgery between the patients with GA and RA.

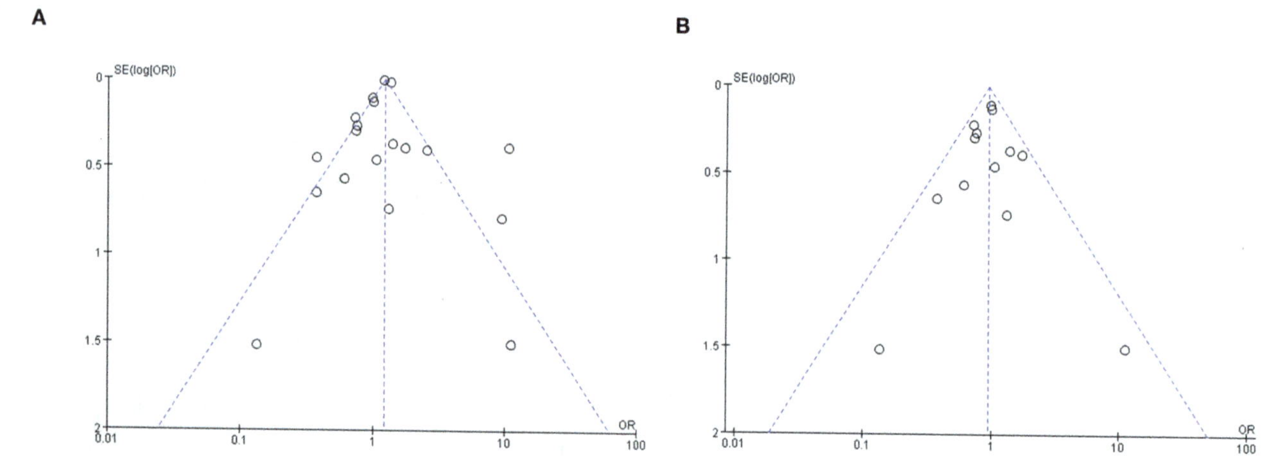

FIGURE 3 | The funnel plots of all included trials: the considerable heterogeneity of included trials **(A)** and lowering heterogeneity through six trials exclusion **(B)**.

GA and RA (OR = 1.12, 95% CI: [1.00, 1.25], $I^2 = 80\%$, p for effect = 0.05) (**Figure 5**).

The subgroup analyses according to study designs, male percentage (≥50 and <50%), mean (or median) age gaps (≥80, 70–80, 60–70, and <60 years), and anesthesia methods in RA group (neuraxial anesthesia and PNB) demonstrated the significant difference in retrospective articles (OR = 1.23, 95% CI: [1.08, 1.39], p for effect = 0.001) (**Figure 6**), male percentage <50% (OR = 1.26, 95% CI: [1.09, 1.46], p for effect = 0.002) (**Figure 7**), age gap between 60 and 70 years (OR = 1.20, 95% CI: [1.07, 1.35], p for effect = 0.002) (**Figure 8**), and neuraxial anesthesia (OR = 1.15, 95% CI: [1.01, 1.31], p for effect = 0.03) (**Figure 9**). However, we did not obtain statistical difference in the subgroups in prospective studies (OR = 0.91, 95% CI: [0.55, 1.49], p for effect = 0.70) (**Figure 6**), male percentage ≥ 50% (OR = 0.96, 95% CI: [0.82, 1.12], p for effect = 0.60) (**Figure 7**), age gaps ≥ 80 years (OR = 0.98, 95% CI: [0.61, 1.57], p for effect = 0.93), 70–80 years (OR = 1.93, 95% CI: [0.66, 5.60], p for effect

Study or Subgroup	GA Events	GA Total	RA Events	RA Total	Weight	Odds Ratio M-H, Fixed, 95% CI
Abe 2020	1017	11049	69	747	26.4%	1.00 [0.77, 1.29]
Ahn 2019	5828	25593	12733	70696	0.0%	1.34 [1.30, 1.39]
Bilge 2015	37	224	9	26	0.0%	0.37 [0.15, 0.90]
Casati 2003	9	15	8	15	0.7%	1.31 [0.31, 5.58]
Chew 2021	0	164	0	298		Not estimable
Choi 2020	142	9921	209	14458	37.7%	0.99 [0.80, 1.23]
Cook 1986	6	51	9	50	1.8%	0.61 [0.20, 1.85]
Ehsani 2020	14	47	2	47	0.0%	9.55 [2.03, 44.89]
Ellard 2014	73	396	24	104	7.0%	0.75 [0.45, 1.27]
Ilango 2016	84	167	88	151	10.3%	0.72 [0.47, 1.13]
Krenk 2012	0	22	0	203		Not estimable
Li 2019	4	42	0	47	0.1%	11.10 [0.58, 212.68]
Liu 2014	15	72	23	145	2.7%	1.40 [0.68, 2.87]
Memtsoudis 2019	28933	1003196	13579	559152	0.0%	1.19 [1.17, 1.22]
Nawi 2021	46	158	10	52	2.4%	1.73 [0.80, 3.73]
Parker 2015	0	164	3	158	0.8%	0.14 [0.01, 2.64]
Shin 2020	17	118	8	58	2.1%	1.05 [0.43, 2.60]
Slor 2011	18	60	171	466	6.1%	0.74 [0.41, 1.33]
Song 2019	165	2538	7	1073	0.0%	10.59 [4.95, 22.64]
Song 2021	24	69	12	69	0.0%	2.53 [1.14, 5.61]
Tzimas 2018	4	33	10	37	1.9%	0.37 [0.10, 1.33]
Total (95% CI)		**22432**		**16989**	**100.0%**	**0.95 [0.83, 1.08]**
Total events	1435		632			

Heterogeneity: $Chi^2 = 13.82$, df = 12 (P = 0.31); $I^2 = 13\%$
Test for overall effect: Z = 0.77 (P = 0.44)

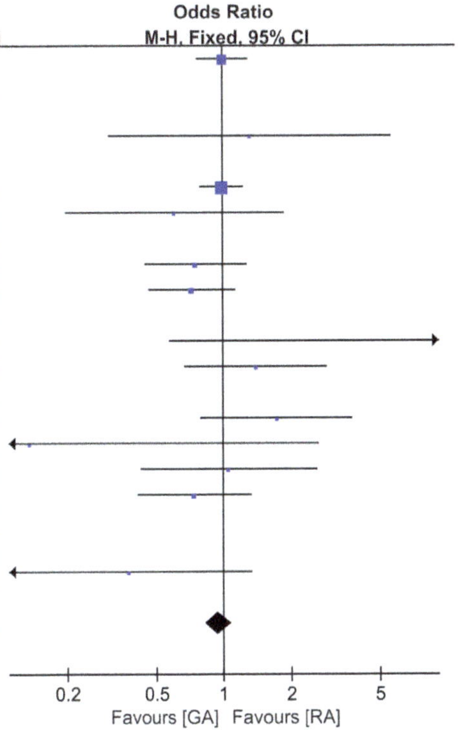

FIGURE 4 | The pooled result of POD incidence in surgical patients with GA and RA after sensitivity analysis.

Study or Subgroup	GA Events	GA Total	RA Events	RA Total	Weight	Odds Ratio M-H, Random, 95% CI
Abe 2020	1017	11049	69	747	11.0%	1.00 [0.77, 1.29]
Ahn 2019	5828	25593	12733	70696	26.3%	1.34 [1.30, 1.39]
Bilge 2015	37	224	9	26	1.5%	0.37 [0.15, 0.90]
Casati 2003	9	15	8	15	0.6%	1.31 [0.31, 5.58]
Chew 2021	0	164	0	298		Not estimable
Choi 2020	142	9921	209	14458	13.3%	0.99 [0.80, 1.23]
Cook 1986	6	51	9	50	0.0%	0.61 [0.20, 1.85]
Ehsani 2020	14	47	2	47	0.5%	9.55 [2.03, 44.89]
Ellard 2014	73	396	24	104	3.8%	0.75 [0.45, 1.27]
Ilango 2016	84	167	88	151	5.0%	0.72 [0.47, 1.13]
Krenk 2012	0	22	0	203		Not estimable
Li 2019	4	42	0	47	0.0%	11.10 [0.58, 212.68]
Liu 2014	15	72	23	145	2.1%	1.40 [0.68, 2.87]
Memtsoudis 2019	28933	1003196	13579	559152	26.7%	1.19 [1.17, 1.22]
Nawi 2021	46	158	10	52	1.9%	1.73 [0.80, 3.73]
Parker 2015	0	164	3	158	0.1%	0.14 [0.01, 2.64]
Shin 2020	17	118	8	58	1.4%	1.05 [0.43, 2.60]
Slor 2011	18	60	171	466	3.2%	0.74 [0.41, 1.33]
Song 2019	165	2538	7	1073	0.0%	10.59 [4.95, 22.64]
Song 2021	24	69	12	69	1.8%	2.53 [1.14, 5.61]
Tzimas 2018	4	33	10	37	0.7%	0.37 [0.10, 1.33]
Total (95% CI)		**1051468**		**646882**	**100.0%**	**1.12 [1.00, 1.25]**
Total events	36261		26958			

Heterogeneity: $Tau^2 = 0.01$; $Chi^2 = 73.84$, df = 15 (P < 0.00001); $I^2 = 80\%$
Test for overall effect: Z = 1.94 (P = 0.05)

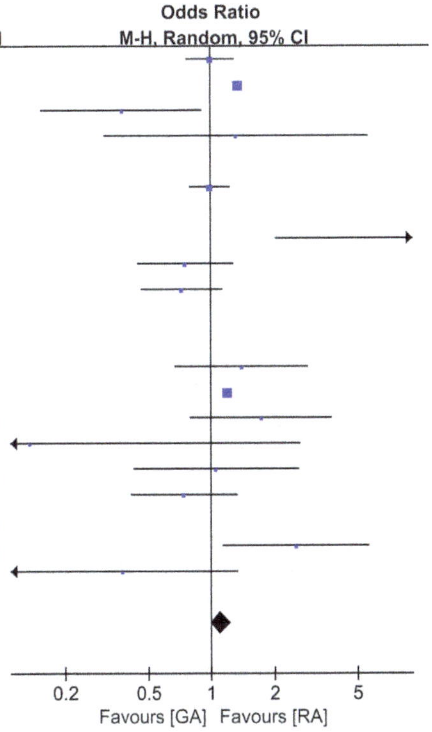

FIGURE 5 | The pooled result of POD incidence in surgical patients with GA and RA after excluding the studies without the information on preoperative cognitive or neuropsychological assessment.

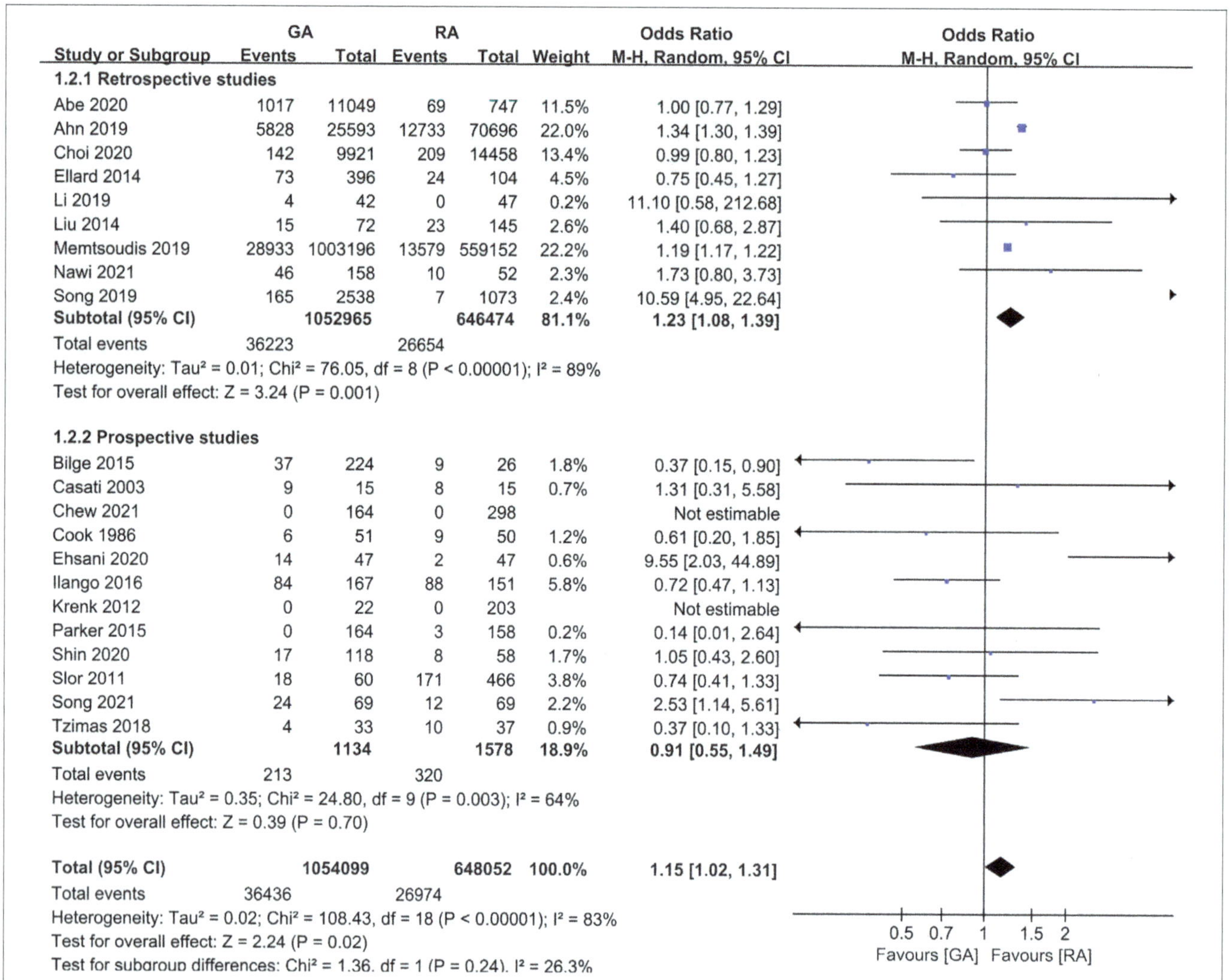

FIGURE 6 | The subgroup analysis according to study designs (retrospective and prospective).

= 0.23), <60 years (OR = 0.67, 95% CI: [0.26, 1.71], p for effect = 0.40) (**Figure 8**), and PNB group (OR = 1.64, 95% CI: [0.70, 3.87], p for effect = 0.26) (**Figure 9**).

DISCUSSION

Although this meta-analysis concluded that compared with RA, the incidence of POD significantly increased in GA patients, we did not obtain the positive result after solving the high heterogeneity of included trials and excluded the trials that did not provide the information on preoperative cognitive or neuropsychological assessment, respectively. Besides, subgroup analyses showed the statistical difference in retrospective studies, studies with male percentage <50%, studies with a mean (or median) age gap 60–70 years, and studies with neuraxial anesthesia group in RA group. However, we did not obtain the considerable difference in POD occurrence between the patients with GA and RA in the trials of prospective designs, the male percentage ≥ 50%, patients with another mean (or median) age gaps except 60–70 years, and patients undergoing PNB in the RA group.

Although the mechanisms of POD occurrence are complex and currently unclear, some studies have exhibited its possible pathogeneses. Severe neuroinflammation may be a main cause of POD in patients undergoing cardiac or non-cardiac surgery (38, 39). The serum S100A2 is a pro-inflammatory factor associated with POD and also a biomarker indicating neural injury according to a clinical study, and maybe an effective predictor of POD (40). Increasing perioperative plasma cortical level is considered as another mechanism of POD occurrence due to its related neuron apoptosis in the hippocampal region (41, 42). Besides, plasma neurofilament light level is also a predictor of POD, independent of changes in inflammation. Elevated plasma neurofilament light level is correlated with reduced hippocampal volume and fractional anisotropy of white matter (43). Furthermore, the preoperative neurotransmitter imbalances

Study or Subgroup	GA Events	GA Total	RA Events	RA Total	Weight	Odds Ratio M-H, Random, 95% CI
3.1.1 Male proportion ⩾50%						
Abe 2020	1017	11049	69	747	11.5%	1.00 [0.77, 1.29]
Choi 2020	142	9921	209	14458	13.4%	0.99 [0.80, 1.23]
Cook 1986	6	51	9	50	1.2%	0.61 [0.20, 1.85]
Ellard 2014	73	396	24	104	4.5%	0.75 [0.45, 1.27]
Subtotal (95% CI)		**21417**		**15359**	**30.6%**	**0.96 [0.82, 1.12]**
Total events	1238		311			
Heterogeneity: Tau² = 0.00; Chi² = 1.63, df = 3 (P = 0.65); I² = 0%						
Test for overall effect: Z = 0.52 (P = 0.60)						
3.1.2 Male proportion<50%						
Ahn 2019	5828	25593	12733	70696	22.0%	1.34 [1.30, 1.39]
Bilge 2015	37	224	9	26	1.8%	0.37 [0.15, 0.90]
Casati 2003	9	15	8	15	0.7%	1.31 [0.31, 5.58]
Chew 2021	0	164	0	298		Not estimable
Ehsani 2020	14	47	2	47	0.6%	9.55 [2.03, 44.89]
Ilango 2016	84	167	88	151	5.8%	0.72 [0.47, 1.13]
Krenk 2012	0	22	0	203		Not estimable
Li 2019	4	42	0	47	0.2%	11.10 [0.58, 212.68]
Liu 2014	15	72	23	145	2.6%	1.40 [0.68, 2.87]
Memtsoudis 2019	28933	1003196	13579	559152	22.2%	1.19 [1.17, 1.22]
Nawi 2021	46	158	10	52	2.3%	1.73 [0.80, 3.73]
Parker 2015	0	164	3	158	0.2%	0.14 [0.01, 2.64]
Shin 2020	17	118	8	58	1.7%	1.05 [0.43, 2.60]
Slor 2011	18	60	171	466	3.8%	0.74 [0.41, 1.33]
Song 2019	165	2538	7	1073	2.4%	10.59 [4.95, 22.64]
Song 2021	24	69	12	69	2.2%	2.53 [1.14, 5.61]
Tzimas 2018	4	33	10	37	0.9%	0.37 [0.10, 1.33]
Subtotal (95% CI)		**1032682**		**632693**	**69.4%**	**1.26 [1.09, 1.46]**
Total events	35198		26663			
Heterogeneity: Tau² = 0.02; Chi² = 97.10, df = 14 (P < 0.00001); I² = 86%						
Test for overall effect: Z = 3.11 (P = 0.002)						
Total (95% CI)		**1054099**		**648052**	**100.0%**	**1.15 [1.02, 1.31]**
Total events	36436		26974			
Heterogeneity: Tau² = 0.02; Chi² = 108.43, df = 18 (P < 0.00001); I² = 83%						
Test for overall effect: Z = 2.24 (P = 0.02)						
Test for subgroup differences: Chi² = 6.36, df = 1 (P = 0.01), I² = 84.3%						

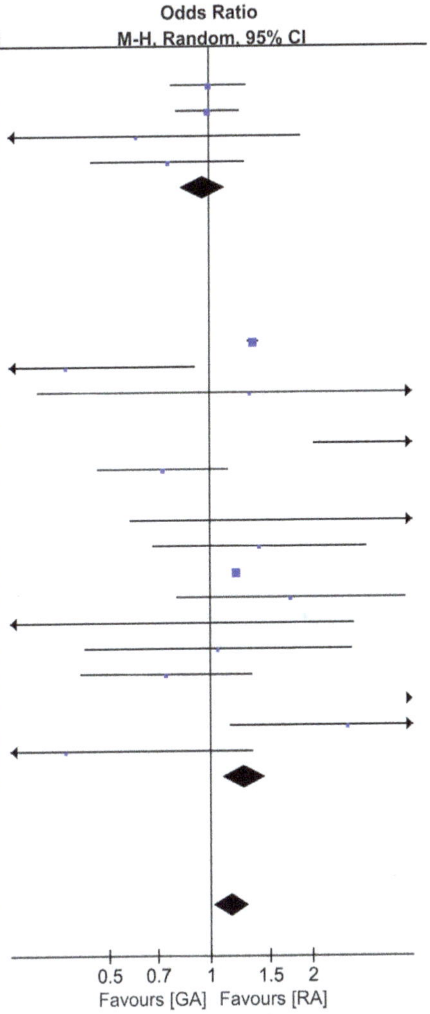

FIGURE 7 | The subgroup analysis according to the male percentage (≥50 and <50%).

occurred in POD patients, such as increased dopamine and glutamate, and decreased glutamine, which potentially increase the fragility of the brain (44). Due to the complex and unclear mechanism of POD, currently, the main method to decrease POD incidence is the intervention of its perioperative risk factors, like preoperative fasting, temperature control, blood pressure management, perioperative sleep improvement, moderate anesthesia depth, and perfect analgesia (7).

General anesthesia can affect the individual conscious state through complex molecular biological mechanisms, including ligand-gated ionotropic receptors, like γ-aminobutyric acid, glutamate, and acetylcholine receptors, and then intervene synaptic transmission between neurons (45). However, the specific mechanism of action of general anesthetics is still elusive. According to animal and clinical studies, GA-related varieties of consciousness and cognition are reversible and transient (46, 47). But some studies exhibited that GA or general anesthetics could produce neural toxicities, and be associated with short- or long-term cognitive dysfunction, and the extent of cognitive defect was proportional to the duration of anesthesia (48, 49). The volatile anesthetics may be a critical risk factor of neural injury through elevating the neural injury biomarkers total tau, neurofilament light, and tau phosphorylation (50, 51). Additionally, GA can increase frontal slow-wave activity, and impaired functional connectivity on diffusion tensor imaging, which may be associated with POD occurrence (52). Besides, GA may disturb the postoperative sleep structure of patients, thereby resulting in POD (53). Therefore, more patients undergoing GA theoretically tend to develop POD. Interestingly, compared with RA, the patients receiving GA did not show significant POD incidence according to some studies (11).

In this meta-analysis, although the pooled result of all included trials demonstrated that POD incidence was higher in surgical patients undergoing GA than RA, the consistent result did not be obtained after solving the high heterogenicity of included trials. Besides, the pooled result

Study or Subgroup	GA Events	GA Total	RA Events	RA Total	Weight	Odds Ratio M-H, Random, 95% CI
2.1.1 Mean age ≥80 years						
Casati 2003	9	15	8	15	0.7%	1.31 [0.31, 5.58]
Ilango 2016	84	167	88	151	5.8%	0.72 [0.47, 1.13]
Nawi 2021	46	158	10	52	2.3%	1.73 [0.80, 3.73]
Parker 2015	0	164	3	158	0.2%	0.14 [0.01, 2.64]
Shin 2020	17	118	8	58	1.7%	1.05 [0.43, 2.60]
Subtotal (95% CI)		**622**		**434**	**10.8%**	**0.98 [0.61, 1.57]**
Total events	156		117			
Heterogeneity: $Tau^2 = 0.08$; $Chi^2 = 5.59$, df = 4 (P = 0.23); $I^2 = 28\%$						
Test for overall effect: Z = 0.08 (P = 0.93)						
2.1.2 Mean age 70-80 years						
Chew 2021	0	164	0	298		Not estimable
Li 2019	4	42	0	47	0.2%	11.10 [0.58, 212.68]
Liu 2014	15	72	23	145	2.6%	1.40 [0.68, 2.87]
Slor 2011	18	60	171	466	3.8%	0.74 [0.41, 1.33]
Song 2019	165	2538	7	1073	2.4%	10.59 [4.95, 22.64]
Song 2021	24	69	12	69	2.2%	2.53 [1.14, 5.61]
Tzimas 2018	4	33	10	37	0.9%	0.37 [0.10, 1.33]
Subtotal (95% CI)		**2978**		**2135**	**12.1%**	**1.93 [0.66, 5.60]**
Total events	230		223			
Heterogeneity: $Tau^2 = 1.43$; $Chi^2 = 42.59$, df = 5 (P < 0.00001); $I^2 = 88\%$						
Test for overall effect: Z = 1.20 (P = 0.23)						
2.1.3 Mean age 60-70 years						
Abe 2020	1017	11049	69	747	11.5%	1.00 [0.77, 1.29]
Ahn 2019	5828	25593	12733	70696	22.0%	1.34 [1.30, 1.39]
Cook 1986	6	51	9	50	1.2%	0.61 [0.20, 1.85]
Ehsani 2020	14	47	2	47	0.6%	9.55 [2.03, 44.89]
Ellard 2014	73	396	24	104	4.5%	0.75 [0.45, 1.27]
Krenk 2012	0	22	0	203		Not estimable
Memtsoudis 2019	28933	1003196	13579	559152	22.2%	1.19 [1.17, 1.22]
Subtotal (95% CI)		**1040354**		**630999**	**62.0%**	**1.20 [1.07, 1.35]**
Total events	35871		26416			
Heterogeneity: $Tau^2 = 0.01$; $Chi^2 = 46.57$, df = 5 (P < 0.00001); $I^2 = 89\%$						
Test for overall effect: Z = 3.05 (P = 0.002)						
2.1.4 Mean age<60 years						
Bilge 2015	37	224	9	26	1.8%	0.37 [0.15, 0.90]
Choi 2020	142	9921	209	14458	13.4%	0.99 [0.80, 1.23]
Subtotal (95% CI)		**10145**		**14484**	**15.2%**	**0.67 [0.26, 1.71]**
Total events	179		218			
Heterogeneity: $Tau^2 = 0.37$; $Chi^2 = 4.43$, df = 1 (P = 0.04); $I^2 = 77\%$						
Test for overall effect: Z = 0.84 (P = 0.40)						
Total (95% CI)		**1054099**		**648052**	**100.0%**	**1.15 [1.02, 1.31]**
Total events	36436		26974			
Heterogeneity: $Tau^2 = 0.02$; $Chi^2 = 108.43$, df = 18 (P < 0.00001); $I^2 = 83\%$						
Test for overall effect: Z = 2.24 (P = 0.02)						
Test for subgroup differences: $Chi^2 = 2.88$, df = 3 (P = 0.41), $I^2 = 0\%$						

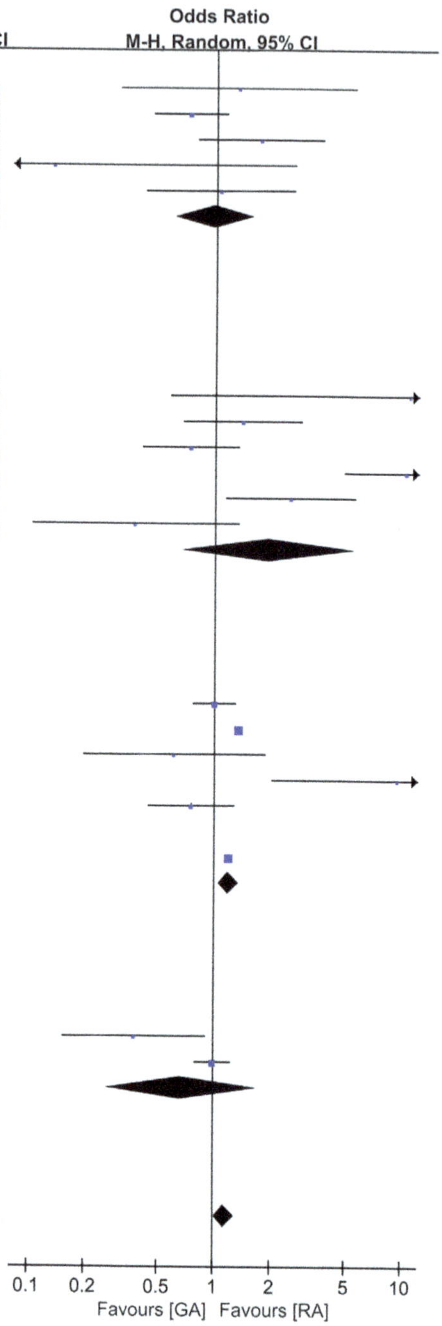

FIGURE 8 | The subgroup analysis according to mean (or median) age gaps (≥80 years, 70–80 years, 60–70 years, and <60 years).

from retrospective studies was positive, while the prospective ones were negative. Given that the retrospective studies have a higher incidence of selection and recall biases, we are not yet sure whether GA is associated with higher POD incidence than RA (54). Additionally, preoperative cognitive function or neuropsychological state of patients considerably affects their POD incidence. In this meta-analysis, all trials provided the cognitive or neuropsychological baseline information without statistical difference between GA and RA groups except for three articles (23, 28, 35). We excluded the three trials and found that GA did not significantly increase the POD incidence of patients compared with RA.

Subgroup analyses of this meta-analysis also exhibited unexpected results. According to previous studies, both male gender and advanced age are risk factors of POD occurrence (55, 56). Interestingly, in this meta-analysis, the pooled result of

Study or Subgroup	GA Events	GA Total	RA Events	RA Total	Weight	Odds Ratio M-H, Random, 95% CI
1.4.1 GA and PNB						
Abe 2020	1017	11049	69	747	11.3%	1.00 [0.77, 1.29]
Ellard 2014	73	396	7	31	1.8%	0.77 [0.32, 1.87]
Liu 2014	15	72	23	145	2.6%	1.40 [0.68, 2.87]
Song 2019	165	2538	2	425	0.7%	14.71 [3.63, 59.52]
Subtotal (95% CI)		**14055**		**1348**	**16.4%**	**1.64 [0.70, 3.87]**
Total events	1270		101			
Heterogeneity: Tau² = 0.59; Chi² = 17.50, df = 3 (P = 0.0006); I² = 83%						
Test for overall effect: Z = 1.13 (P = 0.26)						
1.4.2 GA and neuraxial anesthesia						
Ahn 2019	5828	25593	12733	70696	21.9%	1.34 [1.30, 1.39]
Bilge 2015	37	224	9	26	1.8%	0.37 [0.15, 0.90]
Casati 2003	9	15	8	15	0.7%	1.31 [0.31, 5.58]
Chew 2021	0	164	0	298		Not estimable
Choi 2020	142	9921	209	14458	13.3%	0.99 [0.80, 1.23]
Cook 1986	6	51	9	50	1.1%	0.61 [0.20, 1.85]
Ehsani 2020	14	47	2	47	0.6%	9.55 [2.03, 44.89]
Ellard 2014	73	396	17	73	3.5%	0.74 [0.41, 1.36]
Ilango 2016	84	167	88	151	5.7%	0.72 [0.47, 1.13]
Krenk 2012	0	22	0	203		Not estimable
Li 2019	4	42	0	47	0.2%	11.10 [0.58, 212.68]
Memtsoudis 2019	28933	1003196	13579	559152	22.1%	1.19 [1.17, 1.22]
Nawi 2021	46	158	10	52	2.3%	1.73 [0.80, 3.73]
Parker 2015	0	164	3	158	0.2%	0.14 [0.01, 2.64]
Shin 2020	17	118	8	58	1.7%	1.05 [0.43, 2.60]
Slor 2011	18	60	171	466	3.7%	0.74 [0.41, 1.33]
Song 2019	165	2538	5	648	1.7%	8.94 [3.66, 21.86]
Song 2021	24	69	12	69	2.2%	2.53 [1.14, 5.61]
Tzimas 2018	4	33	10	37	0.9%	0.37 [0.10, 1.33]
Subtotal (95% CI)		**1042978**		**646704**	**83.6%**	**1.15 [1.01, 1.31]**
Total events	35404		26873			
Heterogeneity: Tau² = 0.02; Chi² = 93.13, df = 16 (P < 0.00001); I² = 83%						
Test for overall effect: Z = 2.19 (P = 0.03)						
Total (95% CI)		**1057033**		**648052**	**100.0%**	**1.15 [1.02, 1.30]**
Total events	36674		26974			
Heterogeneity: Tau² = 0.02; Chi² = 108.99, df = 20 (P < 0.00001); I² = 82%						
Test for overall effect: Z = 2.26 (P = 0.02)						
Test for subgroup differences: Chi² = 0.63, df = 1 (P = 0.43), I² = 0%						

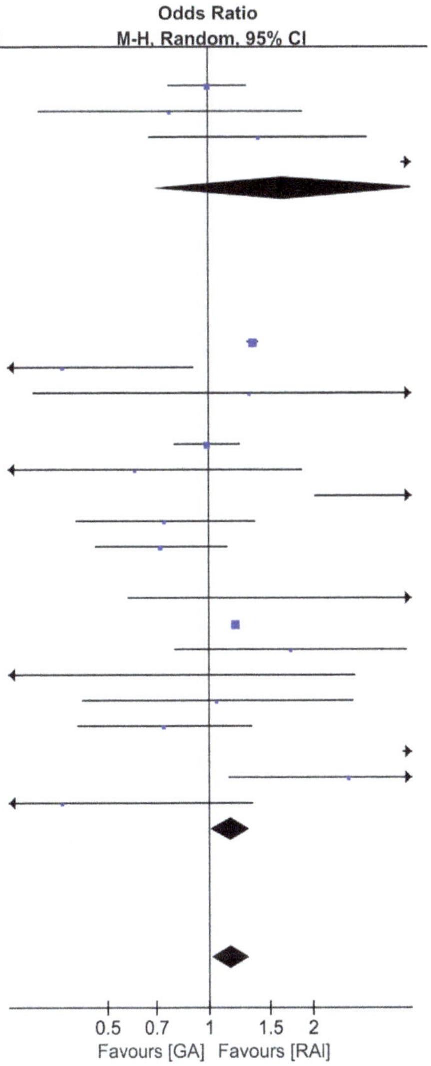

FIGURE 9 | The subgroup analysis according to anesthesia methods in the RA group (neuraxial anesthesia and PNB).

trials with a higher male percentage (≥50%) was not significant in POD incidence between patients with GA and RA, meanwhile, the advanced age did not exhibit a considerable difference in POD occurrence in patients between GA and RA, either. We consider the possible reasons, including the following ones: (1) The POD occurrence in female gender may be more susceptible to the modes of anesthesia; (2) the number of included trials in subgroup of male percentage ≥50% is too small to prove the result; (3) the patients aged 60–70 years are more affected by anesthesia modes in POD occurrence; (4) the subgroup of mean (or median) age gap of 60–70 years included the retrospective studies with large sample size of patients, while the sample size of patients in other mean (or median) age gaps is relatively smaller, respectively. Besides, we obtained the significant result in POD incidence in the subgroup of neuraxial anesthesia. The more studies and larger sample size may be the main cause of this result. The potential reasons above mentioned also need to be further proved in the updated meta-analysis with increasing number of high-quality studies in this field.

There are several limitations in this meta-analysis. Firstly, over 90% of patients are from retrospective studies, which may result in unreliable outcomes due to the selection and recall biases and data loss. Secondly, emergency surgery has been identified as a risk factor of POD (57), however, most of the included trials with patients undergoing both urgent and selective operations did not provide the specific number of urgent and selective patients, which may impact the results. Thirdly, most of the included studies did not clarify whether sedative drugs were used during surgery in the RA group, which might be another factor in interfering with the results. Fourthly, the type and/or dose of general anesthetics varied in the GA group among the included trials, which also is a cause of the uncertain results.

CONCLUSION

In this systematic review and meta-analysis, we did not confirm that GA was associated with a higher incidence of POD in surgical patients when compared with RA. The pooled result should be updated by cumulative high-quality studies in the future.

AUTHOR CONTRIBUTIONS

XZ and MY independently performed the screening process for titles and abstracts and were responsible for extracting the data. HW and JM performed the screening process for full texts. LZ and HW independently assessed the quality of included studies. HW, LZ, and FY were responsible for adjusting data discrepancies. HW conducted the statistical analysis and made the figures and tables. XZ prepared the manuscript. FY and ZW supervised the whole process and ensured the effectiveness of the meta-analysis. All authors have read and approved the submission of the final manuscript.

ACKNOWLEDGMENTS

The authors would like to thank Dr. Yang Wang (Department of Biostatistics, the Chinese Academy of Medical Sciences, Fuwai Hospital, China) for his help with statistical data management.

SUPPLEMENTARY MATERIAL

Supplementary Figure 1 | Risk of bias graph: review authors' judgements about each risk of bias item presented as percentages across all included studies.

Supplementary Figure 2 | Risk of bias summary: review authors' judgements about each risk of bias item for each included study.

Supplementary Table 1 | The guidelines of the 2009 PRISMA (Preferred Reporting Items for Systematic reviews and Meta-analyses).

Supplementary Table 2 | Bias risk of observational studies (retrospective and prospective) by the Newcastle-Ottawa Quality Assessment Scale.

REFERENCES

1. Lipowski ZJ. Delirium (acute confusional states). *JAMA.* (1987) 258:1789–92. doi: 10.1001/jama.258.13.1789
2. Raats JW, van Eijsden WA, Crolla RM, Steyerberg EW, van der Laan L. Risk factors and outcomes for postoperative delirium after major surgery in elderly patients. *PLoS One.* (2015) 10:e0136071. doi: 10.1371/journal.pone.0136071
3. Munk L, Andersen G, Møller AM. Post-anaesthetic emergence delirium in adults: incidence, predictors and consequences. *Acta Anaesthesiol Scand.* (2016) 60:1059–66. doi: 10.1111/aas.12717
4. Avidan MS, Maybrier HR, Abdallah AB, Jacobsohn E, Vlisides PE, Pryor KO, et al. Intraoperative ketamine for prevention of postoperative delirium or pain after major surgery in older adults: an international, multicentre, double-blind, randomised clinical trial. *Lancet.* (2017) 390:267–75. doi: 10.1016/S0140-6736(17)31467-8
5. Saczynski JS, Marcantonio ER, Quach L, Fong TG, Gross A, Inouye SK, et al. Cognitive trajectories after postoperative delirium. *N Engl J Med.* (2012) 367:30–9. doi: 10.1056/NEJMoa1112923
6. Luger MF, Muller S, Kammerlander C, Gosch M, Luger TJ. Predictors of postoperative cognitive decline in very old patients with hip fracture: a retrospective analysis. *Geriatr Orthop Surg Rehabil.* (2014) 5:165–72. doi: 10.1177/2151458514548577
7. Jin Z, Hu J, Ma D. Postoperative delirium: perioperative assessment, risk reduction, and management. *Br J Anaesth.* (2020) 125:492–504. doi: 10.1016/j.bja.2020.06.063
8. Bilotta F, Lauretta MP, Borozdina A, Mizikov VM, Rosa G. Postoperative delirium: risk factors, diagnosis and perioperative care. *Minerva Anestesiol.* (2013) 79:1066–76.
9. Lee U, Mashour GA, Kim S, Noh GJ, Choi BM. Propofol induction reduces the capacity for neural information integration: implications for the mechanism of consciousness and general anesthesia. *Conscious Cogn.* (2009) 18:56–64. doi: 10.1016/j.concog.2008.10.005
10. Pavel MA, Petersen EN, Wang H, Lerner RA, Hansen SB. Studies on the mechanism of general anesthesia. *Proc Natl Acad Sci U S A.* (2020) 117:13757–66. doi: 10.1073/pnas.2004259117
11. Zheng X, Tan Y, Gao Y, Liu Z. Comparative efficacy of Neuraxial and general anesthesia for hip fracture surgery: a meta-analysis of randomized clinical trials. *BMC Anesthesiol.* (2020) 20:162. doi: 10.1186/s12871-020-01074-y
12. Moher D, Liberati A, Tetzlaff J, Altman DG; PRISMA Group. Preferred reporting items for systematic reviews and meta-analyses: the PRISMA statement. *PLoS Med.* (2009) 6:e1000097. doi: 10.1371/journal.pmed.1000097
13. Stang A. Critical evaluation of the Newcastle-Ottawa scale for the assessment of the quality of nonrandomized studies in meta-analyses. *Eur J Epidemiol.* (2010) 25:603–5. doi: 10.1007/s10654-010-9491-z
14. Koster G, Wetterslev J, Gluud C, Zijlstra JG, Scheeren TW, van der Horst IC, et al. Effects of levosimendan for low cardiac output syndrome in critically ill patients: systematic review with meta-analysis and trial sequential analysis. *Intensive Care Med.* (2015) 41:203–21. doi: 10.1007/s00134-014-3604-1
15. Aziz O, Athanasiou T, Darzi A. Minimally invasive conduit harvesting: a systematic review. *Eur J Cardiothorac Surg.* (2006) 29:324–33. doi: 10.1016/j.ejcts.2005.11.032
16. Chen P, Wu X, Wang Z, Li Z, Tian X, Wang J, et al. Effects of levosimendan on mortality in patients undergoing cardiac surgery: a systematic review and meta-analysis. *J Card Surg.* (2018) 33:322–9. doi: 10.1111/jocs.13716
17. Abe H, Sumitani M, Matsui H, Aso S, Inoue R, Fushimi K, et al. Comparing outcomes after peripheral nerve block versus general anesthesia for lower extremity amputation: a nationwide exploratory retrospective cohort study in Japan. *Reg Anesth Pain Med.* (2020) 45:399–404. doi: 10.1136/rapm-2019-101208
18. Ahn EJ, Kim HJ, Kim KW, Choi HR, Kang H, Bang SR. Comparison of general anaesthesia and regional anaesthesia in terms of mortality and complications in elderly patients with hip fracture: a nationwide population-based study. *BMJ Open.* (2019) 9:e029245. doi: 10.1136/bmjopen-2019-029245
19. Bilge EÜ, Kaya M, Senel GÖ, Ünver S. The incidence of delirium at the postoperative intensive care unit in adult patients. *Turk J Anaesthesiol Reanim.* (2015) 43:232–9. doi: 10.5152/TJAR.2015.93798
20. Casati A, Aldegheri G, Vinciguerra E, Marsan A, Fraschini G, Torri G. Randomized comparison between sevoflurane anaesthesia and unilateral spinal anaesthesia in elderly patients undergoing orthopaedic surgery. *Eur J Anaesthesiol.* (2003) 20:640–6. doi: 10.1097/00003643-200308000-00009

21. Chew D, Sethi E, Sim YE, Tan PYB, Abdullah HR, Bin Johri MN, et al. Postoperative delirium following total joint arthroplasties in a multi-ethnic population - a prospective observational study. *Knee.* (2021) 32:103–11. doi: 10.1016/j.knee.2021.08.009
22. Choi EJ, Choi YJ, Lee SW, Choi YM, Ri HS, Park JY, et al. Effect of anesthetic method on incidence of delirium after total hip replacement arthroplasty in South Korea: a population-based study using National Health Insurance claims data. *Korean J Anesthesiol.* (2020) 73:36–43. doi: 10.4097/kja.19091
23. Cook PT, Davies MJ, Cronin KD, Moran P. A prospective randomised trial comparing spinal anaesthesia using hyperbaric cinchocaine with general anaesthesia for lower limb vascular surgery. *Anaesth Intensive Care.* (1986) 14:373–80. doi: 10.1177/0310057X8601400409
24. Ehsani R, Djalali Motlagh S, Zaman B, Sehat Kashani S, Ghodraty MR. Effect of general versus spinal anesthesia on postoperative delirium and early cognitive dysfunction in elderly patients. *Anesth Pain Med.* (2020) 10:e101815. doi: 10.5812/aapm.101815
25. Ellard L, Katznelson R, Wasowicz M, Ashworth A, Carroll J, Lindsay T, et al. Type of anesthesia and postoperative delirium after vascular surgery. *J Cardiothorac Vasc Anesth.* (2014) 28:458–61. doi: 10.1053/j.jvca.2013.12.003
26. Ilango S, Pulle RC, Bell J, Kuys SS. General versus spinal anaesthesia and postoperative delirium in an orthogeriatric population. *Australas J Ageing.* (2016) 35:42–7. doi: 10.1111/ajag.12212
27. Krenk L, Rasmussen LS, Hansen TB, Bogø S, Søballe K, Kehlet H. Delirium after fast-track hip and knee arthroplasty. *Br J Anaesth.* (2012) 108:607–11. doi: 10.1093/bja/aer493
28. Li Z, Long H, Huang F, Zhang Y, Xu J, Wang X. Impact of epidural versus general anesthesia on major lumbar surgery in elderly patients. *Clin Spine Surg.* (2019) 32:E7–E12. doi: 10.1097/BSD.0000000000000708
29. Liu JL, Wang XL, Gong MW, Mai HX, Pei SJ, Yuan WX, et al. Comparative outcomes of peripheral nerve blocks versus general anesthesia for hip fractures in geriatric Chinese patients. *Patient Prefer Adherence.* (2014) 8:651–9. doi: 10.2147/PPA.S61903
30. Memtsoudis S, Cozowicz C, Zubizarreta N, Weinstein SM, Liu J, Kim DH, et al. Risk factors for postoperative delirium in patients undergoing lower extremity joint arthroplasty: a retrospective population-based cohort study. *Reg Anesth Pain Med.* (2019) 44:934–43. doi: 10.1136/rapm-2019-100700
31. Nawi SNM, Wong B, Edwards S, Loh X, Maddison J. A retrospective observational study on the types of anaesthesia in hip fracture surgery. *J Perioper Pract.* (2021). doi: 10.1177/17504589211006020. [Epub ahead of print].
32. Parker MJ, Griffiths R. General versus regional anaesthesia for hip fractures. A pilot randomised controlled trial of 322 patients. *Injury.* (2015) 46:1562–6. doi: 10.1016/j.injury.2015.05.004
33. Shin S, Kim SH, Park KK, Kim SJ, Bae JC, Choi YS. Effects of anesthesia techniques on outcomes after hip fracture surgery in elderly patients: a prospective, randomized, controlled trial. *J Clin Med.* (2020) 9:1605. doi: 10.3390/jcm9061605
34. Slor CJ, de Jonghe JF, Vreeswijk R, Groot E, Ploeg TV, van Gool WA, et al. Anesthesia and postoperative delirium in older adults undergoing hip surgery. *J Am Geriatr Soc.* (2011) 59:1313–9. doi: 10.1111/j.1532-5415.2011.03452.x
35. Song KJ, Ko JH, Kwon TY, Choi BW. Etiology and related factors of postoperative delirium in orthopedic surgery. *Clin Orthop Surg.* (2019) 11:297–301. doi: 10.4055/cios.2019.11.3.297
36. Song Y, Liu Y, Yuan Y, Jia X, Zhang W, Wang G, et al. Effects of general versus subarachnoid anaesthesia on circadian melatonin rhythm and postoperative delirium in elderly patients undergoing hip fracture surgery: a prospective cohort clinical trial. *EBioMed.* (2021) 70:103490. doi: 10.1016/j.ebiom.2021.103490
37. Tzimas P, Samara E, Petrou A, Korompilias A, Chalkias A, Papadopoulos G. The influence of anesthetic techniques on postoperative cognitive function in elderly patients undergoing hip fracture surgery: general vs spinal anesthesia. *Injury.* (2018) 49:2221–6. doi: 10.1016/j.injury.2018.09.023
38. Kazmierski J, Banys A, Latek J, Bourke J, Jaszewski R. Raised IL-2 and TNF-α concentrations are associated with postoperative delirium in patients undergoing coronary-artery bypass graft surgery. *Int Psychogeriatr.* (2014) 26:845–55. doi: 10.1017/S1041610213002378
39. Hirsch J, Vacas S, Terrando N, Yuan M, Sands LP, Kramer J, et al. Perioperative cerebrospinal fluid and plasma inflammatory markers after orthopedic surgery. *J Neuroinflammation.* (2016) 13:211. doi: 10.1186/s12974-016-0681-9
40. Li QH, Yu L, Yu ZW, Fan XL, Yao WX, Ji C, et al. Relation of postoperative serum S100A12 levels to delirium and cognitive dysfunction occurring after hip fracture surgery in elderly patients. *Brain Behav.* (2019) 9:e01176. doi: 10.1002/brb3.1176
41. Kazmierski J, Banys A, Latek J, Bourke J, Jaszewski R. Cortisol levels and neuropsychiatric diagnosis as markers of postoperative delirium: a prospective cohort study. *Crit Care.* (2013) 17:R38. doi: 10.1186/cc12548
42. van der Beek EM, Wiegant VM, Schouten WG, van Eerdenburg FJ, Loijens LW, van der Plas C, et al. Neuronal number, volume, and apoptosis of the left dentate gyrus of chronically stressed pigs correlate negatively with basal saliva cortisol levels. *Hippocampus.* (2004) 14:688–700. doi: 10.1002/hipo.10213
43. Casey CP, Lindroth H, Mohanty R, Farahbakhsh Z, Ballweg T, Twadell S, et al. Postoperative delirium is associated with increased plasma neurofilament light. *Brain.* (2020) 143:47–54. doi: 10.1093/brain/awz354
44. Han Y, Zhang W, Liu J, Song Y, Liu T, Li Z, et al. Metabolomic and lipidomic profiling of preoperative CSF in elderly hip fracture patients with postoperative delirium. *Front Aging Neurosci.* (2020) 12:570210. doi: 10.3389/fnagi.2020.570210
45. Hao X, Ou M, Zhang D, Zhao W, Yang Y, Liu J, et al. The effects of general anesthetics on synaptic transmission. *Curr Neuropharmacol.* (2020) 18:936–65. doi: 10.2174/1570159X18666200227125854
46. Hambrecht-Wiedbusch VS, LaTendresse KA, Avidan MS, Nelson AG, Phyle M, Ajluni RE, et al. General anesthesia does not have persistent effects on attention in rodents. *Front Behav Neurosci.* (2019) 13:76. doi: 10.3389/fnbeh.2019.00076
47. Mashour GA, Palanca BJ, Basner M, Li D, Wang W, Blain-Moraes S, et al. Recovery of consciousness and cognition after general anesthesia in humans. *Elife.* (2021) 10:e59525. doi: 10.7554/eLife.59525
48. Perouansky M. General anesthetics and long-term neurotoxicity. *Handb Exp Pharmacol.* (2008) 182:143–57. doi: 10.1007/978-3-540-74806-9_7
49. Wang B, Zhu C, Zhang N, Li L, Sun L, Xu J. Nampt/RelB pathway protects learning and memory ability in aged rats after general anesthesia with sevoflurane and nitrous oxide. *Int J Clin Exp Pathol.* (2018) 11:293–303.
50. Zuo Z. Are volatile anesthetics neuroprotective or neurotoxic? *Med Gas Res.* (2012) 2:10. doi: 10.1186/2045-9912-2-10
51. McGuigan S, Evered L, Scott DA, Silbert B, Zetterberg H, Blennow K. Comparing the effect of xenon and sevoflurane anesthesia on postoperative neural injury biomarkers: a randomized controlled trial. *Med Gas Res.* (2022) 12:10–7. doi: 10.4103/2045-9912.324591
52. Tanabe S, Mohanty R, Lindroth H, Casey C, Ballweg T, Farahbakhsh Z, et al. Cohort study into the neural correlates of postoperative delirium: the role of connectivity and slow-wave activity. *Br J Anaesth.* (2020) 125:55–66. doi: 10.1016/j.bja.2020.02.027
53. Luo M, Song B, Zhu J. Sleep disturbances after general anesthesia: current perspectives. *Front Neurol.* (2020) 11:629. doi: 10.3389/fneur.2020.00629
54. Talari K, Goyal M. Retrospective studies - utility and caveats. *J R Coll Physicians Edinb.* (2020) 50:398–402. doi: 10.4997/JRCPE.2020.409
55. Wang H, Guo X, Zhu X, Li Y, Jia Y, Zhang Z, et al. Gender differences and postoperative delirium in adult patients undergoing cardiac valve surgery. *Front Cardiovasc Med.* (2021) 8:751421. doi: 10.3389/fcvm.2021.751421
56. Poeran J, Cozowicz C, Zubizarreta N, Weinstein SM, Deiner SG, Leipzig RM, et al. Modifiable factors associated with postoperative delirium after hip fracture repair: an age-stratified retrospective cohort study. *Eur J Anaesthesiol.* (2020) 37:649–58. doi: 10.1097/EJA.0000000000001197
57. Koebrugge B, van Wensen RJ, Bosscha K, Dautzenberg PL, Koning OH. Delirium after emergency/elective open and endovascular aortoiliac surgery at a surgical ward with a high-standard delirium care protocol. *Vascular.* (2010) 18:279–87. doi: 10.2310/6670.2010.00052

26

Alternative Therapies for the Prevention of Postoperative Nausea and Vomiting

Nicoleta Stoicea[1], Tong J. Gan[2], Nicholas Joseph[1,3], Alberto Uribe[1], Jyoti Pandya[1], Rohan Dalal[4] and Sergio D. Bergese[1,5]*

[1] Department of Anesthesiology, The Ohio State University Wexner Medical Center, Columbus, OH, USA, [2] Department of Anesthesiology, Stony Brook University Medical Center, Stony Brook, NY, USA, [3] Department of Neuroscience, The Ohio State University, Columbus, OH, USA, [4] Department of Psychology, The Ohio State University, Columbus, OH, USA, [5] Department of Neurological Surgery, The Ohio State University Wexner Medical Center, Columbus, OH, USA

***Correspondence:**
Nicoleta Stoicea
nicoleta.stoicea@osumc.edu

Postoperative nausea and vomiting (PONV) is a complication affecting between 20 and 40% of all surgery patients, with high-risk patients experiencing rates of up to 80%. Recent studies and publications have shed light on the uses of alternative treatment for PONV through their modulation of endogenous opioid neuropeptides and neurokinin ligands. In addition to reducing PONV, hypnosis was reported to be useful in attenuating postoperative pain and anxiety, and contributing to hemodynamic stability. Music therapy has been utilized to deepen the sedation level and decrease patient anxiety, antiemetic and analgesic requirements, hospital length of stay, and fatigue. Isopropyl alcohol and peppermint oil aromatherapy have both been used to reduce postoperative nausea. With correct training in traditional Chinese healing techniques, acupuncture (APu) at the P6 acupoint has also been shown to be useful in preventing early PONV, postdischarge nausea and vomiting, and alleviating of pain. Electro-acupuncture (EAPu), as with APu, provided analgesic and antiemetic effects through release and modulation of opioid neuropeptides. These non-pharmacological modalities of treatment contribute to an overall patient wellbeing, assisting in physical and emotional healing.

Keywords: postoperative nausea and vomiting, acupuncture, acupressure, hypnosis, alternative medicine

POSTOPERATIVE NAUSEA AND VOMITING

Postoperative nausea and vomiting (PONV) is a complication affecting between 20 and 40% of all surgery patients, with high-risk patients experiencing rates of up to 80% (1–3). This condition severely affects patient satisfaction, with postoperative vomiting (POV) ranking above postoperative pain in least-desirable outcome. Moreover, while postoperative nausea (PON) is responsible for increasing patient anxiety, POV can cause more serious complications, including hematoma, dehydration, aspiration, and esophageal damage (1). For maxillofacial surgical patients, POV is responsible for wound dehiscence and bleeding, leading to further complications (1). In addition to these PONV-precipitated problems, emetic episodes can delay patient discharge from the post-anesthesia care unit by at least 20 min, with a residual group of patients experiencing severe PONV and requiring unplanned hospitalization (1, 3, 4).

NEUROPHYSIOLOGY

Stimulation of vestibular nuclei (VNU), area postrema (AP), and vagal afferent fibers from the gastrointestinal tract, project to the nucleus of the solitary tract (NST), with output pathways to local brain stem areas responsible for the vomiting reflex. NST sends projections to the mid- and fore-brain center responsible for the perception of nausea. Importantly, the AP's capillaries are not surrounded by astrocytes and other glial cells comprising the blood–brain barrier (BBB), thus allowing input from toxins, metabolites, and drugs such as opioids, circulating within the systemic blood flow. The AP can then release serotonin, dopamine, acetylcholine, histamine, and neurokinin-1 ("substance-P") to the NST as well as the reticular formation. Anesthesia is thought to modulate PONV by binding to the ionotropic 5-hydroxytryptamine type 3 (5-HT_3) receptors within the AP and VAF, in addition to binding the solitary tract nucleus directly. Perioperative opioid administration has the potential to produce nausea and vomiting through binding to the μ-opioid receptor within the AP and NTS (5, 6).

RISK FACTORS

Several risk factors exist for both PON and POV. Among them are: female gender, type of surgery, use of nitrous oxide, history of PONV or motion sickness, and perioperative opioid use. Female gender is widely considered to be the greatest risk factor for PON, but not for POV, with females experiencing three to four times the PON rate of male counterparts (1–3). Abdominal and ear, nose, and throat procedures are considered "high-risk" for PONV along with breast surgery, though the latter is believed to be due in part to the female gender. Interestingly, smoking status has been shown to decrease PONV in a manner dependent upon the time since the last cigarette. Whether the protective nature of smoking against PONV is due to nicotine in the tobacco or other chemical content has yet to be established. PONV also seems to be more prevalent in younger patients, especially those whose siblings or parents have experienced PONV (1–3). Iqbal et al. found that PONV steadily rose in prevalence for age 0–3, and thereafter decreased until age 14 when the prevalence again peaked. The authors then noted a steady decrease in PONV risk by around 10% per decade of life (3).

Postoperative opioid consumption also has a significant effect on the rate of PONV, Roberts et al. finding a consistent 6.0% POV reduction when postoperative opioid dose was reduced by half. The study also concluded that postoperative opioid dose escalation increased POV logarithmically ($r^2 = 0.98$, $P < 0.01$) (7). Per Apfel et al., postoperative opioid use might be the single strongest predictor of PONV, with no difference between morphine and piritramide use postoperatively (8). Pierre et al. found patients with a previous history of PONV or motion sickness were four times more likely to experience PONV again, if opioids were required after the procedure (9). A consensus guideline developed by Gan et al. also found postoperative opioid use to be one of the most likely independent predictors of PONV. The guideline also suggested the contribution of alternative medicine to PONV and pain management (10).

ANTIEMETICS

Antiemetics have widely been used to manage PONV and are commonly given both as treatment and prophylaxis for at-risk patients. Several anti-emetic pharmacological classes are available including histamine antagonists, muscarinic acetylcholine antagonists, dopamine antagonists, corticosteroids, 5-HT_3 antagonists, and tachykinin 1 antagonists. 5-HT_3 receptor antagonists are the most commonly used type of antiemetic, with ondansetron being the most prescribed type. Droperidol, a selective dopamine receptor antagonist, dexamethasone, a corticosteroid, transdermal scopolamine, a non-selective, muscarinic acetylcholine receptor antagonist, and the newer 5-HT_3 antagonist, palonosetron, have all been used to treat PONV (5).

ALTERNATIVE THERAPIES

Since 1784, when a commission from The Royal Academy of Science concluded that "imagination" was behind the treatment introduced by Franz Anton Mesmer to heal patients, alternative medicine has evolved rapidly, alongside mainstream medicine (11). For the past two centuries, hypnosis, relaxation imagery, music therapy, aromatherapy, acupressure (Apr), acupuncture (APu), and electroacupuncture (EAPu) have been studied and used mainly for anesthesia and analgesia in medical and surgical procedures. Recent studies and publications have shed light on the uses of alternative treatment for PONV, through their modulation of endogenous opioid neuropeptides and neurokinin ligands (12, 13).

Hypnosis Therapy

At the end of the nineteenth century, Charcot demonstrated hypnosis on hysterical patients. His work was refuted by many contemporary scientists but recognized by renown psychiatrists like Sigmund Freud (1885) and Pierre Janet (14). Differing from its popular media portrayal, hypnosis has been used in the perioperative clinical settings to alleviate both postoperative pain and PONV (15). During hypnosis therapy, the caregiver, trained in hypnotic techniques, offers concentration strategies to the patient during the *induction* phase. These strategies allow the patient to more easily enter subsequent states of narrowed awareness. During the next stage of hypnosis, referred to as *deepening*, the hypnotist attempts to deepen the trance with imagery and memory recall with a focus on relaxation. During this trance state, known as *dissociation*, the patient experiences a separation of behavioral components, when, in a dream-like state, he or she becomes an observer while re-experiencing autobiographical memories. In this state, the hypnotist makes suggestions to reinforce feelings of relaxation and well-being, incompatible with pain or vomiting (12, 16). In a pediatric case report published in 2007, Mackenzie and Frawley described a four session hypnotherapy process used to treat PONV in a 6-year-old boy undergoing multiple esophageal dilation interventions. During these sessions, the patient received the suggestion that he had a "button in his brain" able to turn chewing, gagging, or nausea, ON or OFF. Nurses were instructed not to act in anticipation of a retching event (holding a kidney dish). The report noted a significant reduction and eventual cessation of PONV symptoms in this child (16). In a larger, randomized study of 100 thyroidectomy patients, Eberhart et al. played a tape recording of therapeutic suggestions intraoperatively. The study found a PONV rate reduction from 85.7% in the control group, to 47.2% in the treatment group. A substantial reduction in antimetic pharmacological requirements was reported as a result of this intervention (30.6 versus 68.6%). Studies in other populations have similarly found positive results with hypnosis for PONV (15). In addition to reducing PONV, hypnosis was reported to be useful in attenuating postoperative pain, anxiety, and contributing to hemodynamic stability (12). While the exact neuro-pathway by which hypnosis provides relief of PONV has yet to be fully elucidated, the area of the brain activated in a hypnotic state are known through positron emission tomography (PET) and magnetic resonance imaging studies. Utilizing PET imaging, Faymonville et al. found acute changes in both temporal lobes, basal forebrain areas, the parietal lobe, the precentral gyrus, the prefrontal cortex, insular, and cingulate cortices. Importantly, the medial parietal cortex demonstrated greatly reduced activity, similar to the decreases seen during unconsciousness, coma, general anesthesia, and rapid eye and non-rapid eye movement sleep. The anterior cingulate cortex (Brodmann area 24) was strongly activated during hypnotic trance. This area is known to be innervated by a wide variety of opioid, dopaminergic, seretonergic, noradrenergic, neurokinin 1, and other peptidic pathways. Hypnotic activation of the insulae and anterior cingulate cortex has been consistently shown during pain states. Crosstalk between these two structures and the midbrain and thalamus may provide descending pain inhibition through modification of the pain threshold and perception of pain intensity. The clinically observed analgesic effects of hypnosis may be thus explained through these pathways (12).

Guided Imagery and Relaxation Therapy

Guided imagery is a highly personalized form of therapy wherein patients create a relaxing imagery scenario to relieve anxiety and pain. The most frequently encountered scenarios were linked to nature, a trip, family, the patient's home, or a personal hobby or skill. Guided muscle relaxation may also be used prior to the patient envisioning his or her scenario to further relaxation. A recent meta-analysis performed by Sing and Dalmar in 2014 found that guided imagery intervention is effective for reducing anxiety and pain in surgical patients (17). A randomized study of elective colorectal surgery patients reported a perioperative reduction of opioid consumption by 50%. Such therapy is cost-effective and may be instituted as a complementary method of analgesic and anxiolytic care (18).

Music Therapy

In addition to hypnotic therapy, music therapy has been utilized to deepen the sedation level and decrease patient anxiety, antiemetic and analgesic requirements, hospital length of stay, and fatigue (18, 19). A randomized, controlled study of 35 patients undergoing surgeries with spinal anesthesia and patient-controlled intravenous propofol sedation found a significant reduction in propofol use for the group exposed to music during surgery compared to the control group (18). Other studies found no benefit to music therapy, or reduced anxiolytic effect as compared with drug therapy. Thus, this form of therapy's effectiveness is a subject of contention within the literature. Kliempt et al. utilized both hypnotic suggestion and synchronized hemispheric sound during surgery, as did Nilsson et al. (19). The therapy utilized two sounds, one per ear, with a difference in frequency of 1–30 Hz. The beats are generally imperceivable by the patient but may aid in synchronizing activity between the two hemispheres of the brain (20). Both studies noted a statistically significant reduction in analgesic usage. Nilsson also reported a decrease in the number of patients fatigued at discharge (19). However, no differences in the PONV rates between groups (interventional versus control) were noted. The exact mechanism by which music exerts its positive effects has yet to be conclusively determined. Lin linked heightened levels of growth hormone, and decreased levels of epinephrine and interleukin-6, with lower heart rates, blood pressure, and stress levels in patients exposed to music. Music may produce these changes through immune system mediator interactions with the pituitary gland, hypothalamus, and medulla (18, 21).

Aromatherapy

Another form of adjuvant PONV therapy is aromatherapy, adopted from the traditional use of herbal medicine to treat a wide variety of ailments. Isopropyl alcohol and peppermint oil have both been used previously in studies to reduce PONV. The oil or alcohol is administered with a cotton swab placed under the nares and costs around $0.01 dollar per swab, one of aromatherapy's benefits. Another benefit is a rapid patient response, which has been shown to be faster than the response to 4 mg ondansetron (21). Success of aromatherapy in treating nausea has differed amongst studies, even in similar populations. Merritt et al. found no difference in the rate of PONV with aromatherapy in ambulatory surgery patients, while Anderson and Gross found significant reduction in a similar surgical populations (21, 22). Of interest, Anderson and Gross found no difference between the interventional groups receiving alcohol, peppermint oil, and the placebo saline group. The authors suggested that patient anticipation of PONV symptom alleviation may be responsible for the positive effects of aromatherapy more so than any pharmacodynamic effect elicited from oil or alcohol use (22). Tate noted significant benefit to aromatherapy in gynecological patients, where Ferruggiari found no significant benefit in a general population of female surgical patients (21, 23). Wang et al. found limited efficacy of aromatherapy when treating PONV in pediatric patients. Further studies are necessary to better elucidate the benefits of aromatherapy; however, the American Society of PeriAnesthesia Nurses (ASPAN) *2006 Evidence-Based Clinical Practice Guidelines for the Prevention and/or Management of PONV* noted that the benefits of such therapy equal the risks. A 2012 Cochrane Library review also recognized aromatherapy as generally effective (21, 24).

Acupressure

Acupressure is believed to function by increasing release of β-endorphins from the hypothalamus into the cerebrospinal fluid, along with modulating serotonin transmission via serotonergic and norepinephrinergic system mechanisms. Signal transduction from the dermis to the hypothalamus occurs through Aβ and Aδ afferent sensory fibers leading into the spinal dorsal horn (9). As β-endorphins are believed to have antiemetic effects, there is a clear neurobiological basis for APu's antiemetic effects. Majholm et al. studied the use of acupressure applied at the P6 acupoint, located two cuns (4 cm) proximal to the transverse crease between the tendons of the carpi radialis and palmaris longus. The study found the wristbands to have no antiemetic effect against placebo. Additionally, the study reported mild side effects in a third of the study sample, namely redness, tenderness, and swelling (13). Turgot et al. reported more favorable results in female patients undergoing gynecological procedures. The study found a statistically significant reduction in PONV with the addition of bilaterally applied acupressure wristbands (25). The method of reducing PONV may be more feasible than either APu or EAPu due to the short amount of time necessary to treat each patient, with no special training needed for wristband application.

Acupuncture

With correct training in traditional Chinese healing techniques, APu at the same P6 acupoint has been shown to be useful in preventing early PONV, postdischarge nausea and vomiting, and alleviating postoperative pain (26, 27). Korinenko et al. presented a randomized, controlled study wherein both the incidence as well as the severity of PON after cardiac surgery was reduced significantly by pre-operative APu. Lee and Done demonstrated APu to prevent PONV as effectively as antiemetic therapy (22). Use of APu was also shown to increase the time to the first postoperative opioid medication use in total hip arthroplasty and abdominal surgery patients (28, 29). As opioids have been linked to opioid-induced nausea and vomiting, the dual antiemetic and analgesic properties of APu seem particularly favorable in the surgical setting, reducing side effects and costs (30). APu does present mild risks. White et al. compiled side effects seen in 32,000 APu consultations within the UK. The authors concluded that mild bleeding and needle pain were the only common complications of APu (26). These findings suggest that only bleeding disorders and extreme anticoagulation therapy should be considered contraindications for prophylactic APu therapy. Further studies are needed to determine whether pre-operative, interoperative, or postoperative APu is most effective at attenuating PONV.

Electro-Acupuncture

In 1767 at the Middlesex Hospital of London, a special "apparatus" was used to treat patients with electricity. In his book written in 1892, Steavenson mentioned the therapeutic use of electricity at Guy's Hospital of London around the turn of the century (31). The EAPu practitioner does not have to be as precise when using this method with newer, needleless techniques and a larger area of stimulation (32). New devices such as the ITO ES 130 (ITO Co. LTD., Tokyo, Japan), induce an electrical current in an APu needle, placed at the P6 accupoint. A second needle, placed at a neutral point acts as the grounding electrode, allowing for current to flow through the skin. As with APu, EAPu provides analgesic and antiemetic effects through release of opioid neuropeptides and modulation of the serotonergic, norepinephrinergic, tachykininergic, and endogenous endorphin systems (29, 33). Huang et al. reported a decrease in PONV ($P = 0.044$) corresponding to a transcutaneous electrical acupoint stimulation at 100 Hz, and a lower postoperative visual analgesia score ($P = 0.047$) with frequencies of 2/100 Hz. Reduced visual analgesia scores may in turn be responsible for a decrease in postoperative opioid consumption, known as one of the four major risk factors for PONV (9, 34). High versus low frequency electrical stimulus seems to function differently within the brain. Ji-Sheng Han, noted lesioning of the arcuate nucleus in the hypothalamus eliminated the analgesic effects of low but not high frequency EAPu whereas lesioning of the parabrachial nuclei eliminated high but not low frequency EAPu analgesia. The review also stated that low frequency stimulated opioid neuropeptides mainly bound μ and δ opioid receptors where high frequency stimulated opioid peptides primarily bound κ opioid receptors (29, 33). In clinical trials, Hoffman et al. implemented EAPu therapy for PONV in children between the ages of 4 and 18 years during the postoperative period. The study saw significant reduction in PON (60% in the treatment arms versus 85% in the control arm). POV was not significantly reduced (29). This study demonstrated the feasibility of EAPu in the perioperative setting to reduce PON risk.

In 2014, Yeoh reported that the use of EAPu in laproscopic surgery patients might be a useful, non-pharmacologic intervention for preventing PONV for up to 12 h in adult surgical populations (35).

A study performed at Duke University Medical Center using EAPu stimulation or ondansetron versus placebo for the prevention of PONV concluded that electrostimulation or ondansetron administration encountered the same degree of patient satisfaction and was more effective than placebo (36).

CONCLUSION

Alternative therapies offer attractive methods for managing PONV. However, with the exception of APu and EAPu, there is limited evidence supporting the efficacy of complimentary therapy in clinical practice. In order to expand alternative, complementary therapy in the clinical setting, more prospective clinical trials need to be conducted. These non-pharmacological modalities of treatment contribute to an overall patient wellbeing, assisting in physical and emotional healing. Our review of alternative medicine publications conclude that non-medical therapies for PON and POV should be used in addition to medical therapies, rather than as a substitute.

AUTHOR CONTRIBUTIONS

NS, NJ, and RH participated in a review of the literature. NS and NJ prepared the body of the manuscript. TG, AU, JP, RH, and SB contributed significantly to the critical review of the text. All authors read and approved the final form of the manuscript.

REFERENCES

1. Phillips C, Brookes CD, Rich J, Arbon J, Turvey TA. Postoperative nausea and vomiting following orthognathic surgery. *Int J Oral Maxillofac Surg* (2015) **44**(6):745–51. doi:10.1016/j.ijom.2015.01.006
2. Obrink E, Jildenstal P, Oddby E, Jakobsson JG. Post-operative nausea and vomiting: update on predicting the probability and ways to minimize its occurrence, with focus on ambulatory surgery. *Int J Surg* (2015) **15**:100–6. doi:10.1016/j.ijsu.2015.01.024
3. Iqbal IM, Spencer R. Postoperative nausea and vomiting. *Anaesth Intens Care Med* (2012) **13**(12):613–6. doi:10.1016/j.mpaic.2012.09.012
4. Apfel CC, Korttila K, Abdalla M, Kerger H, Turan A, Vedder I, et al. A factorial trial of six interventions for the prevention of postoperative nausea and vomiting. *N Engl J Med* (2004) **350**(24):2441–51. doi:10.1056/NEJMoa032196
5. Horn CC, Wallisch WJ, Homanics GE, Williams JP. Pathophysiological and neurochemical mechanisms of postoperative nausea and vomiting. *Eur J Pharmacol* (2014) **722**(1):55–66. doi:10.1016/j.ejphar.2013.10.037
6. Flaminia C, Alessandra R, Ilenia M, Consalvo M. Non-analgesic effects of opioids: opioid-induced nausea and vomiting: mechanisms and strategies for their limitation. *Curr Pharm Des* (2012) **18**(37):6043–52. doi:10.2174/138161212803582540
7. Roberts GW, Bekker TB, Carlsen HH, Moffatt CH, Slattery PJ, McClure AF. Postoperative nausea and vomiting are strongly influenced by postoperative opioid use in a dose-related manner. *Anesth Analg* (2005) **101**(5):1343–8. doi:10.1213/01.ANE.0000180204.64588.EC
8. Apfel CC, Stoecklein K, Lipfert P. PONV: a problem of inhalational anaesthesia? *Best Pract Res Clin Anaesthesiol* (2005) **19**(3):485–500. doi:10.1016/j.bpa.2005.03.001
9. Pierre S, Benais H, Pouymayou J. Apfel's simplified score may favourably predict the risk of postoperative nausea and vomiting. *Can J Anaesth* (2002) **49**(3):237–42.
10. Gan TJ, Diemunsch P, Habib AS, Kovac A, Kranke P, Meyer TA, et al. Consensus guidelines for the management of postoperative nausea and vomiting. *Anesth Analg* (2014) **118**(1):85–113. doi:10.1213/ANE.0000000000000002
11. Franklin B, Majault MJ, Le Roy JB, Sallin CL, Bailly JS, D'Arcet J, et al. Report of the commissioners charged by the King with the examination of animal magnetism. 1784. *Int J Clin Exp Hypn* (2002) **50**(4):332–63. doi:10.1080/00207140208410109
12. Faymonville ME, Boly M, Laureys S; Brain Imaging in Neurosciences – An Interdisciplinary Approach. Functional neuroanatomy of the hypnotic state. *J Physiol Paris* (2006) **99**:463–9. doi:10.1016/j.jphysparis.2006.03.018
13. Majholm B, Møller AM. Acupressure at acupoint P6 for prevention of postoperative nausea and vomiting: a randomised clinical trial. *Eur J Anaesthesiol* (2011) **28**(6):412–9. doi:10.1097/EJA.0b013e32833f6f42
14. Aguayo J. Charcot and Freud: Some implications of late 19th century French psychiatry and poliltics for the origins of psychoanalysis. *Psychoanal Contemp Thought* (1986) **9**:223–60.
15. Gurgevich S. Clinical hypnosis and surgery. *Alternative Med Alert* (2003) **6**:10.
16. Mackenzie A, Frawley GP. Preoperative hypnotherapy in the management of a child with anticipatory nausea and vomiting. *Anaesth Intensive Care* (2007) **35**(5):784–7.
17. Singh M, Dalmar A. Use of guided imagery for reduction of painand anxiety and improved quality of sleep in patients undergoing surgery: a review and meta-analysis. *J Patient Centered Res Rev* (2014) **1**:146.
18. Mason, Keira P. *Pediatric Sedation Outside of the Operating Room: A Multispecialty International Collaboration*. New York: Springer (2015). doi:10.1007/978-1-4939-1390-9_32
19. Nilsson U, Rawal N, Uneståhl LE, Zetterberg C, Unosson M. Improved recovery after music and therapeutic suggestions during general anaesthesia: a double-blind randomised controlled trial. *Acta Anaesthesiol Scand* (2001) **45**(7):812–7. doi:10.1034/j.1399-6576.2001.045007812.x
20. Dabu-Bondoc S, Drummond-Lewis J, Gaal D, McGinn M, Caldwell-Andrews AA, Kain ZN. Hemispheric synchronized sounds and intraoperative anesthetic requirements. *Anesth Analg* (2003) **97**(3):772–5. doi:10.1213/01.ANE.0000076145.83783.E7
21. Mamaril ME, Windle PE, Burkard JF. Prevention and management of postoperative nausea and vomiting: a look at complementary techniques. *J Perianesth Nurs* (2006) **21**(6):404–10. doi:10.1016/j.jopan.2006.09.007
22. Anderson LA, Gross JB. Aromatherapy with peppermint, isopropyl alcohol, or placebo is equally effective in relieving postoperative nausea. *J Perianesth Nurs* (2004) **19**(1):29–35. doi:10.1016/j.jopan.2003.11.001
23. Ferruggiari L, Ragione B, Rich ER, Lock K. The effect of aromatherapy on postoperative nausea in women undergoing surgical procedures. *J Perianesth Nurs* (2012) **27**(4):246–51. doi:10.1016/j.jopan.2012.01.013
24. Hines S, Steels E, Chang A, Gilshenan K. Aromatherapy for treatment of postoperative nausea and vomiting: a Cochrane systematic review. *Int J Evid Based Healthc* (2009) **7**(3):211. doi:10.1002/14651858.CD007598.pub2
25. Turgot S, Ozalp G, Dikmen S, Savli S, Tuncel N, Kadiogullari N. Acupressure for postoperative nausea and vomiting in gynaecological patients receiving patient-controlled analgesia. *Eur J Anesthesiol* (2006) **24**:87–91. doi:10.1017/S0265021506001190
26. Holmér PP, Wengström Y. Acupuncture prior to surgery to minimise postoperative nausea and vomiting: a systematic review. *J Clin Nurs* (2012) **21**:13–4. doi:10.1111/j.1365-2702.2012.04114.x
27. Al-Sadi M, Newman B, Julious SA. Acupuncture in the prevention of postoperative nausea and vomiting. *Anaesthesia* (1997) **52**(7):658–61. doi:10.1111/j.1365-2044.1997.143-az0147.x
28. Chen C-C, Yang C-C, Hu C-C, Shih H-N, Chang Y-H, Hsieh P-H. Acupuncture for pain relief after total knee arthroplasty. *Reg Anesth Pain Med* (2014) **40**(1):31–6. doi:10.1097/AAP.0000000000000138
29. Rusy LM, Hoffman GM, Weisman SJ. Electroacupuncture prophylaxis of postoperative nausea and vomiting following pediatric tonsillectomy with or without adenoidectomy. *Anesthesiology* (2002) **96**(2):300–5.
30. Smith HS, Laufer A. Opioid induced nausea and vomiting. *Eur J Pharmacol* (2014) **722**:67–78. doi:10.1016/j.ejphar.2013.09.074
31. Steavenson WE. *Medical Electricity*. Philadelphia, PA: P. Blakiston, Son & Company (1892). 3 p.
32. Available from: http://www.acupuncturetoday.com/abc/electroacupuncture.php
33. Han J-S. Acupuncture: neuropeptide release produced by electrical stimulation of different frequencies. *Trends Neurosci* (2003) **26**:1. doi:10.1016/S0166-2236(02)00006-1
34. Huang S, Peng WP, Tian X, Liang H, Jia Z, Lo T, et al. Effects of transcutaneous electrical acupoint stimulation at different frequencies on perioperative anesthetic dosage, recovery, complications, and prognosis in video-assisted thoracic surgical lobectomy: a randomized, double-blinded, placebo-controlled trial. *J Anesth* (2015). doi:10.1007/s00540-015-2057-1
35. Yeoh AH, Tang SSP, Abdul N, Wan Mat WR, Said S, Che Hassan MR, et al. Effectiveness of P6 Acupoint Electrical Stimulation in Preventing Postoperative Nausea and Vomiting Following Laparoscopic Surgery. *Tubitak gov tr* (2014).
36. Gan TJ, Jiao KR, Zenn M, Georgiade G. A randomized controlled comparison of electro-acupoint stimulation or ondansetron versus placebo for the prevention of postoperative nausea and vomiting. *Anesth Analg* (2004) **99**(4):1070–5. doi:10.1213/01.ANE.0000130355.91214.9E

27

Preventing Ventilator-Associated Lung Injury: A Perioperative Perspective

*Satoshi Kimura, Nicoleta Stoicea, Byron Rafael Rosero Britton, Muhammad Shabsigh, Aly Branstiter and David L. Stahl**

Department of Anesthesiology, The Ohio State University Wexner Medical Center, Columbus, OH, USA

***Correspondence:**
David L. Stahl
david.stahl@osumc.edu

Introduction: Research into the prevention of ventilator-associated lung injury (VALI) in patients with acute respiratory distress syndrome (ARDS) in the intensive care unit (ICU) has resulted in the development of a number of lung protective strategies, which have become commonplace in the treatment of critically ill patients. An increasing number of studies have applied lung protective ventilation in the operating room to otherwise healthy individuals. We review the history of lung protective strategies in patients with acute respiratory failure and explore their use in patients undergoing mechanical ventilation during general anesthesia. We aim to provide context for a discussion of the benefits and drawbacks of lung protective ventilation, as well as to inform future areas of research.

Methods: We completed a database search and reviewed articles investigating lung protective ventilation in both the ICU and in patients receiving general anesthesia through May 2015.

Results: Lung protective ventilation was associated with improved outcomes in patients with acute respiratory failure in the ICU. Clinical evidence is less clear regarding lung protective ventilation for patients undergoing surgery.

Conclusion: Lung protective ventilation strategies, including low tidal volume ventilation and moderate positive end-expiratory pressure, are well established therapies to minimize lung injury in critically ill patients with and without lung disease, and may provide benefit to patients undergoing general anesthesia.

Keywords: lung protective ventilation, low tidal volume ventilation, ventilator-induced lung injury, ventilator-associated lung injury, acute respiratory distress syndrome, general anesthesia

INTRODUCTION

Atelectasis is a common adverse effect of general anesthesia associated with both hypoxemia and postoperative respiratory complications (1–3). Mechanical ventilation (MV) may be used to combat atelectasis by prescribing relatively large tidal volumes (V_T) [up to 15 mL/kg predicted body weight (PBW)] (4, 5). However, we now know that using high V_T ventilation in the intensive care unit (ICU) increases mortality (6), and that MV itself can cause lung injury, through a process referred to as ventilator-induced lung injury (VILI) (7). VILI occurs through a number of different mechanisms.

Barotrauma, defined as pulmonary injury from elevated transpulmonary pressures, was the first widely recognized element of VILI (7, 8). Since it was subsequently demonstrated that humans could generate high airway pressures without causing lung injury, clinical focus shifted to volutrauma, hyperaeration caused by high V_T leading to lung injury (7, 8). Conversely, atelectrauma occurs when tidal ventilation at low airway pressures causes cyclic opening and collapse of unstable lung units (7, 9). This repeated cycling generates disruptive forces on the alveolar basement membranes and augments lung injury (7). Since the early 1990s, numerous studies have shown that MV can trigger the release of pro-inflammatory cytokines and the recruitment of neutrophils (10–13). This biological reaction in response to mechanical forces is known as biotrauma (8, 9, 14, 15).

Clinically, it can be difficult to delineate MV as the precise cause of lung injury. Therefore, when lung injury is concurrent to, but not necessarily caused by, MV, the term ventilator-associated lung injury (VALI) is used (7). The potentially detrimental effects of MV were recognized as early as 1960s (16) when canine studies demonstrated that lung overdistension resulted in an absence of surfactant and subsequent atelectasis (17). Attempts to prevent lung overdistention by therapeutically reducing V_T in humans in the ICU became feasible with acceptance of permissive hypercapnia (18).

Over the past 15 years, studies of patients with acute respiratory failure have resulted in the development of a number of lung protective strategies applied to minimize VALI. These strategies include low V_T to limit volutrauma, higher positive end-expiratory pressure (PEEP) to prevent atelectrauma, and recruitment maneuvers (i.e., application of temporary high airway pressures to reinflate collapsed lung units) (19). The successful application of these strategies in acute respiratory failure has led to increased interest in applying these principles to other patient populations. What remains controversial is whether the principles of lung protective ventilation derived from ICU patients with acute respiratory failure have applicability to otherwise healthy patients in the operating room.

MATERIALS AND METHODS

A systematic literature search was performed to identify clinical studies of lung protective ventilation strategies. We searched PubMed, EMBASE, and the Cochrane Library from inception to May 2015 with restriction to human studies published in English using a combination of standardized search terms and keywords to cover the topics of acute lung injury, acute respiratory distress syndrome (ARDS), MV, lung protective ventilation, low V_T ventilation, and general anesthesia. We reviewed articles that investigated the effects of lung protective ventilation strategies. We included randomized controlled trials (RCT), cohort, cross-sectional, and before-and-after studies. References of all studies were inspected for additional articles that were not identified by the electronic database search. We removed non-human studies, case reports, abstracts, and any other study where the full text was unavailable. Additionally, we excluded studies that specifically examined one-lung ventilation.

RESULTS

Origin of Lung Protective Strategies: Patients with ARDS and Acute Respiratory Failure in the ICU

In 1998, Amato et al. described a lung protective strategy, which included a V_T of <6 mL/kg, PEEP above the lower inflection point, and permissive hypercapnia, was associated with improved survival at 28 days, an improved rate of weaning from MV, and a lower rate of barotrauma in patients with ARDS (20). In 2000, The Acute Respiratory Distress Syndrome Network reported that lower V_T (6 mL/kg of PBW) resulted in decreased mortality and increased ventilator-free days compared with V_T of 12 mL/kg of PBW (6). An increase of 1 mL/kg PBW in initial V_T has been associated with a 23% increase in ICU mortality risk (21). In patients without ARDS, a retrospective cohort study demonstrated the use of large V_T was the main risk factor associated with the development of lung injury (odds ratio 1.3 for each milliliter/kilogram above 6 mL/kg PBW, $p < 0.001$) (22). And a prospective study conducted by the same group concluded that initial ventilator settings of high V_T (odds ratio 2.6 for $V_T > 700$ mL) and high peak airway pressure (odds ratio 1.6 for peak airway pressure >30 cmH_2O) were associated with the development of ARDS in patients without ARDS at the onset of MV (23).

Lung Protective Ventilation during General Anesthesia in Operating Room

Although lung protective ventilation strategies are widely used in the ICU, it remains unclear if these strategies can be directly translated into use in the operating room. Respiratory complications are low in patients undergoing general anesthesia, unlike the ICU (24). Therefore, it may take a much larger number of patients to improve outcomes using lung protective strategies, and there are risks associated with lung protective ventilation, including increased alveolar collapse (25), increased right ventricular afterload (26), hypercapnia and respiratory acidosis (27), and worsened metabolic acidosis (27). Studies on intraoperative MV can be divided into those that target surrogate markers of lung inflammation/injury, clinical outcomes, or systemic reviews and meta-analyses. We examine these studies to better understand the risks and benefits of lung protective ventilation in the operating room (**Table 1**).

Lung Protective Ventilation, Pulmonary Biomarkers, and Lung Mechanics

Inflammatory biomarkers can be used as surrogate outcomes for lung inflammation or injury in patients receiving MV. For example, one RCT compared 40 patients undergoing elective coronary artery bypass grafting (CABG) receiving high V_T/low PEEP or low V_T/high PEEP (28). After 6 h of MV, interleukin (IL)-6 and IL-8 levels were elevated in bronchoalveolar lavage (BAL) fluid and plasma in patients who received higher V_T/low PEEP, suggesting alveolar lung inflammation (28). The attenuation of IL-8, but not IL-6 levels by lung protective ventilation has been replicated in other surgical patients undergoing cardiopulmonary bypass (29) as well as elective surgery (30) but not in major abdominal, thoracic (31), or spinal surgery (32). IL-10 has

TABLE 1 | Randomized controlled trials comparing lung protective strategies with low tidal volumes to conservative ventilation in operating room.

Type of surgery	Source	Patients' population	Lung protective ventilation (V_T)	Conservative ventilation (V_T)	Primary outcome
Cardiac surgery	Chaney et al. (36)	Adults patients undergoing elective on-pump CABG surgery (n = 25)	6 mL/kg with 5 cmH_2O of PEEP (n = 12)	12 mL/kg with 5 cmH_2O of PEEP (n = 13)	Pulmonary mechanics
	Koner et al. (34)	Adult patients undergoing elective on-pump CABG grafting surgery (n = 44)	6 mL/kg with 5 cmH_2O of PEEP (n = 15)	10 mL/kg with 5 cmH_2O of PEEP (n = 14) or zero PEEP (n = 15)	TNF-α and IL-6 levels
	Zupancich et al. (28)	Adult patients undergoing elective on-pump CABG surgery (n = 40)	8 mL/kg with 10 cmH_2O of PEEP (n = 20)	10–12 mL/kg with 2–3 cmH_2O of PEEP (n = 20)	IL-6 and IL-8 in BAL fluid and plasma
	Reis Miranda et al. (29)	Adult patients undergoing elective on-pump CABG or valve surgery (n = 62)	4–6 mL/kg with 10 cmH_2O of PEEP during (n = 22) or after (n = 18) surgery	6–8 mL/kg (n = 22) with 5 cmH_2O of PEEP	IL-6, IL-8, IL-10, TNF-α, and interferon-γ
	Sundar et al. (43)	Adult patients undergoing elective cardiac surgery (n = 149)	6 mL/kg with PEEP according to ARDS Network investigators (6) (n = 75)	10 mL/kg with PEEP according to ARDS Network investigators (6) (n = 74)	Time to extubation
Abdominal surgery	Wrigge et al. (31)	Adult patients undergoing major abdominal surgery (n = 30)	6 mL/kg with 10 cmH_2O of PEEP (n = 15)	12 or 15 mL/kg with zero PEEP (n = 15)	TNF, IL-1, IL-6, IL-8, IL-10, and IL-12
	Weingarten et al. (37)	Adult patients aged >65 years undergoing major open abdominal surgery under general anesthesia (n = 40)	6 mL/kg with 12 cmH_2O of PEEP and recruitment maneuvers (n = 20)	10 mL/kg with no PEEP and no recruitment maneuvers (n = 20)	Oxygenation, pulmonary mechanics, hemodynamic stability
	Treschan et al. (40)	Adult patients undergoing elective upper abdominal surgery lasting ≥3 h under combined general and epidural anesthesia (n = 101)	6 mL/kg with 5 cmH_2O of PEEP (n = 50)	12 mL/kg with 5 cmH_2O of PEEP (n = 51)	Lung function
	Severgnini et al. (38)	Adult patients undergoing elective open abdominal surgery ≥2 h (n = 55)	7 mL/kg with 10 cmH_2O of PEEP and recruitment maneuvers (n = 28)	9 mL/kg with zero PEEP (n = 27)	Modified Clinical Pulmonary Infection Score, gas exchange, and pulmonary functional tests
	Futier et al. (5)	Adults patients at intermediate to high risk of pulmonary complications undergoing major abdominal surgery (n = 400)	6–8 mL/kg with 6–8 cmH_2O of PEEP and recruitment maneuvers (n = 200)	10–12 mL/kg with no PEEP and no recruitment maneuvers (n = 200)	A composite of major pulmonary and extrapulmonary complications occurring by day 7 after surgery
Others	Cai et al. (39)	Adults patients aged 20–50 years with body mass index undergoing elective excision of intracranial lesions (n = 16)	6 mL/kg without PEEP (n = 8)	10 mL/kg without PEEP (n = 8)	Atelectasis (by CT and ABG)
	Memtsoudis et al. (32)	Adult patients undergoing elective lumbar decompression and fusion in prone position under general anesthesia (n = 26)	6 mL/kg with 8 cmH_2O of PEEP (n = 13)	12 mL/kg with zero PEEP (n = 13)	Plasma levels of IL-6 and IL-8, and urinary levels of desmosine
	Choi et al. (33)	Adult patients undergoing a surgical procedure ≥5 h (n = 40)	6 mL/kg with 10 cmH_2O of PEEP (n = 21)	12 mL/kg without PEEP (n = 19)	Markers of coagulation and fibrinolysis
	Wolthuis et al. (30)	Adult patients undergoing a surgical procedure ≥5 h (n = 40)	6 mL/kg with 10 cmH_2O of PEEP (n = 21)	12 mL/kg without PEEP (n = 19)	Polymorphonuclear cell influx, changes in levels of inflammatory markers, and nucleosomes in BAL fluid and/or blood
	Determann et al. (35)	Adult patients undergoing a surgical procedure ≥5 h (n = 40)	6 mL/kg with 10 cmH_2O of PEEP (n = 21)	12 mL/kg without PEEP (n = 19)	Local and systemic levels of Clara cell protein

V_T, tidal volumes; CABG, coronary artery bypass grafting; PEEP, positive end-expiratory pressure; TNF, tumor necrosis factor; IL, interleukin; BAL, bronchoalveolar lavage; CPB, cardiopulmonary bypass; ARDS, acute respiratory distress syndrome; CT, computed tomography; ABG, arterial blood gas.

a similarly mixed profile in response to lung protective MV (29). High V_T/zero end-expiratory pressure (ZEEP) MV does appear to lead to procoagulant activation in the alveolar space (33). Many other inflammatory markers, including tumor necrosis factor-alpha (TNF-α), interferon (IFN)-γ, IL-1, IL-1α, IL-1β, IL-6, IL-12, macrophage inflammatory protein 1α, and macrophage inflammatory protein 1β, or other markers of lung epithelial injury have not been demonstrated to change in response to lung protective ventilation (29–31, 34, 35).

Other studies have demonstrated improved perioperative pulmonary mechanics as a surrogate outcome. One single-center RCT included 25 patients undergoing elective CABG showed a greater reduction in both dynamic and static lung compliance in patients receiving conventional MV, suggesting lung protective MV resulted in improved pulmonary mechanics (36). RCTs in abdominal surgery had varied results showing improved (37), unchanged (38, 39), and degraded (40) pulmonary mechanics in patients receiving lung protective MV. An improvement in the partial pressure of arterial oxygen (PaO_2)/Fraction of inspired oxygen (FiO_2) ratio in abdominal surgery patients appears to reflect the use of recruitment maneuvers more than any particular lung protective strategy (37, 40).

Lung Protective Ventilation and Clinical Outcomes

Several retrospective studies have investigated the association between MV strategies in the operating room and clinical outcomes. A retrospective evaluation of patients admitted to the ICU with postoperative hypoxemic respiratory failure, requiring MV, showed that a high V_T to ideal body weight (IBW) ratio was an independent risk factor for the development of ARDS (41). While a retrospective study of billing data for over 69,000 patients undergoing non-cardiac surgery did not show any effect of V_T on postoperative respiratory complications (24). Another retrospective study of more than 29,000 patients reported that V_T of 6–8 mL/kg IBW were associated with a significant increase in 30-day mortality compared with V_T of 8–10 mL/kg IBW (hazard ratio 1.6, $p = 0.0002$) (42). The authors hypothesized that the increased mortality may be related to the combination of lower V_T and low PEEP (≤5 cmH_2O) (42).

Prospective RCTs of MV in the operating room have specifically targeted high-risk surgical groups, primarily cardiac and abdominal surgery patients. One single-center RCT investigated duration of intubation for cardiac surgery patients by comparing ventilation with low vs. high V_T ventilation. A higher proportion of patients were extubated 6 h postoperatively in the low V_T group (37.3 vs. 20.3%; $p = 0.02$) and fewer patients in the low V_T group required re-intubation (0.3 vs. 9.5%; $p = 0.03$) (43). In two RCTs of patients undergoing open abdominal surgery, lower V_T ventilation combined with PEEP and recruitment maneuvers decreased respiratory complications as measured by two different postoperative pulmonary complication scores when compared to higher V_T ventilation with ZEEP and no recruitment maneuvers (5, 38). The IMPROVE trial also found that patients receiving lung protective ventilation and recruitment maneuvers had decreased postoperative non-invasive ventilation and intubation requirements (5.0 vs. 17.0%, $p = 0.001$), and shorter length of hospital stay (mean difference, −2.45 days, $p = 0.006$) (5). However, in 101 patients undergoing upper abdominal surgery who were randomized to low V_T ventilation (6 mL/kg PBW) with 5 cmH_2O PEEP or to higher V_T ventilation (12 mL/kg PBW) also with 5 cmH_2O PEEP, there was no significant difference in postoperative pulmonary complications (40). In the largest prospective multicenter RCT, conducted by the Protective Ventilation (PROVE) Network Investigators, 900 patients were allocated either to a high level of PEEP (12 cmH_2O) with recruitment maneuvers (higher PEEP group) or a low level of PEEP (≤2 cmH_2O) without recruitment maneuvers (lower PEEP group) while receiving 8 mL/kg V_T (PROVHILO trial). In this study, postoperative pulmonary and extrapulmonary complications were not significantly different between the two groups although hypotension happened more frequently in the higher PEEP group (relative risk 1.29; $p = 0.0016$) and those in the higher PEEP group had a greater need for vasopressors than those in the lower PEEP group (relative risk 1.20; $p = 0.0016$) (44). The results of these trials suggest an important interaction between V_T and PEEP affecting clinical outcomes.

Lung Protective Ventilation Meta-Analyses

The recently updated Cochrane meta-analysis evaluated 12 studies with 1012 participants comparing specifically low vs. high V_T ventilation in the operating room (45). They found no difference in 30-day mortality (risk ratio (RR) 0.79, 95% confidence interval (CI) 0.40-1.54), but the low V_T cohort did show a decrease in postoperative pneumonia and a decreased requirement for both invasive and non-invasive postoperative ventilation (45). Decreased rates of pulmonary infection have been confirmed by other meta-analyses of lung protective ventilation (including interventions in addition to low V_T) (46–48). These additional meta-analyses also failed to demonstrate a mortality benefit to intraoperative lung protective ventilation (46, 47).

Lung Protective Ventilation in Anesthetic Practice

While the data to support lung protective ventilation in the operating room remains unclear, it is worthwhile to examine the current state of anesthetic practice regarding MV. One cross-sectional analysis of intraoperative ventilation during elective abdominal surgery in the United States showed that ventilator settings were non-uniform and ventilation with V_T > 10 mL/ kg PBW is still common (17.5%). BMI ≥30, female gender, and height <165 cm may predispose certain patients to receive large V_T during general anesthesia as providers likely overestimate PBW in this patient group (49). Despite the high prevalence of high V_T ventilation in the operating room, a targeted study of the management of hypoxemic patients (defined by P/F ratio) in the operating room found V_T, and peak inspiratory pressure (PIP) have been decreasing annually while PEEP has been increasing (50). Unfortunately, worsened hypoxemia (lower P/F ratio) correlated most closely with higher FiO_2 and PIP, suggesting that patients who would most benefit from lung protective ventilation are not receiving it (50). Investigators in Australia performed an audit in 272 patients undergoing general anesthesia for three consecutive days in 2013. They showed that a median V_T was 9.5 mL/ kg PBW, suggesting that the practice of MV in the operating room does not always reflect recent studies (51). There are several ongoing studies investigating variation of MV setting within/between centers (52)[1].

DISCUSSION

The translation of research from the ICU to the operating room can be difficult for several reasons. Patients receiving MV in the

[1] IVENT. International Survery on VENTilation Practice (iVENT). In: PROVEnet [Internet]. Available from: https://sites.google.com/site/iventsurvey/.

operating room during general anesthesia commonly lack the derangements in gas exchange and pulmonary mechanics seen in the ICU. While general anesthesia does induce atelectasis, the atelectasis is well-tolerated and relatively short-lived (1–3). Rates of respiratory complications remain low in most populations and the short duration of MV likely affects lung compliance less than a prolonged course of ventilation in ICU. Furthermore, ICU patients are more likely to have comorbid illnesses, such as cardiovascular instability and shock, acid–base abnormalities, and pro-inflammatory states, such as sepsis, which affect the goals of MV.

Based on published ICU data, studies of lung protective ventilation in the operating room generally have used 6–8 mL/kg PBW as low V_T ventilation (**Table 1**), which may not be the ideal V_T for surgical patients (42). Furthermore, studies in the perioperative setting have used low V_T combined with PEEP and/or recruitment maneuvers as the lung protective strategies. Although low V_T ventilation is clearly an important factor of the lung protective ventilation (53), it is still unclear how we should combine these "lung protective strategies," including PEEP and recruitment maneuvers, into a unified best practice for MV in the operating room (44). A subsequent ongoing international multicenter RCT, aims to compare a ventilation strategy using higher levels of PEEP with recruitment maneuvers to one using lower levels of PEEP without recruitment maneuvers in obese patients at risk of postoperative pulmonary complications[2]. This study design hints at the holy grail for intraoperative ventilation: targeted interventions for specific patients. While still heterogeneous themselves, patients with acute respiratory failure and ARDS in the ICU are substantially more homogeneous than the morass of patients undergoing general anesthesia in the operating room. This heterogeneity may, in part, explain the disparate findings in previous studies. However, as we gain a better understanding of the risks and benefits of the various aspects of lung protective strategies, we can more effectively target-specific patient populations for intervention.

[2]Technische Universität Dresden. Protective Ventilation with Higher Versus Lower PEEP during General Anesthesia for Surgery in Obese Patients (PROBESE). In: ClinicalTrials.gov [Internet]. Available from: http://clinicaltrials.gov/show/NCT02148692.

CONCLUSION

As lung protective strategies, including low V_T ventilation, higher PEEP, and/or recruitment maneuvers, continue to evolve, they may also provide benefit to patients undergoing general anesthesia. Larger trials of specific ventilator strategies across different populations are required to evaluate different lung protective strategies and their interaction with different groups of surgical patients to clarify the benefit or harm of lung protective ventilation in the operating room. Furthermore, we need investigations into current practice strategies of clinical anesthesiologists, in order to help shape how new data are applied in the operating room.

AUTHOR CONTRIBUTIONS

SK made contributions to conception and design, participated in drafting the article, and revised it critically for important intellectual content. NS participated in drafting the article and revised it critically for important intellectual content. BB participated in drafting the article and revised it critically for important intellectual content. MS participated in drafting the article and revised it critically for important intellectual content. AB participated in drafting the article and revised it critically for important intellectual content. DS made contributions to conception and design, participated in drafting the article, and revised it critically for important intellectual content.

REFERENCES

1. Duggan M, Kavanagh BP. Pulmonary atelectasis: a pathogenic perioperative entity. *Anesthesiology* (2005) 102(4):838–54. doi:10.1097/00000542-200504000-00021
2. Gunnarsson L, Tokics L, Gustavsson H, Hedenstierna G. Influence of age on atelectasis formation and gas exchange impairment during general anaesthesia. *Br J Anaesth* (1991) 66(4):423–32. doi:10.1093/bja/66.4.423
3. Edmark L, Kostova-Aherdan K, Enlund M, Hedenstierna G. Optimal oxygen concentration during induction of general anesthesia. *Anesthesiology* (2003) 98(1):28–33. doi:10.1097/00000542-200301000-00008
4. Bendixen HH, Hedley-Whyte J, Laver MB. Impaired oxygenation in surgical patients during general anesthesia with controlled ventilation. A concept of atelectasis. *N Engl J Med* (1963) 269:991–6. doi:10.1056/NEJM196311072691901
5. Futier E, Constantin JM, Paugam-Burtz C, Pascal J, Eurin M, Neuschwander A, et al. A trial of intraoperative low-tidal-volume ventilation in abdominal surgery. *N Engl J Med* (2013) 369(5):428–37. doi:10.1056/NEJMoa1301082
6. The Acute Respiratory Distress Syndrome Network. Ventilation with lower tidal volumes as compared with traditional tidal volumes for acute lung injury and the acute respiratory distress syndrome. *N Engl J Med* (2000) 342(18):1301–8. doi:10.1056/NEJM200005043421801
7. Kuchnicka K, Maciejewski D. Ventilator-associated lung injury. *Anaesthesiol Intensive Ther* (2013) 45(3):164–70. doi:10.5603/AIT.2013.0034
8. Oeckler RA, Hubmayr RD. Ventilator-associated lung injury: a search for better therapeutic targets. *Eur Respir J* (2007) 30(6):1216–26. doi:10.1183/09031936.00104907
9. Gattinoni L, Protti A, Caironi P, Carlesso E. Ventilator-induced lung injury: the anatomical and physiological framework. *Crit Care Med* (2010) 38(10 Suppl):S539–48. doi:10.1097/CCM.0b013e3181f1fcf7
10. Tremblay L, Valenza F, Ribeiro SP, Li J, Slutsky AS. Injurious ventilatory strategies increase cytokines and c-fos m-RNA expression in an isolated rat lung model. *J Clin Invest* (1997) 99(5):944–52. doi:10.1172/JCI119259
11. von Bethmann AN, Brasch F, Nusing R, Vogt K, Volk HD, Muller KM, et al. Hyperventilation induces release of cytokines from perfused mouse lung. *Am J Respir Crit Care Med* (1998) 157(1):263–72. doi:10.1164/ajrccm.157.1.9608052
12. Imanaka H, Shimaoka M, Matsuura N, Nishimura M, Ohta N, Kiyono H. Ventilator-induced lung injury is associated with neutrophil infiltration, macrophage activation, and TGF-beta 1 mRNA upregulation in rat lungs. *Anesth Analg* (2001) 92(2):428–36. doi:10.1097/00000539-200102000-00029
13. Tsuno K, Miura K, Takeya M, Kolobow T, Morioka T. Histopathologic pulmonary changes from mechanical ventilation at high peak airway pressures. *Am Rev Respir Dis* (1991) 143(5 Pt 1):1115–20. doi:10.1164/ajrccm/143.5_Pt_1.1115
14. Whitehead T, Slutsky AS. The pulmonary physician in critical care * 7: ventilator induced lung injury. *Thorax* (2002) 57(7):635–42. doi:10.1136/thorax.57.7.635

15. Uhlig S. Ventilation-induced lung injury and mechanotransduction: stretching it too far? *Am J Physiol Lung Cell Mol Physiol* (2002) 282(5):L892–6. doi:10.1152/ajplung.00124.2001
16. Greenfield LJ, Ebert PA, Benson DW. Atelectasis and surface tension properties of lung extracts following positive pressure ventilation and overinflation. *Surg Forum* (1963) 14:239–40.
17. Greenfield LJ, Ebert PA, Benson DW. Effect of positive pressure ventilation on surface tension properties of lung extracts. *Anesthesiology* (1964) 25:312–6. doi:10.1097/00000542-196405000-00009
18. Hickling KG, Henderson SJ, Jackson R. Low mortality associated with low volume pressure limited ventilation with permissive hypercapnia in severe adult respiratory distress syndrome. *Intensive Care Med* (1990) 16(6):372–7. doi:10.1007/BF01735174
19. Zambon M, Vincent JL. Mortality rates for patients with acute lung injury/ARDS have decreased over time. *Chest* (2008) 133(5):1120–7. doi:10.1378/chest.07-2134
20. Amato MB, Barbas CS, Medeiros DM, Magaldi RB, Schettino GP, Lorenzi-Filho G, et al. Effect of a protective-ventilation strategy on mortality in the acute respiratory distress syndrome. *N Engl J Med* (1998) 338(6):347–54. doi:10.1056/NEJM199802053380602
21. Needham DM, Yang T, Dinglas VD, Mendez-Tellez PA, Shanholtz C, Sevransky JE, et al. Timing of low tidal volume ventilation and intensive care unit mortality in acute respiratory distress syndrome. A prospective cohort study. *Am J Respir Crit Care Med* (2015) 191(2):177–85. doi:10.1164/rccm.201409-1598OC
22. Gajic O, Dara SI, Mendez JL, Adesanya AO, Festic E, Caples SM, et al. Ventilator-associated lung injury in patients without acute lung injury at the onset of mechanical ventilation. *Crit Care Med* (2004) 32(9):1817–24. doi:10.1097/01.CCM.0000133019.52531.30
23. Gajic O, Frutos-Vivar F, Esteban A, Hubmayr RD, Anzueto A. Ventilator settings as a risk factor for acute respiratory distress syndrome in mechanically ventilated patients. *Intensive Care Med* (2005) 31(7):922–6. doi:10.1007/s00134-005-2625-1
24. Ladha K, Vidal Melo MF, McLean DJ, Wanderer JP, Grabitz SD, Kurth T, et al. Intraoperative protective mechanical ventilation and risk of postoperative respiratory complications: hospital based registry study. *BMJ* (2015) 351:h3646. doi:10.1136/bmj.h3646
25. Kallet RH, Siobal MS, Alonso JA, Warnecke EL, Katz JA, Marks JD. Lung collapse during low tidal volume ventilation in acute respiratory distress syndrome. *Respir Care* (2001) 46(1):49–52.
26. Viitanen A, Salmenpera M, Heinonen J. Right ventricular response to hypercarbia after cardiac surgery. *Anesthesiology* (1990) 73(3):393–400. doi:10.1097/00000542-199009000-00005
27. Wrigge H, Uhlig U, Baumgarten G, Menzenbach J, Zinserling J, Ernst M, et al. Mechanical ventilation strategies and inflammatory responses to cardiac surgery: a prospective randomized clinical trial. *Intensive Care Med* (2005) 31(10):1379–87. doi:10.1007/s00134-005-2767-1
28. Zupancich E, Paparella D, Turani F, Munch C, Rossi A, Massaccesi S, et al. Mechanical ventilation affects inflammatory mediators in patients undergoing cardiopulmonary bypass for cardiac surgery: a randomized clinical trial. *J Thorac Cardiovasc Surg* (2005) 130(2):378–83. doi:10.1016/j.jtcvs.2004.11.061
29. Reis Miranda D, Gommers D, Struijs A, Dekker R, Mekel J, Feelders R, et al. Ventilation according to the open lung concept attenuates pulmonary inflammatory response in cardiac surgery. *Eur J Cardiothorac Surg* (2005) 28(6):889–95. doi:10.1016/j.ejcts.2005.10.007
30. Wolthuis EK, Choi G, Dessing MC, Bresser P, Lutter R, Dzoljic M, et al. Mechanical ventilation with lower tidal volumes and positive end-expiratory pressure prevents pulmonary inflammation in patients without preexisting lung injury. *Anesthesiology* (2008) 108(1):46–54. doi:10.1097/01.anes.0000296068.80921.10
31. Wrigge H, Uhlig U, Zinserling J, Behrends-Callsen E, Ottersbach G, Fischer M, et al. The effects of different ventilatory settings on pulmonary and systemic inflammatory responses during major surgery. *Anesth Analg* (2004) 98(3):775–81, table of contents. doi:10.1213/01.ANE.0000100663.11852.BF
32. Memtsoudis SG, Bombardieri AM, Ma Y, Girardi FP. The effect of low versus high tidal volume ventilation on inflammatory markers in healthy individuals undergoing posterior spine fusion in the prone position: a randomized controlled trial. *J Clin Anesth* (2012) 24(4):263–9. doi:10.1016/j.jclinane.2011.08.003
33. Choi G, Wolthuis EK, Bresser P, Levi M, van der Poll T, Dzoljic M, et al. Mechanical ventilation with lower tidal volumes and positive end-expiratory pressure prevents alveolar coagulation in patients without lung injury. *Anesthesiology* (2006) 105(4):689–95. doi:10.1097/00000542-200610000-00013
34. Koner O, Celebi S, Balci H, Cetin G, Karaoglu K, Cakar N. Effects of protective and conventional mechanical ventilation on pulmonary function and systemic cytokine release after cardiopulmonary bypass. *Intensive Care Med* (2004) 30(4):620–6. doi:10.1007/s00134-003-2104-5
35. Determann RM, Wolthuis EK, Choi G, Bresser P, Bernard A, Lutter R, et al. Lung epithelial injury markers are not influenced by use of lower tidal volumes during elective surgery in patients without preexisting lung injury. *Am J Physiol Lung Cell Mol Physiol* (2008) 294(2):L344–50. doi:10.1152/ajplung.00268.2007
36. Chaney MA, Nikolov MP, Blakeman BP, Bakhos M. Protective ventilation attenuates postoperative pulmonary dysfunction in patients undergoing cardiopulmonary bypass. *J Cardiothorac Vasc Anesth* (2000) 14(5):514–8. doi:10.1053/jcan.2000.9487
37. Weingarten TN, Whalen FX, Warner DO, Gajic O, Schears GJ, Snyder MR, et al. Comparison of two ventilatory strategies in elderly patients undergoing major abdominal surgery. *Br J Anaesth* (2010) 104(1):16–22. doi:10.1093/bja/aep319
38. Severgnini P, Selmo G, Lanza C, Chiesa A, Frigerio A, Bacuzzi A, et al. Protective mechanical ventilation during general anesthesia for open abdominal surgery improves postoperative pulmonary function. *Anesthesiology* (2013) 118(6):1307–21. doi:10.1097/ALN.0b013e31829102de
39. Cai H, Gong H, Zhang L, Wang Y, Tian Y. Effect of low tidal volume ventilation on atelectasis in patients during general anesthesia: a computed tomographic scan. *J Clin Anesth* (2007) 19(2):125–9. doi:10.1016/j.jclinane.2006.08.008
40. Treschan TA, Kaisers W, Schaefer MS, Bastin B, Schmalz U, Wania V, et al. Ventilation with low tidal volumes during upper abdominal surgery does not improve postoperative lung function. *Br J Anaesth* (2012) 109(2):263–71. doi:10.1093/bja/aes140
41. Hughes CG, Weavind L, Banerjee A, Mercaldo ND, Schildcrout JS, Pandharipande PP. Intraoperative risk factors for acute respiratory distress syndrome in critically ill patients. *Anesth Analg* (2010) 111(2):464–7. doi:10.1213/ANE.0b013e3181d8a16a
42. Levin MA, McCormick PJ, Lin HM, Hosseinian L, Fischer GW. Low intraoperative tidal volume ventilation with minimal PEEP is associated with increased mortality. *Br J Anaesth* (2014) 113(1):97–108. doi:10.1093/bja/aeu054
43. Sundar S, Novack V, Jervis K, Bender SP, Lerner A, Panzica P, et al. Influence of low tidal volume ventilation on time to extubation in cardiac surgical patients. *Anesthesiology* (2011) 114(5):1102–10. doi:10.1097/ALN.0b013e318215e254
44. PROVE Network Investigators for the Clinical Trial Network of the European Society of Anaesthesiology, Hemmes SN, Gama de Abreu M, Pelosi P, Schultz MJ. High versus low positive end-expiratory pressure during general anaesthesia for open abdominal surgery (PROVHILO trial): a multicentre randomised controlled trial. *Lancet* (2014) 384(9942):495–503. doi:10.1016/S0140-6736(14)60416-5
45. Guay J, Ochroch EA. Intraoperative use of low volume ventilation to decrease postoperative mortality, mechanical ventilation, lengths of stay and lung injury in patients without acute lung injury. *Cochrane Database Syst Rev* (2015) 12:CD011151. doi:10.1002/14651858.CD011151.pub2
46. Gu WJ, Wang F, Liu JC. Effect of lung protective ventilation with lower tidal volumes on clinical outcomes among patients undergoing surgery: a meta-analysis of randomized controlled trials. *CMAJ* (2015) 187(3):E101–9. doi:10.1503/cmaj.141005
47. Tao T, Bo L, Chen F, Xie Q, Zou Y, Hu B, et al. Effect of protective ventilation on postoperative pulmonary complications in patients undergoing general anaesthesia: a meta-analysis of randomised controlled trials. *BMJ Open* (2014) 4(6):e005208. doi:10.1136/bmjopen-2014-005208
48. Hemmes SN, Serpa Neto A, Schultz MJ. Intraoperative ventilatory strategies to prevent postoperative pulmonary complications: a meta-analysis. *Curr Opin Anaesthesiol* (2013) 26(2):126–33. doi:10.1097/ACO.0b013e32835e1242
49. Fernandez-Bustamante A, Wood CL, Tran ZV, Moine P. Intraoperative ventilation: incidence and risk factors for receiving large tidal volumes during general anesthesia. *BMC Anesthesiol* (2011) 11:22. doi:10.1186/1471-2253-11-22

50. Blum JM, Fetterman DM, Park PK, Morris M, Rosenberg AL. A description of intraoperative ventilator management and ventilation strategies in hypoxic patients. *Anesth Analg* (2010) 110(6):1616–22. doi:10.1213/ANE.0b013e3181da82e1
51. Karalapillai D, Weinberg L, Galtieri J, Glassford N, Eastwood G, Darvall J, et al. Current ventilation practice during general anaesthesia: a prospective audit in Melbourne, Australia. *BMC Anesthesiol* (2014) 14:85. doi:10.1186/1471-2253-14-85
52. Hemmes SN, de Abreu MG, Pelosi P, Schultz MJ. ESA clinical trials network 2012: LAS VEGAS – local assessment of ventilatory management during general anaesthesia for surgery and its effects on postoperative pulmonary complications: a prospective, observational, international, multicentre cohort study. *Eur J Anaesthesiol* (2013) 30(5):205–7. doi:10.1097/EJA.0b013e32835fcab3
53. Guldner A, Kiss T, Serpa Neto A, Hemmes SN, Canet J, Spieth PM, et al. Intraoperative protective mechanical ventilation for prevention of postoperative pulmonary complications: a comprehensive review of the role of tidal volume, positive end-expiratory pressure, and lung recruitment maneuvers. *Anesthesiology* (2015) 123(3):692–713. doi:10.1097/ALN.0000000000000754

Permissions

All chapters in this book were first published by Frontiers; hereby published with permission under the Creative Commons Attribution License or equivalent. Every chapter published in this book has been scrutinized by our experts. Their significance has been extensively debated. The topics covered herein carry significant findings which will fuel the growth of the discipline. They may even be implemented as practical applications or may be referred to as a beginning point for another development.

The contributors of this book come from diverse backgrounds, making this book a truly international effort. This book will bring forth new frontiers with its revolutionizing research information and detailed analysis of the nascent developments around the world.

We would like to thank all the contributing authors for lending their expertise to make the book truly unique. They have played a crucial role in the development of this book. Without their invaluable contributions this book wouldn't have been possible. They have made vital efforts to compile up to date information on the varied aspects of this subject to make this book a valuable addition to the collection of many professionals and students.

This book was conceptualized with the vision of imparting up-to-date information and advanced data in this field. To ensure the same, a matchless editorial board was set up. Every individual on the board went through rigorous rounds of assessment to prove their worth. After which they invested a large part of their time researching and compiling the most relevant data for our readers.

The editorial board has been involved in producing this book since its inception. They have spent rigorous hours researching and exploring the diverse topics which have resulted in the successful publishing of this book. They have passed on their knowledge of decades through this book. To expedite this challenging task, the publisher supported the team at every step. A small team of assistant editors was also appointed to further simplify the editing procedure and attain best results for the readers.

Apart from the editorial board, the designing team has also invested a significant amount of their time in understanding the subject and creating the most relevant covers. They scrutinized every image to scout for the most suitable representation of the subject and create an appropriate cover for the book.

The publishing team has been an ardent support to the editorial, designing and production team. Their endless efforts to recruit the best for this project, has resulted in the accomplishment of this book. They are a veteran in the field of academics and their pool of knowledge is as vast as their experience in printing. Their expertise and guidance has proved useful at every step. Their uncompromising quality standards have made this book an exceptional effort. Their encouragement from time to time has been an inspiration for everyone.

The publisher and the editorial board hope that this book will prove to be a valuable piece of knowledge for researchers, students, practitioners and scholars across the globe.

List of Contributors

Wei Gao, Lan Yang, Ruini Du, Ge Wang, Bingyu Liu, Yajuan Li, Shanshan Zhang and Qiang Wang
Department of Anesthesiology, Center for Brain Science, The First Affiliated Hospital of Xi'an Jiaotong University, Xi'an, China

Linzhong Zhang
Department of Anesthesiology, Second Hospital of Shanxi Medical University, Taiyuan, China

Xuechang Han
Department of Anesthesiology, The First Affiliated Hospital, College of Clinical Medicine of Henan University of Science and Technology, Luoyang, China

Lai Wei
Department of Anesthesiology, Hunan Provincial People's Hospital, Changsha, China

Jie Fang
Department of Anesthesiology, The First Affiliated Hospital of Henan University of Chinese Medicine, Zhengzhou, China

Xiaqing Zhang
Department of Anesthesiology, Affiliated Hospital of Shaanxi University of Chinese Medicine, Xianyang, China

Jiaqiang Zhang
Department of Anesthesiology, Henan Provincial People's Hospital, Zhengzhou, China

Haiyun Wang
Department of Anesthesiology, The Third Central Hospital of Tianjin, Tianjin, China

Qi Zhou
Department of Anesthesiology, The First Hospital of Hunan University of Chinese Medicine, Changsha, China

Chenggang Wang
Department of Anesthesiology, Shanxi Traditional Chinese Medicine Hospital, Taiyuan, China

Wenting Chen
Department of Anesthesiology, Shuguang Hospital Affiliated to Shanghai University of Traditional Chinese Medicine, Shanghai, China

Xinli Ni
Department of Anesthesiology, General Hospital of Ningxia Medical University, Yinchuan, China

Po-Liang Cheng and Yu-Han Jiang
Department of Medical Research, Taichung Veterans General Hospital, Taichung, Taiwan
Precision Medicine Center, Taichung Veterans General Hospital, Taichung, Taiwan

Hsin-Hua Chen
Division of General Internal Medicine, Department of Internal Medicine, Taichung Veterans General Hospital, Taichung, Taiwan
Big Data Center, Chung Hsing University, Taichung, Taiwan
Department of Industrial Engineering and Enterprise Information, Tunghai University, Taichung, Taiwan
Rong Hsing Research Centre for Translational Medicine, Institute of Biomedical Science, Chung Hsing University, Taichung, Taiwan

Tzu-Hung Hsiao
Department of Medical Research, Taichung Veterans General Hospital, Taichung, Taiwan
Precision Medicine Center, Taichung Veterans General Hospital, Taichung, Taiwan
Department of Public Health, Fu Jen Catholic University, New Taipei City, Taiwan
Institute of Genomics and Bioinformatics, National Chung Hsing University, Taichung, Taiwan

Chen-Yu Wang
Department of Critical Care Medicine, Taichung Veterans General Hospital, Taichung, Taiwan
Department of Nursing, Hung Kuang University, Taichung, Taiwan

Chieh-Liang Wu
Department of Industrial Engineering and Enterprise Information, Tunghai University, Taichung, Taiwan
Department of Critical Care Medicine, Taichung Veterans General Hospital, Taichung, Taiwan
Department of Computer Science, Tunghai University, Taichung, Taiwan
Department of Automatic Control Engineering, Feng Chia University, Taichung, Taiwan
Artificial Intelligence Workshop, Taichung Veterans General Hospital, Taichung, Taiwan

Tai-Ming Ko
Department of Biological Science and Technology, National Chiao Tung University, Hsinchu, Taiwan
Department of Biological Science and Technology, National Yang Ming Chiao Tung University, Hsinchu, Taiwan
Institute of Bioinformatics and Systems Biology, National Chiao Tung University, Hsinchu, Taiwan
Institute of Biomedical Sciences, Academia Sinica, Taipei, Taiwan

Wen-Cheng Chao
Department of Critical Care Medicine, Taichung Veterans General Hospital, Taichung, Taiwan
Department of Medical Research, Taichung Veterans General Hospital, Taichung, Taiwan
Department of Computer Science, Tunghai University, Taichung, Taiwan
Department of Automatic Control Engineering, Feng Chia University, Taichung, Taiwan
Big Data Center, Chung Hsing University, Taichung, Taiwan

Fang-Yu Yen, Wen-Kuei Chang, Shih-Pin Lin and Kuang-Yi Chang
Department of Anesthesiology, Taipei Veterans General Hospital, Taipei, Taiwan
School of Medicine, National Yang Ming Chiao Tung University, Taipei, Taiwan

Tzu-Ping Lin
School of Medicine, National Yang Ming Chiao Tung University, Taipei, Taiwan
Department of Urology, Taipei Veterans General Hospital, Taipei, Taiwan

Vincent Compère and Thomas Clavier
Department of Anaesthesiology and Intensive Care, Rouen University Hospital, Rouen, France
Normandie Université, UNIROUEN, INSERM U982, Mont-Saint-Aignan, France

Emmanuel Besnier, Bertrand Dureuil and Thomas Elie
Department of Anaesthesiology and Intensive Care, Rouen University Hospital, Rouen, France

Nicolas Byhet
Department of Anaesthesiology, Dieppe General Hospital, Dieppe, France

Florent Lefranc
Department of Anaesthesiology, Hôpital privé de l'estuaire, Le Havre, France

Frederic Jegou and Nicolas Sturzenegger
Department of Anaesthesiology, Clinique du Cèdre, Bois-Guillaume, France

Jean Baptiste Hardy
Department of Anaesthesiology, Evreux General Hospital, Evreux, France

Ming Wu
Department of Critical Care Medicine and Hospital Infection Prevention and Control, Health Science Center, The Second People's Hospital of Shenzhen, First Affiliated Hospital of Shenzhen University, Shenzhen, China
Department of Critical Care Medicine, General Hospital of Southern Theatre Command of Peoples Liberation Army, Guangzhou, China

Conglin Wang
Department of Critical Care Medicine, General Hospital of Southern Theater Command of PLA, Guangzhou, China
The First School of Clinical Medicine, Southern Medical University, Guangzhou, China

Zheying Liu
Department of Critical Care Medicine, General Hospital of Southern Theatre Command of Peoples Liberation Army, Guangzhou, China

Zhifeng Liu
Department of Critical Care Medicine, General Hospital of Southern Theatre Command of Peoples Liberation Army, Guangzhou, China
Key Laboratory of Hot Zone Trauma Care and Tissue Repair of Peoples Liberation Army, General Hospital of Southern Theatre Command of Peoples Liberation Army, Guangzhou, China
The First School of Clinical Medicine, Southern Medical University, Guangzhou, China

Caimu Wang, Qijiang Chen, Ping Wang, Weisheng Jin, Chao Zhong, Zisheng Ge and Kangmin Xu
General Intensive Care Unit, Ninghai First Hospital, Ningbo, China

Longxiang Su, Huaiwu He, Dawei Liu and Yun Long
Department of Critical Care Medicine, State Key Laboratory of Complex Severe and Rare Diseases, Peking Union Medical College Hospital, Chinese Academy of Medical Science and Peking Union Medical College, Beijing, China

Pan Pan
College of Pulmonary and Critical Care Medicine, Chinese PLA General Hospital, Beijing, China

Michiel T. U. Schuijt and David M. P. van Meenen
Department of Intensive Care, Amsterdam UMC, Location AMC, Amsterdam, Netherlands

Ignacio Martin-Loeches
Department of Clinical Medicine, Trinity Centre for Health Sciences, Multidisciplinary Intensive Care Research Organization (MICRO), St James's Hospital, Dublin, Ireland

Guido Mazzinari
Department of Anaesthesiology and Critical Care, Hospital Universitario y Politecnico la Fe, Valencia, Spain
Perioperative Medicine Research Group, Instituto de Investigación Sanitaria la Fe, Valencia, Spain

Marcus J. Schultz
Department of Intensive Care and Laboratory of Experimental Intensive Care and Anesthesiology (L•E•I•C•A), Amsterdam UMC, Amsterdam, Netherlands
Mahidol-Oxford Tropical Medicine Research Unit (MORU), Mahidol University, Bangkok, Thailand
Nuffield Department of Medicine, University of Oxford, Oxford, United Kingdom

Frederique Paulus
Department of Intensive Care and Laboratory of Experimental Intensive Care and Anesthesiology (L•E•I•C•A), Amsterdam UMC, Amsterdam, Netherlands
Center of Expertise Urban Vitality, Faculty of Health, Amsterdam University of Applied Sciences, Amsterdam, Netherlands
ACHIEVE, Centre of Applied Research, Amsterdam University of Applied Sciences, Faculty of Health, Amsterdam, Netherlands

Ary Serpa Neto
Department of Intensive Care, Amsterdam UMC, Location AMC, Amsterdam, Netherlands
Australian and New Zealand Intensive Care Research Centre (ANZIC-RC), Monash University, Melbourne, VIC, Australia
Department of Intensive Care, Austin Hospital, Melbourne, VIC, Australia
Data Analytics Research and Evaluation (DARE) Centre, Austin Hospital, Melbourne, VIC, Australia
Department of Critical Care, Melbourne Medical School, University of Melbourne, Melbourne, VIC, Australia
Department of Critical Care Medicine, Hospital Israelita Albert Einstein, São Pãulo, Brazil

Cuiyu Xie, Caihui Zhang and Hao Sun
Department of Anesthesiology, The First Affiliated Hospital of Anhui Medical University, Hefei, China

Yao Lu
Department of Anesthesiology, The First Affiliated Hospital of Anhui Medical University, Hefei, China
Ambulatory Surgery Center, The First Affiliated Hospital of Anhui Medical University, Hefei, China

Chiao-Yi Lin
Graduate Institute of Physiology, College of Medicine, National Taiwan University, Taipei, Taiwan
Department of Anesthesiology, Hsinchu MacKay Memorial Hospital, Hsinchu, Taiwan

Wen-Ting Tseng
Graduate Institute of Physiology, College of Medicine, National Taiwan University, Taipei, Taiwan

Yao-Yin Chang
Department of Electrical Engineering, Graduate Institute of Biomedical Electronics and Bioinformatics, National Taiwan University, Taipei, Taiwan

Mong-Hsun Tsai
Graduate Institute of Biotechnology, College of Bioresources and Agriculture, National Taiwan University, Taipei, Taiwan
Bioinformatics and Biostatistics Core, Center of Genomic and Precision Medicine, National Taiwan University, Taipei, Taiwan

Eric Y. Chuang
Bioinformatics and Biostatistics Core, Center of Genomic and Precision Medicine, National Taiwan University, Taipei, Taiwan
Graduate Institute of Biomedical Electronics and Bioinformatics, College of Electrical Engineering and Computer Science, National Taiwan University, Taipei, Taiwan
College of Biomedical Engineering, China Medical University, Taichung, Taiwan

Tzu-Pin Lu
Bioinformatics and Biostatistics Core, Center of Genomic and Precision Medicine, National Taiwan University, Taipei, Taiwan
Graduate Institute of Epidemiology and Preventive Medicine, College of Public Health, National Taiwan University, Taipei, Taiwan

Liang-Chuan Lai
Graduate Institute of Physiology, College of Medicine, National Taiwan University, Taipei, Taiwan
Bioinformatics and Biostatistics Core, Center of Genomic and Precision Medicine, National Taiwan University, Taipei, Taiwan

Anyi Lu
Department of Anesthesiology, Guangdong Cardiovascular Institute & Guangdong Provincial People's Hospital, Guangdong Academy of Medical Sciences, Guangzhou, China
College of Medicine, Shantou University, Shantou, China

Yingxian Ye, Jiaqi Hu, Ning Wei and Jinfeng Wei
Department of Anesthesiology, Guangdong Cardiovascular Institute & Guangdong Provincial People's Hospital, Guangdong Academy of Medical Sciences, Guangzhou, China

Bimei Lin
Department of Operation Room, Guangdong Cardiovascular Institute & Guangdong Provincial People's Hospital, Guangdong Academy of Medical Sciences, Guangzhou, China

Sheng Wang
Department of Anesthesiology, Guangdong Cardiovascular Institute & Guangdong Provincial People's Hospital, Guangdong Academy of Medical Sciences, Guangzhou, China
Department of Anesthesiology, Linzhi People's Hospital, Linzhi, China

Eizo Watanabe
Department of Emergency and Critical Care Medicine, Chiba University Graduate School of Medicine, Chiba, Japan
General Medical Science, Chiba University Graduate School of Medicine, Chiba, Japan

Osamu Takasu and Teruo Sakamoto
Department of Emergency and Critical Care Medicine, Kurume University School of Medicine, Kurume, Japan

Youichi Teratake and Masahiko Hatano
Biomedical Research Center, Chiba University, Chiba, Japan

Toshiaki Ikeda
Division of Critical Care and Emergency Medicine, Tokyo Medical University Hachioji Medical Center, Hachioji, Japan

Nobuya Kitamura
Department of Emergency and Critical Care Medicine, Kimitsu Chuo Hospital, Kisarazu, Japan

Goichi Honda
Medical Affairs Department, Asahi Kasei Pharma Corporation, Tokyo, Japan

Benjamin Mayer
Institute for Epidemiology and Medical Biometry, Ulm Universtiy, Ulm, Germany

Joji Kotani
Division of Disaster and Emergency Medicine, Department of Surgery Related, Kobe University Graduate School of Medicine, Kobe, Japan
Department of Emergency, Disaster and Critical Care Medicine, Hyogo College of Medicine, Nishinomiya, Japan

Masaaki Ohmori, Ayako Teratani and Shigeto Oda
Department of Emergency and Critical Care Medicine, Chiba University Graduate School of Medicine, Chiba, Japan

E. Marion Schneider
Division of Experimental Anesthesiology, University Hospital Ulm, Ulm, Germany

Xiuxia Bao, Yeke Zhu and Xianhui Kang
Department of Anesthesiology, The First Affiliated Hospital, Zhejiang University School of Medicine, Hangzhou, China

Tao Liu
Department of Anesthesiology, The First People' Hospital of Huzhou, Huzhou, China

Haorong Feng
Department of Anesthesiology, South Taihu Hospital of Huzhou, Huzhou, China

Yingying Wu
Department of Anesthesiology, Huzhou Fourth Hospital, Huzhou, China

Xianghe Wang
Department of Anesthesiology, The 98th Clinical College of People's Liberation Army (PLM), Anhui Medical University, Huzhou, China

Li Zhong
Department of Critical Care Medicine, The First Affiliated Hospital, Guizhou University of Chinese Medicine, Guiyang, China

Jingjing Ji
Department of Critical Care Medicine, General Hospital of Southern Theater Command of PLA, Guangzhou, China

Antonella Cotoia, Paola Sara Mariotti, Claudia Ferialdi, Pasquale Del Vecchio, Renata Beck and Gilda Cinnella
Department of Medical and Surgical Sciences, Anesthesia and Intensive Care Unit, University of Foggia, Foggia, Italy

Simona Zaami
Department of Anatomical, Histological, Forensic, and Orthopedic Science, Sapienza University of Rome, Rome, Italy

Seyyed-Hadi Ghamari, Mohsen Abbasi-Kangevari, Nasim Zamani, Hossein Hassanian-Moghaddam and Ali-Asghar Kolahi
Social Determinants of Health Research Center, Shahid Beheshti University of Medical Sciences, Tehran, Iran

Zhaoyang Li
Department of Intensive Care Medicine, The First Affiliated Hospital of Nanjing Medical University, Nanjing, China

Tingwen Shen
The Health Management Center, The First Affiliated Hospital of Nanjing Medical University, Nanjing, China

Yi Han
Department of Geriatric Intensive Care Medicine, The First Affiliated Hospital of Nanjing Medical University, Nanjing, China

Christel M. A. Valk
Department of Intensive Care and Laboratory of Experimental Intensive Care and Anesthesiology (L·E·I·C·A), Amsterdam UMC, Amsterdam, Netherlands

Claudio Zimatore
Department of Intensive Care and Laboratory of Experimental Intensive Care and Anesthesiology (L•E•I•C•A), Amsterdam UMC, Amsterdam, Netherlands
Department of Emergency and Organ Transplantation, University of Bari Aldo Moro, Bari, Italy

Charalampos Pierrakos
Department of Intensive Care and Laboratory of Experimental Intensive Care and Anesthesiology (L•E•I•C•A), Amsterdam UMC, Amsterdam, Netherlands
Department of Intensive Care, Centre Hospitalier Universitaire Brussels, Brussels, Belgium

Chaisith Sivakorn
Department of Clinical Tropical Medicine, Mahidol University, Bangkok, Thailand

Jutamas Dechsanga
Division of Pulmonary and Critical Care, Department of Medicine, Chonburi Hospital, Chonburi, Thailand

Lieuwe D. J. Bos
Department of Intensive Care and Laboratory of Experimental Intensive Care and Anesthesiology (L•E•I•C•A), Amsterdam UMC, Amsterdam, Netherlands
Department of Pulmonology, Amsterdam UMC, Amsterdam, Netherlands

Salvatore Grasso
Department of Emergency and Organ Transplantation, University of Bari Aldo Moro, Bari, Italy

Ludo Beenen
Department of Radiology, Amsterdam UMC, Amsterdam, Netherlands

Luigi Pisani
Department of Intensive Care and Laboratory of Experimental Intensive Care and Anesthesiology (L•E•I•C•A), Amsterdam UMC, Amsterdam, Netherlands
Mahidol-Oxford Tropical Medicine Research Unit (MORU), Mahidol University, Bangkok, Thailand
Anaesthesia and Intensive Care Unit, Miulli Regional Hospital, Acquaviva delle Fonti, Italy

Yongtao Sun, Linlin Huang, Lingling Xu and Min Zhang
Department of Anesthesiology, The First Affiliated Hospital of Shandong First Medical University & Shandong Provincial Qianfoshan Hospital, Shandong Institute of Anesthesia and Respiratory Critical Medicine, Jinan, China

Yuelan Wang
Department of Anesthesiology, The First Affiliated Hospital of Shandong First Medical University & Shandong Provincial Qianfoshan Hospital, Shandong Institute of Anesthesia and Respiratory Critical Medicine, Jinan, China
Department of Anesthesiology, Shandong First Medical University, Jinan, China

Yongle Guo
Department of Anesthesiology, Shandong First Medical University, Jinan, China

Tsai-Jung Wang and Chun-Te Huang
Department of Critical Care Medicine, Taichung Veterans General Hospital, Taichung, Taiwan
Division of Nephrology, Department of Internal Medicine, Taichung Veterans General Hospital, Taichung, Taiwan

Kai-Chih Pai
College of Engineering, Tunghai University, Taichung, Taiwan
Cloud Innovation School, Tunghai University, Taichung, Taiwan

Li-Ting Wong
Department of Medical Research, Taichung Veterans General Hospital, Taichung, Taiwan

Minn-Shyan Wang
Department of Critical Care Medicine, Taichung Veterans General Hospital, Taichung, Taiwan
Artificial Intelligence Workshop, Taichung Veterans General Hospital, Taichung, Taiwan

Chun-Ming Lai
College of Engineering, Tunghai University, Taichung, Taiwan

Cheng-Hsu Chen
Division of Nephrology, Department of Internal Medicine, Taichung Veterans General Hospital, Taichung, Taiwan

Tao Wang, Dongxu Zhou and Penglin Ma
Critical Care Medicine Department, Guiqian International General Hospital, Guiyang, China

Zhongheng Zhang
Department of Emergency Medicine, Sir Run Run Shaw Hospital, Zhejiang University School of Medicine, Hangzhou, China

Takeshi Wada
Division of Acute and Critical Care Medicine, Department of Anesthesiology and Critical Care Medicine, Hokkaido University Faculty of Medicine, Sapporo, Japan

Atsushi Shiraishi
Emergency and Trauma Center, Kameda Medical Center, Kamogawa, Japan

Satoshi Gando
Division of Acute and Critical Care Medicine, Department of Anesthesiology and Critical Care Medicine, Hokkaido University Faculty of Medicine, Sapporo, Japan
Department of Acute and Critical Care Medicine, Sapporo Higashi Tokushukai Hospital, Sapporo, Japan

Kazuma Yamakawa
Department of Emergency Medicine, Osaka Medical and Pharmaceutical University, Takatsuki, Japan

Seitaro Fujishima
Center for General Medicine Education, Keio University School of Medicine, Tokyo, Japan

Daizoh Saitoh
Division of Traumatology, Research Institute, National Defense Medical College, Tokorozawa, Japan

Shigeki Kushimoto
Division of Emergency and Critical Care Medicine, Tohoku University Graduate School of Medicine, Sendai, Japan

Hiroshi Ogura
Department of Traumatology and Acute Critical Medicine, Osaka University Graduate School of Medicine, Suita, Japan

Toshikazu Abe
Department of Emergency and Critical Care Medicine, Tsukuba Memorial Hospital, Tsukuba, Japan
Health Services Research and Development Center, University of Tsukuba, Tsukuba, Japan

Toshihiko Mayumi
Department of Emergency Medicine, School of Medicine, University of Occupational and Environmental Health, Kitakyushu, Japan

Junichi Sasaki
Department of Emergency and Critical Care Medicine, Keio University School of Medicine, Tokyo, Japan

Naoshi Takeyama
Advanced Critical Care Center, Aichi Medical University Hospital, Nagakute, Japan

Ryosuke Tsuruta
Advanced Medical Emergency & Critical Care Center, Yamaguchi University Hospital, Ube, Japan

Kiyotsugu Takuma
Emergency & Critical Care Center, Kawasaki Municipal Hospital, Kawasaki, Japan

Shin-ichiro Shiraishi
Department of Emergency and Critical Care Medicine, Aizu Chuo Hospital, Aizu, Japan

Yasukazu Shiino
Department of Acute Medicine, Kawasaki Medical School, Kurashiki, Japan

Taka-aki Nakada
Department of Emergency and Critical Care Medicine, Chiba University Graduate School of Medicine, Chiba, Japan

Kohji Okamoto
Department of Surgery, Center for Gastroenterology and Liver Disease, Kitakyushu City Yahata Hospital, Kitakyushu, Japan

Yuichiro Sakamoto
Emergency and Critical Care Medicine, Saga University Hospital, Saga, Japan

Akiyoshi Hagiwara
Center Hospital of the National Center for Global Health and Medicine, Tokyo, Japan

Satoshi Fujimi and Yutaka Umemura
Division of Trauma and Surgical Critical Care, Osaka General Medical Center, Sumiyoshi, Japan

Yasuhiro Otomo
Trauma and Acute Critical Care Center, Medical Hospital, Tokyo Medical and Dental University, Tokyo, Japan

Tianyang Hu and Zhao Qiao
Department of Cardiology, The Second Affiliated Hospital, Chongqing Medical University, Chongqing, China

Ying Mei
Health Management Center, The Second Affiliated Hospital, Chongqing Medical University, Chongqing, China

Marcell Virág and Máté Rottler
Medical School, Institute for Translational Medicine, University of Pécs, Pécs, Hungary
Department of Anesthesiology and Intensive Therapy, Szent György University Teaching Hospital of Fejér County, Székesfehérvár, Hungary
Doctoral School of Clinical Medicine, University of Szeged, Szeged, Hungary

Klementina Ocskay and Balázs Horváth
Medical School, Institute for Translational Medicine, University of Pécs, Pécs, Hungary

Ágnes Sárkány
Department of Anesthesiology and Intensive Therapy, Szent György University Teaching Hospital of Fejér County, Székesfehérvár, Hungary

Tamás Leiner
Medical School, Institute for Translational Medicine, University of Pécs, Pécs, Hungary
Anaesthetic Department, Hinchingbrooke Hospital, North West Anglia National Health Service (NHS) Foundation Trust, Huntingdon, United Kingdom

Daniel Adam Blanco and Alexa Vasquez
CytoSorbents Europe, Berlin, Germany

László Bucsi
Szent György University Teaching Hospital of Fejér County, Székesfehérvár, Hungary

Zsolt Molnár
Medical School, Institute for Translational Medicine, University of Pécs, Pécs, Hungary
Doctoral School of Clinical Medicine, University of Szeged, Szeged, Hungary
CytoSorbents Europe, Berlin, Germany
Department of Anesthesiology and Intensive Therapy, Poznan University of Medical Sciences, Poznan, Poland
Department of Anesthesiology and Intensive Therapy, Semmelweis University, Budapest, Hungary

Xianlin Zhu, Min Yang, Junying Mu and Zaiping Wang
Department of Anesthesiology, The Central Hospital of Enshi Tujia and Miao Autonomous Prefecture, Enshi City, China

Liang Zhang
Department of Anesthesiology, Chongqing Hospital of Traditional Chinese Medicine, Chongqing, China

Hongbai Wang and Fuxia Yan
Department of Anesthesiology, Fuwai Hospital, Chinese Academy of Medical Sciences and Peking Union Medical College, Beijing, China

Tong J. Gan
Department of Anesthesiology, Stony Brook University Medical Center, Stony Brook, NY, USA

Nicholas Joseph
Department of Anesthesiology, The Ohio State University Wexner Medical Center, Columbus, OH, USA
Department of Neuroscience, The Ohio State University, Columbus, OH, USA

Rohan Dalal
Department of Psychology, The Ohio State University, Columbus, OH, USA

Sergio D. Bergese
Department of Anesthesiology, The Ohio State University Wexner Medical Center, Columbus, OH, USA
Department of Neurological Surgery, The Ohio State University Wexner Medical Center, Columbus, OH, USA

Satoshi Kimura, Nicoleta Stoicea, Alberto Uribe and Jyoti Pandya, Byron Rafael Rosero Britton, Muhammad Shabsigh, Aly Branstiter and David L. Stahl
Department of Anesthesiology, The Ohio State University Wexner Medical Center, Columbus, OH, USA

Index

A

Abdominal Distension, 153-154

Abdominal Hernia, 153

Acupressure, 218-222

Acupuncture, 2-3, 9-10, 218-219, 221-222

Acute Kidney Injury, 36, 38-40, 43, 54, 100-101, 117, 135-136, 139-141, 159-160, 166-167, 188, 190-191, 195, 201, 203

Alternative Medicine, 218-219, 221

Analgesia, 2-3, 9, 21-27, 53-54, 72, 78, 89, 92, 103, 168, 171, 173-174, 206, 213, 219, 221-222

Anesthesia, 1, 3, 5-7, 9, 21-27, 29-34, 71-78, 89, 93, 103-104, 106, 110, 119-126, 133, 152-156, 173-174, 205-210, 212-213, 215-217, 219-220, 223-228

Antiemetic Drugs, 2, 7, 75

Atelectasis, 223-225, 227-228

Autoimmune Disease, 12-13, 15

Axillary Temperature, 119, 125

Azasetron, 71-77

B

Blood Cell Count, 112, 114-116, 136, 138

Bupivacaine, 22, 79-80, 82-87

C

Cardiac Surgery, 33, 57, 88-93, 173, 201, 203, 212, 216, 221, 225-226, 228

Cardiopulmonary Bypass, 34, 88-90, 92-93, 225, 228

Cardiopulmonary Interaction, 56, 59

Catecholamines, 7, 120, 198

Cholecystectomy, 5-6, 8, 77

Circulatory Protection, 55-56

Clinical Tasks, 29-34

Coronavirus, 12, 56, 61-62, 69-70, 127, 134, 145, 150-151, 197, 203

Cumulative Fluid Balance, 158-159, 163-164, 166

Cytokine, 43, 54, 95, 197-198, 201-203, 228

Cytosorb, 197-199, 201-203

D

Dexmedetomidine, 3, 44-48, 50, 52-54, 71-78, 89, 154, 174

Diaphragm, 58, 102-111

Disease Severity, 67, 116, 136, 142, 158, 198

E

Epidural Analgesia, 21, 25, 27

Exertional Heatstroke, 35, 43, 112-113, 116

G

General Anesthesia, 1, 3, 6, 9, 22, 26, 72, 78, 89, 104, 106, 110, 124-125, 205-208, 213, 216-217, 220, 223-228

H

Heart Diseases, 88

Hemidiaphragmatic Excursion, 102-103, 106-107

Hemoadsorption, 197-203

Hyperthyroidism, 153

Hypnosis, 218-220, 222

I

Immunocompetent Patients, 11-16

Immunoparalysis, 12, 15, 17, 19-20

Immunosuppressants, 11-13, 15

In-hospital Mortality, 46, 48, 50, 135-142, 151, 161, 166, 176-177, 179, 181-183, 187-191, 194, 202

Inflammatory Markers, 45, 198, 217, 225, 228

Intensive Care Unit, 12-13, 19, 33, 35, 38-39, 44, 50, 54, 62, 89, 94, 118-119, 133-134, 137, 142-145, 147, 150-151, 159, 161, 164, 167, 171-174, 188-191, 195, 197-199, 208-209, 216, 223

K

Kidney Function, 36, 129, 135, 138, 140, 142

L

Laryngeal Mask, 152-154, 157

Lidocaine, 22, 26, 79-80, 82-87, 104, 152, 154

Lung Injury, 20, 55-56, 59-60, 62, 69, 163, 166, 223-224, 227-228

Lung Protective Ventilation, 56, 223-224, 226-228

M

Mechanical Ventilation, 44-46, 50, 53-60, 62, 69-70, 90, 111, 128, 131, 134, 146, 149-151, 160, 164, 168-169, 171-172, 197-199, 202, 223, 227-229

Meta-analysis, 9-10, 26-28, 44, 48, 50, 52-54, 60, 78, 91-93, 101, 125, 134, 159, 163, 166, 173-174, 185, 187, 195, 203, 205-206, 209, 212-216, 220, 222, 226, 228

Metabolic Features, 12, 15, 18

Morbidly Obese Patients, 152-154, 156-157

Mortality, 11-13, 15-17, 19, 21, 24, 26-27, 35-42, 44-46, 48, 50-54, 61-69, 77, 88, 90-92, 94-98, 100, 112-113, 115, 117, 130-131, 134-151, 156, 158-168, 171-172, 176-177, 179-183, 187-191, 194-195, 198-199, 202-204, 216, 223-224, 226, 228

Motion Sickness, 7-8, 74, 219

N

Nausea, 1-7, 9-10, 71-78, 154, 218-222

Neuraxial Anesthesia, 123, 205-210, 215

Non-gastrointestinal Surgery, 1-3, 6

Nutritional Obesity, 153-154

O

Obstructive Sleep Apnea, 153-154, 156

Organ Dysfunction, 12, 16, 45, 100-101, 135-136, 142, 167, 169, 187, 194-195

P

Pain Score, 7, 73, 92, 169

Pathway Analyses, 11-12, 14

Perioperative Management, 25, 88-89

Perioperative Period, 6, 21, 125, 152, 154

Peripheral Nerve Block, 205-206, 208, 216

Phosphate Levels, 135, 141-143

Polymorphisms, 94-95, 97-98, 100

Postoperative Delirium, 205, 208, 216-217

Postoperative Nausea, 1-2, 6, 9-10, 71-72, 74-78, 218, 222

Postoperative Opioid, 8, 77, 219, 221-222

Prognosis, 23, 28, 35-36, 40, 43, 58, 83, 113-114, 116, 129, 131, 134-136, 141-142, 186-188, 193, 195, 205-206, 222

Prognostic Capacity, 144-145, 147-149

Propensity Score Matching, 95-97, 187-188, 190-193

Psychological Support, 3, 6-7

Pulmonary Function, 102-111, 228

Pulse Pressure, 55-60

R

Regional Anesthesia, 26-27, 173, 205-206, 208

Remifentanil, 3, 5, 72, 74-75, 77-78, 154

Renal Cell Carcinoma, 21-22, 24, 27-28

Renal Transplant, 13, 15

Rhabdomyolysis, 35-36, 38, 41-43

S

Sedation, 3, 5, 9, 44-48, 50-54, 63, 73, 77, 168-174, 218, 220, 222

Sepsis, 11-20, 28, 36, 43-46, 48, 50-54, 94-101, 116, 118, 135-143, 160-161, 163-167, 171, 177, 186-188, 192, 194-195, 227

Septic Shock, 12, 15-17, 19-20, 45-46, 48, 50-54, 57, 96-97, 99-101, 118, 135-136, 142, 165-167, 187-191, 193-196, 198, 201, 203

T

Thyroidectomy, 71-73, 75, 77-78, 153, 220

Tracheal Intubation, 45, 152, 154-157

U

Urine Output, 36, 63, 187-193, 195

V

Vasopressor Use, 135-138, 140-142

Visual Analog Scale, 2, 6, 73, 75, 121, 125